LOCAL FLAPS IN FACIAL RECONSTRUCTION

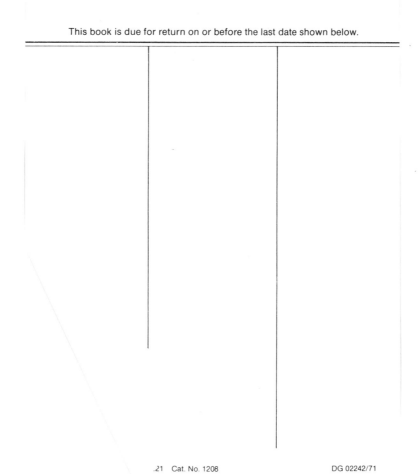

LOCAL FLAPS IN FACIAL RECONSTRUCTION

SHAN RAY BAKER, M.D., F.A.C.S.
PROFESSOR AND CHIEF, SECTION OF FACIAL PLASTIC AND RECONSTRUCTIVE SURGERY,
DEPARTMENT OF OTOLARYNGOLOGY
DIRECTOR, CENTER FOR FACIAL COSMETIC SURGERY
UNIVERSITY OF MICHIGAN
ANN ARBOR, MICHIGAN

NEIL A. SWANSON, M.D.
PROFESSOR AND INTERIM CHAIRMAN, DEPARTMENT OF DERMATOLOGY
PROFESSOR, DEPARTMENT OF OTOLARYNGOLOGY
DIRECTOR, DIVISION OF DERMATOLOGIC SURGERY
OREGON HEALTH SCIENCES UNIVERSITY
PORTLAND, OREGON

WITH *1,290* ILLUSTRATIONS

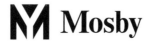 Mosby

St. Louis Baltimore Berlin Boston Carlsbad Chicago London Madrid
Naples New York Philadelphia Sydney Tokyo Toronto

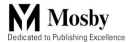
Mosby
Dedicated to Publishing Excellence

Editor: Robert Hurley
Associate Developmental Editor: Christine Pluta
Project Manager: Linda Clarke
Project Supervisor: Vicki Hoenigke
Designer: Sheliah Barrett
Manufacturing Supervisor: Karen Lewis
Cover art: Ellen Dawson

Copyright © 1995 by Mosby–Year Book, Inc.

Printed in the United States of America
Composition by The Clarinda Company
Printing/binding by Maple Vail

Mosby–Year Book, Inc.
11830 Westline Industrial Drive
St. Louis, Missouri 63146

Library of Congress Cataloging in Publication Data

Local flaps in facial reconstruction / [edited by] Shan Ray Baker,
  Neil A. Swanson.
       p.   cm.
    Includes bibliographical references and index.
    ISBN 0-8016-6925-1 (alk. paper)
    1. Facial flaps.   2. Face--Surgery.   3. Surgery, Plastic.
  I. Baker, Shan R.   II. Swanson, Neil A. (Neil Azel), 1949-
    [DNLM: 1. Surgical Flaps.   2. Face--surgery.   3. Surgery, Plastic.
  WE 705 L812 1995]
  RD523.L63   1995
  617.5'20592--dc20
  DNLM/DLC
  for Library of Congress   94-38851
                                                                  CIP

95 96 97 98 / 9 8 7 6 5 4 3 2 1

CONTRIBUTORS

ROBERT E. ADHAM, M.D.
Blount Memorial Hospital
Maryville, Tennessee

EUGENE L. ALFORD, M.D.
Assistant Professor, Department of Otolaryngology
  and Human Communication
Baylor College of Medicine
The Methodist Hospital
St. Luke's Hospital
Houston, Texas

RICHARD L. ANDERSON, M.D.
Professor, Division of Ophthalmic Plastic Reconstructive and Orbital Surgery
University of Utah
Salt Lake City, Utah

LOUIS C. ARGENTA, M.D.
Professor and Chairman
Bowman Gray School of Medicine
Professor and Chairman
North Carolina Baptist Hospital
Winston-Salem, North Carolina

DENNIS R. BANDUCCI, M.D.
Assistant Professor of Surgery
Pennsylvania State University
Director, Plastic Surgery Clinic
The Milton S. Hershey Medical Center
Hershey, Pennsylvania

FERDINAND F. BECKER, M.D.
Courtesy Clinical Assistant Professor
University of Florida College of Medicine
Active Staff, Department of Surgery
Indian River Memorial Hospital
Vero Beach, Florida

DAVID A. BRAY, M.D.
Associate Professor of Surgery, Division of Head and
  Neck Surgery
University of California, Los Angeles
Los Angeles, California

MARC D. BROWN, M.D.
Assistant Professor of Dermatology and
  Otolaryngology
Director, Mohs Surgery and Cutaneous Oncology
Strong Memorial Hospital
University of Rochester
Rochester, New York

RICHARD E. BROWNLEE, M.D.
Assistant Professor, Department of Otolaryngology
University of Florida
Shands Teaching Hospital
Gainesville, Florida

PAUL J. BYORTH, M.D.
Chief Resident, Department of Otolaryngology-Head
  and Neck Surgery
University of California, Davis, Medical Center
Sacramento, California

MACK L. CHENEY, M.D.
Assistant Professor of Otolaryngology
Harvard Medical School
Director of Facial Plastic and Reconstructive Surgery
Massachusetts Eye and Ear Infirmary
Boston, Massachusetts

TED A. COOK, M.D., F.A.C.S.
Associate Professor
Director, Facial Plastic and Reconstructive Surgery
Department of Otolaryngology/Head and Neck
  Surgery
Oregon Health Sciences University
Portland, Oregon

LEONARD M. DZUBOW, M.D.
Associate Professor of Dermatology
University of Pennsylvania School of Medicine
Hospital of the University of Pennsylvania
Philadelphia, Pennsylvania

PATRICK M. FLAHARTY, M.D.
Assistant Professor, Division of Ophthalmic Plastic
Reconstructive and Orbital Surgery
University of Utah
Salt Lake City, Utah

JOHN L. FRODEL, M.D.
Assistant Professor
Director, Division of Facial Plastic and Reconstructive
  Surgery
Department of Otolaryngology-Head and Neck
  Surgery
Johns Hopkins Medical Institutions
Baltimore, Maryland

TIMOTHY W. FROST, M.D.
Gerald Champion Memorial Hospital
Alamogordo, New Mexico

RICHARD G. GLOGAU, M.D.
Clinical Associate Professor of Dermatology
University of California, San Francisco
San Francisco, California

GEORGE S. GODING, JR., M.D.
Assistant Professor
University of Minnesota
Hennepin County Medical Center
Minneapolis, Minnesota

ANN F. HAAS, M.D.
Assistant Professor, Department of Dermatology
University of California, Davis, School of Medicine
University of California, Davis, Medical Center
Sacramento, California

DAVID B. HOM, M.D.
Assistant Professor
University of Minnesota School of Medicine
Division of Facial Plastic and Reconstructive Surgery
Department of Otolaryngology
University of Minnesota Hospital
Hennepin County Medical Center
Minneapolis, Minnesota

TIMOTHY M. JOHNSON, M.D.
Assistant Professor of Dermatology, Otorhino-
  laryngology, and Plastic Surgery
University of Michigan Medical School
Co-Director, Cutaneous Surgery and Oncology Unit
University of Michigan Medical Center
Ann Arbor, Michigan

WAYNE F. LARRABEE, JR., M.D.
Clinical Professor, Department of Otolaryngology
  Head and Neck Surgery
University of Washington
Staff
Swedish Hospital
Children's Hospital
Seattle, Washington

DAVID J. LEFFELL, M.D.
Associate Professor of Dermatology
Yale School of Medicine
Chief, Dermatologic Surgery
Yale-New Haven Hospital
New Haven, Connecticut

ERNEST K. MANDERS, M.D.
Professor of Surgery and Pediatrics
Pennsylvania State University
Chief, Division of Plastic and Reconstructive Surgery
The Milton S. Hershey Medical Center
Hershey, Pennsylvania

FREDERICK J. MENICK, M.D.
Clinical Associate Professor and Chief of Plastic
  Surgery
Arizona Health Science Center
University of Arizona
University Medical Center
Tucson, Arizona

LLOYD B. MINOR, M.D.
Assistant Professor, Department of Otolaryngology–
  Head and Neck Surgery
John Hopkins University
Baltimore, Maryland

BRUCE R. NELSON, M.D.
Assistant Professor of Dermatology, Otorhino-
  laryngology, and Plastic Surgery
University of Michigan Medical School
Co-Director, Cutaneous Surgery and Oncology Unit
University of Michigan Medical Center
Ann Arbor, Michigan

WILLIAM R. PANJE, M.D.
Clinical Professor and Director
Head and Neck Reconstruction and Skull Base Surgery
Rush Medical College-Rush University
Director, Head and Neck Reconstruction and Skull
    Base Surgery
Rush-Presbyterian-St. Luke's Medical University
Good Samaritan Hospital
Rush North Shore Medical Center
Ingalls Memorial Hospital
Chicago, Illinois

BHUPENDRA C. K. PATEL, M.D., F.R.C.S.,
F.C.OPHTH.
Assistant Professor, Division of Ophthalmic Plastic
    Reconstructive and Orbital Surgery
University of Utah
Salt Lake City, Utah

VITO C. QUATELA, M.D.
Associate Professor of Facial Plastic Surgery
University of Rochester Medical Center
Strong Memorial Hospital
Rochester, New York

GREGORY J. RENNER, M.D.
Associate Professor of Surgery, Division of
    Otolaryngology
American Cancer Society Professor of Clinical
    Oncology
University of Missouri, Columbia
Full Time Staff (Attending)
University of Missouri Hospital and Clinics
Ellis Fischel Cancer Center
Consulting Staff
Truman Memorial VA Hospital
Columbia, Missouri

BROCK D. RIDENOUR, M.D.
Assistant Professor and Director, Division of Facial
    Plastic Surgery
Washington University School of Medicine
Attending Surgeon
Barnes Hospital
Jewish Hospital
St. Louis, Missouri

STUART J. SALASCHE, M.D.
Associate Professor
Arizona Health Science Center
Tucson, Arizona

KEVIN A. SHUMRICK, M.D.
Associate Clinical Professor
University of Cincinnati College of Medicine
Director, Division of Facial Plastic Surgery and
    Maxillofacial Trauma
University of Cincinnati Medical Center
Cincinnati, Ohio

RONALD J. SIEGLE, M.D.
Associate Professor of Clinical Otolaryngology
Ohio State University
Director, Cutaneous Oncology and Dermatologic
    Surgery
Ohio State University Hospitals
Arthur G. James Cancer Hospital and Research
    Institute
Columbus, Ohio

JONATHAN M. SYKES, M.D.
Assistant Professor, Department of Otolaryngology-
    Head and Neck Surgery
University of California, Davis, Medical Center
Sacramento, California

J. REGAN THOMAS, M.D.
Assistant Clinical Professor of Otolaryngology
Washington University School of Medicine
Director, Facial Plastic Surgery Center
St. Louis, Missouri

TOM D. WANG, M.D., F.A.C.S.
Assistant Professor
Oregon Health Sciences University
Portland, Oregon

JOHN A. ZITELLI, M.D.
Adjunct Clinical Associate Professor of Dermatology
Jefferson Medical College
Shadyside Hospital
Pittsburgh, Pennsylvania

This textbook is dedicated to John Lawrence Kemink (1949-1992), a surgeon with the ability to give hearing to those who could not hear. Husband, father, teacher, friend. You will be missed, but not forgotten.

PREFACE

This textbook presents an in-depth discussion of the use of local flaps for reconstruction of the face, scalp, and neck. It is designed to be a "working man's" manual for reconstruction of the head and neck, providing practical and effective methods of repairing primarily cutaneous defects in a variety of sizes, configurations, and locations. It is unique in that the contributors are from a variety of surgical specialties, including plastic surgery, otolaryngology, ophthalmology, and dermatology. The authors are individuals who we believe have exceptional knowledge and experience using local flaps in facial reconstruction and are some of the more respected surgeons in their respective specialties.

We are fully cognizant of the political and philosophical differences among the various surgical specialties involved in facial reconstruction, but it is important that we attempt to set aside any conflicts, disagreements, and differences in an effort to promote an interchange of ideas and knowledge that would be both educational for physicians and beneficial to patient care. This textbook represents an excellent example of mutual respect among a diverse group of surgeons. Several surgical specialties have expertise in various aspects of facial reconstruction, and we have attempted to draw on their collective talent.

This work represents the culmination of 16 years of cooperative interaction between the editors. During this interval, we have shared the care of over a thousand patients, which we believe was to their benefit. This cooperative arrangement facilitated the interchange of knowledge and experience which led to a hybrid of surgical approaches for the repair of facial cutaneous defects. The benefit of this cross fertilization of ideas was the source of our desire to edit a textbook that fosters such interchange of reconstructive surgical experience. Perhaps this book will foster more cooperative interchanges between specialties? The people who gain the most are our patients.

Shan R. Baker, M.D., F.A.C.S.
Neil A. Swanson, M.D.

CONTENTS

LOCAL FLAPS IN FACIAL RECONSTRUCTION

Section I

Flaps of the Face and Neck

1

ANATOMY OF THE SKIN

Timothy M. Johnson

Bruce R. Nelson

INTRODUCTION

The skin is a complex organ system that is essential for all mammalian life. It may be viewed as a double-layered sheath that covers the surface of the body. The outer layer of skin is known as the epidermis, and the inner layer is called the dermis. The dermis is attached to the subcutaneous fat and underlying musculature by fibrous insertions. Important adnexal structures such as hair follicles, sebaceous glands, sweat glands, immune cells, nerves, and vessels are present in the skin (Fig. 1-1). The skin as an organ system is a dynamic, metabolic, and immunologic tissue responsible for many important physiologic properties. A complete understanding of anatomy is the cornerstone of surgery. In addition, an awareness of cutaneous anatomy is essential to an understanding of the human body's functional, social, and esthetic relationship with its environment.[1-3] The purpose of this chapter is to provide a basic knowledge of the normal anatomy of the skin. Possession of such knowledge will rebut those who say most surgeons cannot tell the difference between the epidermis and the dermis, yet cut through these layers on a daily basis.

GENERAL CHARACTERISTICS

Skin is highly variable from one person to another and varies regionally within the same individual with respect to color, consistency, texture, thickness, and content of hair and sebaceous glands. Skin may be divided into smooth non–hair-bearing (glabrous) and hair-bearing (nonglabrous) areas. Almost all skin is hair-bearing. Skin is the heaviest human organ, weighing approximately 3.79 kg.[4] As a tissue, skin ranks fourth heaviest, behind fat, bone, and muscle. The largest organ in surface area, the lung, measures about 4.2 m^2 on expiration[2]; in comparison, the skin measures approximately 1.7 m^2 in surface area.[5]

Considerable variation in skin thickness, elastic fibers, and content of adnexal structures exists with respect to anatomic region, age, and sex. An appreciation of these variations is clinically important for wound healing and esthetics. These variations play an integral role in the definition of esthetic units, boundaries, and junctions. The surgeon must apply knowledge of these factors to determine the best reconstructive option during flap or graft surgery. Careful examination of the skin enables determination of the best tissue match for esthetic reconstruction. Discrepancies in the thickness of skin edges should be noticed and corrected before closure for exact reapproximation of the edges. The best donor site for a full-thickness skin graft is determined by an examination of all potential donor sites with respect to skin thickness, color, texture, and content of hair follicles and sebaceous glands. Careful examination of the skin before surgery may uncover several clues that may influence the outcome. Individuals with fair skin, light hair, and blue eyes may develop postoperative scars that remain pink for an extended period. Persons with dark skin, hair, and eyes may develop scars after surgery that remain pigmented for an extended time. An assessment of previous scars and keloids should be made. Individuals who are double-jointed, can touch their tongue to their nose (Gorlin's sign), demonstrate hyperextensibility of the elbows and knees, and have lax skin and anterior hooding of the navel may be at higher risk of developing widened scars. Patients with common skin conditions such as atopic dermatitis, psoriasis, and unusually dry skin may have high counts of staphylococcal organisms on their skin, which increases their risk for wound infections. In essence, basic knowledge of skin anatomy is used daily in reconstructive surgery.

Figure 1-1   **Schematic vertical cross section of skin.**

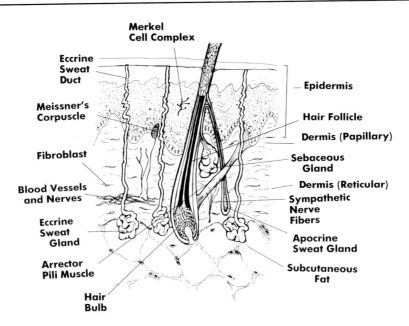

Aging is characterized by numerous changes in the skin. The epidermis becomes atrophic, or thinned, with loss of normal cell structure and maturation. The dermis also may thin as collagen bundles become homogenized and basophilic and ground substance accumulates within the dermis.[6] The leathery appearance results in part from clumping and build up of dermal elastic fibers. Many of these changes can be corrected and reversed in varying degrees with modalities ranging from topical tretinoin (Retin-A) to chemical peel to dermabrasion. (Figs. 1-2 to 1-5). The elements that make up the skin are discussed next.

EPIDERMIS

The epidermis, the most superficial layer of skin, is a keratinizing stratified squamous epithelium. The pilosebaceous unit, eccrine, and apocrine sweat glands all arise from this layer. Four distinct cell types comprise this layer: keratinocytes, melanocytes, Langerhans cells, and Merkel cells. The predominant cell type is the keratinocyte, which makes up about 80% of the cells in the epidermis. Four clearly defined layers are contained in the epidermis: basal cell (stratum basale), prickle cell (stratum spinosum), granular cell (stratum granulosum), and keratin (stratum corneum) (Fig. 1-6). The basal layer is the deepest layer in the epidermis. It is composed of a single germinative layer of basophilic columnar and cuboidal cells. These cells divide and migrate superficially to the next layer, the prickle cell layer. This layer, which is several cells thick, is com-

posed of polygonal cells with abundant eosinophilic cytoplasm. Small spiny desmosonal attachments between the prickle cells are evident under light microscopy. As the prickle cells migrate superficially, they differentiate to the granular cell layer. This layer, usually one to four cells thick, is composed of cells with deeply basophilic keratohyalin granules. Further maturation occurs in the outermost stratum corneum. The keratinocytes in this layer lose their nuclei and appear flattened to form plates of keratin, which are shed as dead skin. Total epidermal turnover time from the basal layer to the stratum corneum is approximately 30 days. The thickness of the epidermis is generally about 0.075 to 0.15 mm. The epidermis is thin at birth, becomes thicker at puberty and in early adulthood, and thins in the fifth to sixth decades of life.

Melanocytes

Melanocytes, of neural crest origin, are found in the basal layer. The ratio of melanocytes to basal cells ranges from 1:4 to 1:10. These cells are cuboidal, with clear cytoplasm and eccentrically located, crescent-shaped nuclei. The function of melanocytes is to produce protective melanin pigment. The melanocyte is a dendritic cell with stellate projections. The melanin is packaged in the form of melanosomes, which are transported through the stellate dendritic projections to the surrounding keratinocytes in the prickle cell layer. The prickle cells engulf the melanosomes and distribute the pigment in an umbrellalike distribution over the keratinocyte nucleus (Fig. 1-7). This is nature's

Figure 1-2 Aged sun-damaged skin characterized by actinic lentigines, solar elastoses, and actinic keratoses.

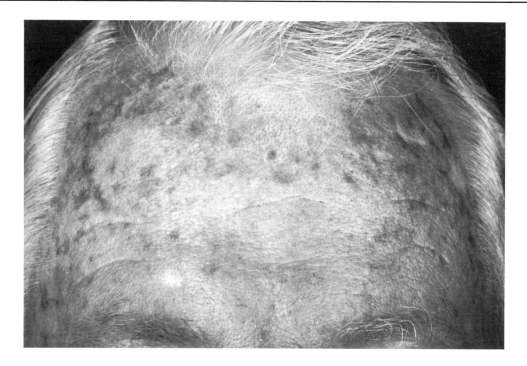

Figure 1-3 Marked improvement of solar skin changes 3 months after dermabrasion.

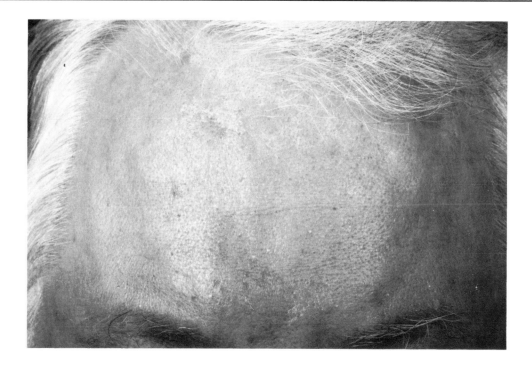

Figure 1-4   Skin biopsy specimen obtained from patient in Fig. 1-3 before dermabrasion demonstrates clumping and disarray of elastic fibers in papillary dermis. Clumped elastic fibers are darkly stained with Verhoeff–van Gieson stain.

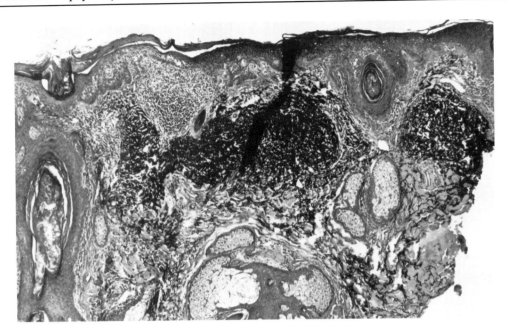

Figure 1-5   Skin biopsy specimen from patient in Fig. 1-4 at 3 months after dermabrasion demonstrates absence of clumped dermal elastic fibers.

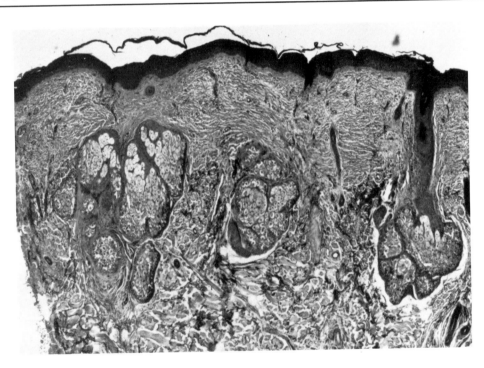

Figure 1-6   Layers of epidermis.

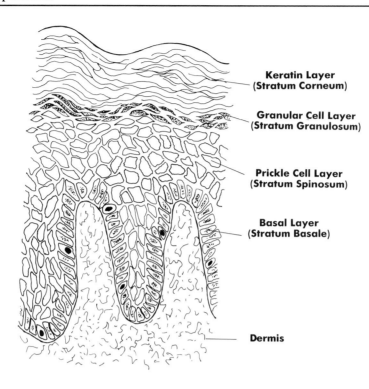

Keratin Layer
(Stratum Corneum)

Granular Cell Layer
(Stratum Granulosum)

Prickle Cell Layer
(Stratum Spinosum)

Basal Layer
(Stratum Basale)

Dermis

Figure 1-7   Melanocytes in basal layer *(arrow)* send stellate dendritic projections to surrounding cells in basal and prickle cell layers. These keratinocytes engulf melanosomes from the dendritic projections and distribute pigment in an umbrellalike distribution over the cell nuclei, protecting the nuclei from ultraviolet radiation.

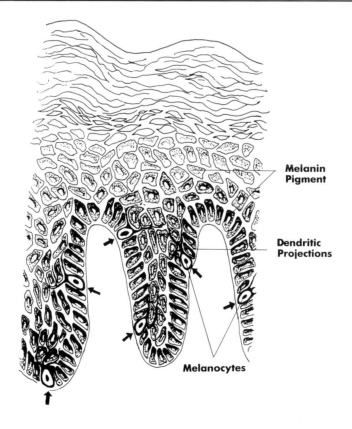

Melanin
Pigment

Dendritic
Projections

Melanocytes

way of protecting the nuclei of the keratinocytes from ultraviolet radiation. This partly explains why people with less pigmentation are at greater risk for development of cutaneous malignant tumors. The number of melanocytes does not differ between races. The active packaging of melanosomes is greater in pigmented skin and accounts for the darker skin color seen in pigmented patients. In vitiligo, melanocytes are completely absent. In albinism, melanocytes are present but lack the enzyme tyrosinase. Without tyrosinase, tyrosine cannot be transformed into melanin. Tyrosinase activity and melanocyte density decreases with age.[7,8]

Langerhans Cells

Langerhans cells are found in the suprabasilar epidermis, mainly in the prickle cell layer and in the dermis. These cells function as mediators of immunologic responses in the skin. They are difficult to identify without special staining or electron microscopy. They may be seen with supravital reactions (methylene blue), gold-chloride stain, enzymatic adenosine triphosphatase, and immunohistochemical anti-immune response-associated (Ia) antibodies. Surface markers for Fc, C3, and Ia antigens are present on these cells. With the use of electron microscopy, cytoplasmic organelles known as Birbeck's granules are seen. Under light microscopy the cells resemble melanocytes. As on melanocytes, dendritic projections are present. These dendritic processes are capable of capturing and processing antigens within the skin. The antigen then may be presented to skin lymphocytes. The Langerhans cell is a bone marrow derived immunocompetent cell that participates in delayed hypersensitivity and skin allograft reactions, whose number increases markedly during these reactions. The number of Langerhans cells decreases following exposure to ultraviolet radiation. This may play a role in skin carcinogenesis with respect to the skin's immune system. The number of Langerhans cells also decreases with age.[9]

Merkel Cells

Merkel cells are found in the epidermis and dermis in close association with peripheral nerve endings. The origin of this cell type is unknown. These cells may aggregate to form tactile corpuscles associated with myelinated peripheral nerves. Although they are thought to be slowly adapting touch receptors, solitary Merkel cells have an unclear function. Merkel cells, like Langerhans cells, are difficult to identify with light microscopy. With electron microscopy, membrane-bound dense core granules may be found. These granules are similar to neurosecretory granules of cells of the amine precursor uptake and decarboxylation (APUD) system of the body.[10] Merkel cell tumors may arise from these cells.

BASEMENT MEMBRANE ZONE (DERMOEPIDERMAL JUNCTION)

The epidermis is attached to the dermis by the basement membrane zone (Fig. 1-8). With light microscopy, this zone is identified as a thin pink band that stains positive with periodic acid-Schiff (PAS) stain. This complex zone provides mechanical support to the epidermis and acts as a barrier to chemicals and other substances. Tonofilaments within the basal cell condense and attach to an electron-dense thickening known as the attachment plaque at the inferior aspect of the basal cell plasma membrane. This is called the hemidesmosome. The hemidesmosomes are firmly anchored to the underlying lamina densa (basal lamina) through connecting anchoring filaments in the lamina lucida (clear zone). The lamina densa is attached to the underlying dermis by anchoring fibrils and dermal microfibril bundles. Anchoring fibrils are composed of type VII collagen. These fibrils are absent in new scars and are decreased in sun-exposed skin.[11] These fibrils are degraded by collagenase. Ultraviolet light may stimulate keratinocytes to produce interleuken-1, which in time may stimulate collagenase. Topical tretinoin increases the density of anchoring fibrils, possibly by inhibiting collagenase.[12,13] The basement membrane zone is contiguous from the epidermis around hair follicles and sweat ducts into the dermis.

EPIDERMAL APPENDAGES

Pilosebaceous Unit

The pilosebaceous unit includes the sebaceous gland, hair shaft, hair follicle, arrector pili muscle, and sensory end organ (Fig. 1-9). This structure has motor and sensory function and is responsible for production of hair and sebum (oil). On the scalp, the follicular component is predominant, resulting in thick, dense terminal hair. On the temples and forehead, the hair consists of fine, thin vellus hair. On the nasal tip, the sebaceous component predominates and is enlarged, resulting in a characteristic skin quality. The complete pilosebaceous unit is absent on mucous membranes. Reepithelialization of partial-thickness wounds occurs not only from the wound edges but also from the follicles, sweat ducts, and sebaceous glands.

Figure 1-8   Basement membrane zone anatomy (dermoepidermal junction).

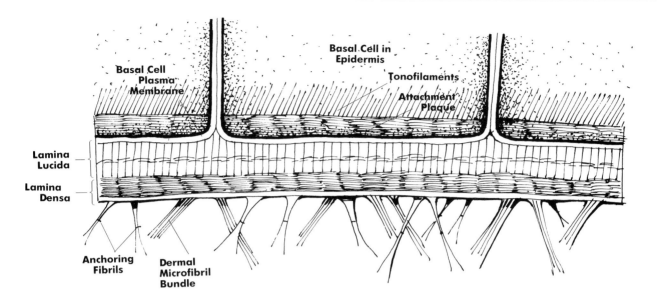

Figure 1-9   Pilosebaceous unit. Hair follicle layers are shown in vertical and cross section.

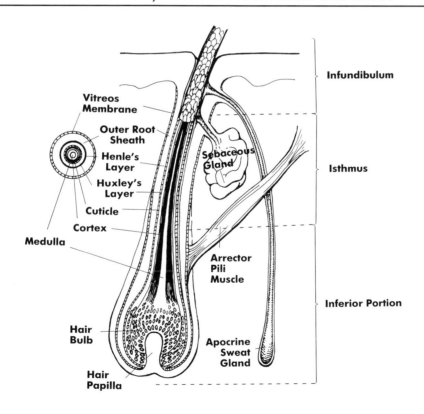

Sebaceous Glands

Sebaceous glands are unilobular or multilobular structures that connect to the infundibulum of the hair follicle by a squamous epithelial duct. Each lobule consists of a peripheral cuboidal or flattened germinative cell layer. These cells give rise to a central lipid-laden vacuolated cell population with characteristic clear to foamy cytoplasm. The glands secrete sebum into the sebaceous duct, to the follicle, and onto the surface of the skin. Sebum, a lipid oily mixture, provides emollients to the hair and skin.

Sebaceous glands enlarge and become functionally active during puberty. They are found everywhere on the body except the palms and soles and are most abundant on the face, chest, back, and scalp. The secretion of sebum is influenced by androgens and estrogens and is associated with acne. These glands may enlarge considerably in middle-aged and elderly persons, producing yellow papular lesions known as sebaceous hyperplasia. The sebaceous glands appear to arise independently in certain locations. They are named Fordyce spots when they occur on the lips and meibomian glands when they are on the eyelids.

Hair Follicle

The hair follicle is a complex structure, with several distinct layers (Figs. 1-9, 1-10). The follicle develops as an oblique downward proliferation of epidermal cells with an intact basement membrane, which extends into the underlying dermis and subcutaneous fat. This forms the external root sheath of the hair follicle. The hair bulb lies at the base of the follicle. This germinative cell layer gives rise to the inner root sheath and the hair shaft. Melanocytes in the hair bulb determine hair color by giving rise to melanosomes within the cortex of the hair shaft. The distal hair bulb surrounds the connective tissue hair papilla as an arch. The hair papilla is a specialized mesenchymal structure that has a rich vascular supply and abundant nerve endings.

The hair follicle consists of three portions known as the infundibulum, isthmus, and inferior portion. The superficial portion, the infundibulum, extends from the skin surface to the opening of the sebaceous duct into the follicle. The middle portion, the isthmus, extends from the follicular opening of the sebaceous duct to the insertion of the arrector pilus muscle into the follicle. The inferior portion of the follicle lies below the follicular insertion of the arrector pilus muscle.

The mature hair follicle is encased by a vascular connective tissue sheath separated from the external root sheath by the basement membrane. In the infundibulum, the external root sheath consists of all layers of the epidermis. Distal to the follicular opening of the sebaceous duct, the external root sheath consists of a markedly vacuolated prickle cell layer. The cells are vacuolated due to the presence of glycogen. The internal root sheath and hair shaft are derived from the germinative hair matrix in the bulb. The internal root sheath consists of three distinct layers. Henle's layer is most peripheral and is one cell thick. Huxley's layer is in the middle and is two cells thick. The cuticle is central and consists of imbricated flattened cells. The cuticular cells form overlapping ridges or grooves where sebum is deposited and gives luster to hair. The hair shaft consists of the cuticle, cortex, and medulla. The central medulla is absent in lanugo and vellus hairs. The cuticle of the shaft is joined with the cuticle of the internal root sheath, functioning as one structure.

Hair growth occurs in three cyclical phases called anagen, catagen, and telogen (Fig. 1-11). The anagen or growth phase develops as the inferior portion of the follicle grows downward to form a fully developed hair bulb and papilla. The catagen or involutional phase develops by upward movement of the inferior portion of the follicle to the level of the follicular attachment of the arrector pilus muscle. An epithelial column surrounded by a connective tissue band can be identified in the path of upward movement. In the telogen or resting phase, the inferior portion of the follicle is lost. The hair cycle is different in various anatomic regions. In the human scalp, on average, 84% of hairs are in anagen, 1% are in catagen, and 13% are in telogen.[14,15] The follicular epithelium lying in the dermis provides an additional source of germinative cells for reepithelialization of partial-thickness wounds. The follicular dermal extension of the epidermis also allows epidermal diseases such as Bowen's disease (squamous cell carcinoma in situ) to extend into the dermis. This may result in a higher recurrence rate if superficial treatment methods do not destroy the follicular downward extension of the disease process.

Arrector Pilus Muscles and Sensory Nerves

The arrector pilus muscle inserts into the perifollicular connective tissue sheath at the junction of the isthmus and inferior portion of the follicle. This small muscle extends obliquely and upward into the papillar dermis. Sympathetic contraction of this muscle makes the hair "stand up" as it is pulled from an oblique position to a vertical position. This results in cutis anserina, or goose bumps. Sensory nerves are located around the isthmus and inferior portion of the hair follicle. These nerves are stimulated as a touch receptor when the hairs are touched.

Figure 1-10   Vertical section of normal hair showing layers of the hair follicle.

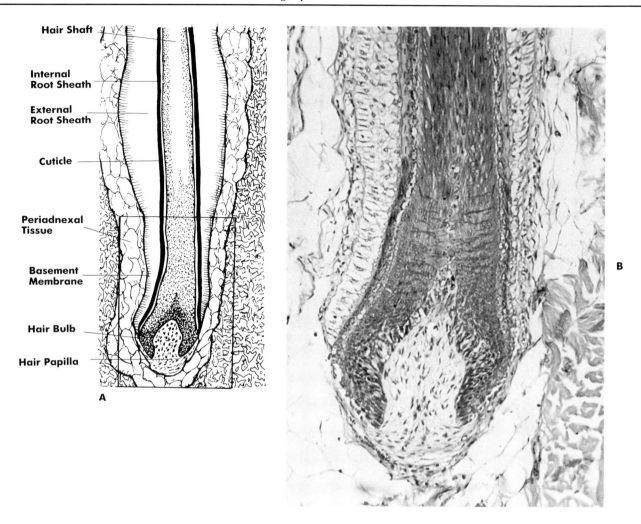

Hair Shaft

Internal
Root Sheath

External
Root Sheath

Cuticle

Periadnexal
Tissue

Basement
Membrane

Hair Bulb

Hair Papilla

A

B

Figure 1-11   Hair growth cycle proceeding from anagen to catagen and then telogen phase. In anagen inferior portion of follicle grows downward, forming fully developed hair bulb and papilla. Catagen phase develops by upward movement of inferior portion of follicles to the level of arrector pilus muscle attachment. Epithelial column can be identified in path of upward movement. In telogen, inferior portion of follicle is lost.

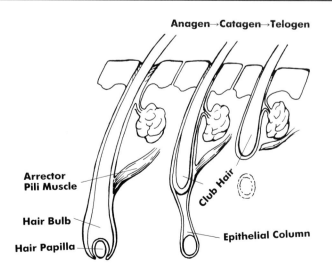

Anagen→Catagen→Telogen

Arrector
Pili Muscle

Club Hair

Hair Bulb

Epithelial Column

Hair Papilla

Eccrine Glands

Eccrine glands are distributed almost everywhere on the skin except the mucous membranes. These sweat-producing glands are particularly dense on the palms, soles, axillae, and forehead. The eccrine unit is composed of a coiled secretory gland, a coiled and straight dermal duct, and a coiled intraepidermal duct. The secretory gland is located in the deep reticular dermis or subcutaneous fat. The glandular lumen is surrounded by an inner layer of clear and dark secretory cells and an outer layer of contractile myoepithelial cells. The gland is innervated by nerve fibers, which are stimulated by thermal, mental, and gustatory stimuli. The dermal duct is predominantly straight and consists of a double layer of basophilic cuboidal cells. The dermal duct ascends upward to the coiled intraepidermal duct, which opens directly to the skin surface. The duct modifies the composition of sweat, which consists of water, sodium, chloride, potassium, urea, and lactate at a pH ranging from 4.0 to 6.8.

Apocrine Glands

Apocrine glands are distributed primarily in the axillae and groin but also on the eyelids (Moll's glands) and the external auditory canal (ceruminous glands). These glands produce an odorless secretion, which has an unknown function and which becomes odorous due to cutaneous microorganisms. Apocrine glands, like sebaceous glands, enlarge and become active at puberty.

The apocrine unit consists of a secretory gland and a duct that connects to the hair follicle or directly to the skin surface. The secretory gland lies in the deep reticular dermis or superficial fat and consists of an outer layer of myoepithelial cells and an inner layer of columnar or cuboidal eosinophilic cells. The inner layer of cells secrete droplets into the lumun by decapitation secretion. These glands are larger than eccrine glands and are innervated by nerves that may be stimulated by external stimuli such as excitement or fear. The apocrine duct ascends upward through the dermis and usually connects to the infundibulum of the hair follicle superior to the sebaceous duct. The duct may also bypass the follicle and directly empty onto the surface of the skin.

DERMIS

The dermis represents the inner layer of skin between the epidermis and subcutaneous fat. This fibrous connective-tissue matrix is made up of collagen, elastic tissue, and ground substance. Dispersed throughout the dermis are epidermal appendages, blood vessels, nerves, and cells, including fibroblasts, mononuclear cells, and mast cells. The dermis is divided into the relatively thin, superficial papillary dermis and the thicker, deep reticular dermis. There is great regional variation in thickness of the dermis, ranging from less than 1 mm on the eyelid, to 1.5 mm on the temple, 2.5 mm on the scalp, and greater than 4 mm on the back.[2] The dermis is thin at birth, increases in thickness until the fourth or fifth decade, then decreases. Men usually have a thicker dermis than do women.

Collagen

Collagen is a complex protein made up of collagen fibers synthesized by fibroblasts in the dermis. The mechanical strength and extensibility of the skin greatly depends on dermal collagen fibers. Collagen types I and III make up the majority of dermal collagen. Type I collagen is most abundant and found predominantly as thick broad bands in the reticular dermis. Type III collagen makes up the fine collagen fibers located primarily in the papillary dermis. Types IV and VII collagen are located primarily at the basement membrane. Ferrous iron and vitamin C are required for collagen synthesis.[2] The content of skin collagen decreases by 1% per year throughout adulthood.[16] This may be due to decreased collagen synthesis, increased collagen degradation rate by collagenase, or both. Topical tretinoin may affect aging skin and wound healing by inhibition of dermal collagenase.

Elastic Tissue

Elastic fibers in the dermis are primarily responsible for the recoil and elastic properties of the skin. The normal fibers are not readily seen on skin biopsy without the aid of elastic tissue stains such as the Verhoeff-van Gieson stain, which stains elastic tissue black. With the use of special stains, the elastic fibers in the papillary dermis are seen to be thin and tend to run perpendicular to the skin surface, whereas those in the reticular dermis are seen to be thicker and tend to run parallel to the skin surface. Elastic fibers in the dermis are synthesized primarily by fibroblasts. Like collagen, elastic tissue is in a continuous state of synthesis and degradation by elastase. Elastic tissue is composed of a protein elastin and a microfibrillar matrix that contains fibrillin, a glycoprotein, and other components. The amino acids desmosine and isodesmosine are unique to elastin protein.[17,18] Elastic fibers tend to thicken and form clumps in the papillary dermis in sun-damaged skin. These fragmented clumps of abnormal elastic tissue disappear following chemical peel or dermabrasion. (See Figs. 1-4 and 1-5.)

Ground Substance

Fibrous connective tissue and cellular constituents are embedded in ground substance. Ground substance is composed primarily of fibronectin and the glycosaminoglycans hyaluronic acid, chondroitin-4-sulfate, and dermatan sulphate. In the dermis the ground substance is synthesized by fibroblasts, and possibly mast cells and smooth-muscle cells, and appears as fine mucinous stroma on skin biopsy. Ground substance plays a role in skin hydration and helps to preserve the tensile elasticity of compressed skin by redistributing the pressure forces. Relative dehydration in the skin due to displacement of ground substance is partly responsible for the phenomenon termed mechanical creep. Mechanical creep plays a role in the physiologic factors of immediate intraoperative tissue expansion.[19]

Cellular Components

The chief cell in the dermis is the fibroblast. This metabolic dynamic cell is important for many functions of the skin. It is abundant in the papillary dermis and scant in the reticular dermis, and it plays a major synthetic role in wound healing and production of collagen, elastin, and ground substance. It also behaves as a contractile cell during wound contraction. The number of fibroblasts in the skin decreases with age.

Mast cells are found perivascularly and in the papillary dermis. These cells may contribute to synthesis of ground substance and may be abundant in scars. The histamine released by mast cells may account for the frequent symptom of pruritus in hypertrophic scars and keloids because these scars often contain numerous mast cells.

Nerve Supply

A rich nerve supply to the skin consisting of free nerve endings and specialized nerve end organs permits the body to accurately interpret the continuous bombardment of stimuli received from the external environment (Fig. 1-12). Free sensory and autonomic nerve endings from the peripheral nervous system arborize up to the basement membrane zone.

The sensory nerves relay sensations of pain, temperature, pressure, and proprioception. Specialized receptors include Meissner's corpuscles, pacinian corpuscles, and Merkel cell complexes. The Merkel cell neural-cellular complex is in the epidermis and responds to touch. Meissner's corpuscles, located in the papillary dermal papillae, mediate fine touch sensation. Pacinian corpuscles, located deeper in the subcutaneous tissue, mediate deep pressure and possibly vibration. Free

Figure 1-12   Nerve supply to skin.

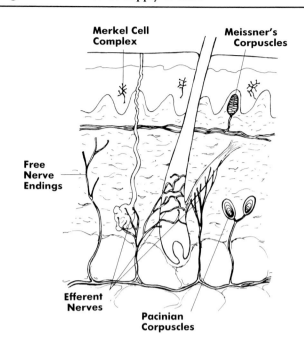

Figure 1-13   Vascular supply to skin. Superficial and deep vascular plexus provides nourishment to skin and adnexal structures.

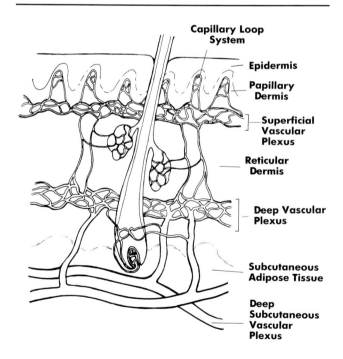

nerve endings in the dermis are primarily responsible for the appreciation of temperature, pruritus, and pain. The efferent nerves in the dermis innervate blood vessels and appendageal structures. Stimulation of these nerves regulates cutaneous vascular and appendageal function.

Vascular Supply

Soft-tissue surgery on the head and neck usually heals particularly well due to a rich vascular supply. The blood flow in the skin is directed toward the more metabolically active epidermis via the dermal papillae, hair papillae, and adnexal structures. Two vascular plexuses connected by communicating vessels are present in the reticular dermis (Fig. 1-13). The deep vascular plexus lies at the junction of the dermis and subcutaneous fat. This deep plexus receives its vascular supply from the deep subcutaneous perforating vessels. Arterioles from the deep vascular plexus supply the skin appendages, pilosebaceous units, and the superficial vascular plexus located in the superior aspect of the reticular dermis. The superficial vascular plexus gives rise to a rich capillary loop system in the superficial dermal papillae in the papillary dermis. This loop system is adjacent to the epidermis, and it provides nutrients to the metabolically active epidermis by diffusion. The dermis also contains a lymphatic system that resembles the vascular plexuses.

SUMMARY

A basic knowledge of skin anatomy is required to fully understand skin tissue match, tissue stretch, skin thickness and elasticity, wound contraction, and other concepts used on a daily basis by surgeons who perform local flap reconstructive surgery.

REFERENCES

1. Whitaker DC: Skin anatomy and physiology. In Janusz editor: *Local flaps and free skin grafts in head and neck reconstruction.* St Louis, 1992, Mosby Year Book, Inc.

2. Berrnett RG: *Cutaneous structure, function, and repair.* In Klein A, editor: *Fundamentals of cutaneous surgery.* St Louis, 1988, Mosby Year Book, Inc.

3. Mckee PH: *Normal histology of the skin.* In Jowell M and Smillie L, editors: *Physiology of the skin.* Philadelphia, 1989, JB Lippincott.

4. Goldsmith LA: My organ is bigger than your organ. *Arch Dermatol* 126:301, 1990.

5. Montagna W and Parakkal PF: *Structure and function of the skin,* ed 3, New York, 1974, Academic Press, Inc.

6. Braverman IM and Fonferko E: Studies in cutaneous aging: II. The microvasculature. *J Invest Dermatol* 78:444, 1982.

7. Gilchrest BA, Blog FB, Szabo G: Effects of aging and chronic sun exposure on melanocytes in human skin. *J Invest Dermatol* 73:141, 1979.

8. Hu F: Aging of melanocytes. *J Invest Dermatol* 73:70, 1979.

9. Thiers BH, Maize JC, Spicer SS et al: The effect of aging and chronic sun exposure on human Langerhans cell populations. *J Invest Dermatol* 82:223, 1984.

10. Winkelmann RK: The Merkel cell system and a comparison between it and the neurosecretory or APUD cell system. *J Invest Dermatol* 69:41, 1977.

11. Tidman MJ, Eady RA: Ultrastructure morphometry of normal human dermal-epidermal junction: the influence of age, sex, and body region on lamina and nonlaminar components. *J Invest Dermatol* 83:448, 1984.

12. Woodley DT, Zelickson AS, Briggaman RA et al: Treatment of photoaged skin with topical tretinoin increases epidermal-dermal anchoring fibrils. *JAMA* 263:3057, 1990.

13. Zelickson AS, Mottaz JH, Weiss JS et al: Topical tretinoin in photoaging: an ultrastructural study. *J Cutan Aging Cos Dermatol* 1:41, 1988.

14. Kligman AM: The human hair cycle. *J Invest Dermatol* 33:307, 1959.

15. Barman JM, Astore I, Pecoraro V: The normal trichogram of the adult. *J Invest Dermatol* 44:223, 1965.

16. Shuster S, Black MM, McVitie E: The influence of age and sex on skin thickness, skin collagen and density. *Br J Dermatol* 93:639, 1975.

17. Sandberg LB, Soskel NT, Leslie JG: Elastin structure, biosynthesis, and relation to disease states. *N Engl J Med* 304:566, 1981.

18. Cotta-Pereira G, Guetta RF, Bittencourt-Sanpaio S: Oxytalan, elaunin, and elastic fibers in the human skin. *J Invest Dermatol* 66:143, 1976.

19. Johnson TM, Brown MD, Sullivan MJ et al: Immediate intraoperative tissue expansion. *J Am Acad Dermatol* 22:283, 1990.

2

SKIN FLAP PHYSIOLOGY

George S. Goding, Jr.

David B. Hom

INTRODUCTION

The creation of a cutaneous flap applies specific stresses to otherwise normal skin. These stresses include local tissue trauma and reduced neurovascular supply to the affected tissue. The extent to which skin can survive these injuries is a reflection of the anatomic and physiologic characteristics of skin as well as the cutaneous response to injury. Knowledge of these principles has led to improved skin flap survival by means of flap design and flap delay. Increase of cutaneous flap survival by minimization of the deleterious physiologic effects of flap transposition is an area of active research.

PHYSIOLOGIC CHARACTERISTICS OF SKIN

The skin serves as a sensory and protective organ. The thick epidermal layers are largely impermeable to gases and to most liquids. Because of this, many agents that could result in beneficial effects are ineffective when they are applied to intact skin. Preservation of sensation in transferred cutaneous flaps is desirable, but its physiologic effect on flaps is unclear.

The blood supply to the skin serves two important functions. It provides nutritional support and a thermoregulatory mechanism for the body. Primarily because of its thermoregulatory function, the rate of blood flow through the skin is one of the most variable in the body. When skin is at normal temperatures, the amount of blood flowing through the skin (0.25 L/m^2 of body surface area) is approximately 10 times the flow required for nutritional support.[1] Blood flow can increase up to seven times this value with maximal vasodilatation. When the body is exposed to extreme cold, blood flow can be reduced to levels that are marginal for cutaneous nutrition.

The nutrient capillary network in the reticular dermis and the arteriovenous shunts in the more superficial papillary dermis[2] perform the two functions of the cutaneous circulation. The amount of blood flow to the skin depends ultimately on arteriolar pressure and flow. Under conditions of adequate systemic vascular pressure, however, arterioles act as preshunt and precapillary sphincters that regulate the flow through each vascular network.[3]

The sphincters in the two vascular systems respond to different stimuli (Fig. 2-1). The precapillary sphincter, which controls the amount of nutritive blood flow to the skin, responds to local hypoxemia and increased metabolic byproducts by dilation.[4,5] Under these conditions the blood flow is increased (e.g., in reactive hyperemia). The preshunt sphincters are involved in regulating the changes in blood flow that affect thermoregulation and systemic blood pressure.[2,6] Release of norepinephrine by the postganglionic sympathetic fibers results in contraction of the preshunt sphincters. This diverts blood away from the skin surface, where heat loss can occur. With increased body temperature, the sympathetic vasoconstrictor impulses decrease, allowing for greater blood flow to the skin.[1]

Vasodilation can also occur with excessive body temperature. Local release of acetylcholine by sympathetic nerve fibers may cause vasodilation by directly affecting vasodilator fibers or acting through the release of the potent vasodilator bradykinin from the sweat glands. The cutaneous circulation is also extremely sensitive to circulating norepinephrine and epinephrine. Even in areas of skin that have lost their sympathetic innervation, a mass discharge of the sympathetic system will still result in intense vasoconstriction in the skin.[1]

Figure 2-1 Precapillary (▲) and preshunt (■) sphincters in skin. Precapillary sphincter regulates nutritive blood flow to skin and responds to locally produced stimuli. Preshunt sphinters are involved in thermoregulation and are affected by sympathetic stimuli from the central nervous system.

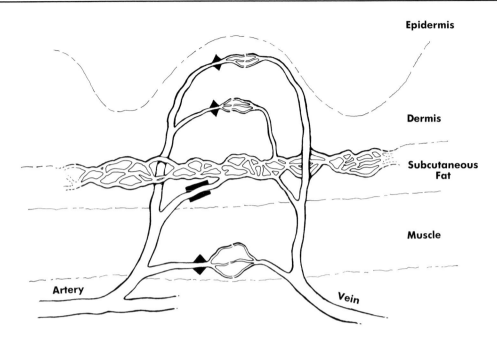

NEUROVASCULAR SUPPLY TO LOCAL SKIN FLAPS

Blood vessels travel by one of two main routes to terminate in the cutaneous circulation. Musculocutaneous arteries pass through the overlying muscle to which they provide nutrition, and septocutaneous[7] arteries (also referred to as direct cutaneous arteries) travel through fascial septa, which divide the muscular segments (Fig. 2-2).

The cutaneous portion of septocutaneous arteries typically runs parallel to the skin surface, providing nutrition to a large area of skin. Septocutaneous arteries typically have a pair of veins accompanying them and run above the superficial muscular fascia.[8] The more common musculocutaneous arteries leave the muscle and enter the subcutaneous tissue to supply a smaller region of skin.

Septocutaneous and musculocutaneous arteries empty into a diffuse interconnecting vascular network of dermal and subdermal plexuses. This network provides a redundancy in the vascular supply to the skin. A collateral blood supply supports the vascular territory of each musculocutaneous artery. Lymphatic vessels form a plexus running parallel and deep to the network of blood capillaries.[9] The lymphatic capillaries end in blind sacs and conduct extracellular fluid back into the bloodstream.

The neural supply to the skin originates from both

Figure 2-2 Depiction of varying pathways to skin that define musculocutaneous (MC) and septocutaneous (SC) arteries.

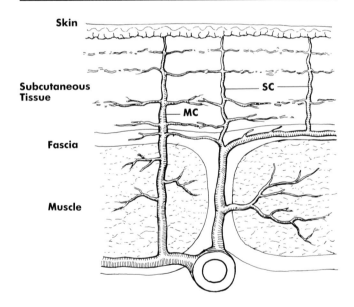

sensory nerves and sympathetic nerves. The sensory nerves are distributed in segmental fashion, forming dermatomes, and participate in the skin's protective function. The postganglionic terminals of cutaneous sympathetic nerves contain the neurotransmitter norepinephrine and are found in the area of cutaneous arterioles.[1,10,11]

Figure 2-3   Classification of skin flaps based on vascular supply. A, Random. B, Arterial cutaneous. C, Fasciocutaneous. D, Musculocutaneous.

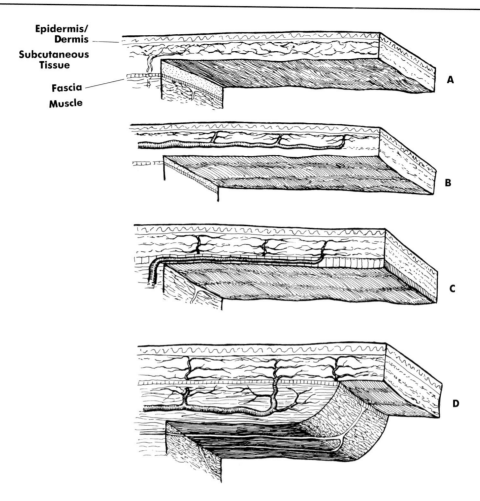

VASCULAR DESIGN OF COMMON LOCAL SKIN FLAPS IN THE HEAD AND NECK

The vascular supply to a flap is critical to its survival and is the basis of one classification system of flaps (Fig. 2-3).[12] Local flaps in the head and neck are primarily random or arterial cutaneous.

Random Cutaneous Flaps

The blood supply to a random cutaneous flap is derived from musculocutaneous arteries near the base of the flap. Blood is delivered to the tip of the flap by the interconnecting subdermal plexus. The random cutaneous flap is commonly used in local flap reconstruction and can be rotated, transposed, advanced, or tubed.

Length-to-width ratios of random cutaneous flaps have been recommended for various areas of the body.

These differences reflect a regional variation of the neurovascular supply to the skin. Such a description can serve as a guide in designing random cutaneous flaps but should not imply that a wider flap would extend survival length.[12]

Arterial Cutaneous Flaps

Arterial cutaneous flaps (also called axial pattern flaps) typically have an improved survival length compared with random cutaneous flaps. This advantage results from the incorporation of a septocutaneous artery within its longitudinal axis. An island flap is an arterial flap with a pedicle consisting of nutrient vessels without the overlying skin. Island flaps can be useful to increase flexibility and reduce pedicle bulk in certain reconstructive procedures.

Use of arterial cutaneous flaps is limited by the availability of direct cutaneous arteries. An example of an arterial cutaneous flap used in facial reconstruction is the midforehead flap based on the supratrochlear artery.

The surviving length of arterial flaps is related to length of the included septocutaneous artery. Survival beyond the arterial portion of the flap is based on the subdermal plexus and is essentially a random cutaneous extension of the flap. Flap necrosis secondary to ischemia can be said to occur only in the random portion of the flap (because destruction of the arterial pedicle makes the entire flap random).

PHYSIOLOGIC CHANGES AFTER SKIN FLAP ELEVATION

Some changes detrimental to skin survival occur when a cutaneous flap is created. That flap survival occurs at all is a testimony to the minimal nutritional requirements of skin. The primary insults that affect flap survival are impaired vascular supply and the resultant ischemia. In the presence of adequate blood flow, survival of the complete flap occurs. Nerve section and inflammation influence flap survival primarily by affecting blood flow. The formation of new vascular channels between the transposed flap and the recipient bed also influence flap survival.

Impairment of Vascular Supply

Partial interruption of the vascular supply to the skin is the most obvious and critical change that occurs with elevation of a cutaneous flap. This interruption results in a local decrease in perfusion pressure to the skin. In arterial or myocutaneous flaps, the blood supply to the skin overlying the vascular pedicle is usually adequate.[13] In random flaps or random extensions of flaps, the decrease in perfusion pressure becomes more pronounced with increasing distance from the base of the flap.[14,15] When perfusion is reduced in one area of a random flap, the adjacent vascular territories supplied by a separate perforating vessel can provide a low-pressure blood supply through the subdermal plexus (Fig. 2-4). Since the nutritional requirements of skin are relatively low, several vascular territories can be compromised before necrosis will result.

The survival length of the random portion of the flap depends on the physical properties of the supplying vessels (intravascular resistance) and the perfusion pressure.[14] When the perfusion pressure drops below the critical closing pressure of the arterioles in the subdermal plexus, nutritional blood flow ceases, and flap necrosis occurs. In the past, random cutaneous flaps were often designed relative to a desired length-to-width ratio, that is, a wider base was needed to successfully transfer a longer flap. The wider random flap includes additional vessels only with the same perfusion pressure. The relationship between perfusion pressure and critical closing pressure is not altered, and no change in survival length occurs[12,16] (Fig. 2-5).

Myers[17] has emphasized that "fresh flaps are always both viable and ischemic." Depending on the degree of ischemia and the amount of time before recovery of nutrient blood flow, the flap will either die or recover. In the pig model, arterial and random flaps can tolerate an average of 13 hours of total avascularity and remain viable.[18] In flaps with reduced perfusion, this time is probably much longer.

In surviving flaps, blood flow gradually increases. If the flap is in a favorable recipient site, a fibrin layer forms within the first 2 days. Neovascularization of the

Figure 2-4   Vascular territories in skin flap. Multiple perforating vessels exist and are interconnected at periphery of their vascular territory. When some of these vessels are cut, blood supply can be replaced from nearby perforating vessels and then tissue necrosis does not occur.

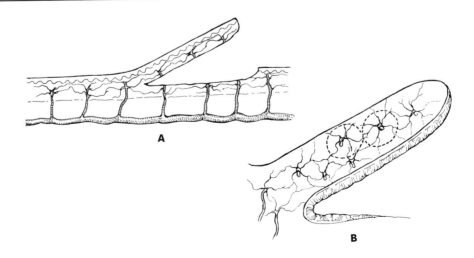

A

B

flap begins 3 to 7 days after flap transposition. Early neovascularization has been detected at 4 days in the pig and rabbit models[19,20] and at 3 days in the rat model.[21] Revascularization adequate for division of the flap pedicle has been demonstrated by 7 days in animal models and man.[19,22,23]

During revascularization, vascular endothelial cells play a major role in the formation of new vessels. Normally, endothelial cells are in a quiescent state; however, when stimulated by angiogenic growth factors, these cells can dramatically proliferate. This normally occurs only under certain conditions, such as wound healing and ovulation.

Beginning with an angiogenic stimulus, the angiogenic process involves a number of discrete yet overlying steps (Fig. 2-6). Initially, the vessels become dilated and permeable with retraction of the endothelial cells and a decrease in endothelial junctions. The basement membrane is then dissolved by proteases and the

endothelial cells migrate from the vascular wall toward the angiogenic stimulus. Behind the leading front of migrating endothelial cells, endothelial cell replication begins forming a capillary sprout that elongates toward the angiogenic source. The nearby capillary sprouts then anastomose to each other and form capillary loops. As capillary loops and sprouts continue, the loops become patent and form new blood vessels. These blood vessels differentiate and lay down basement membrane that consists of type IV collagen, laminin, and proteoglycans. Pericytes and fibroblasts then migrate to the capillary loop sites.[24]

With the continued presence or absence of the angiogenic stimulus, substantial remodeling, regression, and rearrangement of the new capillaries occur.[24] Some capillaries join preexisting flap vessels (inosculation), but the majority of revascularization appears to involve direct ingrowth of recipient vessels into the flap[25] (Fig. 2-7). New capillaries can grow toward an angiogenic source at a mean rate of 0.2 mm/day. When the angiogenic stimulus is discontinued, the capillary vessels regress and eventually disappear within weeks. Angiogenic growth factors can stimulate capillary growth over distances of 2 to 5 mm.[26]

To prevent an uncontrollable cascade of neovascularization, mechanisms to inhibit angiogenesis are believed to exist. Evidence suggests that pericytes can suppress endothelial growth by direct contact.[27] Thus, the physiologic response of angiogenesis may be analogous to the blood coagulation pathway that must be maintained at a constant steady state of control. In soft-tissue wound repair, macrophages, lymphocytes, mast cells, and platelets are involved in the release of various factors that modulate angiogenesis.[24] Tissues that are particularly high in angiogenic factors are bovine brain,[28] corpus luteum,[29] retina,[30] salivary

Figure 2-5 **Fallacy of the length-to-width ratio. Slope of decreasing perfusion pressure versus flap length does not change with incorporation of additional vessels (flap A versus flap B) with same perfusion pressure. Flap necrosis occurs when perfusion pressure falls below critical closing pressure of capillary bed.**

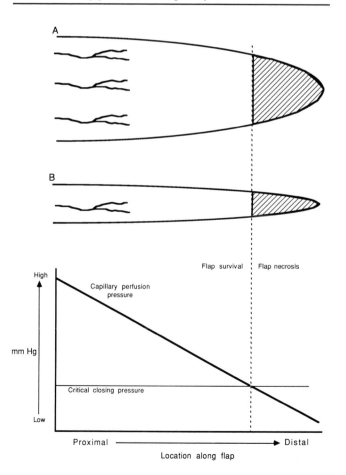

Figure 2-6 **Steps in angiogenesis. A, Initial stimulus with retraction of endothelial cells and thinning of basement membrane. B, Migration of endothelial cells and formation of capillary sprout. C, Formation of capillary loops, which become patent to form new blood vessels.**

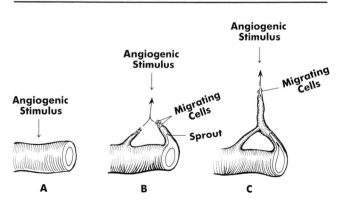

Figure 2-7   Cross section of flap demonstrating direct ingrowth (A) versus inosculation (B).

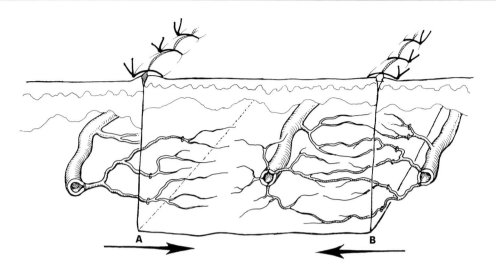

glands,[31] and lymphatic tissues.[32] Benign and malignant tumors are other potential sources of angiogenic growth factors.

The venous outflow from the skin also is impaired with flap elevation. Venous flow can occur through the subdermal plexus or by venous channels that accompany the feeding artery in the pedicle. Complete venous occlusion in the early postelevation period may be more damaging to flap survival than inadequate arterial supply.[33] Fortunately, the subdermal plexus alone is often adequate to provide adequate venous outflow. Care must be taken, however, to preserve venous outflow in flaps that are pedicled solely on the feeding vessels.

Impairment of lymphatic drainage also occurs with flap elevation. Reduction of the cutaneous lymphatic drainage results in an increase in interstitial fluid pressure, which is compounded by increased leakage of intravascular protein associated with inflammation. The resulting edema can decrease capillary perfusion by increasing the intravascular resistance.

Nerve Section

Both cutaneous and sympathetic nerves are severed in the process of flap elevation. While loss of sensation may limit the usefulness of the flap after transfer, adrenergic denervation has implications for flap survival. When a sympathetic nerve is divided, catecholamines are released from the nerve terminal and the mechanism for catecholamine reuptake is eliminated.[34-36] A local hyperadrenergic state exists, which produces vasoconstriction mediated by α-adrenergic receptors in the cutaneous vasculature.

The vasoconstricting effect of sympathectomy further reduces the total flap's blood flow,[37,38] which

already has been diminished by division of supplying vessels. This negatively affects the ratio of perfusion pressure to the critical closing pressure of the arterioles in the subdermal plexus. A greater proportion of the distal flap is excluded from the blood supply and necrosis becomes more likely. The stored transmitter is depleted within 24 to 48 hours,[35,39] and blood flow increases as the concentration of norepinephrine declines.[38] In critical areas of the flap, however, the time to recovery of nutrient blood flow may be delayed sufficiently to produce additional necrosis.

Inflammation and Prostaglandins

The surgical trauma associated with a newly raised flap results in an inflammatory response. Histamine, serotonin, and kinins are released into the extracellular compartment after flap elevation, increasing the permeability of the microcirculation. The result is an increase in the concentration of proteins and cells within the extracellular space. The presence of nonbacterial inflammation that begins a few days before flap elevation has been shown to improve flap survival.[40,41] This is presumably the result of an increase in local blood flow. The inflammation created during flap elevation, however, may have deleterious effects due to the resultant edema.

The action of the primary mediators of the inflammatory response (histamine, serotonin, and kinins) is short-lived. After kinin formation and in the presence of complement, injured cells synthesize prostaglandins. Prostaglandins play an important role in the later stages of the inflammatory reaction while simultaneously initiating the early phases of injury repair.

Prostaglandins are derived from essential fatty acids that are incorporated in membrane phospholipids (Fig.

Figure 2-8 Synthesis of prostaglandins and thromboxanes and their general effects in the cutaneous circulation.

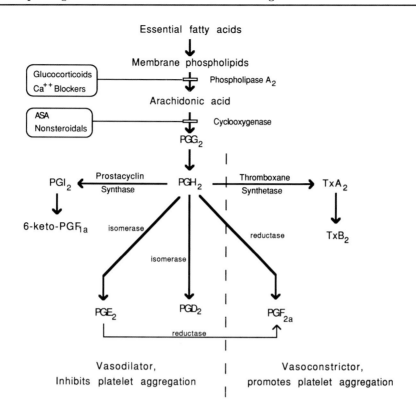

2-8). Activation of phospholipases results in the production of prostaglandin H_2 (PGH_2) by cyclooxygenase. Prostaglandin E_1 (PGE_1) and prostaglandin E_2 (PGE_2) can be synthesized from prostaglandin H_2 by isomerases in the vascular endothelium. Both PGE_1 and PGE_2 produce vasodilation. Prostaglandin D_2 (PGD_2) is also formed by an isomerase reaction and is the principal cyclooxygenase product of the mast cell. Its effects on the cutaneous microvasculature are similar to PGE_1. Prostacyclin (PGI_2) is a vasodilating agent and inhibitor of platelet aggregation that is derived from PGH_2 through the action of prostacyclin synthase. In the skin, PGI_2 is primarily produced in the endothelial cells of blood vessels.[42,43]

Thromboxane synthetase converts PGH_2 into thromboxane A_2 and is primarily located in the platelets. Its effects include vessel constriction and promotion of platelet aggregation.[44] Prostaglandin F_{2a} (PGF_{2a}) is derived from PGH_2 by a reductase reaction. A marked increase in resistance is seen in cutaneous arteries, arterioles, and venules in the presence of PGF_{2a}.[45]

The synthesis of prostaglandins and thromboxane can be altered by pharmacologic manipulation. The action of phospholipase A_2 can be inhibited by drugs that reduce the availability of Ca^{++}. Glucocorticoids also affect phospholipase A_2 activity by inducing the synthesis of a protein that inhibits the enzyme.[46]

Aspirin and other nonsteriodal antiinflammatory medications interfere with the cyclooxygenase enzyme and inhibit the synthesis of PGH_2.

Prostacyclin levels were found to peak 7 days after elevation of a porcine flank flap.[42] Elevation of a bipedicled dorsal flap in rats resulted in elevated levels of PGE_2, PGF_{2a}, and thromboxane B_2, with a return to near-normal levels by day 7. Conversion to a single pedicle flap ("delay") resulted in a blunted production of thromboxane and an elevated PGE_2 level. Elevation of a single-pedicle flap in the same model showed an elevation of PGE_2, PGF_{2a}, and thromboxane B_2 levels that was greater and more prolonged than seen with surgical delay.[47] Prostaglandins clearly play a role in the inflammatory response after flap surgery. Whether these changes in prostaglandin levels represent a cause or a side effect of the observed phenomenon remains to be demonstrated.

Reperfusion (Free Radicals)

Return of blood flow to a flap that is ischemic due to excessive release of norepinephrine occurs in approximately 12 hours. With norepinephrine depletion and continued inflammatory response, blood flow can reach a maximum at 24 hours.[38,48] When oxygen becomes available with reperfusion, an additional menace to flap survival is produced, the free radical. This

Figure 2-9   Possible mechanism for formation of oxygen free radicals during reperfusion after ischemia and subsequent reduction of superoxide radical.

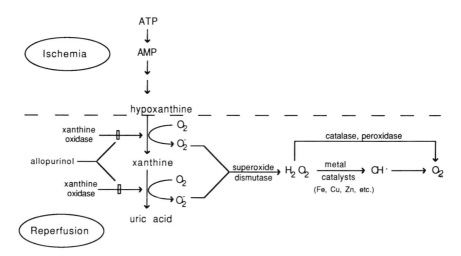

byproduct of reperfusion can cause damage at both the cellular and subcellular levels,[49,50] contributing to postischemic tissue necrosis.

Free radicals are extremely reactive compounds because of an unpaired electron in their outer orbitals. Oxygen free radicals are formed by the sequential univalent reduction of molecular oxygen. The superoxide anion radical (O_2^-) is formed by the addition of a single electron to molecular oxygen. Superoxide is a byproduct of adenosine triphosphate production in the mitochondria and other oxidation reduction reactions.[50] Polymorphonuclear cells are a second source of superoxide radicals that are released in response to bacterial inflammation.[51]

A major source of free radicals in ischemic tissue is the enzyme xanthine oxidase[52] (Fig. 2-9). With ischemia, high-energy phosphate compounds are converted to hypoxanthine, which accumulates in the tissues. When oxygen becomes available with reperfusion, xanthine oxidase catalyzes the conversion of hypoxanthine into uric acid and produces superoxide in the process. This reaction is an important mechanism in ischemic tissue injury in skin flaps.[53]

WOUND HEALING

The acute physiologic consequences of skin flap creation as it affects blood flow are of primary importance in the determination of early flap viability. Other mechanisms, however, play an equally important role in proper wound healing of the flap and help determine the flap's ultimate outcome. These additional mechanisms include the four cascades (clotting, compliment, kinin, and plasminogen), collagen formation,

and collagen degradation. Optimal flap wound healing depends on a well-orchestrated interplay of all of these processes.

Over the last decade, the role of peptide growth factors in soft-tissue wound healing has gained more attention. These signal proteins contribute to flap wound healing by controlling the recruitment and proliferation of cells (endothelial, epithelial, and fibroblast), which modulate the formation of new vessels, collagen, epithelium, and matrix (Fig. 2-10).

ATTEMPTS TO ALTER SKIN FLAP VIABILITY

Kerrigan[54] outlined extrinsic and intrinsic causes of skin flap failure. Extrinsic reasons for flap necrosis are those that do not result from the design of the raised flap. Examples include systemic hypotension, infection, and pedicle compression. These factors can often be overcome in the clinical situation. The primary intrinsic factor that affects flap survival is inadequate blood flow. Numerous experimental attempts have been made to influence flap microcirculation and/or decrease the deleterious effects of inadequate blood flow to the flap (Fig. 2-11). The most successful attempt has been flap delay.

Research Methods

A large amount of literature is available on the physiologic characteristics of skin flaps. The results of several studies give conflicting results. Experimental results are often difficult to interpret because of variation in choice of animal model, timing of treat-

Figure 2-10 Role of peptide growth factors.

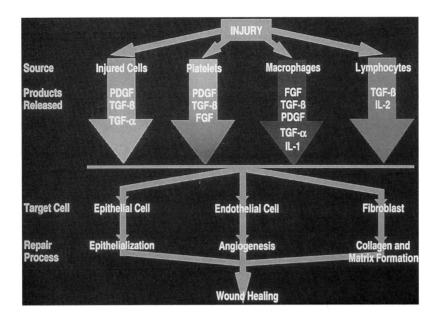

Figure 2-11 Experimental attempts to affect flap survival.

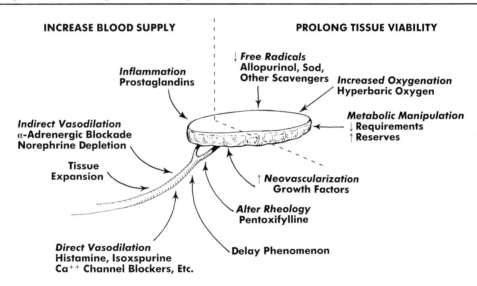

ment, route of drug administration, method of data collection, and repeatability of the study.[55] Standardization of research methods would help resolve some of these difficulties.

Two basic experimental designs have been used to investigate the consequences of a vascular insult on a surgical flap. In one design the blood supply to a flap was interrupted for varying amounts of time by occluding or otherwise interrupting flow through the vascular pedicle. The maximum amount of ischemic time that the flap can survive in the experimental and control groups was determined. This design has been used for investigation of the no-reflow phenomenon

and ischemia tolerance. The second design involved flaps with a random extension in which the effects of an experimental manipulation on flap survival or flap blood flow was compared with a control. From this basic framework a number of animal models and methods to assess blood flow and survival have been developed in attempts to alter skin flap viability.

Delay

Four facts are accepted about the delay phenomenon: (1) the phenomenon requires surgical trauma, (2) a large percentage of the neurovascular supply to the flap must be eliminated, (3) delay results in increased flap survival at the time of tissue transfer, and (4) the beneficial effects can last up to 6 weeks in humans.[56] There are three theories regarding the mechanism of delay: (1) delay improves blood flow, (2) delay conditions tissue to ischemia,[57] and (3) delay closes arteriovenous shunts.[58] Most recent reports support a mechanism that results in increased circulation to the flap.

Sympathetic denervation causing depletion of norepinephrine within the flap is one mechanism thought to play a role in the increase of blood flow to a delayed flap. Release of norepinephrine occurs soon after flap elevation, and norepinephrine stores are largely depleted in the first 24 to 48 hours.[35,39] After catecholamine depletion, a relative state of sympathectomy develops but the vasculature to the flap has an increased sensitivity to the effects of adrenergic drugs (a hyperadrenergic state).[34] Pang et al[38] theorized that a change in the vasoactivity of the small arteries allowed delivery of more blood to the distal portion of the flap. During elevation of the bipedicled flap, there is a release of vasoconstrictive substances (norepinephrine, thromboxane, and serotonin). Necrosis is not seen during the first stage of delay because the bipedicled flap has an ample blood supply. During the delay period, catecholamine depletion occurs and there is a recovery from the hyperadrenergic state. Conversion of the delayed flap to a single pedicle is not accompanied by the same degree of vasoconstriction, resulting in improved blood flow and increased survival.[59]

Development of vascular collaterals and reorientation of the major vascular channels is another mechanism to increase blood flow to the distal portion of the single pedicle flap.[60-62] Longitudinal flow also is enhanced by vasodilating substances released by inflammation and mild ischemia.[63] Pang et al[59] hypothesized that the depletion of vasoconstricting substances played a role in the early stage of delay and that locally released vasodilating substances were involved in the later stages (see box below).

Mechanisms of improvement of blood flow by the delay phenomenon

- Depletion of vasoconstricting substances
- Formation of vascular collaterals and reorientation of vascular channels
- Stimulation of an inflammatory response
- Release of vasodilating substances

Increase of Blood Supply

Indirect Vasodilators The intense vasoconstriction associated with release of norepinephrine after flap elevation would seem to hinder flap survival. As discussed above, one of the benefits of flap delay seems to be depletion of norepinephrine before creation of the flap to be transferred. If this vasoconstriction could be blocked or reversed, the duration and severity of distal flap ischemia should be lessened. The result would be increased flap survival without the need for delay.

Several anesthetic agents have vasoactive properties and may influence flap survival. Because general anesthetics are often used during the creation of larger flaps, any potential effects on flap survival are important. Isoflurane, a sympatholytic vasodilator, was found to significantly improve flap survival compared with nitrous oxide, which induces vasoconstriction.[64]

Investigators have attempted to produce a "pharmacologic delay" by suppressing the catecholamine-induced vasoconstriction seen after flap elevation. Methods have included administration of α-adrenergic blocking agents and depletion of norepinephrine stores, but both methods have had mixed results and have resulted in systemic toxicity.

Direct Vasodilators Direct vasodilators such as histamine, hydralazine, and topical dimethylsulfoxide have showed both a beneficial effect and no effect on skin flap survival.[55] Isoxsuprine is a phenylethylamine derivative of epinephrine and has α-adrenergic receptor antagonistic and β-adrenergic receptor agonistic properties that result in relaxation of vascular smooth muscle. Isoxsuprine was found to increase blood flow in the area of the dominant artery in porcine myocutaneous and arterial flaps; unfortunately, no improvement in blood flow was seen in the distal random portion of the flaps or in flap survival.[63,65] The smaller vessels in the distal random portion of a flap were theorized to have a different sensitivity to vasodilator drugs than do muscular or axial arteries. Manipulation of these distal vascular channels appears to be critical in the improvement of flap survival.

Experiments that investigated the effects of other direct vasodilators have given either mixed results or have yet to be confirmed. Studies have attempted to increase skin flap survival with calcitonin gene-related peptide,[66,67] calcium channel blockers,[68-70] topical nitroglycerin,[71,72] and topical dimethyl sulfoxide.[73,74] The failure of direct vasodilators to reproducibly increase flap survival indicates that mechanisms other than direct arterial dilation are important in survival of the ischemic flap.

Neovascularization Neovascularization can be potentially accelerated with angiogenic growth factors to improve flap viability. Increased flap survival and vascularity were seen when an endothelial cell growth factor was applied in a sustained release fashion to accelerate peripheral neovascularization in compromised flaps.[75,76]

Alteration of Rheology In a homogeneous fluid that exhibits equal shear stress at different rates of shear, flow in a vessel can be approximated by the Poiseuille equation [1]:

$$Q = \frac{\Delta P * r^4 * \pi}{1 * 8 * \eta}$$

where:
Q = flow in a vessel
ΔP = pressure gradient
r^4 = the fourth power of the vessel radius
l = vessel length
η = viscosity

Although blood is not a newtonian fluid, the qualitative relationships in the equation remain. In larger vessels the radius is a dominant factor, but in the capillary microcirculation viscosity becomes more important. By a decrease in the viscosity of blood, it may be possible to increase flow to the distal random portion of the newly raised flap and beneficially affect flap survival. Viscosity is influenced by the hematocrit, serum proteins, temperature, and red blood cell deformability and aggregation as well as other factors.[77] Each of these factors can be potentially manipulated with a resultant change in viscosity.

Pentoxifylline and low-viscosity whole-blood substitutes (Fluosol-DA) also will lower viscosity. Pentoxifylline is a hemorrheologic agent that results in increased red blood cell deformability[78] and decreased platelet aggregability.[77] When given 7 to 10 days before flap elevation, pentoxifylline has increased flap survival in porcine dorsal flank flaps[79] and the rat dorsal flap.[77] Beneficial effects with limited preoperative dosing of pentoxifylline, however, have not been uniform.[80,81] Fluosol-DA administration has also failed to consistently increase flap survival.[82,83]

Inflammation The surgical trauma associated with a newly raised or delayed flap results in an inflammatory response. This response results in a local increase in blood flow that could benefit flap survival. Improved flap survival has been shown with different methods for creation of an inflammatory response before flap creation.[40,84,85] These studies demonstrate that the inflammatory response can be a stimulus for "delay" without sympathectomy or vascular division.

The mechanism by which inflammation produces a beneficial effect appears to involve the products of cyclooxygenase metabolism of arachadonic acid. On the other hand, cyclooxygenase inhibitors such as indomethacin and ibuprofen have been shown to increase skin flap viability.[86,87] Glucocorticoids, which inhibit phospholipase A_2 activity, have also increased flap survival in some studies.[88-90] Administration of prostaglandins that cause vasodilation and decrease platelet aggregation tend to increase survival of experimental flaps.[91-93] Blocking thromboxane A_2 synthesis has had mixed results.[44,94]

Tissue Expansion Tissue expansion has been demonstrated to increase the size of the transferred flap in experimental animals and in humans. Examination of expanded skin in the guinea pig has shown an increase in the thickness[95] and mitotic activity[96] of the epidermal layer, a finding that indicates epidermal proliferation. Blood flow in expanded tissue is greater than in skin overlying a noninflated expander 1 hour after creation of a pedicled flap in the porcine model.[97] The increased blood flow to expanded skin when compared to delay seems to be short-lived.[98,99] Apart from the early changes seen with expander manipulation, the flap viability and blood flow in expanded skin appear to be similar to those seen in delayed flaps.[100]

Prolonged Viability

Protection Against Harmful Agents The formation of free radicals with reperfusion and the return of molecular oxygen to ischemic tissue has been a recent focus of experiments attempting to improve flap survival. This research has focused on decrease in the production of free radicals and employment of agents that remove free radicals (free radical scavengers) from the immediate environment.

Administration of allopurinol (a xanthine oxidase inhibitor) preoperatively prevents the increased xanthine oxidase activity seen with acute flap elevation.[101] Improved survival of dorsal rat flaps has been accomplished when allopurinol was given at high doses,[102,103] but lower doses had no effect. The high doses required have led to concern about the use of allopurinol to increase flap survival in the clinical setting.

A number of free radical scavengers are available to protect the tissues from destruction by free radicals. Superoxide dismutase (SOD), an intracellular free radical scavenger, catalyzes the conversion of superoxide to hydrogen peroxide (H_2O_2) and molecular oxygen. When given systemically, SOD is an effective scavenger of the superoxide radical regardless of its source.[53] SOD treatment has resulted in improved flap survival[103-105] and increased tolerance to ischemia in rat abdominal flaps.[106,107] Improved flap survival has also been demonstrated with a number of other naturally occurring compounds with free radical scavenging properties. These include deferoxamine,[108] vitamin E, vitamin A, vitamin C, glutathione,[109] various amino acids,[110] and amino acid derivatives.[111]

The hydrogen peroxide formed by the dismutation of superoxide is not particularly harmful. In the presence of chelated metal complexes, however, hydrogen peroxide can be converted into a hydroxyl radical (OH·) by the Fenton or Haber-Weiss reaction (see Fig. 2-9).[112] The hydroxyl radical is much more reactive and may be responsible for much of the damage inflicted by oxygen free radicals.[50] The presence of a hematoma under a flap may decrease flap survival by increasing the available iron, which acts as a catalyst in the formation of free radicals.[113]

Increase of Tolerance of Ischemia

Increased oxygenation Improvement in flap survival with hyperbaric oxygen treatment has been documented in the rat model.[114,115] Hyperbaric oxygen treatment, however, increases blood oxygen-carrying capacity by at most 20%.[114] A greater effect of hyperbaric oxygen treatment may be that it increases oxygen diffusion from surrounding perfused tissue to the ischemic portion of the flap.[116] Increased flap survival occurs with treatments that use 21% hyperbaric oxygen, which implies that increased oxygen could be delivered with an increase in pressure alone.[117] A treatment delay of 24 hours or longer after elevation of rat dorsal flaps results in little benefit from hyperbaric oxygen.[118,119] An experiment using a porcine model was less successful in improvement of flap survival.[120]

Metabolic manipulation Decreasing the metabolic requirements or increasing the metabolic reserves of skin are additional strategies to increase flap survival. These approaches are based on the idea that flap necrosis occurs when tissue metabolic demand is greater than what the blood supply can deliver. An effective way to reduce metabolic activity and delay necrotic changes is to decrease temperature, but improvement in flap survival is not seen with this method.[121,122]

IMPAIRED FLAPS

Smoking tobacco is associated with an increased chance of flap necrosis in facelift operations.[123] Exposure to tobacco smoke resulted in increased flap necrosis of dorsal flaps in rats[124] and hamsters.[125] The deleterious effects of nicotine appear to increase with prolonged exposure.[126] The mechanism whereby tobacco or nicotine produces decreased flap survival is unknown but may involve direct endothelial damage, vasoconstriction secondary to catecholamine release, or local concentrations of prostaglandins.

Radiation has been shown to be deleterious to flap survival in some studies[127,128] but not in others.[119,129,130] The reason for this discrepancy is probably because of differences in the radiation regimen administered (that is, radiation dosage, fractionation, and surgical timing with respect to the radiation). Radiation treatment results in endarteritis obliterans and altered wound healing. Despite prior radiation, the delay phenomenon continues to improve flap survival.[131] Flap neovascularization is delayed but not eliminated after radiation.[132] The use of angiogenic growth factors has the potential to increase the viability of irradiated skin flaps by means of accelerating revascularization.[76]

SUMMARY

The blood flow required for nutritional support of the skin is dramatically less than what is available to carry out its thermoregulatory function. This allows skin to survive a compromise of its blood supply during creation of local flaps. The surviving length of a particular flap depends on the relationship between the intravascular perfusion pressure and the critical closing pressure of the arterioles in the subdermal plexus. Appropriate flap design is the most critical factor in maintenance of adequate intravascular perfusion pressure and avoidance of tissue necrosis.

During the first 48 hours after a flap is raised, the transferred tissue must survive a number of hazards. The arteriolar closing pressure is increased by catecholamine released from divided sympathetic nerves within the tissue. An inflammatory response begins the process of wound healing but may also impair blood flow with the formation of tissue edema. The increased oxygen supply available with reperfusion results in the formation of free radicals that can further damage tissue. Beyond the first few days, neovascularization and wound healing lessen the surviving flap's dependence on the pedicle.

Attempts to improve flap survival have involved improving flap design, altering the early physiologic impairment of blood flow, and increasing tissue resistance to ischemia. Surgical delay is the most effective intervention. Pharmacologic manipulations designed to improve blood flow or increase tissue tolerance of ischemia have not achieved the significant and reproducible results required for incorporation into common clinical use. Research is ongoing to expand the boundaries of local flap reconstruction.

REFERENCES

1. Guyton A: *Textbook of medical physiology*, ed 5. Philadelphia, 1976, WB Saunders Co.

2. Sherman J: Normal arteriovenous anastomoses. *Medicine* 42:247, 1963.

3. Greene N: Physiology of sympathetic denervation, *Ann Rev Med* 13:87, 1962.

4. Grange H, Goodman A, Grange N: Role of resistance and exchange vessels in local microvascular control of skeletal muscle oxygenation in the dog, *Circ Res* 38:379, 1976.

5. Wideman M, Tuma R, Mayorvitz H: Defining the precapillary sphincter. *Microvasc Res* 12:71, 1976.

6. Folkow B: Role of the nervous system in the control of vascular tone, *Circulation* 21:760, 1960.

7. Daniel RK, Kerrigan CL: *Principles and physiology of skin flap surgery*. In McCarthy, JG, editor: *Plastic surgery*, vol 1. Philadelphia, 1990, WB Saunders Co.

8. Webster JP: Thoraco-epigastric tubed pedicles, *Surg Clin North Am* 17:145, 1937.

9. Bloom W and Fawcett DW: *A textbook of histology*. Philadelphia, 1975, WB Saunders Co.

10. Anden N, Carlsson A, Haggendal J: Adrenergic mechanisms, *Ann Rev Pharmacol* 9:119, 1969.

11. Mellander S, Johansson B: Control of resistance, exchange, and capacitance functions in the peripheral circulation, *Pharmacol Rev* 20:117, 1968.

12. Daniel RK: *The anatomy and hemodynamics of the cutaneous circulation and their influence on skin flap design*. In Grabb WC, Myers MB, editors: *Skin flaps*, Boston, 1975, Little, Brown & Co.

13. Gottrup F, Oredsson S, Price DC, et al: A comparative study of skin blood flow in musculocutaneous and random-pattern flaps, *J Surg Res* 37:443, 1984.

14. Cutting CA: Critical closing and perfusion pressures in flap survival, *Ann Plast Surg* 9:524, 1982.

15. Landis E: Microinjection studies of capillary permeability, *Am J Physiol* 82:217, 1927.

16. Milton S: Fallacy of the length-width ratio, *Br J Plast Surg* 57:502, 1971.

17. Myers B: Understanding flap necrosis, *Plast Reconstr Surg* 78:813, 1986 (editorial).

18. Kerrigan C, Daniel R: Critical ischemia time and the failing skin flap, *Plast Reconstr Surg* 69:986, 1982.

19. Tsur H, Daniller A, and Strauch B: Neovascularization of skin flaps: route and timing, *Plast Reconstr Surg* 66:85, 1980.

20. Verlander E: Vascular changes in a tubed pedicle: V. an experimental study, *Acta Chir Scand* Suppl 322:1, 1964.

21. Gatti J, LaRossa D, Brousseau D, et al: Assessment of neovascularization and timing of flap division, *Plast Reconstr Surg* 73:396, 1984.

22. Cummings C, Trachy R: Measurement of alternative blood flow in the porcine panniculus carnosus myocutaneous flap, *Arch Otolaryngol* 111:598, 1985.

23. Klingenstrom P and Nylen B: Timing of transfer of tubed pedicles and cross flaps, *Plast Reconstr Surg* 37:1, 1966.

24. Furcht LT: Critical factors controlling angiogenesis: cell products, cell matrix, and growth factors, *Lab Invest* 55:505, 1986.

25. Smahel J: *The healing of skin grafts*. In Montandon D, editor: *Clinics in plastic surgery*, Philadelphia, 1977, WB Saunders Co.

26. Folkman J: How is blood vessel growth regulated in normal and neoplastic tissue? *Cancer* Res 46:467, 1986.

27. D'Amore PA: *The role of growth factors and cell-cell communication in the control of angiogenesis*. In Cederholm-Williams SA, Ryan TJ, Lydon MJ, editors: *Fibrinolysis and angiogenesis in wound healing*. Princeton, NJ, 1987, Excerpta Medica.

28. Maciag T, Cerundolo S, Ilsley S, et al: An endothelial cell growth factor, *Proc Natl Acad Sci* 76:5674-5678, 1979.

29. Gospodarowicz D, Thakoral KK: Production of a corpus luteum angiogenic factor responsible for the proliferation of capillaries and revascularization of the corpus luteum, *Proc Natl Acad Sci USA* 75:874, 1978.

30. Federman JL, Brown JC, Felberg NT, et al: Experimental ocular angiogenesis, *Am J Ophthalmol* 89:231, 1980.

31. Huffman H, McAustan B, Robertson D, et al: An endothelial growth stimulating factor from salivary glands, *Exp Cell Res* 102:269, 1976.

32. Amerbuch R, Kuban L, Sidley Y: Angiogenesis induction by tumors, embryonic tissues and lymphocytes, *Cancer Res* 36:3435, 1976.

33. Su CT, Im MJ, Hoopes JE: Tissue glucose and lactate following vascular occlusion in island skin flaps, *Plast Reconstr Surg* 70:202, 1982.

34. Pearl R: A unifying theory of the delay phenomenon: recovery from the hyperadrenergic state, *Ann Plast Surg* 7:102, 1981.

35. Palmer B: Sympathetic denervation and reinnervation of cutaneous blood vessels following surgery, *Scand J Plast Reconstr Surg* 4:93, 1970.

36. Jurell G, Norberg K, and Palmer B: Surgical denervation of the cutaneous blood vessels, *Acta Physiol Scand* 74:511, 1968.

37. Kerrigan C, Daniel R: Skin flap research: a candid view, *Plast Reconstr Surg* 13:383, 1984.

38. Pang C, Neligan C, Forrest C, et al: Hemodynamics and vascular sensitivity to circulating norepinephrine in normal skin and delayed and acute random skin flaps in the pig, *Plast Reconstr Surg* 78:75, 1986.

39. Jurell G: Adrenergic nerves and the delay phenomenon, *Ann Plast Surg* 17:497, 1986.

40. Liston S: Nonbacterial inflammation as a means of enhancing skin flap survival, *Laryngoscope* 94:1075, 1984.

41. Macht S, and Frazier W: The role of endogenous bacterial flora in skin flap survival, *Plast Reconstr Surg* 65:50, 1980.

42. Hauben D, Aijlstra F: Prostacyclin formation in delayed pig flank flaps, *Ann Plast Surg* 13:304, 1984.

43. Kaley G, Hintze T, Panzenbeck M, et al: *Role of prostaglandins in microcirculatory function*, In Neri GG, et al, editors: *Advances in prostaglandin, thromboxane, and leukotriene research*, Vol. 12, 1985. New York, 1985, Raven Press.

44. Kay S, Green C: The effect of a novel thromboxane synthetase inhibitor dazegrel (UK38485) on random pattern skin flaps in the rat, *Br J Plast Surg* 39:361, 1986.

45. Nakano J: *General pharmacology of prostaglandins*. In Cuthbert MF, editor: *The prostaglandins*, Philadelphia, 1973, JB Lippincott Co.

46. Campbell WB: *Lipid-derived autacoids: eicosanoids and platelet-activating factor*. In Gilman AG, Rall TW, Nies AS, et al, editors: *Goodman and Gilman's the pharmacologic basis of therapeutics*, New York, 1990, Pergamon Press.

47. Murphy R, Lawrence W, Robson M, et al: Surgical delay and arachidonic acid metabolites: evidence for an inflammatory mechanism: an experimental study in rats, *Br J Plast Surg* 38:272, 1985.

48. Sasaki G, Pang C: Hemodynamics and viability of acute neurovascular island skin flaps in rats, *Plast Reconstr Surg* 65:152, 1980.

49. Mulliken J, Im M: The etiologic role of free radicals in hematoma-induced flap necrosis. *Plast Reconstr Surg* 77:802, 1986 (discussion).

50. Southorn P, Powis D: Free radicals in medicine: I. Chemical nature and biologic reactions. *Mayo Clin Proc* 63:381, 1988.

51. Babior B, Kipnes R, Curnutte J: Biological defence mechanisms: the production by leukocytes of superoxide, a potential bactericidal agent, *J Clin Invest* 52:741, 1973.

52. McCord J: Oxygen-derived free radicals in postischemic tissue injury, *N Engl J Med* 312:159, 1985.

53. McCord J: Improved survival of island flaps after prolonged ischemia by perfusion with superoxide dismutase, *Plast Reconstr Surg* 77:643, 1986 (discussion).

54. Kerrigan CL: Skin flap failure: pathophysiology, *Plast Reconstr Surg* 72:766, 1983.

55. Kerrigan C, Daniel R: Pharmacologic treatment of the failing skin flap, *Plast Reconstr Surg* 70:541, 1982.

56. Pearl R: The delay phenomenon: why the fuss? *Ann Plast Surg* 13:307, 1984.

57. McFarlane RM, Heagy FC, Radin S, et al: A study of the delay phenomenon in experimental pedicle flaps, *Plast Reconstr Surg* 35:245, 1965b.

58. Reinisch JF: The pathophysiology of skin flap circulation: the delay phenomenon, *Plast Reconstr Surg* 54:585, 1974.

59. Pang C, Forrest C, Neligan P, et al: Augmentation of blood flow in delayed random skin flaps in the pig: effect of length of delay period and angiogenesis, *Plast Reconstr Surg* 78:68, 1986.

60. Cutting C, Bardach J, Tinseth F: Haemodynamics of the delayed skin flap: a total blood flow study, *Br J Plast Surg* 34:133, 1981.

61. Guba A: Study of the delay phenomenon in axial pattern flaps in pigs, *Plast Reconstr Surg* 63:550, 1979.

62. Suzuki S, Isshiki N, Ohtsuka M, et al: Experimental study on "delay" phenomenon in relation to flap width and ischaemia, *Br J Plast Surg* 41:389, 1988.

63. Pang C, Neligan P, Nakatsuka T, et al: Pharmacologic manipulation of the microcirculation in cutaneous and myocutaneous flaps in pigs, *Clin Plast Surg* 12:173, 1985.

64. Dohar J, Goding G, Azarshin K: The effects of inhalation anesthetic agents on survival in a pig random skin flap model, *Arch Otolaryngol* 118:37, 1992.

65. Neligan P, Pang C, Nakatsuka T, et al: Pharmacologic action of isoxsuprine in cutaneous and myocutaneous flaps, *Plast Reconstr Surg* 75:363, 1985.

66. Kjartansson J, Dalsgaard C: Calcitonin gene related peptide increases survival of a musculocutaneous critical flap in the rat, *Eur J Pharmacol* 142:355, 1987.

67. Knight K, Martin T, Coe S, et al: Effect of the vasodilator peptides calcitonin gene-related peptide and atriopeptin on rabbit microvascular blood flow: preliminary communication, *Br J Plast Surg* 41:147, 1988.

68. Hira M, Tajima S, Sano S: Increased survival length of experimental flap by calcium antagonist nifedipine, *Ann Plast Surg* 24:45, 1990.

69. Miller A, Falcone R, Nappi J, et al: The lack of effect of nifedipine on failing skin flaps, *J Dermatol Surg Oncol* 11:612, 1985.

70. Nichter L, Sobieski M: Efficacy of verapamil in salvage of failing random skin flaps, *Ann Plast Surg* 21:242, 1988.

71. Nichter L, Sobieski M, Edgerton M: Efficacy of topical nitroglycerin for random-pattern skin-flap salvage, *Plast Reconstr Surg* 75:847, 1985.

72. Rohrich R, Cherry G, Spira M: Enhancement of skin-flap survival using nitroglycerin ointment, *Plast Reconstr Surg* 73:943, 1984.

73. Arturson G, Khanna N: The effects of hyperbaric oxygen, dimethyl sulfoxide, and complamim on the survival of experimental skin flaps, *Scand J Plast Reconstr Surg* 4:8, 1970.

74. Myers M, Donovan W: *Augmentation of tissue oxygen by dimethyl sulfoxide and hydrogen peroxide.* In Bruley C and Dicher H, editors: *Oxygen transport to tissue: instrumentation, methods, and psychology.* New York, 1973, Plenum Press.

75. Hom D, Assefa G: The effects of endothelial cell growth factor on vascular compromised skin flaps, *Arch Otolaryngol Head Neck Surg* 118:624, 1992.

76. Hom D, Assefa G, Song C: Endothelial cell growth factor: application to irradiated soft tissue, *Laryngoscope,* 103:165, 1993.

77. Roth A, Briggs P, Jones E, et al: Augmentation of skin flap survival by parenteral pentoxifylline. *Br J Plast Surg* 41:515, 1988.

78. Ehrly A: Improvement of the flow properties of blood: a new therapeutic approach in occlusive arterial disease, *Angiology* 27:188, 1976.

79. Yessenow R, Maves M: The effects of pentoxifylline on random skin flap survival, *Arch Otolaryngol Head Neck Surg* 115:179, 1989.

80. Chu B, Deshmukh N: The lack of effect of pentoxifylline on random skin flap survival, *Plast Reconstr Surg* 83:315, 1989.

81. Hodgson R, Brummett R, Cook T: Effects of pentoxifylline on experimental skin flap survival. *Arch Otolaryngol Head Neck Surg* 113:950, 1987.

82. Chowdary R, Berkower A, Moss M, et al: Fluorocarbon enhancement of skin flap survival in rats, *Plast Reconstr Surg* 79:98, 1987b.

83. Ramasastry S, Waterman P, Angel M, et al: Effect of fluosol-DA (20%) on skin flap survival in rats, *Ann Plast Surg* 15:436, 1985.

84. Kami T, Yoshmura Y, Nakajima T, et al: Effects of low-power diode lasers on flap survival, *Ann Plast Surg* 14:278, 1985.

85. Lawrence W, Murphy R, Robson M, et al: Prostanoid derivatives in experimental flap delay with formic acid, *Br J Plast Surg* 37:602, 1984.

86. Robson M, DelBeccaro E, Heggers J: The effects of prostaglandins on the dermal microcirculation after burning and the inhibition of the effect by specific pharmacological agents, *Plast Reconstr Surg* 63:781, 1979.

87. Sasaki G, Pang C: Experimental evidence for involvement of prostaglandins in viability of acute skin flaps: effects on viability and mode of action, *Plast Reconstr Surg* 67:335, 1981.

88. Kristensen J, Wadskov S, Henriksen O: Dose-dependent effect of topical corticosteroids on blood flow in human cutaneous tissue, *Acta Derm Venereol* 58:145, 1978.

89. Mendelson B, Woods J: Effect of corticosteroids on the surviving length of skin flaps in pigs, *Br J Plast Surg* 31:293, 1978.

90. Mes L: Improving flap survival by sustained cell metabolism within ischemic cells: a study using rabbits, *Plast Reconstr Surg* 65:56, 1980.

91. Reus W, Murphy R, Heggers J, et al: Effect of intraarterial prostacyclin on survival of skin flaps in the pig: biphasic response, *Ann Plast Surg* 13:29, 1984.

92. Silverman DG, Brousseau DA, Norton KJ, et al: The effects of a topical PGE_2 analogue on global flap ischemia in rats, *Plast Reconstr Surg* 84:794, 1989.

93. Suzuki S, Isshiki N, Ogawa Y, et al: Effect of intravenous prostaglandin E1 on experimental flaps, *Ann Plast Surg* 19:49, 1987.

94. Ono I, Ohura T, Murazumi M, et al: A study on the effectiveness of a thromboxane synthetase inhibitor (OKY-046) in increasing survival length of skin flaps, *Plast Reconstr Surg* 86:1164, 1990.

95. Austad E, Pasyk K, McClatchey K, et al: Histomorphic evaluation of guniea pig skin and soft tissue after controlled tissue expansion, *Plast Reconstr Surg* 70:704, 1982.

96. Francis A, Marks R: Skin stretching and epidermopoiesis, *Br J Exp Pathol* 58:35, 1977.

97. Marks M, Burney R, Mackenzie J, et al: Enhanced capillary blood flow in rapidly expanded random pattern flaps, *J Trauma* 26:913, 1986.

98. Goding G, Cummings C, Trachy R: Tissue expansion and cutaneous blood flow, *Laryngoscope* 98:1, 1988.

99. Ricciardeli E, Goding G, Bright D, et al: Acute blood flow changes in rapidly expanded and adjacent skin, *Arch Otolaryngol Head Neck Surg* 115:182, 1989.

100. Sasaki G, Pang C: Pathophysiology of skin flaps raised on expanded pig skin. *Plast Reconstr Surg* 74:59, 1984.

101. Im M, Shen W, Pak C, et al: Effect of allopurinol on the survival of hyperemic island skin flaps, *Plast Reconstr Surg* 73:276, 1984.

102. Angel M, Ramasastry S, Swartz W, et al: Augmentation of skin flap survival with allopurinol, *Ann Plast Surg* 18:494, 1987.

103. Pokorny A, Bright D, Cummings C: The effects of allopurinol and superoxide dismutase in a rat model of skin flap necrosis, *Arch Otolaryngol Head Neck Surg* 115:207, 1989.

104. Freeman TJ, Maisel RH, Goding GS, et al: Inhibition of endogenous superoxide dismutase with diethyldithiocarbamate in acute island skin flaps, *Otolaryngol Head Neck Surg* 103:938, 1990.

105. Zimmerman T, Sasaki G, Khattab S: Improved ischemic island skin flap survival with continuous intraarterial infusion of adenosine triphosphate-magnesium chloride and SOD: a rat model, *Ann Plast Surg* 18:218, 1987.

106. Marzella L, Jesudass R, Manson P, et al: Functional and structural evaluation of the vasculature of skin flaps after ischemia and reperfusion, *Plast Reconstr Surg* 81:742, 1988.

107. Sagi A, Ferder M, Levens D, et al: Improved survival of island flaps after prolonged ischemia by perfusion with superoxide dismutase, *Plast Reconstr Surg* 77:639, 1986.

108. Angel M, Narayanan K, Swartz, W et al: Deferoxamine increases skin flap survival: additional evidence of free radical involvement in ischaemic flap surgery, *Br J Plast Surg* 39:469, 1986.

109. Hayden R, Paniello R, Yeung C, et al: The effect of glutathione and vitamins A, C, and E on acute skin flap survival, *Laryngoscope* 97:1176, 1987.

110. Paniello R, Hayden R, and Bello S: Improved survival of acute skin flaps with amino acids as free radical scavengers, *Arch Otolaryngol Head Neck Surg* 114:1400, 1988.

111. Kim YS, Im MJ, Hoopes JE: The effect of a free-radical scavenger, N-2-mercaptopropionylglycine, on the survival of skin flaps, *Ann Plast Surg* 25:18, 1990.

112. Del Mastro R: An approach to free radicals in medicine and biology. *Acta Physiol Scand.* Suppl 492:153, 1980.

113. Angel M; Narayanan K, Swartz W, et al: The etiologic role of free radicals in hematoma-induced flap necrosis, *Plast Reconstr Surg* 77:795, 1986.

114. Kernahan D, Zingg W, Kay C: The effects of hyperbaric oxygen on the survival of experimental skin flaps, *Plast Reconstr Surg* 36:19, 1965.

115. Perrins D: *The effect of hyperbaric oxygen on ischemic skin flaps.* In Grabb W, Myers MB, editors: *Skin flaps.* Boston, 1975, Little, Brown & Co.

116. Cutting C: *Skin flap physiology.* In Cummings C, editor: *Otolaryngology Head and Neck Surgery.* St Louis, 1986, Mosby–Year Book.

117. Tan C, Im M, Myers R, et al: Effect of hyperbaric oxygen and hyperbaric air on survival of island skin flaps, *Plast Reconstr Surg* 73:27, 1984.

118. Jurell G and Kaijser L: The influence of varying pressure and duration of treatment with hyperbaric oxygen on the survival of skin flaps: an experimental study, *Scand J Plast Reconstr Surg* 7:25, 1973.

119. Nemiroff P, Merwin G, Brant T, et al: Effects of hyperbaric oxygen and irradiation on experimental skin flaps in rats, *Otolaryngol Head Neck Surg* 93:485, 1985.

120. Caffe H, Gallagher T: Experiments on the effects of hyperbaric oxygen on flap survival in the pig, *Plast Reconstr Surg* 81:954, 1988.

121. Goding G, Cummings C, Bright D: *Effects of local hypothermia on the porcine myocutaneous flap.* In Stucker FJ, editor: *Plastic and reconstructive surgery of the head and neck: proceedings of the Fifth International Symposium. American Academy of Facial Plastic and Reconstructive Surgery.* Philadelphia, 1991, BC Decker.

122. Kiehn C, and Desprez J: Effects of local hypothermia on pedicle flap tissue, *Plast Reconstr Surg* 25:349, 1960.

123. Rees T, Liverett D, Guy C: The effect of cigarette smoking on skin flap survival in the face lift patient, *Plast Reconstr Surg* 73:911, 1984.

124. Nolan J, Jenkins R, Kurihata K, et al: The acute effects of cigarette smoke exposure on experimental skin flaps, *Plast Reconstr Surg* 75:544, 1985.

125. Craig S Rees T: The effects of smoking on experimental skin flaps in hamsters, *Plast Reconstr Surg* 75:842, 1985.

126. Forrest C, Pang C, Lindsay W: Dose and time effects of nicotine treatment on the capillary blood flow and viability of random pattern skin flaps in the rat, *Br J Plast Surg* 40:295, 1987.

127. Patterson T, Berry R, Hopewell J, et al: *The effect of radiation in survival of experimental skin flaps.* In Grabb WC and Myers MB, editors: *Skin flaps.* Boston, 1975, Little, Brown & Co.

128. Young CMA, Hopewell JW: The effects of preoperative x-irradiation on the survival and blood flow of pedicle skin flaps in the pig, *Int J Radiation Oncol Biol Phys* 9:865, 1983.

129. Kleiman L, Hasslinger B, Eddy H, et al: The effects of carbocisplatin and radiation on skin flap survival, *Arch Otolaryngol Head Neck Surg* 118:68, 1992.

130. Fisher J, Hurn I, Rudolph R, et al: The effect of delay on flap survival in an irradiated field, *Plast Reconstr Surg* 73:99, 1984.

131. Weisman R, Blumberg A, Brousseau D, et al: Fluorometric assessment of skin flap viability in the rat: effect of radiation therapy, *Otolaryngol Head Neck Surg* 91:151, 1983.

132. Clarke H, Howard C, Pynn B, et al: Delayed neovascularization in free skin flap transfer to irradiated beds in rats, *Plast Reconstr Surg* 75:560, 1985.

3

BIOMECHANICS OF SKIN FLAPS

Brock D. Ridenour

Wayne F. Larrabee, Jr.

INTRODUCTION

There was a time when skin flap design was more art than science. Practitioners devised clever flaps of precise geometric design, but possessed little more than an intuitive understanding of the biomechanical properties of cutaneous tissue. By picking up a skin fold, they could estimate extensibility or judge the relation between tension and blood flow. Flap survival was erratic and unsure, depending on the experience, instinct, and judgment of the individual surgeon. During this period progress in reconstructive surgery occurred primarily by trial and error.

More recently, expanded scientific knowledge has overshadowed the need for art in much of plastic surgery. Today proper skin flap design relies less on instinct and more on science, emphasizing vascular patterns, pathophysiologic characteristics, and the biomechanical features of cutaneous tissue. Because the unique mechanical properties of skin influence blood flow and flap survival, they must be carefully thought about in the design of the local skin flap. The study of soft tissue biomechanics has increased precision and reliability, ensuring the local skin flap as the procedure of choice in small and medium-sized facial defects.

BIOMECHANICAL PROPERTIES OF CUTANEOUS TISSUE

The mechanical properties of a material are described by the relationship that exists between a force applied to a specimen and the resultant deformation of the specimen as a function of time. In engineering these mechanical properties are defined by the quantities *stress* (force per unit of original cross section) and *strain* (change in length divided by the original length). The stress-strain relationship is independent of the dimensions of the specimen and is a property of the material

itself. Uniform engineering materials (titanium) have a linear stress-strain (force-deformation) relationship, such that their mechanical properties can be described by a proportionality constant (C = stress/strain). If the stress-strain relationship does not vary as a function of time, the material is said to be *elastic*.[1]

Unlike many engineering materials, skin is a heterogeneous substance, composed of a network of dissimilar materials. It is a living tissue, capable of proliferation and change in response to a physical stimulus. The extraordinary physical characteristics of skin must serve its adaptive needs. It is not surprising, therefore, that the mechanical properties of cutaneous tissue are unique compared with those of other materials. For simplicity, skin can be said to have three basic mechanical properties: nonlinearity, anisotropy, and viscoelasticity.

Nonlinearity

The mechanical behavior of skin is attributable to its heterogeneous nature. Skin is composed of a series of interrelated networks that are intimately entwined. Structurally important components in the dermis include the collagen fibers, elastic fibers, nerve fibers, capillaries, lymphatics, and ground substance. In skin that is fully relaxed, collagen fibers are distributed throughout the dermis in a seemingly haphazard arrangement. Collagen is woven in a multidirectional array without preferential orientation of thick and thin bundles. Numerous connections between collagen bundles form a continuous network without visible free ends. There are no restrictive attachments among adjacent collagen bundles that seem free to glide, relative to each other. Wavy elastic fibers loop spirally around collagen and attach at multiple points along each bundle. Elastic fibers function as a type of energy storage device, bringing stretched collagen back to a relaxed position. Structural proteins bathe in a medium of interstitial fluid that acts as a lubricant on one

Figure 3-1 Stress-strain curve for isolated skin can be divided into three separate regions. Aged skin deforms under its own weight, shifting apparent origin of curve along X-axis. (From Larrabee WF Jr: Immediate repair of facial defects, *Dermatol Clin* **7**:662, 1989.)

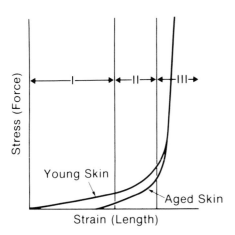

hand and a buffer against too sudden change on the other.

A typical stress-strain curve for isolated skin is shown in Fig. 3-1. The shape of the curve is similar to stress-strain and force-advancement curves obtained from tests on skin flaps[2] and other soft tissues.[1] Judging from its basic form, it is apparent that skin is nonlinear and that its mechanical behavior can be divided into three separate regions: (1) an initial flat section in which considerable extension occurs with little force, (2) an intermediate region of rapid transition, and (3) a terminal portion where little extension is possible despite great increases in applied force. An explanation for the shape of this curve has been formulated, based on histologic examination of the sequential stages of skin extension. During initial deformation randomly oriented collagen and elastic fibers are stretched in the direction of the applied force. Collagen fibers do not bear any burden until some of the bundles are completely straightened.[1] As a result, there is little resistance to initial deformation, and the stress-strain relationship is nearly linear and elastic (region 1). Naturally occurring tensions in the skin and small movements resulting from flexion and extension at joints all correspond to the first portion of the curve.[1] Without such freedom of movement, joint motion would require great muscular effort and skin would act as a restrictive envelope. As deformation progresses, additional collagen fibers are recruited into the load-carrying role, and resistance rises rapidly (region 2). At high-stress loads practically all the dermal collagen fibers are aligned in the direction of the applied force. At this point no further deformation is possible due to the inextensible nature of fully

oriented collagen (region 3). Wholly oriented collagen limits the damage due to large accidental stresses and prevents further deformation, thereby preserving the structural integrity of the epidermis.[1]

As one might expect, the mechanical properties of skin show a marked age dependency. Loss of elastic fibers occurs with age,[1] altering the shape of the stress-strain curve. Degeneration of the elastin network leads to a progressive loss in the elastic recovery of skin. As a result, aged skin deforms under its own weight, modifying the apparent origin of the stress-strain curve (Fig. 3-1). The final phase of deformation is similar for young and aged skin, suggesting that the stiffness of collagen does not change with age.

The stress-strain curve clearly illustrates that skin has a finite capacity for deformation or extension. Wound closure along the terminal portion of the stress-strain curve tests the reserve of the fibrous network and all the tissues entwined within. Taut collagen fibers efface small-caliber blood vessels and obliterate terminal capillaries,[3] increasing the risk of tissue necrosis. In many skin flaps blood supply is already tenuous, and a small increase in tension will result in a critical interruption of distal blood flow. When a random skin flap is raised, its blood supply is limited by the number and caliber of vessels entering at the anatomic base of the flap. Sudden release of stored catecholamines from disrupted nerve endings results in an intense vasoconstriction, which persists from 16 to 32 hours.[4,5] Total blood flow declines precipitously when measured from proximal to distal across the length of a skin flap.[6] Even a modicum of unnecessary tension may further impede blood flow and adequate nutrition.

The effect of tension on blood flow has been shown by observation of blanching tensions[3] and by comparison of tissue survival to wound-closure tensions in animal models.[7] A quantitative description of the relationship between blood flow and wound tension is seen in Fig. 3-2. In this experimental pig model[8] the investigators created a random skin flap 3 cm wide and 6 cm long. Laser Doppler blood flow measurements were recorded at the base of the flap (area 4) and at separate 2-cm intervals, toward the distal tip (area 1). Tension was increased by 50-g increments to maximal tension. Several important observations can be made. First, blood flow is inversely proportional to the distance from the base of the flap. Second, blood flow decreases steadily with increasing tension until a critical value of 200 to 250 g is reached. Beyond this critical tension, there is little decline in flow despite tensions to 900 g. Flow returns to pretension levels immediately after tension is released.[8] Although one cannot commute quantitative data from a pig model to humans, the principal conclusions of this study are consistent

Figure 3-2   Relationship between tension and blood flow in 3-cm-wide and 6-cm-long random skin flap. Measurements were taken at 2-cm intervals from base of flap (area 4) to distal tip (area 1). Flow decreases steadily until critical value of 200 to 250 g is reached. (From Larrabee WF Jr, Holloway GA Jr, Sutton D: Wound tension and blood flow in skin flaps, *Ann Otol Rhinol Laryngol* **93**:114, 1984.)

Figure 3-3   Effect of tension on survival of random-patterned skin flaps. Flaps of intermediate length are sensitive to effects of tension. Flaps closed with less than 250 g of tension tended to survive, whereas flaps closed with greater tension underwent necrosis. (From Larrabee WF Jr, Holloway GA Jr, Sutton D: Wound tension and blood flow in skin flaps, *Ann Otol Rhinol Laryngol* **93**:113, 1984.)

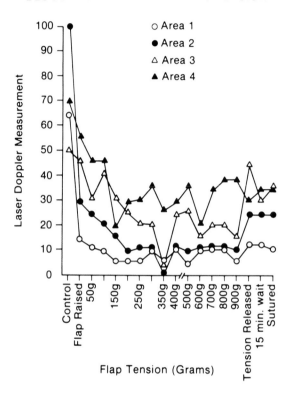

LASER DOPPLER MEASUREMENT OF FLAP BLOOD FLOW WITH INCREASING TENSION

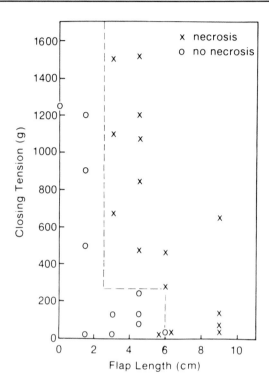

with empirical observation. Increasing tension results in a precipitous decline in blood flow, and the distal aspect of any flap is at the highest risk for necrosis.

Based on the supporting evidence in Fig. 3-2, it seems fair to remark that excess wound-closure tension can result in necrosis, particularly in flaps with border-line viability or impaired microcirculation. Larrabee et al[8] explored this possibility by designing a study to measure the effect of tension on survival in random-patterned skin flaps of equivocal viability. All flaps were created with a base of 3 cm, and the length was varied from 0 to 9 cm. Flaps were elevated in the subcutane-ous plane, superficial to the panniculus carnosus and advanced to close defects of varying size. Closure tension was measured precisely. The result of their study is summarized in Fig. 3-3. Not surprisingly, all flaps greater than 6 cm long underwent some necrosis, irrespective of closure tension. In the random-pat-terned skin flap, the length of the surviving segment was influenced by the number and caliber of blood

vessels that entered the anatomic base of the flap. Distal blood flow required an adequate perfusion pressure and a healthy microcirculation. Even with little or no tension, the longer flaps did not receive sufficient circulation through the cutaneous vascular plexus. Similarly, all flaps shorter than 1.5 cm remained viable, even when closed under excessive tension. In the short skin flap, survival was ensured because of an ample blood supply. Flaps of intermediate length, however, were quite sensitive to the effects of tension. Flaps closed with 250 g of tension or less tended to survive, whereas those closed under greater tension underwent necrosis. In summary, this study affirms the clinical observation that flaps with excellent blood flow can withstand extremes of tension. However, poorly de-signed flaps with inadequate blood flow will usually fail, despite a tension-free closure. Skin flaps with equivocal blood flow are most vulnerable to ischemic injury due to incremental changes in wound-closure tension.

Minor variations in flap design can alter the me-chanical characteristics of cutaneous tissue and change the force necessary for advancement and closure. A properly designed skin flap will minimize wound-closure tension and increase critical blood flow. In like manner, a poorly designed flap risks injury to important nutrient vessels while securing little or no mechanical advantage. Many practical questions concerning proper flap design have already been addressed in the pig model. According to Larrabee and Sutton[2], the rectangular advancement flap should be designed with a length-to-width ratio of at least 1:1. After this point, an increase in the ratio results in a gradual decline in wound-closure tension. Further increases in the length-to-width ratio are not always profitable and may risk necrosis of the distal portion of the flap. There is little advantage in increasing the length-to-width ratio if closure can be achieved along the early portion of the force-advancement curve. Advancement flaps should be designed with use of the minimal length-to-width ratio necessary to effect a low-tension closure. On a facial flap a ratio between 1:1 and 2:1 is ideal; further lengthening may prove necessary to avoid excessive tension but is usually unnecessary. Similarly, animal models have shown little mechanical benefit in extending rotation flaps past 90°.[2] Other considerations such as skin redraping may warrant the use of longer rotation flaps.

The forces that resist skin flap advancement are more complex than we have alluded to thus far. The edge of a skin flap is advanced both to stretch the skin and to overcome resistance between the dermis and underlying tissues.[9] The magnitude of this resistance (shearing force) varies considerably, depending on the site of interest and the age of the patient. Shearing forces can often be reduced by undermining in the subcutaneous plane. With undermining, vertical attachments between the subdermis and dermis are lysed, releasing the skin to slide unrestricted over the subcutaneous tissue. As undermining is increased, the origin of the shearing force is moved away from the edge of the flap and more free skin is available for low-resistance redraping (stretching).

In narrow-based skin flaps the skin mobility and subsequent redraping are commensurate with the extent of undermining. As undermining is increased, the force required to advance the leading edge a constant distance falls exponentially toward zero.[9] This is not intended to imply that extensive undermining beyond the base of the flap is always desirable or even useful. In fact, the vast majority of the benefit from undermining is achieved within the first 1 or 2 cm. Undermining beyond a short distance risks injury to surrounding structures and may compromise blood flow.

In broad-based flaps extensive undermining can result in an unexplained increase in the force necessary for advancement. In an experiment that used a pig model, 2 × 6 = cm elliptical defects were created (Fig.

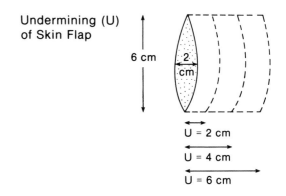

Figure 3-4   A 2 × 6 cm fusiform defect was created and undermined 2, 4, and 6 cm. (From Larrabee WF Jr: Design of local skin flaps. In Thomas JR, editor: American Academy of Ophthalmology HNS Instructional Courses, vol 3. St Louis, 1990, Mosby–Year Book, Inc.)

Figure 3-5   Force required to advance skin flap after undermining 2, 4, and 6 cm. Increasing undermining from 4 to 6 cm had little effect on force necessary for advancement. (From Larrabee WF Jr, Sutton D: Variation of skin stress-strain curves with undermining, *Surg Forum* 32:555, 1981.)

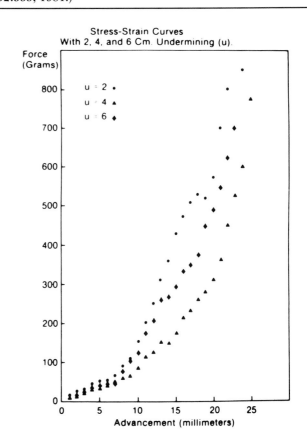

3-4). Undermining was performed to 2 cm, and a stress-strain (force-advancement) curve was created with a calibrated force gauge.[10] Curves were then measured after undermining 4 and 6 cm (Fig. 3-5). Ten series of curves were recorded in four piglets. In general, when undermining was increased from 2 to 4 cm, there was easier advancement of the skin flap (the curve shifted to the right). Increase of undermining from 4 to 6 cm often resulted in little change and sometimes resulted in a paradoxical shift of the curve to the left (more difficult advancement). Three of 10 flaps required more force for wound edge advancement when undermining was performed to 6 cm, compared with 4 cm. In no case did increasing the undermining from 4 to 6 cm result in a substantial decrease in the force required for advancement. Similar results were obtained in an experiment using broad-based flaps of different design.[9] There is not yet a simple explanation for this observed behavior. Rather, it seems apparent that with increased undermining of the broad-based skin flap the shearing force paradoxically increases, overshadowing any benefit obtained from low-resistance redraping of free skin.[9]

Anisotropy

There are enormous individual variations in the extensibility of human skin—differences between the slim and obese, young and old, male and female. The shape of the stress-strain curve (extensibility) is further influenced by edema, inflammation, hormonal conditions, and body height. It is the variation in skin tension within the same individual, however, that is of the most interest to the reconstructive surgeon. The variation in skin tension in different sites of the body is remarkable. On the face the skin is lax around the eyes and in the lateral cheek, and it is taut on the nose, chin, and forehead. Additionally, in each of these locations there are directional considerations for skin movement. The directional (anisotropic) qualities of skin are well known. In most regions of the body there is skin tension in every direction, but the degree of tension is greatest only in one, along the relaxed skin tension lines (RSTLs).[11] An incision made at right angles to the relaxed skin tension lines will gape widely and is much more likely to produce a stretched or hypertrophic scar. Therefore, whenever possible, elliptical excisions should be performed parallel to the RSTLs. This places the maximum closure-tension parallel to the lines of maximal extensibility (LME). The LME run perpendicular to the RSTLs and represent the direction in which closure can be performed with the least tension.[12] Local skin flaps are designed so that donor site closure is parallel to the lines of maximal extensibility.

RSTLs are not to be confused with Langer's lines.

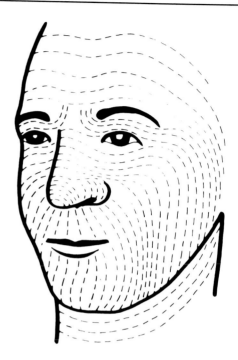

Figure 3-6   Relaxed skin tension lines (RSTLs) of face. In general, lines of maximal extensibility (LME) run perpendicular to relaxed skin tension lines. (From Larrabee WF Jr: Immediate repair of facial defects, *Dermatol Clin* **7**:663, 1989.)

The orientation of Langer's lines are often distinct from the creases formed in living subjects, when the joints are placed in a relaxed position. RSTLs follow the longest and straightest furrows formed when skin is relaxed (Fig. 3-6). They are not visible features of the skin but are derived from the act of pinching the skin and observing the furrows and ridges that form.[11] Whether lines of cutaneous tension (RSTLs) have an anatomic basis is subject to intense controversy. There is some evidence to suggest that when skin tension is preserved at the time of biopsy, the RSTLs are supported by a small number of extracellular support fibers. Although most of the fiber network has an apparent random orientation in the dermis, a small number of straight and thin fiber bundles (collagen and elastin) can be identified parallel to the RSTLs.[13] The predominate orientation of these fibers in the direction of the RSTLs suggests a possible cause-and-effect relationship.

Viscoelasticity

If the stress-strain relationship does not vary as a function of time, the material is said to be elastic. Skin behaves as an elastic substance only during the initial deformation at a low stress level. At higher loads skin shows viscoelastic properties, and strain becomes a function of both load and time. Two time-dependent properties of skin that are routinely employed by surgeons are *creep* and *stress relaxation.*

Creep refers to the increase in strain (change in length/original length) seen when skin is placed under a constant stress (force per unit area). At high-stress loads, a modicum of creep can be achieved in a short time. A small increase in length (strain) occurs, as compressed and straightened collagen fibers displace interstitial fluid that is loosely bound to the extracellular matrix (ground substance). When skin is stretched in the air, it is often possible to see the physical extrusion of fluid from its undersurface.[3] Time is required for fluid to move from one area to another, which explains the time dependence of the process. This mechanism, however, does not adequately explain the dramatic increase in strain that occurs in tissue expansion and in biologic conditions such as pregnancy and chronic obesity.

The first clinical application of tissue expansion was published by Neumann[14] in 1957 and the technique was later reintroduced and improved by Radovan.[15] Although few would refute its clinical utility, considerable debate has ensued regarding the most intriguing theoretical issue involving tissue expansion: Does tissue expansion generate an increase in the population of cells available for tissue transfer? Austad et al[16] proposed that question more than a decade ago: "Is it simply a 'loan,' or truly a 'dividend' of extra tissue?" Austad's work, and the work of others, clearly suggests the latter. Criticism of expansion has centered on the belief that the process may only thin the skin, trading

thickness for surface area. In fact, tissue expansion does result in thinning of the dermis,[16-18] at least initially. However, a mounting body of evidence suggests that over time dermal compensation will take place.

The preservation of epidermal thickness during expansion has been verified by several authors.[16,19] More recent studies by Austad and co-workers[20] and Olenius et al[21] have used tritiated thymidine labeling to illustrate an increase in epidermal mitotic activity in guinea pig and human skin, respectively. Although it is clear that expansion triggers keratinocyte proliferation, the mechanism by which keratinocytes respond to an expanding mass beneath them remains unknown. With use of a pig model, Johnson and colleagues[17] measured a marked increase in total surface area of skin both during and after tissue expansion (Fig. 3-7). It is noteworthy that expanders remained in place for the duration of data collection. Their presence may have provided some degree of ongoing stimulus[22] in addition to limiting the postexpansion shrinkage of tissue. Nonetheless, the experiment clearly demonstrates a marked increase in skin surface area immediately after expansion.

The long-term effects of tissue expansion on the dermis are more difficult to discern. Unequivocally, dermal thickness is reduced both during tissue expansion and for an undefined period thereafter. What is not clear, however, is whether eventual restoration of the normal dermis occurs and by what mechanism. In the study in pigs by Johnson and co-workers[17] dermal thinning persisted for 36 weeks after complete expan-

Figure 3-7   Increase in surface area seen with tissue expansion. Tissue expanders were left implanted during postexpansion period. (From Johnson PE, Kernahan DA, Bauer BS: Dermal and epidermal response to soft-tissue expansion in the pig, *Plast Reconstr Surg* **81:391, 1988.**)

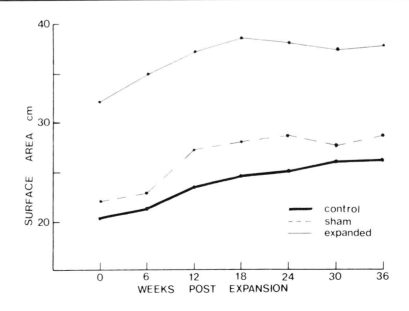

sion (Fig. 3-8). Because tissue expanders remained implanted, direct clinical translation of this data is cautioned. Nonetheless, dermal compensation appears to be slow compared with the rapid proliferative response of the keratinocytes. Such a discrepancy is not encountered in physiologic expansion, as in chronic obesity, in which collagen content and dermal thickness remain uniform.[23] This finding suggests that preservation of the dermis and collagen content is influenced by the mechanism and timing of skin stretch. However, in their study of expanded pig skin, Johnson and colleagues[17] demonstrated convincingly that collagen density does not change during expansion (Fig. 3-9) and that the initial reduction of collagen content becomes insignificant with time (Fig. 3-10). The total collagen content in the expanded surface area was increased at the completion of expander filling and again at 36 weeks after expansion.[17] These data imply that expansion not only results in new tissue for reconstruction but also that the new tissue is created by proliferation at both the dermal and epidermal levels. However, new tissue is not created by rapid (intraoperative) expansion. The clinical efficacy of intraoperative cyclic loading is derived mainly from the effect of increased undermining.[24]

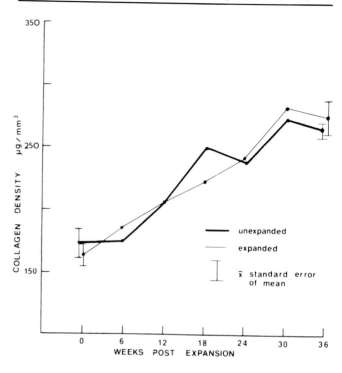

Figure 3-9   Collagen density does not change during tissue expansion. (From Johnson PE, Kernahan DA, Bauer BS: Dermal and epidermal response to soft-tissue expansion in the pig, *Plast Reconstr Surg* **81:394, 1988.**)

Figure 3-8   Dermal thickness following tissue expansion. Persistent thinning is noted 36 weeks after expansion. Tissue expanders were left implanted during postexpansion period. (From Johnson PE, Kernahan DA, Bauer BS: Dermal and epidermal response to soft-tissue expansion in the pig, *Plast Reconstr Surg* **81:393, 1988.**)

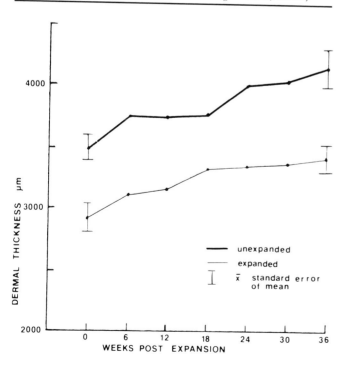

Figure 3-10   Collagen content in each sample is initially decreased in expanded areas, but these differences are not significant at 36 weeks after expansion. (From Johnson PE, Kernahan DA, Bauer BS: Dermal and epidermal response to soft-tissue expansion in the pig, *Plast Reconstr Surg* **81:394, 1988.**)

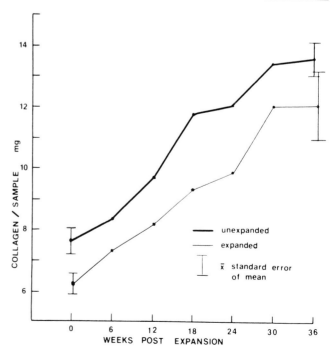

The other time-dependent property of skin that is of clinical significance is stress-relaxation. Stress-relaxation refers to a decrease in stress that occurs when skin is held under tension at a constant strain. Stress-relaxation has been less studied than creep, but the two properties appear to be related. If a flap is closed under excessive tension, a certain amount of relaxation occurs as the tissue *creeps*. Stress-relaxation allows large lesions in inelastic regions to be removed if the principle of serial excision is applied.

SUMMARY

The mechanical properties of cutaneous tissue are unique and must be considered in the design of the local skin flap. The stress-strain curve for skin is nonlinear and determines wound-closure tension, blood flow, and flap survival. Flaps of intermediate length are most sensitive to the effects of tension. Minor variations in skin flap design will avoid excess tension and allow closure along the initial portion of the force-deformation curve. The extent of undermining differs for narrow and broad-based skin flaps. Excess undermining can result in a paradoxical increase in wound-closure tension and may pose a risk of injury to surrounding structures. Because skin is anisotropic, there are directional variations in extensibility. Fusiform excision parallel to the RSTL will place the maximum closure tension in the direction of the LME. Time-dependent properties of skin such as creep and stress-relaxation are clinically useful phenomena that permit tissue expansion and serial excision.

REFERENCES

1. Daly CH, Odland GF: Age-related changes in the mechanical properties of human skin, *J Invest Dermatol* 73:84, 1979.

2. Larrabee WF, Sutton D: The biomechanics of advancement and rotation flaps, *Laryngoscope* 91:726, 1981.

3. Gibson T, Kenedi RM: Biomechanical properties of skin, *Surg Clin North Am* 47:279, 1967.

4. Pearl MR: A unifying theory of the delay phenomenum: recovering from the hyperadrenergic state, *Ann Plast Surg* 7:102, 1981.

5. Jurell G, Hyemdah LP, Fredholm BP: On the mechanism by which antiadrenergic drugs increase survival of critical skin flaps, *Plast Reconstr Surg* 72:518, 1983.

6. Pang CY, Neligan PC, Forrest CR, et al: Hemodynamics and vascular sensitivity to circulating norepinephrine in normal skin and delayed and acute random skin flaps in the pig, *Plast Reconstr Surg* 78:75, 1986.

7. Stell PM: The effects of varying degrees of tension on the viability of skin flaps in pigs, *Br J Plast Surg* 33:371, 1980.

8. Larrabee WF Jr, Holloway GA Jr, Sutton D: Wound tension and blood flow in skin flaps, *Ann Otol Rhinol Laryngol* 93:112, 1984.

9. Cox KW, Larrabee WF Jr: A study of skin flap advancement as a function of undermining, *Arch Otolaryngol* 108:151, 1982.

10. Larrabee WF Jr, Sutton D: Variation of skin stress-strain curves with undermining, *Surg Forum* 32:553, 1981.

11. Borges AF: Relaxed skin tension lines, *Dermatol Clin* 7:169, 1989.

12. Borges AF: The rhombic flap, *Plast Reconstr Surg* 67:458, 1981.

13. Piérard GE, Lapière CM: Microanatomy of the dermis in relation to relaxed skin tension lines and Langer's lines, *Am J Dermatopathol* 9:219, 1987.

14. Neumann C: The expansion of an area of skin by progressive distention of a subcutaneous balloon, *Plast Reconstr Surg* 19:124, 1957.

15. Radovan C: Breast reconstruction after mastectomy using the temporary expander, *Plast Reconstr Surg* 69:195, 1982.

16. Austad ED, Pasyk KA, McClatchey KD et al: Histomorphologic evaluation of guinea pig skin and soft tissue after controlled tissue expansion, *Plast Reconstr Surg* 70:704, 1982.

17. Johnson PE, Kernahan DA, Bauer BS: Dermal and epidermal response to soft-tissue expansion in the pig, *Plast Reconstr Surg* 81:390, 1988.

18. Cherry GW, Austad E, Pasyk K, et al: Increased survival and vascularity of random-pattern skin flaps elevated in controlled, expanded skin, *Plast Reconstr Surg* 72:680, 1983.

19. Squier CA: The stretching of mouse skin in vivo: effect on epidermal proliferation and thickness, *J Invest Dermatol* 74:68, 1980.

20. Austad ED, Thomas SB, Pasyk K: Tissue expansion: dividend or loan? *Plast Reconstr Surg* 78:63, 1986.

21. Olenius M, Dalsgaard CJ, Wickman M: Mitotic activity in expanded human skin, *Plast Reconstr Surg* 91:213, 1993.

22. Austad ED: Dermal and epidermal response to soft-tissue expansion in the pig, *Plast Reconstr Surg* 81:396, 1988 (discussion).

23. Black MM, Bottoms E, Shuster S: Skin collagen and thickness in simple obesity, *Br Med J* 4:149, 1971.

24. Mackay DR, Saggers GC, Kotwal N, et al: Stretching skin: undermining is more important than intraoperative expansion, *Plast Reconstr Surg* 86:722, 1990.

4

Suture Needles and Techniques for Wound Closure

Jonathan Mark Sykes

Paul Joseph Byorth

SELECTION OF SUTURES AND SUTURE NEEDLES

INTRODUCTION

The history of surgery is one of constant progress in wound-closure techniques. This evolution can be followed from ancient times, when pincers of army ants or horsetail hair and sharpened bones were used, to the modern-day swaged needle and suture. Today, one has a myriad of needle types and designs in conjunction with many suture materials that can be used for wound closure. The goals of this chapter are to review the currently available sutures and needles and the significant interactions between sutures, needles, and needle holders to provide a framework for the understanding and selection of appropriate wound-closure materials and methods.

Before selecting suture material for a given wound, one must identify the goals for wound closure. In general, suture closure of a wound is performed so that primary wound healing can occur. In particular, to achieve that goal several basic principles must be followed: (1) the obliteration of dead space, (2) the even distribution of remaining tension along deep suture lines, (3) the maintenance of tensile strength across the wound by the suture until tissue tensile strength is adequate, and (4) the approximation and eversion of the epithelial portion of the closure. All other goals of primary wound closure (i.e., aesthetic and functional concerns) are dependent upon satisfactory performance of the above tasks.

WOUND HEALING

With the goals of wound closure in mind, an understanding of the wound-healing process can assist in obtaining those goals. The wound-healing process has been divided into three phases[1]: (1) lag or inflammatory phase (day 0-5), (2) granulation or fibroplasia phase (day 6-14), and (3) maturation phase (day 15–indefinite).

Lag or Inflammatory Phase (Day 0-5)

This phase begins at the time of incision with an immediate capillary vasoconstriction, followed by vasodilation and increased capillary permeability. A coagulum of fibrin, fibronectin, platelets, and polymorphonuclear leukocytes (PMNs) forms. The platelets and PMNs release vasoactive and trophic factors from cytoplasmic granules over the first 48 hours. Monocytic cells slowly increase in number performing a phagocytic role and are the dominant cells by day 4. Capillary growth occurs at preexisting vessels with endothelial buds directing themselves toward the wound space. Fibroblasts appear by day 4, and reticulin and collagen fibrils can be detected in the wound space. The wound-breaking strength of skin at the end of this phase is minimal (6% of normal skin[2]) and is attributed to the fibrin coagulum.

Granulation or Fibroplasia Phase (Day 6-14)

The hallmark of the granulation phase is the rapid increase in the numbers of fibroblasts migrating into the wound space. These are closely followed by endothelial buds, which acquire a central lumen and differentiate into capillaries, arterioles, and venules. The reticulin and collagen fibrils seen in phase 1 have no connection to the collagen of the wound edges.

Due to collagenolytic activity, the collagen of the wound edge takes on a frayed appearance, and by day 5 or 6 it can be demonstrated that there are interdigitations with collagen of the incisional space. These changes in collagen are responsible for the development of intrinsic mechanical wound tensile strength. The completion of the second phase is characterized by obliteration of the incisional space by fibroblasts, capillaries, macrophages, and collagen bundles. The wound-breaking strength of skin at the end of this phase is minimal to moderate (6% to 14% of normal skin)[1] and is attributed to the newly formed collagen.

Maturation Phase (Day 15-Indefinite)

The beginning of the maturation phase is marked by decreased numbers of fibroblasts end macrophages. The wound becomes much less vascular. Collagen fibers are highly disorganized. A certain degree of remodeling of collagen occurs at this time. Collagen oriented along lines of wound-closure tension remains, and other fibers are removed. New bundles of collagen are laid down, but there is an overall decrease in density of collagen. Wound-breaking strength slowly increases with the passage of time. The wound-breaking strength of skin reaches 45% of normal at day 70, and 50% of normal at day 120.[1] Fascial tissue may take as long as 9 months to regain 75% of normal strength.[1] Under optimal conditions, wound strength never returns to more than 80% that of normal tissue.[2]

The "normal" tissue healing process can be affected by many factors. To assist the primary healing of surgical wounds, one must identify and optimize these patient factors (Table 4-1).

With knowledge of wound healing and an accurate assessment of the location and type of tissues to be repaired, one can begin the suture selection process. With the advent of synthetic materials, the types of suture available have grown and the selection process has become more challenging. One can make decisions more easily if aware of the specific qualities of each suture and the implications for their use.

SUTURE SELECTION

The selection of suture material can be based on a variety of useful characteristics. In order to analyze and select appropriate suture material, definitions of commonly used terms relating to suture material are

Table 4-1   Factors Affecting Wound Healing

Local Factors	General Factors
Blood supply	Age
Denervation	Endocrine function (pancreas, thyroid)
Fluid collection	Drug therapy (antiinflammatory, cytotoxic)
Infection	Sepsis
Previous or concurrent irradiation	Major organ failure (pulmonary, cardial, hepatic, renal)
Mechanical stress	Obesity
Surgical technique	Malignant disease

Modified from Bucknall TE, Ellis H: *Wound healing for surgeons*, East Sussex, England, Bailliere Tindall, 1984.

necessary (see box on p. 41). The ideal suture would lend itself to use in all circumstances (see box on p. 41). Because there are significant differences in local and regional tissue composition and because differing demands may be placed upon the suture material, an ideal suture for all purposes does not exist. By examining the specific characteristics of the "ideal" suture, one can be more discriminating in the selection of appropriate suture material for each given task.

The eventual outcome of wound closure is affected by the amount of initial tissue injury from suture passage. This can be controlled by appropriate needle selection (discussed in the following section) and knowledge of the surface characteristics of the suture. The coefficient of friction of a given suture is determined by the filament type (monofilament, braid, twist), the material composition, and the coating agents used (Fig. 4-1).[3] In general, monofilaments have the lowest coefficient of friction and cause the least amount of tissue injury upon passage. Polypropylene is one of the most "slippery" materials.[4] Coating agents are made of many things. The most common agent is silicone; other materials include beeswax and polymers of suture material (e.g., Polygalactin 370, Polycaprolate). Elasticity of suture can also affect the amount of tissue injury. The optimal elasticity allows for tissue edema and detumescence while maintaining adequate tissue approximation. It is the overtightened suture secondary to tissue edema that causes ischemia with resultant "railroad tracks." Poliglecaprone 25 (Monocryl, Ethicon) and Polybutester (Novafil, Davis & Geck) are two sutures known for their elasticity.

Tissue reaction affects wound outcome by its effects on the healing process. Tissue reaction is determined by the interaction of the suture with the surrounding tissues. This can be due to the material composition or antigenicity of the suture and coating agents or to the physical properties of the suture.

Chromic gut and plain gut are sutures that elicit the

Suture Material: Definition of Terms

Absorbable suture
Undergoes progressive loss of mass or volume (does not correlate with loss of tensile strength)

Breaking strength
Limit of tensile strength at which material (or tissue) failure occurs

Capillarity
Extent to which absorbed fluid is transferred along the strand

Elasticity
A measure of a suture's ability to regain its original form and length after deformation

Fluid absorption
Ability to take up fluid after immersion

Knot pull tensile strength
Breaking strength of a suture material, which can be 10% to 40% weaker after deformation by knot placement

Knot strength
Amount of force necessary to cause a knot to slip, which is directly proportional to the coefficient of static friction and plasticity of a given material

Memory
A suture's inherent capability to return to or maintain its original gross morphologic shape; it is a function of elasticity, plasticity, and diameter

Nonabsorbable suture
Undergoes no significant loss of mass or volume (does not correlate with retention of tensile strength)

Plasticity
A measure of a suture's ability to deform without breaking and to maintain that new form after relief of the deforming force

Straight pull tensile strength
Linear breaking strength of suture material

Suture pullout value
Limit of strength of a particular tissue as measured by the force applied to a loop of suture at which tissue failure occurs

Tensile strength
A material or tissue's ability to resist deformation and breakage

Wound-breaking strength
Limit of tensile strength of a healing wound at which wound separation occurs

Coefficient of friction
A numeric value that quantifies a material's surface characteristics that act to resist motion against another surface

---

Ideal Suture Material Characteristics

Minimal tissue injury or tissue reaction
Ease of handling
High tensile strength
Favorable absorption profile
Resistance to infection

---

most tissue reaction.[5] This is due to the type of digestion of the suture material. Collagen suture, such as chromic gut or plain gut, is absorbed by proteolysis. The source of proteolytic enzymes is PMNs and monocytes. Due to this type of digestion, inflammatory agents are also present and therefore elicit an inflammatory response. Silk, although considered a nonabsorbable material, undergoes significant proteolysis over a 2-year period before becoming stable.[2] Synthetic fibers that are absorbable are digested by simple hydrolysis and are thus much less reactive. Uncoated absorbable monofilament sutures are only minimally less reactive than coated braided absorbables. Nonab-

Figure 4-1 Scanning electron micrograph (40x) of various suture materials; *top left*, silk suture; *top right*, nylon suture; *bottom left*, coated synthetic braided suture (vicryl); *botton right*, chromic gut suture.

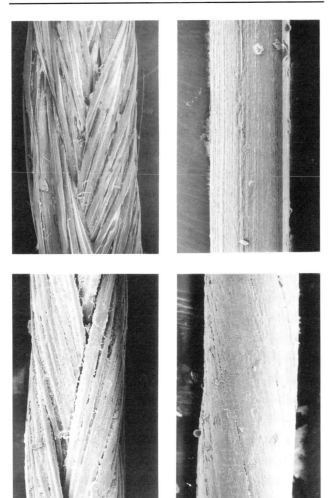

sorbable sutures elicit the least amount of reaction due to material composition.

Tissue reaction secondary to the physical properties of suture can be attributed to the capillarity and fluid absorption profile of the suture. These characteristics are a function of material composition and filament type. Multifilament sutures have the greatest capillarity and tend to absorb fluid.[2] These "wicking" characteristics can be either detrimental or beneficial. The suture may assist in drainage of tissue fluid, or the suture and its tract may act as a pathway for the introduction of pathogens. This may affect the rate of wound infection. If tissue closed with braided sutures becomes infected, the suture tends to harbor bacteria in its interstices and thus may be a poor choice in colonized areas, or areas in which suture must remain for a long period of time.

A suture that is easy to handle is pliable, allows for precise knot tension adjustment, can be securely grasped, and once tied with a minimum of throws, remains secure. The ease with which suture is handled is determined by several characteristics, including suture filament type, diameter, and material composition. In general, braided sutures are the easiest to handle. For any given suture material, a braided filament has the highest coefficient of friction. This allows for an easier grasp of the suture, both in suture-on-hand contact and suture-on-suture contact. The stiffness or memory of a suture is determined by the filament type, material composition, and diameter of the suture. Stiff suture is not easy to handle. For any given suture material, a braided filament is the least stiff. Material composition determines the elasticity and plasticity of a suture. For handling purposes, elasticity makes suture difficult to work with. Knots tend to spring apart, and kinks or bends tend to remain. Plasticity is a helpful quality for suture handling: knots remain more secure, and kinks and bends can be removed from the suture. Silk has been considered the gold standard for overall ease of handling.

Tensile strength is important for the maintenance of tissue approximation. A suture material with high tensile strength allows for the smallest caliber suture to perform the task. Certain limits apply to this principle. When tissue or wound-closure tension is high, at a certain limit a small diameter suture will cut through the tissue. Ideally then, the suture diameter and tensile strength should be well matched, and the suture used should be no stronger than the tissue to be approximated. Suture pullout values quantify tissue strength and can help in suture selection in this aspect (Table 4-2).[1] Surgical steel has the greatest tensile strength available, while silk is the least strong.[1]

The absorption profile of a suture is of importance in that different demands are placed upon suture for different purposes. If suture is to be removed (e.g., nonabsorbable suture used for skin closure), then the absorption profile is relatively unimportant. If the suture is to remain in situ, the amount of foreign body that remains may become important. The suture may become visible, extrude, or become infected. One must know the length of time for which tensile strength is needed and whether the presence of a foreign body will be of significance. These characteristics are determined by the suture material composition and the coating agent.

Standards for suture were first included in the U.S. Pharmacopeia (USP) in 1937. This has provided for some standardization and hence a means for comparison of suture materials. Standards were set so that for each USP size there is a corresponding metric size. To meet the standard for each size, the average strand diameter must remain within defined limits and must meet minimum tensile strength requirements. The USP specifications for suture are listed in three categories: collagen suture (Table 4-3), synthetic absorbable suture (Table 4-4), and nonabsorbable suture (Table 4-5).[6] Upon review of these separate groups, several observations can be made: (1) USP size and metric size do not correlate across all categories (e.g., USP #4-0 chromic and #3-0 nylon are both metric size 2); (2) metric size correlates with limits on average diameter in all categories; (3) metric size does not uniformly relate to suture knot pull tensile strength (e.g., to meet the standard, the minimum tensile strength for #4-0 chromic is 0.77 kgf, while for #4-0 nylon it is 0.95 kgf); and (4) although all sutures must meet class specifications for tensile strength, some suture materials closely approximate the standard and others greatly exceed the standard. Note that many commonly used sutures do not meet USP standards. This is specified on each package. Tables 4-6, 4-7, and 4-8 highlight some of the important characteristics of currently available suture.

In the final analysis, one must identify and prioritize the demands to be placed upon the suture and customize the selection process to fit each clinical situation. In general, recommendations for suture size selection can be made by anatomic region (Table 4-9). More specifically, this determination must include patient tissue factors, patient behavior factors, and the surgeon's technique as variables. To illustrate this point, one can contrast two different wounds in the same anatomic location. Consider a full-thickness traumatic laceration of the lip and a full-thickness defect of the lip after resection of a T_1 lip cancer. These defects are similar in that they both occur in the same anatomic location, are of equally significant aesthetic concern, and may *grossly* appear to be the same defect. The only difference between these wounds may be the amount of tissue loss and therefore the tension under which the wound may be closed. Perhaps the laceration occurred in an otherwise healthy 20-year-old, and the cancer resection patient is a cachectic 85-year-old. Certainly this description conjures up much different impressions. For the lip laceration, a #3-0 chromic suture for the mucosal closure would be adequate. It will form a secure knot and will only remain for a short but adequate period of time. The risk of infection with proper technique is very low. The selection of #3-0 chromic suture for the muscular closure would be appropriate. Certainly the tensile strength and time

Text continued on p. 49.

Table 4-2   **Suture Pullout Values***

Fat	0.2 kg
Muscle	1.27 kg
Skin	1.82 kg
Fascia	3.77 kg

*All pullout values are subject to variation due to anatomic distribution and histologic composition.

Modified from Bucknall TE, Ellis H: *Wound healing for surgeons,* East Sussex, England, Bailliere Tindall, 1984; with permission.

Table 4-3   **USP Specifications for Collagen Suture**

USP Size	Metric Size (gauge no.)	Limits on Average Diameter (mm)		Knot-pull Tensile Strength (kgf)	
		Min.	Max.	Limit on Average Min.	Limit on Individual Strand Min.
9-0	0.4	0.040	0.049	—	—
8-0	0.5	0.050	0.069	0.045	0.025
7-0	0.7	0.070	0.099	0.07	0.055
6-0	1	0.10	0.149	0.18	0.10
5-0	1.5	0.15	0.199	0.38	0.20
4-0	2	0.20	0.249	0.77	0.40
3-0	3	0.30	0.339	1.25	0.68
2-0	3.5	0.35	0.399	2.00	1.04
0	4	0.40	0.499	2.77	1.45
1	5	0.50	0.599	3.80	1.95
2	6	0.60	0.699	4.51	2.40
3	7	0.70	0.799	5.90	2.99
4	8	0.80	0.899	7.00	3.49

From United States Pharmacopeia— National Formulary (USP XXII— NF XVII) USP Convention; with permission.

Table 4-4 USP Specifications for Synthetic Absorbable Suture

USP Size	Metric Size (gauge no.)	Limits on Average Diameter (mm)		Knot-pull Tensile Strength (kgf) (except where otherwise specified)* Limit on Average Min.
		Min.	Max.	
12-0	0.01	0.001	0.009	—
11-0	0.1	0.010	0.019	—
10-0	0.2	0.020	0.029	0.025*
9-0	0.3	0.030	0.039	0.050*
8-0	0.4	0.040	0.049	0.07
7-0	0.5	0.050	0.069	0.14
6-0	0.7	0.070	0.099	0.25
5-0	1	0.10	0.149	0.68
4-0	1.5	0.15	0.199	0.95
3-0	2	0.20	0.249	1.77
2-0	3	0.30	0.339	2.68
0	3.5	0.35	0.399	3.90
1	4	0.40	0.499	5.08
2	5	0.50	0.599	6.35
3 and 4	6	0.60	0.699	7.29
5	7	0.70	0.799	

*The tensile strength of the specific USP size is measured by straight pull.

From United States Pharmacopeia—National Formulary (USP XXII— NF XVII) USP Convention; with permission.

Table 4-5   USP Specifications for Nonabsorbable Surgical Sutures

USP Size	Metric Size (gauge no.)	Limits on Average Diameter (mm)		Limits on Average Knot-pull (except where otherwise specified) *Tensile Strength (kgf)		
		Min.	Max.	Class I Min.	Class II Min.	Class III Min.
12-0	0.01	0.001	0.009	0.001*	—	0.002*
11-0	0.1	0.010	0.019	0.006*	0.005*	0.02*
10-0	0.2	0.020	0.029	0.019*	0.014*	0.06*
9-0	0.3	0.030	0.039	0.043*	0.029*	0.07*
8-0	0.4	0.040	0.049	0.06	0.04	0.11
7-0	0.5	0.050	0.069	0.11	0.06	0.16
6-0	0.7	0.070	0.099	0.20	0.11	0.27
5-0	1	0.10	0.149	0.40	0.23	0.54
4-0	1.5	0.15	0.199	0.60	0.46	0.82
3-0	2	0.20	0.249	0.96	0.66	1.36
2-0	3	0.30	0.339	1.44	1.02	1.80
0	3.5	0.35	0.399	2.16	1.45	3.40 ◀
1	4	0.40	0.499	2.72	1.81	4.76 ◀
2	5	0.50	0.599	3.52	2.54	5.90 ◀
3 and 4	6	0.60	0.699	4.88	3.68	9.11 ◀
5	7	0.70	0.799	6.16	—	11.4 ◀
6	8	0.80	0.899	7.28	—	13.6 ◀
7	9	0.90	0.999	9.04	—	15.9 ◀
8	10	1.00	1.099	—	—	18.2 ◀
9	11	1.100	1.199	—	—	20.5 ◀
10	12	1.200	1.299	—	—	22.8 ◀

Limits on knot-pull tensile strength apply to nonabsorbable surgical suture that has been sterilized. For nonsterile sutures of Class I and Class II, the limits are 25% higher.

*Tensile strength of sizes smaller than USP size 8-0 (metric size 0.4) is measured by straight pull. Tensile strength of sizes larger than USP size 2-0 (metric size 3) of monofilament Class III (metallic) nonabsorbable surgical suture is measured by straight pull.

◀ Silver wire meets the tensile strength values of Class I sutures but is tested in the same manner as Class III sutures.

Class I—composed of silk or synthetic fibers where the coating agent does not significantly affect thickness.

Class II—composed of cotton or linen or synthetic fibers where the coating significantly affects thickness but not strength.

Class III—composed of mono- or multifilament metal wire.

From United States Pharmacopeia—National Formulary (USP XXII—NF XVII) USP Convention; with permission.

Table 4-6   Natural Fibers[4,7,9]

Name	Source	Special Processing	Filament	Relative Tensile Strength*	Tensile Strength Profile†	Absorption Profile	Tissue Reaction‡	Ease of Use§
ABSORBABLE:								
Plain gut	Highly purified (nearly 100%) collagen derived from submucosa of sheep intestines or serosa of beef intestine	None	Twisted "virtual" monofilament	2	75% at 7 days	70 days proteolysis		
Chromic gut		Chromium salt treatment resists breakdown		2	75% at 14 days	90 days proteolysis	5	4
Fast-absorbing gut		Heat treated to speed up degradation		2	75% at 5 days	60-70 days proteolysis		
Plain collagen	Beef achilles tendon	Chromium salt treatment	Twisted "virtual" monofilament		75% at 7 days	70 days proteolysis		
Chromic collagen		Chromium salt treatment			35% at 14 days	90 days proteolysis	4	3
NONABSORBABLE:								
Silk	Silkworm	Coating with beeswax or silicone; dyed	Braided	1	Progressive loss over 1 year	Significant at 2 years proteolysis	4	1 (gold standard)
Cotton	Cotton seed		Twisted	1				2
Linen	Flax seed		Twisted	2				2
Surgical steel			Braided or monofilament	5	Significant loss only if kinked		1	5

*Relative tensile strength scale; 1 = least, 5 = greatest strength. When accompanied by (), indicates relative rank within a relative strength class: (1) = greatest, (5) = least.

†Represents percentage of original dry, out of package tensile strength.

‡Represents relative tissue reaction: 1 = least, 5 = greatest reaction.

§Represents relative overall ease of use: 1 = easiest, 5 = most difficult.

Table 4-7   Absorbable Synthetic[4,7,9]

Name	Source	Special Processing	Filament	Relative Tensile Strength*	Tensile Strength Profile†	Absorption Profile	Tissue Reaction‡	Ease of Use§
Poliglecaprone 25 (Monocryl, Ethicon)	Synthetic copolymer glycolide and caprolate	Undyed	Monofilament	4 (1)	50-60% at 1 wk 20-30% at 2 wk 20% at 3 wk	90-120 days hydrolysis	2	1—very pliable elastic
Polydioxanone (PDSII, Ethicon)	Synthetic polymer polydioxanone	Undyed	Monofilament	4 (4)	70% at 3 wk 50% at 4 wk 25% at 6 wk	180-210 days hydrolysis	2	3
Polygalactin 910 (Vicryl, Ethicon)	Synthetic copolymer glycolide lactide	Dyed violet or undyed, coated galactin 370	Braid	4 (2)	65% at 2 wk 40% at 3 wk 8% at 4 wk	56-70 days hydrolysis	3	2
Polyglycolic acid (Dexon II Dexon''s,'' Davis & Geck)	Synthetic polymer	Dyed or undyed, coated polycaprolate	Braid	4 (3)	65% at 1 wk 35% at 2 wk 5% at 4 wk	90-120 days hydrolysis	3	2
Polyglyconate (Maxon, Davis & Geck)	Synthetic polymer polytrimethylene carbonate	Dyed	Monofilament	4 (1)	75% at 2 wk 50% at 4 wk 25% at 6 wk	180-210 days hydrolysis	2	2

*Relative tensile strength scale: 1 = least, 5 = greatest strength. When accompanied by (), indicates relative rank within a relative strength class: (1) = greatest, (5) = least.

†Represents percentage of original dry, out of package tensile strength.

‡Represents relative tissue reaction: 1 = least, 5 = greatest reaction.

§Represents relative overall ease of use: 1 = easiest, 5 = most difficult.

Table 4-8 Nonabsorbable Synthetic[4,7,9]

Name	Source	Special Processing	Filament	Relative Tensile Strength*	Tensile Strength Profile†	Absorption Profile	Tissue Reaction‡	Ease of Use§
Nylon Dermalon (Davis & Geck) Ethilon (Ethicon)	Synthetic polyamide	Clear or dyed	Monofilament	3	81% at 1 yr 72% at 2 yr 66% at 11 yr	Slow hydrolysis stable at 2 yr	2	2—low coefficient of friction
Nurolon (Ethicon) Surgilon (Davis & Geck)		Dyed, silicone coated	Braided	2	Same as above	Same as above	2$^+$	1
Polybutester Novafil (Davis & Geck)	Synthetic copolyner polyglycol terephthate polytrithylene terephthate	Dyed blue	Monofilament	3	—	None	1	2—very elastic, very low coefficient of friction
Polyester Ticron (Davis & Geck) Ethibond extra (Ethicon)	Synthetic Dacron polyester	Dyed, silicone coated	Braided	3	—	None	2	2
Dacron (Davis & Geck) Mersilene (Ethicon)	Synthetic Dacron polyester	Dyed, uncoated	Braided	2	—	None	2	3
Polypropylene prolene (Ethicon) Surgilene (Davis & Geck)	Synthetic polymer propylene	Dyed blue	Monofilament	2		None	1	3—very low coefficient of friction

*Relative tensile strength scale: 1 = least, 5 = greatest strength. When accompanied by (), indicates relative rank within a relative strength class: (1) = greatest, (5) = least.
†Represents percentage of original dry, out of package tensile strength.
‡Represents relative tissue reaction; 1 = least, 5 = greatest reaction.
§Represents relative overall ease of use: 1 = easiest, 5 = most difficult.

Table 4-9 **A Regional Guide to Suture Selection**

Region	Cutaneous Suture	Subcutaneous/ Fascia Suture	Comments
Eyelid and periorbital	#6-0, #7-0	#4-0, #5-0	Minimal tensile strength requirements Aesthetic concerns at a premium
Nose and pinna	#5-0, #6-0	#4-0, #5-0	Small tensile strength requirements Aesthetic concerns at a premium
Lip and vermillion	#6-0	#3-0, #4-0	Moderate tensile strength requirements due to highly active region Aesthetic concerns at a premium
General facial and anterior neck	#5-0, #6-0 #4-0, #5-0	#3-0, #4-0	Moderate to high tensile strength requirements due to regional mobility Significant aesthetic concerns
Nasal and oral mucosa	#3-0, #4-0	#3-0, #4-0	Moderate tensile strength needed due to tissue mobility May select based on ease or no need for removal No aesthetic concern
Scalp and posterior neck	#3-0, #4-0	#2-0, #3-0	Tensile strength needed for moderately heavy tissue and very mobile region Minimal aesthetic concern
Superior trunk	#2-0, #3-0	#2-0, #3-0	Tensile strength needed for heavy tissues in a relatively mobile area
Major musculocutaneous flaps	#4-0, #5-0	#1-0, #2-0 #3-0	Maximal tensile strength needed because sutures are often under significant tension May require long-term tensile strength

present would be adequate to allow for healing. As the cutaneous portion of the wound could be closed without tension, a #6-0 nylon suture would be a good selection. This would supply adequate tensile strength, cause minimal tissue trauma and tissue reaction, and therefore help to attain the best aesthetic result.

For closure of the resection defect, one knows that there is a much greater chance for wound dehiscence. A #3-0 longer acting absorbable braided suture would be a better choice. This will form a secure knot and remain for an extended period of time. Although a long-acting absorbable monofilament could be selected, the number of throws needed for knot security would surely create a large, irritating foreign body, which could erode into adjacent mucosa. For muscular closure, a braided long-acting or longer acting monofilament absorbable suture may be the best selection. These sutures will maintain tensile strength for an extended period of time so that if wound healing is slow, the wound will be safely approximated until adequate healing can occur. The cutaneous closure may also be under some wound closure tension. Selection of a #5-0 nylon suture may provide more tensile strength for good approximation without sacrificing aesthetic outcome. This is, of course, only one way to approach these wounds. Many different suture types and suturing techniques could be used. The point of this example is that thought *must* go into the suture selection process.

SUTURE NEEDLES

As sutures have evolved, so have the needles on which they have been used. Currently there are many types and sizes of needles available. In order to select a surgical needle, one must begin with a basic understanding of the anatomy of a needle (Fig. 4-2). Suture needles are made from high-grade stainless steel and have three major anatomic sections: a point, a body, and a swage. The point begins at the tip of the needle and ends at the completion of the taper at the maximum diameter of the needle. The body of the needle begins at that point, forms the majority of the length of the needle, and ends at the contour change that marks the beginning of the swage of the needle. The swage extends to the end of the needle, at which point the suture exits from the needle.

The needle point is the "working" end of the needle. The needle type and silicone coating determine the ease with which it passes through tissue. The quality of the stainless steel and the silicone determines the number of passes through tissue with which the ease of passage is maintained.[7,8] There are many types of needle points, of which three are discussed here: taper, conventional cutting, and reverse cutting.

The taper needle point (Fig. 4-3**A**) is round, and its sharpness is determined by the taper ratio and tip angle (Table 4-10).[7] Taper ratios vary from 8:1 to 12:1, and tip angles vary from approximately 20 to 35 degrees. Taper needle points become sharper with higher taper ratios and lower tip angles. The taper point needle penetrates and passes through tissues by stretching the tissues. The taper point needle is used for soft, elastic, and easy-to-penetrate tissues.

Figure 4-2 Schematic diagram of the anatomy of a needle.

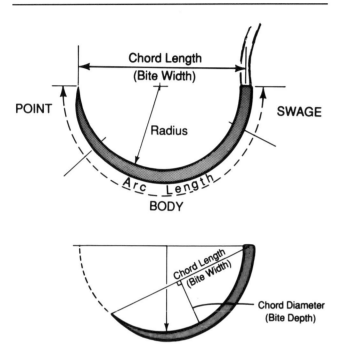

The point of a cutting needle is triangular in shape (Fig. 4-3**B**). The degree of sharpness of this type of needle point is attributed to its three cutting edges. Its taper ratio and tip angle are of less importance. This type of needle penetrates and passes through tissue by cutting a pathway. Conventional cutting needle points have the third cutting edge on the inner curve of the needle. If one exerts upward pressure on this type of needle, it will tend to take a more shallow course or even cut entirely through the tissue bite. This is a surface-seeking needle point. Reverse cutting needle points (Fig. 4-3**C**) have the third cutting edge on the outer curve of the needle. If one exerts downward pressure on this type of needle it will tend to take a deeper course than would be expected due to the curvature of the needle. This is a depth-seeking needle. Cutting needles are used for hard and tough-to-penetrate tissues.

The needle body plays an important role in overall needle performance. Although there is some significant needle-tissue contact at the body of the needle, the most important function of the body is its interaction with the needle holder and its ability to transmit penetrating force to the point. For appropriate suture needle and needle holder selection, an understanding of commonly used terms is necessary (see Table 4-10). For good needle control, the needle body must be held securely between the needle holder jaws. Needle factors affecting this interaction include needle diameter and radius, body geometry, and stainless steel alloy. These factors determine the bending moment, ulti-

Figure 4-3 Schematic diagram of commonly used suture needles. The cross-sectional geometry of the needle point, needle body, and needle swage is shown in the inset drawings. *A*, **Taper needle.** *B*, **Conventional cutting needle.** *C*, **Reverse cutting needle.**

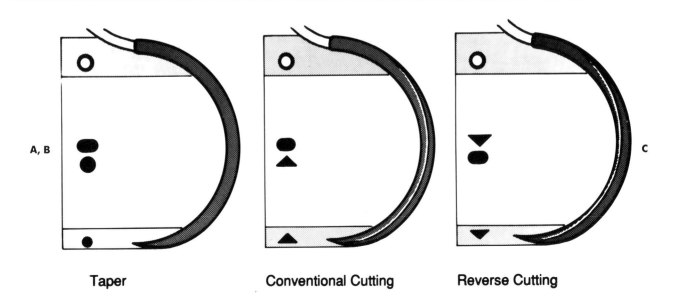

mate moment, yield moment, and needle ductility. The metal alloy and diameter are primary determinants of the needle bending moment and ductility.[8] For any given combination of alloy and diameter, the cross-sectional body geometry can significantly alter the bending moment, ductility, and contact stability with the needle holder jaws.[8] For instance, a flat needle maximizes the contact surface with the needle holder jaws and is very secure (Fig. 4-4). A round-bodied needle, on the other hand, has minimal surface contact with the needle holder jaws and is insecure. However, the configuration of a flat needle minimizes the needle bending moment, while a round needle has more resistance to bending. This concept can be understood by placing a tongue blade flat between one's fingers and bending the blade. If one then places the blade vertically and repeats the maneuver, one will note the difficulty in bending the blade and securely holding the blade. To select the most appropriate needle geometry, one must identify the ease with which the tissue may be penetrated (i.e., the force required for passage of the needle). Most needle bodies are ovoid to maximize the surface contact with the needle holder jaws and yet maintain adequate vertical height for maximum bend-

Table 4-10   **Suture Needle and Needle Holder: Definition of Terms**[8]

Angle of Needle Failure
Angle of deformation at which a needle rapidly loses resistance to plastic deformation.

Bending Moment
Force applied to needle creating angular deformation.

Needle Ductility
Resistance to needle breakage.

Needle Holder Clamping Moment
Force applied to a suture needle by a needle holder. This applied force may cause deformation of a curved needle.

Taper Ratio
Length-to-width ratio of the needle point. A measurement of the sharpness of a needle point.

Tip Angle
Angle described by two straight lines drawn from the tip of the needle toward the body that best match the slightly curved contour of the taper. A measurement of the sharpness of a needle point.

Ultimate Moment
Greatest bending moment at which the limits of nonreversible (plastic) deformation are reached.

Yield Moment
Greatest bending moment at which reversible (elastic) deformation occurs.

Figure 4-4   **Side view of a typical needle holder holding the three different geometric shapes of needle body. This illustrates the increased contact points of an ovoidly shaped needle body. Increased contact points maximize security between the needle holder and the suture needle body.**

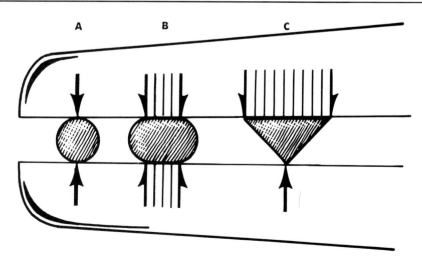

Figure 4-5   Schematic diagram of various suture needle configurations.

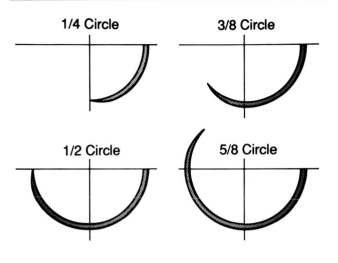

1/4 Circle   3/8 Circle

1/2 Circle   5/8 Circle

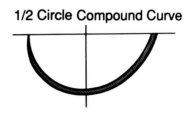

1/2 Circle Compound Curve

ing moment. Selection of a needle body shape is based upon the location and the tissue bite that is to be enclosed by the suture. For the even distribution of tension, the optimal course of a suture through tissue is a semicircular one. It is because of this that the majority of needles are semicircular. Needle body shape for semicircular needles can be described by the radius and fraction (¼, ⅜, ½, ⅝) of a complete circle (Fig. 4-5). A practical means for determining which needle shape is most appropriate for each wound is the use of the chord length (bite width) and radius (bite depth). The appropriate needle chord length can be determined by assessing the distance from the wound edge to the point of needle entry. Assuming that when the needle exits the skin it will be equidistant from the wound edge, then the distance from entry to exit will be the optimum chord length. It should be noted that arc length and *not* chord length is the measurement supplied on suture packages. To select the most appropriate fraction of a circle, the quantity or depth of tissue to be enclosed must be assessed. As the depth of bite increases, the fraction of a complete circle needed increases.

The swage of a needle is the segment at which the needle and the suture material are joined. Before the advent of swaged needles, suture had to be threaded through the eye of a standard needle or onto the eye of a French needle. Swaging of a needle can be achieved by two methods. Channel swaging is performed by employing a press to create a channel in the suture needle. The suture material is then placed into the channel and the channel crimped over the suture to secure it in place. There is no material removed to create a channel, and when crimped into place, the diameter of a channel swage is greater than the diameter of the body of the suture needle. Drill swaging is achieved by creation of a drill hole inside which the suture can be placed. The needle is then crimped to secure the suture. Material is removed in the drilling process, and when crimped, the swage diameter becomes less than the diameter of the body of the needle. The majority of commercially available suture materials are currently available on drill swaged needles.

Only after the selection of an appropriate needle can an appropriate needle holder be selected. The ideal needle holder is well matched to suit the needle size and the amount of force required to firmly secure and drive the needle. Poor selection may lead to difficulty in suture placement or needle deformation and breakage. The needle holder can be considered as two levers that rotate about a common fulcrum. The long end of the lever is the handle, and the short end of the lever is the jaw. Due to the differences in length of the handle and jaw, a mechanical advantage is created. Proportionately, the longer the handle and shorter the jaw, the greater the mechanical advantage. The selection of the needle holder handle and jaw length determines the amount of force exerted upon the needle.[8] The width of the jaw determines how the force is applied to a curved needle. A curved needle contacts the jaws of the needle holder on three points: one point on the outer curvature and two points on the inner curvature. This creates a moment arm, which acts to apply the force to a needle in such a fashion as to flatten the curvature of the needle. This is called the needle holder clamping moment. As the width of the needle holder jaw increases, so does the clamping moment. To select the correct combination of needle holder handle length, jaw length, and jaw width, one must select the clamping moment that is less than the yield moment of the selected needle. Practically speaking, since these numbers are not readily available, needle holder jaw width should be no wider than 30% to 35% of the needle radius (Fig. 4-6), and handle length should be proportionately shorter for smaller needles. If nonreversible deformation of a needle occurs, then the yield moment has been exceeded, and a different needle driver should be selected. Tables 4-11 and 4-12 review commonly used indications for each type needle point and body shape.

Figure 4-6   Schematic diagram of interaction between needle holder and suture needle. *A*, Needle holder of appropriate size. *B*, Needle holder too large for needle shown, which creates inadvertent straightening of the suture needle. *C*, Needle holder too small for needle shown, which allows for needle rotation around long axis of the needle holder.

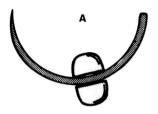 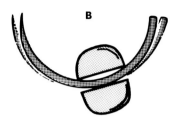 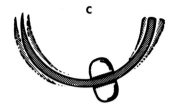

Table 4-11   Needle Point Types and Applications

Type	Application	
Taper	Aponeurosis	Nerve
	Biliary tract	Peritoneum
	Blood vessels	Pleura
	Dura	Subcutaneous fat
	Fascia	Urogenital tract
	Gastrointestinal tract	
	Muscle	
Conventional or reverse cutting	Dermis	
	Ligament	
	Nasal cavity	
	Oral cavity	
	Pharynx	
	Skin	
	Tendon	
Tapercut (tapered cutting point, very sharp)	Bronchus	Periosteum
	Dermis	Pharynx
	Ligament	Sclerotic vessels
	Nasal cavity	Tendon
	Oral cavity	Trachea
	Ovary	Uterus
	Perichondrium	

Note that there is no standardized sizing system or nomenclature for the "generic" suture needle. One must gain an appreciation for the proprietary designations through experience and the assistance of the scrub nurse. Table 4-13 lists some of the more commonly used nomenclature.

Table 4-12   Needle Body Shapes and Applications

Shape	Application	
¼ circle	Eye	
	Microsurgical	
⅜ circle	Aponeurosis	Nerve
	Biliary tract	Perichondrium
	Blood vessel	Periosteum
	Dura	Peritoneum
	Eye	Pleura
	Fascia	Tendon
	Gastrointestinal tract	Urogenital tract
	Muscle	
	Myocardium	
½ circle	Biliary tract	Peritoneum
	Eye	Pharynx
	Gastrointestinal tract	Pleura
	Muscle	Respiratory tract
	Nasal cavity	Skin
	Oral cavity	Subcutaneous fat
	Pelvis	Urogenital tract
⅝ circle	Cerebrovascular system	Urogenital tract
	Nasal cavity	
	Oral cavity	
	Pelvis	
Compound curved ("J" shaped)	Cleft palate repair	
	Eye	
Kieth (straight)	Gastrointestinal tract	Pharynx
	Nasal cavity	Skin
	Oral cavity	Tendon
		Vessels

CONCLUSION

Through the understanding of factors that affect wound healing, one can identify specific properties of sutures and needles that can best assist in closure of a wound. Familiarity with the physical properties and interactions between suture, suture needles, and needle holders can make one a more discriminating and effective surgeon.

Table 4-13   **Commonly Used Nomenclature**

BV	Blood Vessel
TE	Three Eighths
P	Plastic Surgery
PS	Plastic Surgery
CPS	Conventional Plastic Surgery
PC	Precision Cosmetic
OPS	Oculoplastic Surgery
M	Muscle
J	Conjunctiva
FS	For Skin
FSL	For Skin Large
X	Exodontial
KS	Kieth Straight
SC	Straight Cutting
FN	For Tonsil
SH	Small Half
MH	Medium Half
CT	Circle Taper
ST	Straight Taper
CP	Cutting Point
T	Taper
E	Three Eighths
O	One Fourth
SC	Standard Cutting
S	Straight
CTE	Cutting Taper Three-Eighths
PR	Plastic Reconstructive
PRE	Plastic Reconstructive Three-Eighths

REFERENCES

1. Bucknall TE, Ellis H: *Wound healing for surgeons,* East Sussex, England, Bailliere Tindall, 1984.
2. Moy RL, Waldman B, Hein DL: A review of sutures and suturing techniques, *J Dermatol Surg Oncol* 18:785, 1992.
3. Courtesy Arun Gadre.
4. Pham S, Rodeheaver GT, et al: Ease of continuous dermal suture removal, *J Emerg Med* 8:539, 1990.
5. Swanson NA, Tromovitch TA: Suture materials, 1980's: properties, uses, and abuses, *Int J Dermatol* 21:373, 1982.
6. United States Pharmacopeia—National Formulary (USP XXII—NF XVII), USP Convention.
7. Edlich RF, Thacker JG, et al: Past, present, and future for surgical needles and needle holders, *Am J Surg* 166:522, 1993.
8. Edlich RF, Towler MA, et al: Scientific basis for selecting surgical needles and needle holders for wound closure, *Clin Plast Surg* 17:583, 1990.
9. Bourne RB, Bitar H, et al: In vivo comparison of four absorbable sutures: Vicryl, Dexon Plus, Maxon, and PDS, *Can J Surg* 31:1988.

A special thanks to Bill Hoffman, Ethicon, and Diana Andrews, Davis & Geck, for their cooperation and assistance in obtaining much of the proprietary information for their suture products.

TECHNIQUES FOR WOUND CLOSURE

Surgical wounds may be approximated using various methods and materials. These include sutures, skin clips or staples, skin tapes, and wound adhesives. The material and method are chosen based on numerous factors, including the size and location of the wound and the tension across the wound surface. Any material used should hold the wound edges in approximation until sufficient tensile strength is achieved so that the foreign material is not required. This section outlines a variety of methods of wound closure and the rationale for use of specific techniques in specific clinical situations.

BASIC PRINCIPLES

Wound healing represents a complex series of interrelated events that produce successful restoration of tissue integrity. The biochemical and cellular response to wound injury has been carefully researched. A definable sequence of events, starting with wound closure and progressing to repair and remodeling of damaged tissue, has been well described.[1] This ordered process results in a healed wound and a permanent scar.

The surgical goal of most wound closures is to minimize scar formation. Inconspicuous scarring will usually maximize both the aesthetic and functional result. In order to minimize scarring for an individual wound, the surgeon must pay careful attention to many aspects of wound healing in the perioperative period. In particular, these include careful cleansing of the wound, design of closure to minimize wound-closure tension, and meticulous hemostasis and atraumatic technique during closure. Additionally, postoperative wound care to maintain asepsis and provide for drainage of fluid collections is essential. Attention to these perioperative details will maximize the chance for inconspicuous scarring.

PREOPERATIVE CONSIDERATIONS

Proper preparation of both the patient and the surgical wound site are necessary to optimize wound healing. The age and general health of the patient greatly affect the process of healing. Specific local and systemic conditions can alter this process and result in delayed healing. It is important to determine whether primary closure of the wound is indicated. If primary wound closure would predispose to infection, compromise the vascularity of the flap, or compromise the patient functionally, then delayed primary closure or healing by second intention may give the best result.

Systemic conditions that may affect normal healing include peripheral vascular disease, diabetes mellitus, smoking, immunologic compromise, and sepsis. Any systemic disease or condition that causes vasoconstriction of small arterioles may result in decreased perfusion of skin flaps and subsequent abnormal healing. For this reason, it is preferable to treat all disease processes prior to flap reconstruction when possible. This includes treatment of sepsis and control of hyperglycemia preoperatively. Additionally, it is important to urge patients to stop smoking well in advance of elective surgery that involves the use of local flaps. Lawrence and colleagues have demonstrated the detrimental effect of cigarette smoking on flap survival in an experimental study in rats.[2] Rees et al have associated heavy smoking with an increased risk of skin flap necrosis during rhytidectomy.[3] For these reasons, it is preferable for patients to stop smoking for at least 2 weeks before and 3 weeks after elective flap surgery.

Preparation of the surgical wound is very important to successful wound repair. Increased bacterial counts in wounds have been shown to decrease skin graft survival both in humans and in animal experiments. Krizek et al performed quantitative bacterial cultures in wounds awaiting skin grafts.[4] They found that the critical bacterial count was 10^5 organisms per gram of tissue; in wounds with a bacterial count of less than 10^5, the graft survival rate was 94%, while survival rates were only 19% when counts exceeded 10^5. Similar findings have been shown on skin grafts in rabbits.[5] Additionally, Murphy et al have shown the adverse effect of microbial contamination on musculocutaneous and random flaps.[6] For these reasons, careful cleansing and scrubbing of wounds are necessary to reduce microbial skin contaminants. In traumatic wounds, high pressure irrigation has been shown to greatly reduce bacterial counts and enhance wound-closure success.[7] Attention to both local and systemic conditions preoperatively plays a major role in the success rate of any wound closure. If care is taken to eliminate the effects of systemic conditions and mini-

Table 4-14   Wound Closure Methods: Advantages and Disadvantages

Characteristic	Suture	Staple	Tape
Ease of use	−	+	+
Utility	+	−	−
Precision	+	−	−
Speed	−	+	+
Need for anesthesia	−	−	+
Ease of removal	−	+	+
Resistance to infection	−	−	+
Ability to disperse tension	+	+	−

+ = favorable, − = unfavorable.

mize local bacterial contaminants, wound closure can be optimized.

OPERATIVE CONSIDERATIONS

The basic goals of any surgical wound closure are to maximize both the aesthetic and functional result. This is best accomplished by accurately recreating the normal anatomy and minimizing cutaneous scarring.

Surgical wounds may be approximated using various materials and methods. These include suturing, taping, surgical clips or staples, and wound adhesives. All of these methods can lead to excellent results if appropriately selected. The method of closure chosen should minimize wound-closure tension and provide maximum skin eversion. Additionally, any closure technique should pay attention to areas of functional importance, such as the lips and eyelids. If these important functional areas are not accurately recreated, a poor overall aesthetic and functional result may be achieved, despite good cutaneous scarring. By analyzing patient factors, tissue characteristics, orientation to lines of minimal tension, and wound proximity to vital structures, one can arrive at the optimal method for wound closure (Table 4-14).

It is of critical importance to minimize tension across the wound surface because increased tension can result in depressed scar formation. Wound-closure tension can be minimized in several ways, including careful flap design, adequate undermining of tissues, and placement of sufficient deep (fascia, muscle, dermal) sutures (Fig. 4-7). Placement of deep sutures is performed to: (1) minimize wound-closure tension, (2) reduce wound dead space, and (3) provide for wound eversion.[8] Additionally, deep muscle sutures in areas such as the lip or eyelid are important to recreate the normal anatomy and function.

The need for deep sutures is based on the wound

location, depth, and *width.* Wounds located in areas with increased underlying muscular activity or across joint surfaces require deep sutures to minimize skin tension. Wider wounds or those with missing tissue (e.g., after cutaneous lesion removal or trauma) also necessitate layered closure. Deeper wounds often re-

quire layered closure to decrease deadspace and minimize the risk of hematoma formation.

Placement of deep sutures is usually performed in a simple fashion with buried knot placement (see Fig. 4-7). The buried knot allows for wound eversion and lessens the chance that the patient will notice the deep suture, because the knot is farthest from the skin edge. The buried-knot dermal suture should be placed with the suture path being farthest from the skin surface at the wound edge and closest to the skin surface as the suture travels away from the wound edge. It is careful placement of the deep suture layer that produces maximal wound eversion, minimal skin tension, and maximal wound edge approximation.

SUTURE

Suture closure of surgical wounds continues to be the gold standard. Selection of the appropriate suture material, needle type and diameter, and technique for closure contribute to the precision of this method. Primary closure of a wound using suture has the

Figure 4-7   Schematic diagram of deep suture placement. Placement of deep sutures should eliminate dead space and accomplish wound edge approximation and eversion.

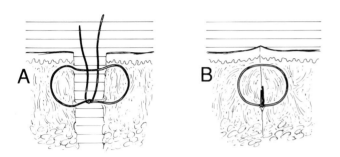

Figure 4-8   *A,* Proper placement of cutaneous suture showing equal distribution of tension along the entire wound edge. This everted surgical wound provides for an aesthetic result at 3 months postoperatively. *B,* Improper placement of cutaneous suture with a surgical bite too far from the skin edge and too superficial. This creates vector forces that are too great in a horizontal direction and produces an inverted wound 3 months postoperatively. *C,* Improper placement of cutaneous suture farther from the skin edge and more superficial in the surgical bite. The force vectors on this wound are greater in a horizontal direction and create more wound inversion 3 months postoperatively. Additionally, permanent suture marks result in areas of pressure necrosis where wound-closure tension is greatest.

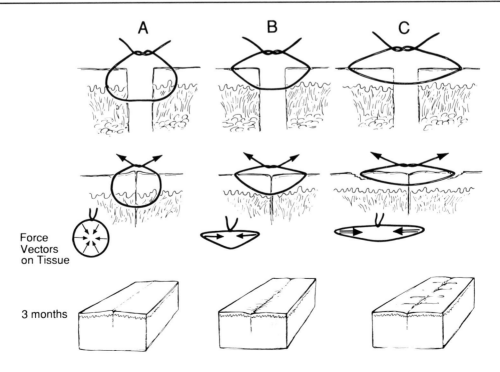

greatest utility of all methods because of its adaptability to each situation. The greatest disadvantage to the use of suture is the time needed for placement.

Cutaneous approximation can be accomplished by various suturing techniques. The technique selected should provide secure approximation and maintenance of wound tensile strength. Since most surgical wounds have achieved only 7% of their final tensile strength by 2 weeks after repair, wound-closure tension should be minimized prior to cutaneous closure.[9] The ideal cutaneous suturing technique should be simple, efficient, and allow precise wound approximation that will eventually produce an aesthetic scar.

It is critically important to minimize wound-closure tension prior to suture closure. This will allow the suture to place an even distribution of force vectors on the skin (Fig. 4-8**A**). If this is properly accomplished, the wound should appear slightly everted at the time of repair and for a few weeks afterward. After further healing and wound contraction occur, the wound edges will flatten and the scar result will be appealing. This is best accomplished by placing the suture close to the wound edge and incorporating a deeper bite into the subcutaneous tissues.

If the tissue incorporated into the cutaneous surgical closure is too superficial and too far from the skin edge, the eventual scar will be less than optimal (Fig. 4-8**B**). In this scenario, the force vectors are greatest perpen-

dicular to the wound edge, and wound-closure tension is increased. The scar appears flat at the time of surgical repair, and as wound contraction occurs, the wound edge inverts and the scar appears depressed.

If the surgical tissue bite is more superficial and even farther from the wound edge, an unsightly scar will usually result (Fig. 4-8**C**). The force vectors and wound-closure tension are even greater, and the suture cuts through the cutaneous layer. These scars also appear depressed secondary to wound edge inversion. Additionally, permanent suture marks perpendicular to the surgical scar may result as the suture material causes pressure necrosis in areas of greatest tension.

A variety of suture techniques are available for cutaneous wound closure. The most common suture method is the *simple interrupted* (Fig. 4-9**A**). It has the advantage of allowing selective adjustments of wound edges in given areas. However, this method is more time-consuming than continuous sutures. The *simple continuous* suture provides secure and rapid wound closure (Fig. 4-9**B**). It is best suited for wounds that do not require significant wound edge adjustments and has the advantage of evenly distributing tension along the entire wound length.

Mattress sutures have the advantage of providing increased wound eversion. The *vertical mattress* suture first incorporates a large bite of tissue placed away from the wound edge and a smaller bite of tissue

Figure 4-9   *A*, **Simple interrupted suture.** *B*, **Simple continuous suture.** *C*, **Horizontal mattress suture.** *D*, **Vertical mattress suture.**

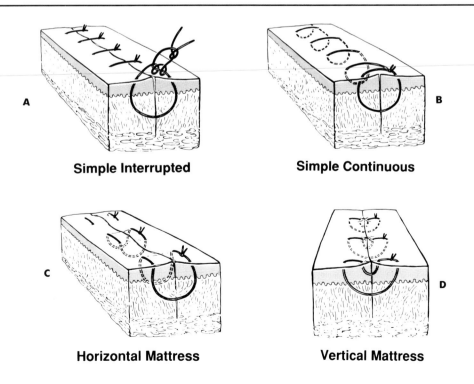

Simple Interrupted   **Simple Continuous**

Horizontal Mattress   **Vertical Mattress**

placed close to the wound edge (Fig. 4-3**C**). This suture decreases dead space and wound-closure tension while providing controlled wound eversion. The *horizontal mattress* suture provides maximal wound eversion by incorporating two bites of tissue in a pursestring manner (Fig. 4-3**D**). This method does not act to decrease dead space. The *intracuticular* or *running intradermal* suture is a technically more challenging method of wound closure but can provide excellent aesthetic scars (Fig. 4-10). Its advantages include ease of suture removal and absence of suture marks. However, wounds closed with this technique may tend

toward wound inversion. The method involves crossing back and forth in the dermal layer without penetrating the cutaneous layer. A loop can be made through the skin along the suture line to facilitate suture removal.

Cutaneous closure using suture has the greatest utility as it allows for selective adjustments in areas of tissue mismatch. This is very important in the use of local skin flaps because recruited tissue frequently differs from recipient tissue in thickness (Fig. 4-11**A**). Suture closure enables one to precisely approximate these tissues and minimize tissue mismatch. In order to alleviate disparities in tissue thickness, deep sutures must be placed to align the dermal-subdermal tissue planes in each wound edge (Fig. 4-11**B** and **C**). Cutaneous closure must then precisely align the epithelial edges by taking a deeper bite in the thinner segment and a more superficial bite in the thicker segment (Fig. 4-11**D** and **E**).

Suture closure of wounds remains the gold standard because of its adaptability, utility, and precision. Meticulous suture closure produces the maximal functional and aesthetic result when correctly applied.

STAPLES

Primary wound closure with surgical staples is a reliable and effective method. The major advantage in using staples for wound closure is decreased operative time. Surgical staples lack the precision needed for skin approximation in many areas (e.g., eyelid margin, vermillion border). Staples cannot be used on delicate

Figure 4-10   *A*, Intracuticular continuous suture. *B*, **Cross-section of a loop of intracuticular continuous suture illustrating placement to achieve maximal wound edge eversion.**

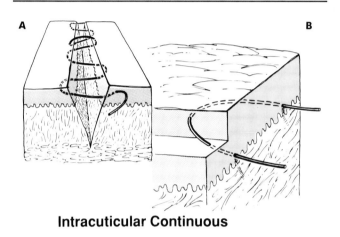

Intracuticular Continuous

Figure 4-11   *A*, **Schematic diagram illustrating two pieces of tissue of unequal thickness.** *B*, *C*, **Placement of deep sutures in mismatched tissue to achieve maximal cutaneous alignment.** *D*, *E*, **Placement of cutaneous sutures in mismatched tissue to achieve maximal cutaneous approximation and tissue eversion.**

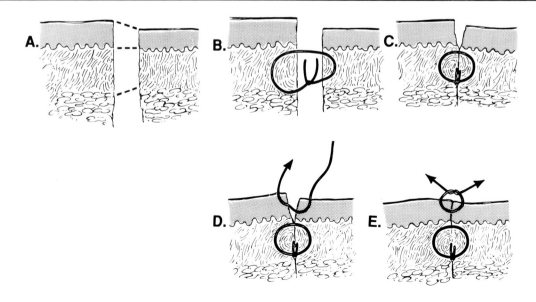

tissues, finely contoured areas, over bony prominences, or on wounds that lie in a concavity. Satisfactory results are difficult to obtain in areas with significant tissue thickness mismatch or in dynamic areas. With an appropriately selected wound, aesthetic outcome and patient comfort are equal to that with sutured closure.[10]

The technique of surgical staple placement requires approximation of the subcutaneous tissues prior to cutaneous closure (Fig. 4-12**A**). Tissue forceps are used to grasp the wound edges. The tissue edges are then approximated and everted while the stapler is gently applied and activated (Fig. 4-12**B**). Staples should be placed at an interval consistent with maintaining wound edge approximation. Failure to approximate and evert the wound edges may lead to wound edge inversion or epithelial overlap. Pressure necrosis and transverse scarring may occur if too much pressure is exerted while activating the stapler. An appropriately placed staple will apply an even force in the transverse direction to approximate the wound edge and maintain eversion of the cutaneous margin (Fig. 4-12**C**).

TAPES

In order to use tape closure effectively, patients must be carefully selected. This closure method is ideal when there is no skin tension and the wound surface is flat. If the wound is superficial, no deep closure may be required prior to the application of surgical tapes. If the wound is deeper, lies perpendicular to the relaxed skin tension lines, or has significant surface tension, surgical tapes should only be used in conjunction with meticulous deep wound closure. The tape acts to maintain (not attain) tissue approximation and cannot be used to overcome inadequate approximation of the deep supporting tissues. The major advantages of tape closure are ease of placement and patient comfort.

Placement of tape for closure should be preceeded by subcutaneous tissue approximation. The wound edges must be thoroughly cleansed. An acrylate skin adhesive is applied to the surrounding skin and allowed to dry until tacky. Tapes are then applied perpendicular to the wound edge under no tension. Slight digital pressure or the use of forceps to approximate or align small gaps may be necessary at times. When applied appropriately, the small amount of remaining wound-closure tension is evenly distributed throughout the entire skin-tape contact surface (Fig. 4-13**A**). However, when the remaining skin tension is significant (e.g., after insufficient deep wound closure), the skin-tape contact surface is inadequate to maintain approximation. This creates shearing forces on the skin surface, which result in epidermolysis and wound edge inversion (Fig. 4-13**B**).

Figure 4-12   *A,* **Deep tissue approximation required prior to placement of surgical staple.** *B,* **Tissue forceps approximating and everting the tissue edge during application of a surgical staple.** *C,* **Appearance of surgical wound after appropriate placement of surgical staple. Note the equal and well-distributed horizontal vector forces on the tissue edge after appropriate placement.**

Surgical Staple Closure

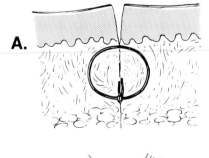

A.

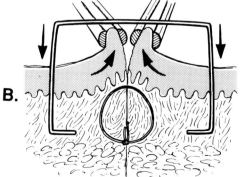

B.

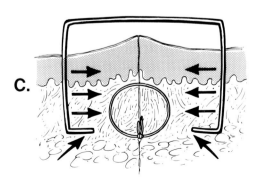

C.

Figure 4-13 *A,* Appropriately selected wound for surgical taping. Adequate deep tissue approximation allows for minimal and well-distributed tension between the surgical tape and skin surface after application. *B,* Poorly selected wound for surgical taping. Inadequate deep tissue closure creates gaping of the surgical wound and increased and poorly distributed tension between the skin surface and surgical tape interface. This creates shearing of the skin surface, which results in wound edge inversion and epidermolysis.

Paper Tape Closure

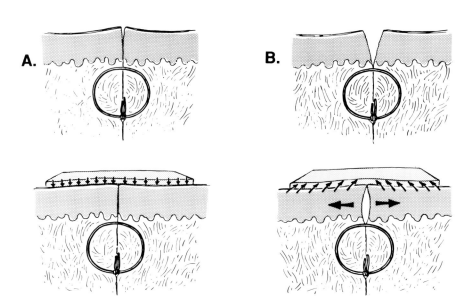

POSTOPERATIVE CONSIDERATIONS

Considerable time as well as energy and effort are expended in preoperative planning and technical execution of a surgical procedure. No less important is the attention paid to caring for the postoperative wound.

Primary closure of a wound requires tissue apposition. Although this may be accomplished intraoperatively, untoward events in the immediate postoperative period may defeat the purpose of primary closure. In addition to meticulous surgical technique, other strategies must be used to avoid complications.

One should consider the use of a compression dressing, bolster, or drain whenever a significant area has been undermined or overlies a concavity. These strategies help to prevent hematoma formation and fluid collection and assist in maintaining deep tissue approximation.

All surgical wounds should be maintained under aseptic conditions for 24 to 48 hours postoperatively. This allows time for the wound to form a fibrin seal, which decreases its susceptibility to infection. When possible, an absorptive occlusive dressing should be used. Antibiotic ointment can be used because although the antibiotic is of questionable benefit, the ointment acts an occlusal barrier.

The wound must be closely monitored for signs of hematoma formation, infection, and necrosis. Frequent meticulous wound care and prompt treatment of complications are essential.

Regardless of the method of wound closure, the sutures, staples, or skin tapes must eventually be removed. One must balance the ongoing need for support of the wound closure with concern for aesthetics. Many factors contribute to the speed with which wounds heal. Preexisting medical conditions, previous radiation, or current medical therapy can significantly retard the healing process. These factors must be taken into account prior to suture removal. Cutaneous sutures can be removed between 4 and 15 days postoperatively. Wounds closed under minimal tension may remain well coapted after early suture removal by virtue of the fibrin seal. In the compromised patient, however, a conservative approach, with later suture or staple removal, will lead to a more satisfactory outcome. The best aesthetic outcome will be obtained if sutures or staples are removed prior to epithelialization of the staple or suture tracts.

Patient counseling prior to hospital discharge can be a powerful adjunct to surgical care. Instructions on wound care, bathing, exercise, sun exposure, and scar massage will help to optimize the surgical outcome and patient satisfaction.

CONCLUSION

The optimal functional and aesthetic result is the goal for both surgeon and patient. Thorough preoperative evaluation, patient selection, and selection of the method for wound closure will lead to more efficient use of time and better control of surgical scarring.

BIBLIOGRAPHY

1. Falcone PA, Caldwell MD: Wound metabolism, *Clin Plast Surg* 17:443, 1990.
2. Lawrence WT, Murphy RC, Robson MC, et al: The detrimental effect of cigarette smoking on flap survival: an experimental study in the rat, *Br J Plast Surg* 37:216, 1984.
3. Rees TD, Liverett DM, Guy GL: The effect of cigarette smoking on skin flap survival in the face-lift patient, *Plast Reconstr Surg* 73:911, 1984.
4. Krizek TJ, Robson MC, Kho E: Bacterial growth and skin graft survival, *Surg Forum* 18:518, 1967.
5. Liedburg NCF, Reiss E, Artz CP: The effect of bacteria on the take of split thickness skin grafts in rabbits, *Ann Surg* 142:92, 1955.
6. Murphy RC, Robson MC, Heggers JP, et al: The effect of microbial contamination on musculocutaneous and random flaps, *J Surg Res* 41:75, 1986.
7. Stevenson TR, Thacker JG, Rodeheaver GT, et al: Cleansing the traumatic wound by high pressure syringe irrigation, *JACEP* 5:17, 1976.
8. Moy RL, Waldman B, Hein D: A review of sutures and suturing techniques, *J Dermatol Surg Oncol* 18:785, 1992.
9. Harris DR: Healing of the surgical wound: I. basic considerations, *J Am Acad Dermatol* 1:197, 1979.
10. Edlich RF, Becker DG, Thacker JG, et al: Scientific basis for selecting staple and tape skin closures, *Clin Plast Surg* 17:571, 1990.

5

CLASSIFICATIONS, DEFINITIONS, AND CONCEPTS IN FLAP SURGERY

Neil A. Swanson

A flap is defined as movement of adjacent skin and subcutaneous tissue from one location to another with a direct vascular supply. This is in contrast to a skin graft, which is the movement of tissue, usually from a distant site, without an intact vascular network. The graft therefore depends upon several factors to form its own vascularity. The purpose of this chapter is to introduce several of the general concepts of flaps, including terminology and classifications, which will be used throughout this book.

TERMINOLOGY

Classically, movement occurs by *advancement, rotation,* or *transposition* of tissue.[1,2] However, over the years I have come to appreciate that there are probably only two basic tissue movements: (1) a *sliding* movement of adjacent tissue from one site to another and (2) a *lifting* movement of tissue, usually across a bridge of normal tissue.

A *primary defect* is the created wound to be closed. In this book, it is usually a wound created by tumor extirpation. However, the wound could also be created by other means, such as trauma. A *secondary defect* is the wound created by tissue movement necessary to close the primary defect (Fig. 5-1). The development of every flap creates a secondary defect. The art of reconstructive surgery is often the design of a flap to place the secondary defect in an appropriate location. With good flap design, the secondary defect is created in an area of loose adjacent tissue that can be easily approximated within correct anatomic boundaries and/or relaxed skin tension lines. In the case of large defects, the secondary defect may need to be closed with a skin graft (Fig. 5-2).

The *primary motion* of a flap is the movement or stress placed on the tissue of the flap in order to close the primary defect. This usually occurs by sliding of tissue (advancement and/or rotation) or by a lifting movement of tissue around a pivotal point (i.e., transposition or interpolation). The *secondary motion* of tissue is the movement or stress, created by performance of the primary motion, placed on the tissue surrounding the primary defect. Therefore, a combination of stresses, both primary and secondary, occurs when transferring a flap (Fig. 5-3). The final stress on tissue, skin lines, and surrounding fixed structures (e.g., eyelids or orifices) is the summation of the primary and secondary motions, or *vector forces.* Therefore, it is important not only to fit the final suture line of the flap within appropriate aesthetic skin lines and boundaries, but also to understand the stresses that are placed on surrounding tissue by the primary and secondary motion of the tissue. If not correctly appreciated, undesired results may occur (Figs. 5-4, 5-5).

Skin has two important properties that enable tissue movement: (1) elasticity and (2) movability. *Elasticity* is the ability of the skin to stretch. Skin in different anatomic sites has different elasticity. Cheek skin, for example, is very elastic. *Movability* refers to the ability of skin to move from one point to another. It is often unrelated to elasticity. For example, temple skin is less movable than cheek skin, although they may be similar in elasticity. The galea aponeurotica causes the scalp and portions of the forehead to be inelastic. Flaps in these areas must be designed with wide arcs in order to accommodate the lack of skin movability.

The *pedicle* of a flap is the area of the flap and adjacent tissue that supplies blood to the flap. A flap should be designed with a pedicle in mind that will provide sufficient vascularity to the flap. Care must be taken not to violate the pedicle during the dissection of a flap. *Delay* is a means of increasing blood supply to the flap. In this case, a flap is designed, and a portion is raised on its vascular pedicle and then sutured back in place for a period of time. At a later date, the entire flap is raised and moved into place. This technique

Figure 5-1   *A*, Tissue movement to close the primary defect creates a secondary defect. *B*, Clinical case showing a primary defect resulting from extirpation of a tumor of the nasal ala. *C*, Transposition of tissue from the cheek to close the primary defect results in a secondary defect, in this case on the cheek. The closure of the secondary defect aligns in the melolabial sulcus.

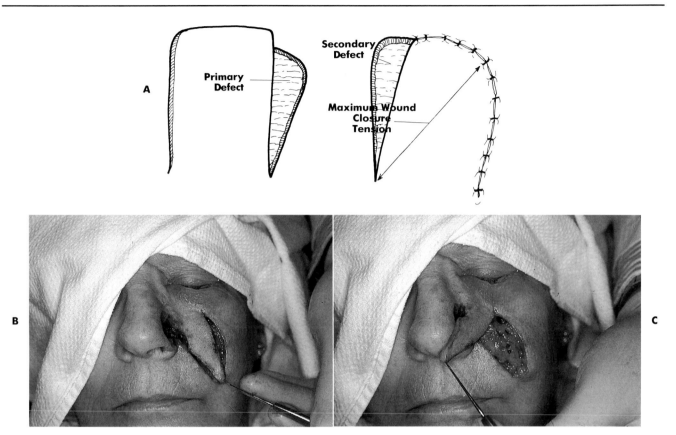

Figure 5-2   *A*, In the majority of the cases, secondary defects can be closed primarily. However, it is sometimes necessary to close the secondary defect using a skin graft. This patient had a recurrent basal cell carcinoma following three previous surgical excisions. Therefore, there was very little tissue mobility on his cheek, so that when the primary defect was closed, it was necessary to place a skin graft to repair the secondary defect. In this case, the donor tissue for the skin graft was the standing cutaneous deformity that resulted from the sliding of tissue into the primary defect. *B*, Three months postoperative.

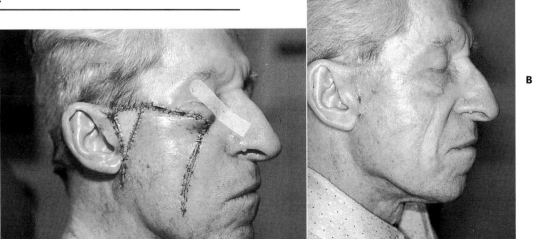

Figure 5-3 *A,* To close this forehead defect with the flap designed, the primary motion is that of transposition. The rhombic flap is outlined and transposed into place. The double arrows illustrate the secondary motion that will occur in the forehead from medial to lateral in response to the transposition of the rhombic flap. In this instance, the secondary motion aided the ability to close the defect. Single arrows indicate area of maximum wound closure tension. *B,* 1 week result at time of suture removal. *C,* This rhombic flap is designed to close the defect created by removing the pigmented lesion. *D,* The secondary motion of this properly designed rhombic flap is exactly parallel to the lateral canthus with little or no distortion of the eyelids.

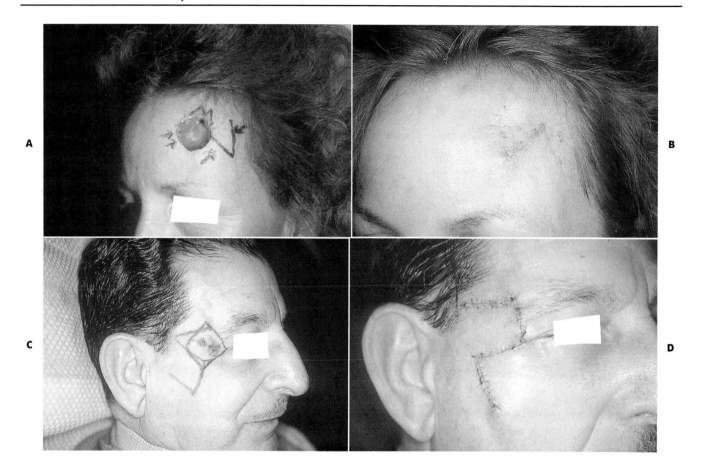

Figure 5-4 *A,* This variation of the rhombic flap is poorly designed. *B,* The secondary motion that resulted from the transpostion of this flap pulled the alar rim up and caused asymmetry.

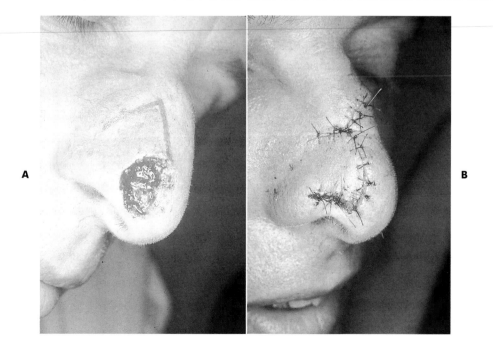

Figure 5-5 *A,* **The dorsal nasal or Reiger flap is a good choice for repair of the nasal defect shown.** *B* **and** *C,* **The sliding flap is executed without difficulty. However, because it was poorly designed, when it was moved into place, the resultant secondary motion resulted in malalignment of the nasal tip. A greater arc should have been designed for the flap so that the secondary motion occurred perpendicular to the nasal tip.**

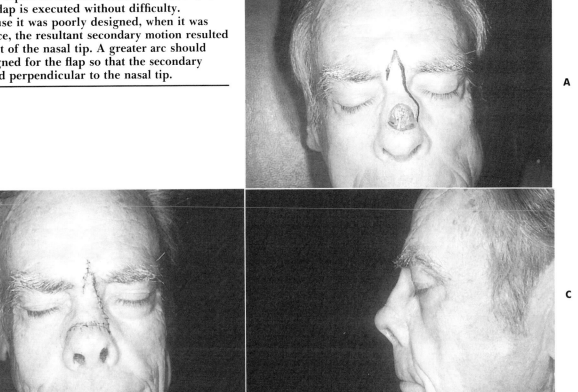

enhances vascularity of the flap as a result of enlargement and realinement of the vasculature in the subdermal plexus of the flap. A *key stitch* is the initial stitch placed to align the flap. With sliding flaps (advancement and/or rotation), the key stitch usually closes the primary defect. With flaps that lift over a bridge of normal tissue (transposition and/or interpolation), the key stitch usually closes the secondary defect. This allows the transposed flap to lie without tension within the primary defect.

The concept of *aesthetic units* and the *borders* representing the areas of interface between these units has become increasingly important in the performance of flap surgery. The face is divided into several aesthetic units with defined borders. These are natural anatomic areas, often with symmetry on the contralateral side, which must be respected (Fig. 5-6). As discussed in many chapters of this textbook, the preferred flap for reconstruction is frequently a flap that can be designed, where possible, within the same aesthetic unit as the defect. Scars are best camouflaged by placing incisions along aesthetic borders. When a defect crosses aesthetic units, it is often best to compartmentalize the repair and design individual flaps to construct the separate

components of the defect that are located within separate aesthetic units. When a single flap must be used to reconstruct a defect that involves more than one aesthetic unit, the outcome is often less than optimal (Fig. 5-7). It is often of benefit to enlarge a defect to fit and/or fill an entire aesthetic unit or subunit and replace the entire unit with a flap of adjacent tissue.

In managing skin cancer, surgical *margins* are important prior to the design of flaps and the movement of tissue. The majority of defects presented in this textbook were created by the removal of a neoplasm. The best-designed reconstruction is a failure if executed before the neoplasm is adequately removed. Surgical margins can be obtained by excision with permanent section control, excision with random frozen section control, or by the use of Mohs micrographic surgery.[3] The majority of defects illustrated in this book were created by the use of Mohs micrographic surgery. Subsequent reconstruction is often accomplished by the Mohs surgeon acting as the reconstructive surgeon or in an interdisciplinary approach in concert with the reconstructive surgeon.[4] This book is not meant to be a treatise on Mohs micrographic

Figure 5-6   *A,* The face is divided into cosmetic units and boundaries. *B,* Cosmetic "subunits" of the nose. *C,* Cosmetic "subunits" of the upper lip. Wherever possible, one should close a defect within a cosmetic unit; crossing cosmetic units can result in less than optimal results.

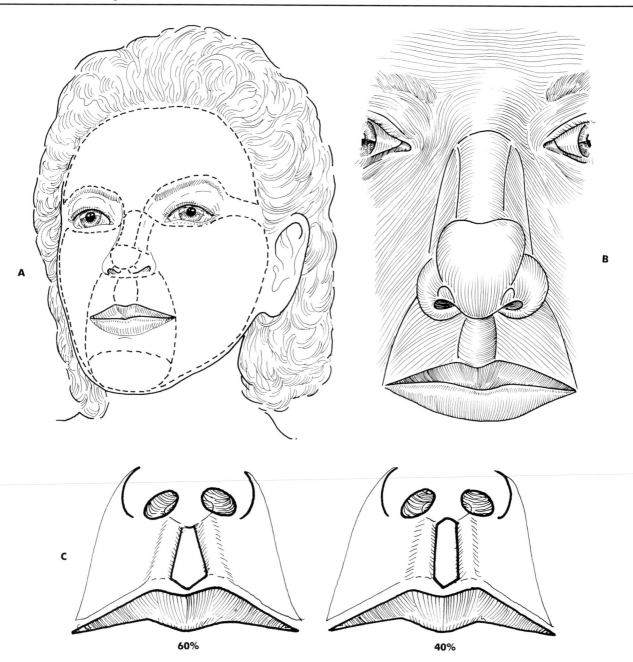

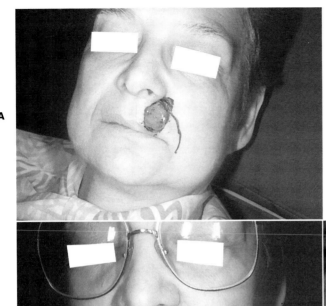

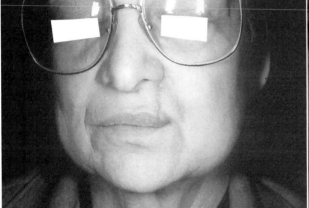

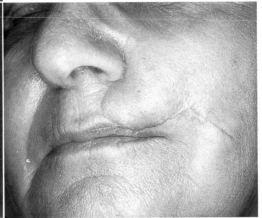

Figure 5-7 Two cases of upper lip repair. *A,* A local flap is designed to close the defect within that cosmetic unit. *B,* Wound closure is confined to one cosmetic unit that is likely to maximize scar camouflage. Result at 1 week. *C,* In this case, tissue was transposed from the cheek across the cosmetic boundary of the melolabial sulcus into the upper lip. This has yielded a less than optimal result.

surgery, but for properly indicated tumors it is the optimal method for obtaining complete marginal control and tumor extirpation. Following Mohs surgery, defects can usually be repaired immediately. However, if there is a concern about adequate margins, there is no harm in postponing reconstruction and waiting for final pathology reports or delaying to observe for recurrence.

FLAP CLASSIFICATION

Flaps have been classified in several ways. The most common methods of classification are by *location, blood supply,* and *tissue movement.*

Flaps classified by *location* are based upon the location of the donor tissue and are either direct or indirect. *Direct flaps* are those where tissue is moved from a site adjacent to or near the primary defect, maintaining attachment to some form of a vascular supply. *Indirect flaps* are those where tissue is harvested with a vascular pedicle from a site remote from the primary defect and transferred either by microvascular surgery or by staged movement of the pedicle to the

recipient site. Based upon *location,* flaps are classified as local, regional, or distant. The vast majority of flaps discussed in this textbook are local. A *local flap* is one where tissue immediately adjacent to the primary defect is harvested to cover that defect. A *regional flap* is one where tissue is harvested as a direct flap from a site removed from the primary defect and not immediately adjacent to it. An example of a regional flap is a deltopectoral flap used to repair a defect of the lip or cheek. *Distant flaps* are usually harvested as microvascular free flaps or staged tubed flaps in which the pedicle is "walked" toward the ultimate recipient site.

A second method of flap classification is based upon *blood supply.* The most commonly discussed are **random** and **axial pattern flaps.** *Random pattern flaps* are flaps based on the rich perforating vascular plexus of the skin (Fig. 5-8). They are not necessarily based on a named blood vessel. *Axial pattern flaps,* on the other hand, are based and dependent upon a named artery for the majority of their blood supply (Fig. 5-9). Most axial pattern flaps have a degree of randomness to the distal portion of the flap. An example of a random pattern flap is the rhombic transposition flap or the melolabial transposition flap (Fig. 5-10). An example of

Figure 5-8   Random pattern flaps are based on the rich subcutaneous and intradermal plexus that supplies vascularity to the skin.

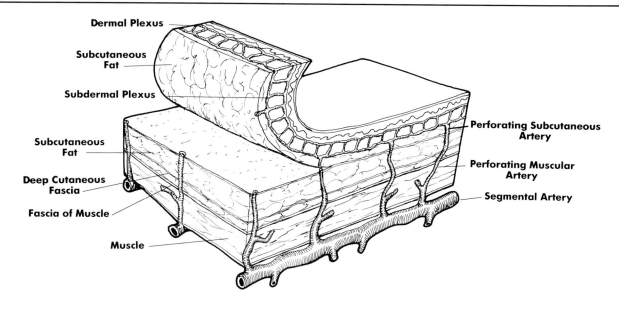

Figure 5-9   Axial pattern flaps are based on a named artery for blood supply. Most axial pattern flaps have a degree of random pattern to the distal portion of the flap.

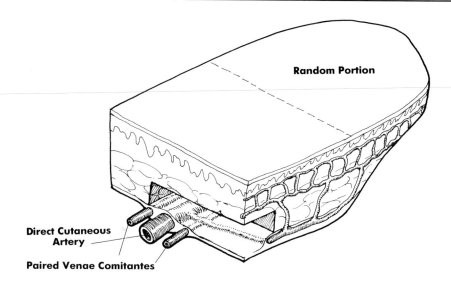

Figure 5-10 *A,* The melolabial transpostion flap is nourished by the rich vasculature of the cheek, and is an example of the random pattern flap. It receives its blood supply from the subcutaneous and intradermal plexus. *B,* Transpostion of the flap. This blood supply is so rich that the flap can be thinned to a great degree when transposed and still maintain its blood supply. *C,* Six months postoperative.

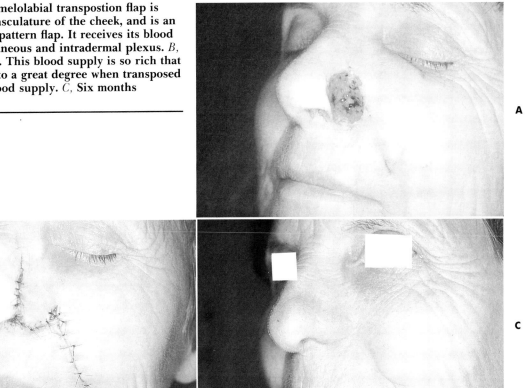

an axial pattern flap is the paramedian forehead flap based on the supratrochlear artery and vein (Fig. 5-11).

A third method of flap classification is based upon *tissue movement.* Classically, the basic movement of tissue is by advancement, rotation, or transposition, and flaps have been referred to as advancement flaps, rotation flaps, or transposition flaps. In the last several years I have found it more useful to classify flaps based upon two types of tissue movement, as (1) sliding flaps and (2) flaps that are transposed across intact skin by moving around a pivotal point. Pivotal flaps share common features of standing cutaneous deformity at the pivotal point and decreased effective length as the flap moves about its pivotal point. They may be sliding (rotation) or lifting (transposition/interpolation). Sliding flaps can move tissue by direct advancement, sliding about a pivotal point (rotation), or a combination of both. I perform very few pure advancement or pure rotation flaps. They exist (i.e., U or H plasty), but most advancement and rotation flaps combine the movements of sliding and pivoting. I have found it more useful to think of them as primarily sliding flaps. With the *sliding flap,* the tissue movement to cover the primary defect leaves a secondary defect that consists principally of wounds of unequal length. The line of

closure of the secondary defect is often designed to be positioned along aesthetic borders and to maximize the width of the pedicle of the flap. The secondary defect is often repaired by the use of tissue sharing techniques, the removal of a triangle of excess tissue along the long arc or limb, or by performing a back-cut (Fig. 5-12). Included in this classification of sliding flaps is the subcutaneous pedicle/advancement flap (Fig. 5-13). These are usually random pattern flaps, although occasionally they may be axial. They are almost always local flaps.

The second type of basic tissue movement is that which pivots about a point and **lifts** a flap across a bridge of normal tissue. These are transposition and interpolation flaps. By definition, these flaps lift over a bridge of intervening tissue to cover a primary defect. The secondary defect is removed from the primary defect, is designed in an appropriate area of loose donor skin, bears the majority of the vector forces of wound closure tension, and is repaired first. A *transposition flap* is a pivotal flap with its base designed adjacent to the defect and transfers tissue across a surface of intact skin in one stage. It is usually a random pattern flap, although occasionally it can be axial. An *interpolation flap* is a pivotal flap with its base removed from the

Figure 5-11   The paramedian forehead flap is an example of an axial pattern flap. It is based on the supratrochlear artery and can be transposed with a very narrow pedicle because of the blood supply emanating from a single vessel. (Courtesy Shan R. Baker, M.D.).

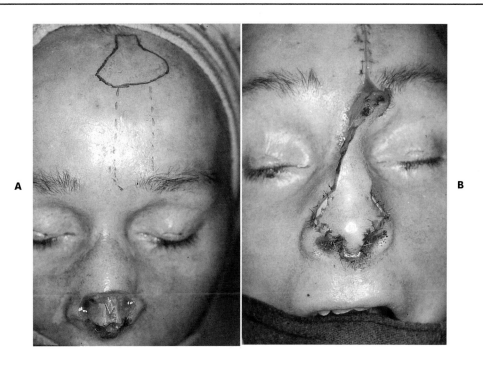

Figure 5-12   This cheek advancement/rotation flap is an example of a sliding flap. *A*, Outline of this flap within cosmetic boundaries. Tissue slides into place to cover a primary defect. The resultant secondary defect is an example of wounds of uneven length, with the inner arc being shorter that the outer arc. This is usually closed by shortening the outer arc by removing a triangle somewhere along that arc (Burow's triangle). *B*, One week postoperative. *C*, One month postoperative.

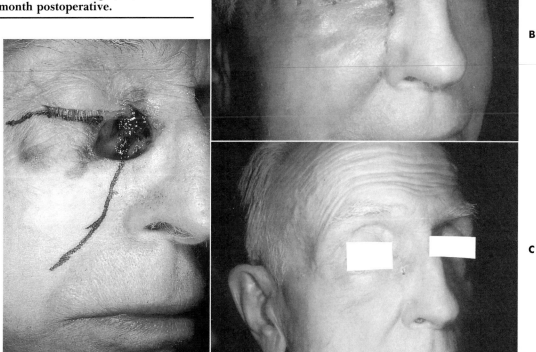

Figure 5-13   The subcutaneous island pedicled flap receives its blood supply from the vascular pedicle directly under the flap; in this case from branches of the labial artery through the vascular pedicle on which the flap is advanced. *A*, Defect after Mohs surgery. *B*, Flap designed. *C*, Flap advanced upon its subcutaneous pedicle donor site closed in V to Y fashion. *D*, Result 2 months postoperative.

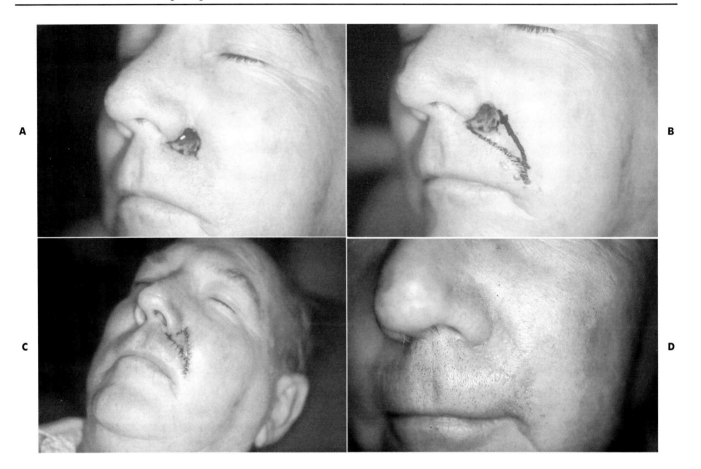

Method of Classifying Flaps

Local Random Pattern
Sliding
   Advancement
   Rotation combination
   Alphabet (O->T, A->T)
Lifting
   Single transposition
   Bilobe transposition
   Rhombic and variations
   Melolabial interpolation
Local Axial Pattern
Sliding
   Reiger
   Island pedicle
Lifting
   Forehead direct
   Forehead interpolation

vicinity of the primary defect and transposes tissue across an adjoining bridge of normal skin to cover the primary defect, leaving the pedicle attached (Fig. 5-14). At a later date, once vascularity to the distal portion of the flap has been assured, the flap is divided in a second procedure. Interpolation flaps are often axial in nature, although they may be random.

Flap classification using a single method can be difficult and confusing. For the sake of this textbook, the vast majority of flaps discussed are local. The box on this page represents my preferred method of classification. Flaps are divided into local random pattern flaps and local axial pattern flaps. Some flaps may bridge this classification because many axial pattern flaps have some degree of randomness. However, this classification has proven helpful in designing and discussing local flaps. Regional and distant flaps are usually axial in nature, and the majority are outside the scope of this textbook.

Figure 5-14 The melolabial interpolation flap transposes tissue across a bridge of normal skin maintaining the blood supply at the pedicle. *A,* Defect following Mohs surgery with interpolation flap incised. *B,* Transposition of the flap with closure of the secondary defect to facilitate motion. *C,* The flap remains attached distally to its random vascular supply. *D,* After approximately 3 weeks the pedicle is transected, once the flap has been vascularized at the recipient site. *E,* Two months following flap inset.

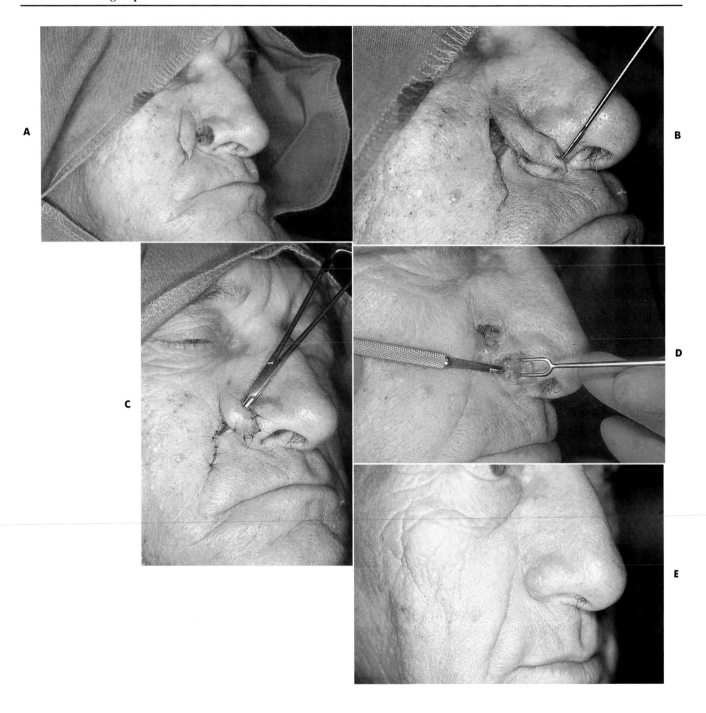

REFERENCES

1. Jackson IT: *Local flaps in head and neck reconstruction*, St Louis, 1985, The CV Mosby Co.
2. Grabb WC, Myers MB, editors: *Skin flaps*, Boston, 1975, Little, Brown.
3. Swanson NA: Mohs surgery: technique, indications, applications, and the future, *Arch Dermatol* 119:761, 1983.
4. Baker SR, Swanson NA: Reconstruction of midfacial defects following surgical management of skin cancer: the role of tissue expansion, *J Dermatol Surg Oncol* 20:133, 1994.

6

ROTATION FLAPS

Ted A. Cook

Richard E. Brownlee

INTRODUCTION

Reconstruction of facial defects is a challenging and often perplexing undertaking. A reconstructive surgeon can no longer ignore form in favor of function and must be able to restore harmony and balance to all facial structures. Competent repair of facial defects requires an intimate knowledge of the anatomy, function, and esthetics of the many different units that collectively make up the face. Possession of a large surgical repertoire of different flaps has little use without an understanding of when, where, why, and how to best use each repair.[1] A review of head and neck anatomy is beyond the scope of this chapter; however, a brief mention of the concepts of esthetic units and relaxed skin tension lines (RSTLs) is warranted in any discussion of reconstruction of cutaneous and subcutaneous facial defects.

The face can be divided into specific areas, or esthetic units, which have common characteristics, such as skin thickness, color, texture, and amount of hair and/or natural anatomic lines, which are commonly known as esthetic borders. As seen in Fig. 6-1, these borders follow familiar landmarks such as eyebrows, melolabial folds, filtral borders, vermilion borders, and hairline. These esthetic units and their junction lines come together to give form and character to what we call the face. These borders also form perfect lines for the creative surgeon to hide an incision when designing flaps for surgical repairs and are particularly useful in the design of rotation flaps.

The RSTLs, as seen in Fig. 6-2, are lines that are intrinsic to the anatomy of facial skin. These lines result from the orientation of collagen fibers of the skin and are obvious in the aging face but are even more important in the young face. Incisions created in these lines will generally heal well; however, incisions at right angles to these lines will heal more slowly and ultimately result in wider scars. Thus, RSTLs create a matrix of lines that can be used to create favorable incisions for the design of rotation flaps.

The basic rotation flap is a simple pivotal flap, which is curvilinear in shape and which rotates around a pivotal point near the defect.[2] The flap is best suited for repair of defects that are triangular. It is designed immediately adjacent to the defect, and thus one side of the defect is the advancing edge of the flap. Design of the classic rotation flap is seen in Fig. 6-3. As with all pivotal flaps, a standing cutaneous deformity will develop at the base of the flap. A Burow's triangle can be removed to facilitate repair of the donor site wound (Fig. 6-4). The vector of greatest wound-closure tension after rotation of the flap is from the pivotal point to a point located on the peripheral circumference of the curvilinear incision (Fig. 6-5). A back cut[3] or

Figure 6-1 Facial esthetic units and nasal esthetic subunits.

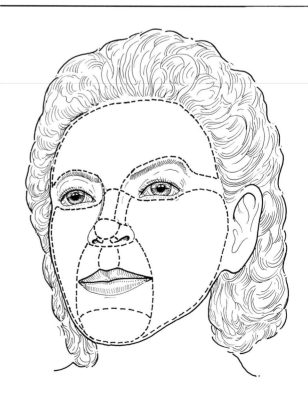

Figure 6-2 RSTLs are intrinsic to anatomy of facial skin.

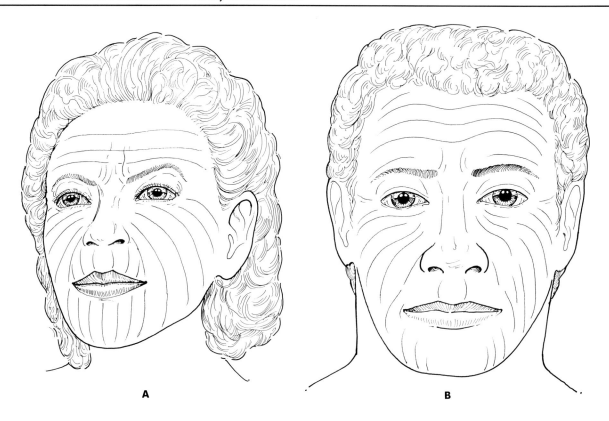

A

B

Figure 6-3 Rotation flaps are pivotal flaps with curvilinear configuration.

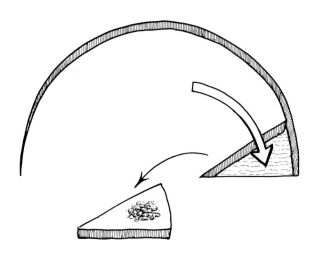

excision of a Burow's triangle[4] at the base of the flap shifts the position of the pivotal point and thus changes the wound-closure tension vector as well as the location of the standing cutaneous deformity.[5-7] The flap when converted to a two-dimensional form would appear as in Fig. 6-6. A problem encountered with rotation flaps

is the unequal length of the flap's border compared with the width of the primary and secondary defects. The classic method to equalize this discrepancy is to excise an equalizing (Burow's) triangle at some point along the curvilinear periphery of the incision (Fig. 6-6, side A), which is equal in length to the width of the base of defect[4] (Fig. 6-6, side C). This results in equalizing the lengths of the two sides of the incision (Fig. 6-6, sides A and B).

Another solution to the problem is to avoid the need for an equalizing triangle by changing the movement of the flap from one that is purely pivotal to the one that is both pivotal and advancement. By advancing the flap while at the same time rotating it through its pivotal point, the surgeon can better equalize the discrepancy (Fig. 6-7). In so doing, the surgeon takes advantage of the distensibility (Fig. 6-8, side B) and the compressibility (Fig. 6-8, side A) of the skin.

Repair is then accomplished by using the principle of halving, by suturing on the bias (Fig. 6-8). An experienced surgeon will learn to suture on the bias from one end of the flap to the other without resorting to planned halving sutures. As a general rule in the design of rotation flaps on the face, side B or the length of the flap itself should be four times the width of the

Figure 6-4   *A,* Burow's triangle can be removed to facilitate repair of the donor site wound. *B,* A standing cutaneous deformity will develop at the base of the flap *(small arrow).*

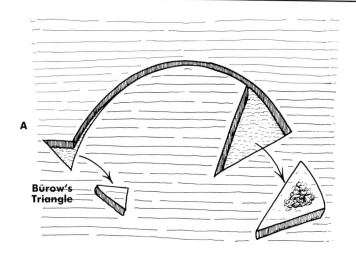

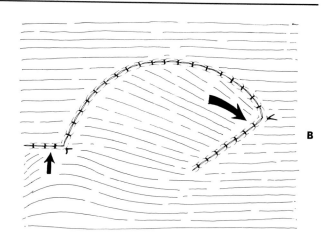

Figure 6-5   Vector of greatest wound-closure tension is from pivotal point to point located on peripheral circumference of curvilinear incision. Back cut or excision of Burow's triangle at base of flap *(inset)* shifts position of pivotal point and thus changes wound-closure tension vector as well as location of standing cutaneous deformity.

Figure 6-6   Design of rotation flap converted to two-dimensional form. Discrepancy between border of rotation flap (side B) and width of primary and secondary defects (side A) is equalized by excision of a triangle of skin (Burow's triangle) at some point along curvilinear periphery of incision (side A), with base equal in width to width at base of defect (side C).

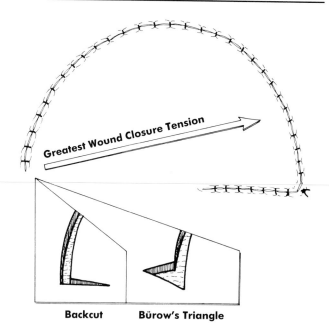

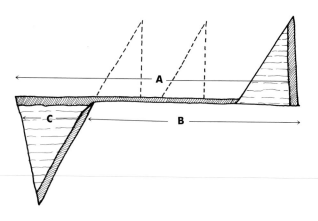

base of the triangular defect (Fig. 6-6, side C). With this 4:1 ratio, excision of a Burow's triangle is usually not necessary.

So that the surgeon can avoid standing cutaneous deformities at the base of the triangular defect, the defect shape ideally should have the proportions of

2:1, height to width (Fig. 6-9). In addition, if the arc of rotation of the flap is to be a completely symmetrical curve, the height of the triangular defect should be 0.5 to 1 times the radius of the curve of the flap (Fig. 6-10). The pure rotation flap is a pivotal flap, but it does of necessity involve some advancement of the pivotal point and thus the base of the pedicle during flap transfer. It is usually random in its vascularity but, depending on the position of the base of the flap, it may be axial in design.

There are many advantages of the rotation flap. The flap has only two sides; thus it does lend itself very well

Figure 6-7   Need for excision of Burow's triangle is often avoided by advancement of distal tip of rotation flap and repair of wound by suturing on the bias.

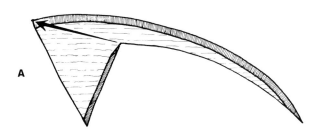

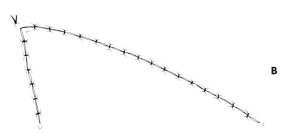

Figure 6-8   *A* and *B*, Surgeon takes advantage of distensibility of side B and compressibility of side A to achieve wound repair without excision of Burow's triangle by advancing and stretching side B to reach most distal edge of defect. *C* and *D*, Wound is repaired by principle of halving sutures.

Figure 6-9   To minimize standing cutaneous deformity that develops at base of rotation flaps, the most ideal configuration of triangular defect for repair has height-to-width ratio of 2:1.

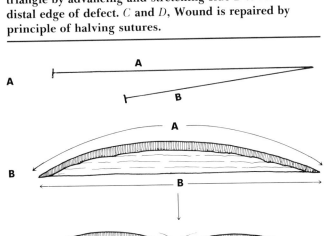

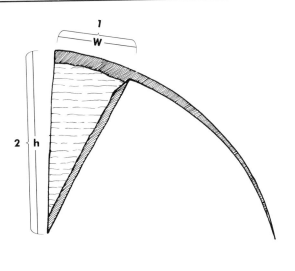

Figure 6-10   For symmetrical rotation flap, ideally, height of triangular defect for repair should be 0.5 to 1 times the radius (r) of curvature of flap.

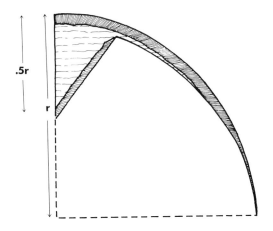

to having both edges placed in borders of esthetic units of the face or into one esthetic border and one RSTL. The flap is broad-based, and therefore its vascularity tends to be reliable. There is great flexibility in design and positioning of the flap.[8-10] Design of the flap so that it is inferiorly based promotes lymphatic drainage and reduces flap congestion and edema. Similarly, arterial and venous disruptions may be minimized and sensory innervation may be maximized by appropriate positioning of the base of the flap. Rotation flaps may be quite large and are particularly useful for reconstruction of sizable defects of the lower area of the cheek and upper part of the neck.

Disadvantages of rotation flaps are few. The defect for which the rotation flap is designed to repair should be triangular or must be modified by trimming normal tissue to create a triangular defect. The nature of the flap creates a right angle at the distal tip, and the surgeon must take care in positioning this tip so that the vascularity of the flap is not compromised. As with all pivotal flaps, rotation flaps develop standing cutaneous deformities at their base, which may not be easily removed without compromising the vascularity of the flap. Thus a second-stage removal of the deformity may be necessary. In addition, like all pivotal flaps, the effective length of the flap becomes progressively less as the flap moves through its arc of rotation, so the flap must be designed large enough to compensate for this phenomenon.

Rotation flaps are useful in all areas of the cheek. Chin reconstruction often can be readily accomplished with rotation flaps, occasionally with two flaps to optimize the use of esthetic borders to camouflage incisions.[9] Large areas of the upper part of the neck may be resurfaced with rotation flaps, recruiting relaxed skin in the lower area of the cheek or neck. Large rotation flaps with the arc of the flap designed along the hairline are quite helpful for repair of temporal and lateral forehead defects. Smaller rotation flaps may be used for repairs in the glabellar area.

Another appropriate use of rotation flaps is repair of scalp defects.[10] The inelasticity of scalp tissue and the spherical shape of the cranium are factors that often require the concomitant use of multiple rotation flaps. Scalp flaps must be large relative to the size of the defect. The general rule of a 4:1 ratio of length of flap to base of defect does not apply well in the scalp because of the inelasticity of scalp tissue. Flap design with a ratio of 6:1 is often required in the scalp. Galeatomies and intraoperative tissue expansion are often helpful in the reconstruction of larger scalp defects even when very large rotation flaps are used.

Rotation flaps are not useful in nasal reconstruction because of the lengthy incision required for rotation flaps and the need to undermine and advance the pivotal point. Small defects over the dorsum of the nose are better repaired with transposition flaps such as bilobed or rhombic flaps or even full-thickness skin grafts. Furthermore, a rotation flap transferred from cheek to the side wall of the nose usually results in an unacceptable cosmetic result because of the bridging across the nasal-facial sulcus. Similarly, pure rotation flaps from the cheek are inappropriate for reconstruction of lip defects because the arc of the flap must extend across the melolabial fold and sulcus. The resulting incision line bridges an esthetic border with concave topography; thus, it is almost impossible to hide the incisions for the flap in esthetic borders.

In summary, the rotation flap is an ideal method to reconstruct medium to large defects of the cheek, neck, forehead, and scalp. When the flap is created as a large lateral inferiorly based flap, it provides a flexible means of transfer of large amounts of tissue. A dependable well-vascularized flap may be used in an irradiated area and in patients who have cutaneous vascular compromise as a result of smoking or diabetes mellitus.

SURGICAL TECHNIQUE

In anticipation of using a rotation flap to repair a facial defect, the surgeon should assess the patient's overall health factors. In our hands this is generally accomplished at the time the patient is first seen, before creation of the defect, which is usually the result of excision of a cutaneous malignant neoplasm by a dermatologic surgeon. Generalized factors such as age, cardiovascular status, smoking history, general and endocrine health status, familial health factors, and drug use are evaluated. Preoperatively, the use of drugs such as aspirin, ibuprofen, anticoagulants, and β-blockers is discontinued or modified in dosage if possible.

In patients with skin cancer who are to undergo tumor excision, emotional stability and self-image are evaluated and a long-term program of psychological support from our nursing services is initiated. Factors relating to the histologic analysis of the skin cancer are discussed with the patient, and consultation may be obtained from the dermatologic surgeon, head and neck oncologic surgeon, and radiation oncologist as indicated. Preexcisional close-up and full-face photographs are obtained. Finally, a complete and open discussion of tumor excision and reconstructive plans is held with the patient and all supportive family members.

Factors such as the possible need for flap revision and dermabrasion are discussed before the first reconstructive surgical procedure. All facial reconstructions with use of rotation flaps are performed in our facial plastic surgery operating room with the use of an anesthesiologist who monitors the patient. In most cases of monitored anesthetic care, midazolam (Versed), fentanyl, or (Propofol) is used. In children, a general endotracheal anesthetic is preferred.

Assessment of possible reconstructive alternatives begins at the first visit and evaluation of the patient. Skin lines are evaluated along with the skin condition, distensibility, and turgor. Flap design is tentatively planned before micrographic excision. After the excision close-up photographs of the resulting skin defect are obtained, and reconstruction is planned for the next day. Rotational flaps are usually designed so that they are inferiorly and laterally based. The margins of the flap are placed in the borders of esthetic units when possible and in RSTLs when esthetic borders are not in the immediate vicinity of the defect. Use of esthetic borders in design of the flap may even necessitate excision of normal skin so that the flap edges are positioned along these borders.

The quintessential large rotation flap is the cervical facial rotation flap used for reconstruction of large cheek defects. In the design of this flap, we attempt whenever possible to use the melolabial and alar-facial sulci as the medial border of the flap. The subciliary margin that continues laterally into the periauricular crease becomes the superior and posterior border of the flap, respectively. After the induction of intravenous analgesia, regional block and local infiltrative anesthesia are accomplished with the use of a mixture of equal parts of 0.5% lidocaine (Xylocaine) and 0.25% bupivacaine (Marcaine) (both solutions contain a 1:200,000 concentration of epinephrine). This mixture is titrated, with nine parts anesthetic mixture to one part sodium bicarbonate solution. Thus, provision is made for a relatively rapid-onset but long-duration anesthetic, allowing the surgeon to use a volume of over 30 ml if required. The titrated solution has neutral pH and thus burns less on injection than does an anesthetic without sodium bicarbonate added. The entire face is then prepared and draped. Methylene blue is used to mark the designed flap and areas adjacent to the defect that will require excision. The back of the scalpel blade is then used to scratch the design of the flap into the skin. The methylene blue then is erased from the surface of the skin before any incisions are made. This "scratched-out" design is more precise than the methylene blue markings, does not smear with sponging, and provides a better appearance of the wound at the end of the procedure.

When micrographic excision has been used to remove a skin tumor, the entire margin of the defect is excised with incisions perpendicular to the skin margin to create a triangular defect, which will allow for rotation of the flap into position. All these excisions are executed before the flap is raised. All incisions are made with a No. 15C scalpel blade on a No. 9 scalpel handle. All incisions are absolutely vertical to skin margin with no beveling whatever. The flap margins are incised, and any skin that must be removed to enable the flap to extend to adjacent esthetic borders or RSTLs is also excised. The flap is handled only by the use of skin hooks and is undermined widely under the base. Additionally, all sides of the donor site and defect are undermined for a distance of at least 2 cm. An exception to this rule is when the borders of the donor site are relatively fixed, such as the melolabial fold, nasofacial groove, or subciliary margin. These borders

are undermined only 4 to 5 mm so that wound edge eversion can occur but without distortion of adjacent facial structures. All undermining is accomplished with sharp dissection in the subdermal fat plane. Meticulous hemostasis is established with monopolar needle-tipped electrocautery.

The flap is then rotated into position with the use of skin hooks for handling, and the size of the standing cutaneous deformity at the base of the flap is assessed before suturing. If any further advancement of the apex of the flap or any modification of the base of the triangular defect is required, it is accomplished before the flap is sutured into position.

We depend on sucuticular sutures, along the entire length of the wound to suspend the flap. The first suture is placed at the flap suspension point, which is the point of greatest wound-closure tension. In the case of large cervical facial rotation flaps, this point is usually near the attachment of the lateral canthus to the periosteum of the orbit. The second subcuticular suture is used to secure the distal tip of the flap. Subcuticular sutures are then sewn along the entire periphery of the flap, every 8 to 10 mm. For subcuticular sutures to support the greatest wound-closure tension points, 4-0 polydiaxanone (PDS) sutures are used, and the remaining subcuticular sutures are 5-0 PDS. All cutaneous closures are accomplished with 6-0 fast-absorbing gut sutures placed in an interrupted or running locked fashion. When flap incisions extend along the preauricular crease or in the postauricular upper cervical area, 5-0 fast-absorbing gut sutures may be substituted. Along the vermilion border inverted or semiburied 5-0 chromic sutures are used. For cutaneous closure in hair-bearing areas of the male face, we prefer 5-0 (Dermalon) to fast-absorbing gut sutures. Drains are not used even with very large flaps.

Postoperatively, a bulk compression dressing is placed over the entire flap and the adjacent areas of the face. Dressings consist of bacitracin ointment and nonadherent (Telfa) bandages over the wound edges and then a layer of loose synthetic polyester (Dacron) upholstery batting held in place by rolls of (Kerlix) strategically placed in a semi-Barton dressing form. This is then covered with layers of 3-inch (Coban), which is stretched to provide a moderate amount of compression over the entire surface of the flap and donor site. This dressing is left in place for 2 days and then replaced with a looser dressing of Kerlix and (Kling) for an additional 2 days. After removal of the dressings, the patient is asked to apply an antibiotic ointment to all wound edges and sutures twice a day. Any residual undissolved skin sutures are carefully trimmed by the sixth postoperative day. When permanent skin sutures are used, they are removed by the fifth postoperative day. Patients are instructed to avoid strenuous exercise for 2 weeks after surgery and are asked to avoid sun and extreme temperature exposures for at least 1 month postoperatively. The patient is given careful follow-up care, and the patient and family members are provided psychological support by physician and nursing staff. Plans for any revisional surgery are discussed. In all instances, at least dermabrasion of the flap is planned 3 to 6 months postoperatively.

The following are examples of the use of rotation flaps for reconstruction of defects in various locations about the face.

CASE EXAMPLES

CASE 1

A 51-year-old man had a 3 × 4 cm healed split-thickness skin graft of the forehead and temporal area. The graft had been placed in an area in which a basal cell carcinoma had been resected 2 years before his consultation. The graft was unchanged over the 2-year interval, and there was no evidence of recurrent tumor. The patient was interested in a better appearance. Examination of the site showed the graft to be depressed (Fig. 6-11) with elevated hypertrophic scarred margins. The surgical challenge was to replace the graft with forehead skin without causing distortion of the brow or hairline and to place as many of the incisions as possible into esthetic borders and RSTLs.

A combined approach was developed with use of a rotation flap based laterally and an advancement flap based medially. Each flap measured 6 cm long and had a width equal to the height of the graft (4 cm). Fig. 6-11**D** shows the repair at 3 months after surgery. No distortion of hairline or brow was noted. The scars that resulted from incisions for the flap were particularly well camouflaged along the hairline and in the horizontal creases of the forehead. The vertical scar was more apparent but was acceptable to the patient. Dermabrasion of the scars was recommended; however, the patient elected not to have this procedure performed.

CASE 2

A 52-year-old woman presented with a defect of her left cheek and upper lip after micrographic surgical excision of a basal cell carcinoma (Fig. 6-12). The medial border of the defect was at the alar-facial sulcus and extended minimally into the upper lip. The challenge was to repair the defect without distortion of the lip or the alar base and to place incisions in esthetic borders and RSTLs. The lateral and vertical dimensions of the defect were, respectively, 5 cm and 3.5 cm.

Figure 6-11 *A,* Healed split-thickness skin graft (3 × 4 cm) of right temple. *B,* Lateral rotation and medial advancement flaps are designed to allow removal of split-thickness skin graft and closure of wound.

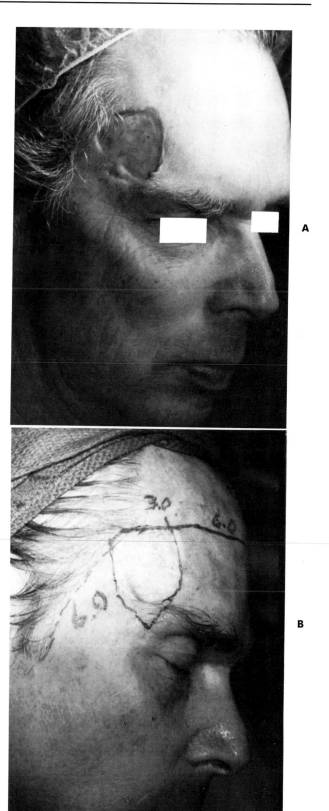

Continued.

Figure 6-11, cont'd.   *C*, Removal of graft and wound closure. *D*, Appearance 3 months postoperatively.

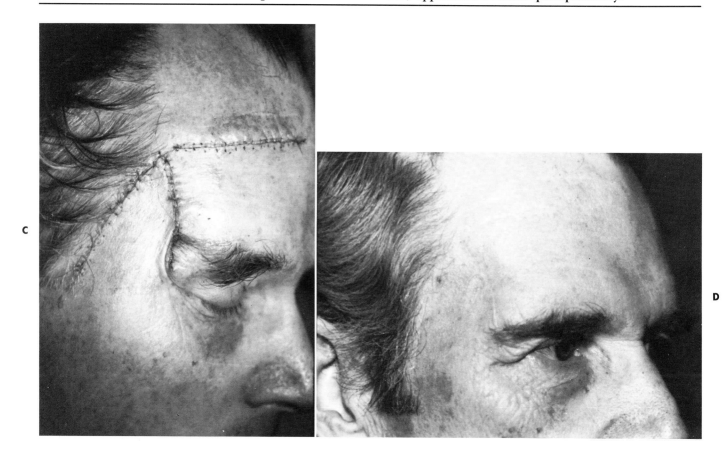

Figure 6-12   *A*, A 3.5 × 5 cm skin defect of medial cheek after excision of basal cell carcinoma.

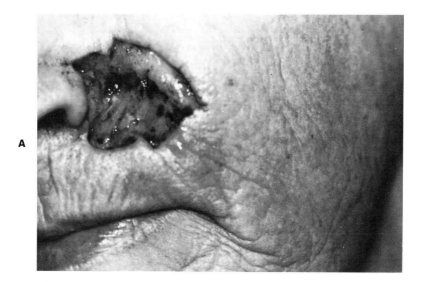

Figure 6-12, cont'd. *B* and *C*, Inferior-based rotation flap is designed to recruit redundant skin from medial cheek. Standing cutaneous deformity is removed in melolabial sulcus. Flap is incised. *D*, Medial border of flap after wound repair lies in melolabial sulcus. *E*, Six months postoperatively, superior scar is apparent.

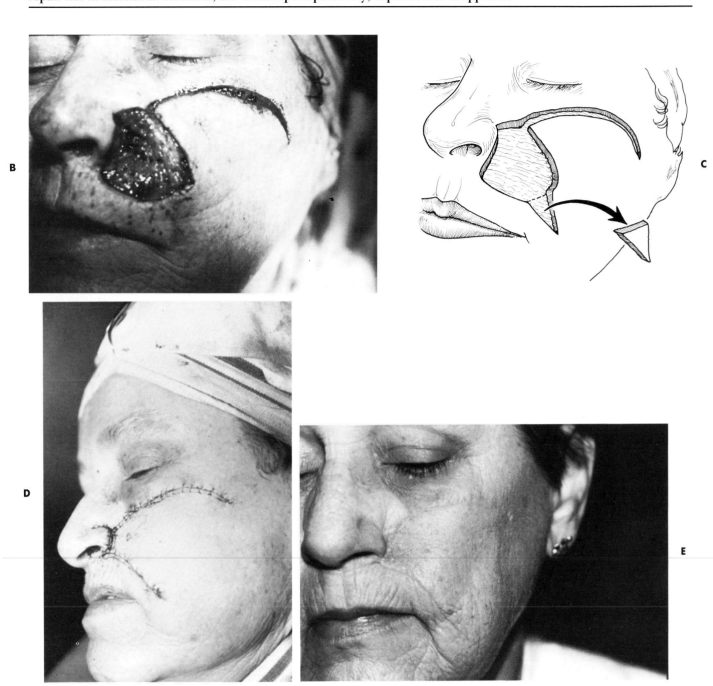

A large inferiorly based rotation flap was incised. The flap was designed to recruit skin from the medial cheek. The medial border of the flap after wound repair lay in the melolabial sulcus. The result at 6 months was satisfactory in terms of lack of distortion of the lip and alar base. Moderate success was achieved in attempts to restore a melolabial fold. The superior aspect of the scar, which resulted from transfer of the flap, was visible because the arc of the flap did not lie in the subciliary line. A better flap design may have been to begin the arc of the flap at the alar-facial sulcus and extend it superiorly along the subciliary line and from there laterally.

Figure 6-13   *A* and *B*, A 6 × 5.5 cm skin defect of medial cheek and upper lip after excision of basal cell carcinoma.

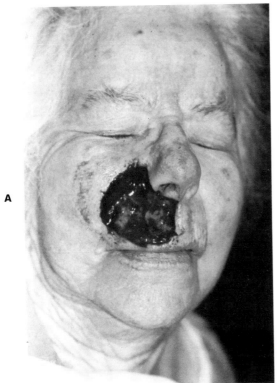

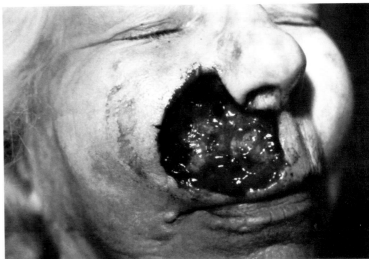

CASE 3

An 84-year-old woman was left with a defect of the cheek and upper lip after micrographic excision of a basal cell carcinoma. The defect consisted of a loss of virtually all of the skin of the right side of the upper lip extending into the nasal alar base and laterally onto the cheek (Fig. 6-13). The orbicularis oris muscle remained intact. The vertical height of the defect was 4.5 cm along the line of the melolabial fold and 6 cm along a line that extended from the vermilion through the alar-facial sulcus. The horizontal dimension of the defect was 5.5 cm.

A large cervical facial rotation flap was designed with an arch of 20 cm. The superior margin of the flap extended from the alar-facial sulcus along the subciliary line laterally to the preauricular crease. Fig. 6-13D

shows the flap after transfer and removal of a standing cutaneous deformity at the lateral aspect of the defect. At 4 months postoperatively, there was no distortion of the lower eyelid or nasal ala. The redundancy of tissue near the oral commissure was the result of inadequate excision of the standing cutaneous deformity. In addition, there was a visible scar along the anterior-inferior margin of the flap near the vermilion and filtrum, where a triangle of normal skin was left. A better result may have been obtained had the remainder of this esthetic subunit been excised and the border of the flap brought to the junction of the filtrum and vermilion. Additionally, much more of the standing cutaneous deformity should have been excised by extension of the excision downward into the melolabial sulcus, which would have assisted in camouflaging the resulting scar.

Figure 6-13, cont'd.   *C*, Large cervical facial rotation flap is designed so that superior border of flap is positioned along subciliary line. *D*, Wound repaired with rotation flap. Standing cutaneous deformity is excised at lateral oral commissure. *E* and *F*, Four months postoperatively there is distortion of oral commissure from inadequate removal of standing cutaneous deformity.

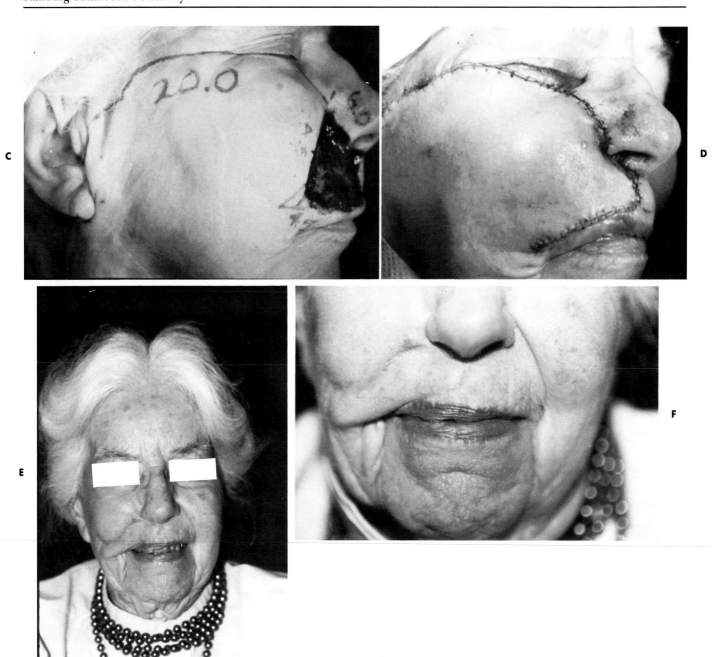

CASE 4

A 46-year-old woman had a lentigo maligna of the left cheek (Fig. 6-14). The lentigo was excised with micrographic control, resulting in a defect 3 cm wide and 7 cm high involving the left lower eyelid and cheek.

An inferiorly based rotation flap was designed with the arc of the flap extending above the lateral canthus to the hairline and along the hairline to the preauricular crease. The standing cutaneous deformity of the flap was trimmed so that the excision was parallel to the melolabial sulcus. At 4 months postoperatively, the results were acceptable to the patient. Dermabrasion was declined by the patient.

Figure 6-14 *A*, Lentigo maligna of left cheek and lower eyelid. *B*, A 7 × 3 cm skin defect of medial cheek and lower eyelid after resection of skin lesion. Rotation flap is designed to reconstruct defect. *C*, Wound repaired. Arch of flap extends above level of lateral canthus, and flap is supported by deep sutures placed in periosteum of lateral orbital rim. Standing cutaneous deformity is excised parallel to melolabial sulcus. *D*, Appearance 4 months postoperatively.

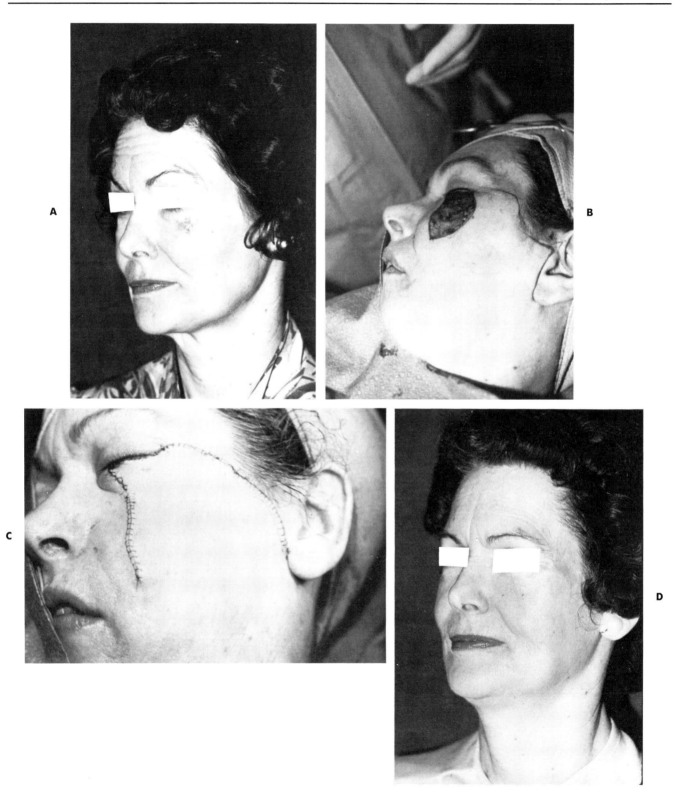

CASE 5

A 62-year-old man was referred for reconstructive surgery. A previous attempt had been made to reconstruct an extensive central facial defect with a microsurgical radial forearm flap after resection of squamous cell carcinoma. The patient also had received a course of postoperative radiotherapy 6 months earlier. The microsurgical flap was edematous and provided a poor color and texture match with the adjacent skin of the cheek and nose (Fig. 6-15). In addition, the patient suffered from an ectropion of the right lower eyelid, and the flap produced redundant subcutaneous tissue and skin in the right cheek and lateral aspect of the nose.

Complete excision of the microsurgical flap was planned. A cheek rotation flap and paramedian forehead flap were used to reconstruct the defect left from removal of the microsurgical flap. The rotation flap was used to repair the cheek component of the defect, and the forehead flap was used to reconstruct the nasal component. The rotation flap was suspended from above the lateral and medial canthis. A photograph 1 month postoperatively showed correction of the extreme preoperative ectropion (not shown). There was a persistent nasocutaneous fistula near the medial canthus, which required repair.

Figure 6-15   *A*, Patient with ectropion of right lower eyelid after resurfacing of large skin defect with microsurgical forearm flap. Flap has provided poor color and texture match with surrounding facial skin. *B*, Complete removal of microsurgical flap is planned. Large rotation cheek flap is designed to resurface cheek component of resulting facial defect.

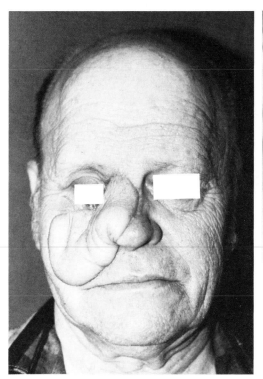

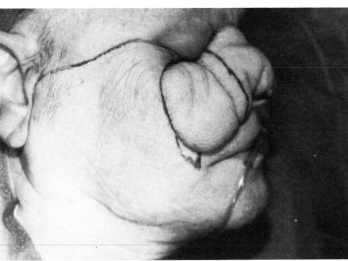

A

B

Continued.

Figure 6-15, cont'd. *C,* Rotation flap is suspended from above medial and lateral canthi. Standing cutaneous deformity is removed in melolabial sulcus. *D,* Paramedian forehead flap is used to resurface nasal component of facial defect. *E,* Appearance 1 month postoperatively.

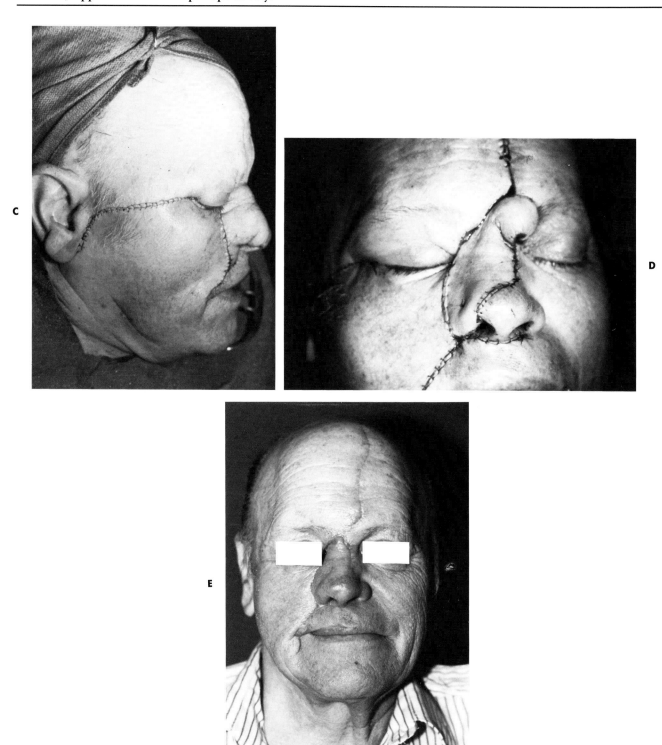

SUMMARY

The rotation flap is an extremely versatile flap. Only two incisions are required to create the flap. Although these incisions are at right angles to one another, it is usually possible to camouflage both in facial esthetic borders or along RSTLs. The flap is extremely dependable because of its very broad base and is thus useful in patients with impaired skin vascularity. Because of the flexibility of design afforded by the simplicity of this procedure, it is easy for the surgeon to design inferiorly based flaps with their attendant advantages of arterial, venous, and lymphatic supplies. Rotation flaps are readily combined with other types of local skin flaps. They are particularly useful in repair of large scalp and medial cheek defects. The flexibility of design inherent in this flap also has made it increasingly helpful for many resurfacing problems.

REFERENCES

1. Baker SR: Options for reconstruction in head and neck surgery. In Cummings CW, Frederickson FM, Harker LA, et al, editors: *Otolaryngology Head and Neck Surgery Update,* vol 1, St Louis, 1989, CV Mosby.
2. Grabb WC, Myers MB: *Skin flaps,* Boston, 1975, Little Brown.
3. Esser JF: Studies in plastic surgery of the face, *Ann Surg* 65:297, 1917.
4. Imre T: *Jidplastik und plastische Operationen und anderer Weichteile des Gesichts,* Budapest, 1928, Stadium Verlag.
5. Larrabee WF Jr, Sutton D: The biomechanics of advancement and rotation flaps, *Laryngoscope* 91:726, 1981.
6. Dzubow LM: Indications for a geometric approach to wound closure following Mohs surgery, *J Dermatol Surg Oncol* 13:480, 1987.
7. Dzubow LM: The dynamics of flap movement: the effect of pivotal restraint on flap rotation and transposition, *J Dermatol Surg Oncol* 13:1348, 1987.
8. Saad MN, Maisels DO: Further applications of the rotation advancement technique, *Br J Plast Surg* 25:116, 1972.
9. Golomb FM: Closure of the circular defect with double rotation flaps and Z-plasties, *Plast Reconstr Surg* 74:813, 1984.
10. Album MJ: Repair of large scalp defect by bilateral rotation flaps, *J Dermatol Surg Oncol* 4:906, 1978.

EDITORIAL COMMENTS

Shan R. Baker

Rotation flaps are pivotal flaps that have a curvilinear configuration. The secondary defect created by the flap represents a transformation and translocation of the primary defect.[1] The geometry of the secondary defect is determined by the size of the flap. The longer the flap, the longer and the more narrow is the secondary defect because the surface area encompassed by the primary defect is equivalent to the surface area of the secondary defect.[1] The narrower the width of the secondary defect, the less is the tension required to close the wound and the less is the secondary movement of tissue adjacent to the defect. Thus, the longer the rotation flap, the less is the wound-closure tension. In addition, the longer the flap length relative to the width of the defect, the less difficult it is to redistribute the standing cutaneous deformity by suturing the incision with use of the rule of halves.

Rotation flaps are designed immediately adjacent to the defect, with the advancing border of the flap representing one of the borders of the defect. Similar to other pivotal flaps, the base of the flap along with its pivotal point are frequently advanced to a limited degree toward the defect during wound closure. This reduces wound-closure tension and often necessitates a smaller flap with less rotation about the pivotal point than when the flap's base is not widely undermined and advanced. The authors note that the distal tip of the flap is also often advanced by stretching the flap to reach the most distal point of the defect. The maneuver of stretching the flap accomplishes two things: (1) It reduces the overall size of the flap required to resurface the defect and (2) it reduces the standing cutaneous deformity by advancing a portion of the deformity peripherally away from the flap's base.

I do not use many rotation flaps for reconstruction of facial defects. This is because frequently the defect is of a size or location that necessitates that the curvilinear configuration of the incision, required to create the flap, cross at right angles to esthetic borders or RSTLs. This results in a poorly camouflaged scar along a portion of the donor site. In my practice the use of rotation flaps on the face is limited to repair of large medial cheek defects, in which the curvilinear incision can be placed along the inferior orbital rim, or defects of the upper forehead, in which the incision for the flap is placed along the hairline. One disadvantage of large rotation flaps in men designed to extend from the infraorbital rim or subciliary line into a preauricular crease is that movement of the flap causes hair-bearing skin of the sideburn to be displaced forward into the non–hair-bearing area of the lower temple.

Rotation flaps work extremely well in repair of defects in the periauricular area where recruitment of the upper posterior cervical skin is necessary. The curvilinear incision is placed adjacent to the earlobe and along the hairline of the postauricular scalp and if necessary can extend along the anterior border of the trapezius muscle. An incision in this area produces favorable scars even though they do not follow RSTLs. A Z-plasty at the base of the flap facilitates closure of the secondary defect. Rotation flaps are the preferred method to repair most scalp defects with use of local tissue. Because of its spherical topography, the scalp accommodates curvilinear incisions well and the flaps can be constructed large without the need to regard RSTLs or esthetic borders. The advantage of large rotation flaps in the repair of scalp defects is that they require less stretch or elasticity compared with smaller flaps to close a given defect. Wound-closure tension also has a wider area of distribution when larger flaps are used; thus the flap donor site is easier to close primarily compared with other types of pivotal flaps.

Reference

1. Dzubow LM: *Facial flaps: biomechanics and regional applications*, Norwalk, Conn, 1990, Appleton & Lange.

EDITORIAL COMMENTS

Neil A. Swanson

The rotation flap is the second of the sliding flaps. As the authors accurately state, the pure rotation flap has a pivotal component to it. However, in my experience there are very few pure rotational flaps. They usually are a combination of motion that includes advancement. The rotation flap, like the advancement flap, depends on the creation of a secondary defect, which basically is managed as wounds of unequal length. The authors present a good discussion of the management of the secondary defect, triangulation or shortening of the arc, or "sewing it out." The important concept is that, when triangulation is necessary, the triangle can be placed anywhere along the arc of the flap so that it is best hidden in RSTLs or hair-bearing skin.

Although the geometry of this flap, as discussed, includes a fairly wide arc in the base of the flap, the arc ends up being adjusted depending on many considerations. At times, the arc needs to be shortened to keep the rotational arc inside a hair-bearing line so as not to rotate hair-bearing tissue to non–hair-bearing skin. On the other hand, the arc may need to be very large for tissue that does not move well or is limited by the galeal facia such as on the scalp or forehead. There are other times when the arc is made large to hide resultant scars within cosmetic lines and boundaries. The cervical-facial rotation flap discussed in detail in the chapter is an example.

Because most defects left after Mohs surgery are circular or oval, a rotation flap is often placed into a circle instead of a triangle. My preference is to rotate the flap first and then triangulate the circle by removing a redundant cutaneous cone. Often I find this cone to be either larger or smaller than I expected. It can also often be removed by widening of the base of the flap.

The rotation flap, as described by the authors, completely closes the primary defect. This results in minimal secondary tissue movement in response to the flap's primary motion and the creation of a larger secondary defect. When used in areas where there is the ability to use secondary motion, the flap does not have to be fully rotated or advanced. A portion of the primary defect can be closed to take advantage of secondary tissue motion or gain. A good way to visualize this is to place a temporary suture through the apex of the flap after it has been cut and fully undermined. The apex of the rotational arc can then be manually rotated through its full arc, allowing the surgeon to appreciate whether there is a need to close the entire primary defect or whether there can be sharing between the primary defect and the secondary defect.

Two important technical points discussed are as follows: (1) The reconstructive surgeon should feel comfortable in enlarging the surgical defect if that is necessary to provide a better esthetic result. Just because margins are clear at a fixed defect size does not mean that normal adjacent skin should not be excised to give a better reconstructive effort. (2) The technique described of scratching skin markings with the back of a scalpel blade is very useful. As discussed, it gives a permanent outline of the flap to be cut and does not wash off with patient scrub preparation or any bleeding during surgery.

There are instances, as with any of the other basic flap types, when multiple rotation flaps are useful. These can be double (the O-Z) or with three or more rotational arcs (pinwheel). Several examples of rotational flaps, both single and multiple, will be given during the discussions of the reconstruction of specific areas of the face.

7

ADVANCEMENT FLAPS

Mark D. Brown

INTRODUCTION

The most basic advancement flap is the simple linear layered closure, which involves undermining and direct advancement of tissue side to side to cover and close a primary defect. This closure does not create a secondary defect and additional incisions are made only for the removal of a standing cutaneous deformity (dog-ear). However, the term *advancement flap* usually refers to a flap created by incisions, which allow for a "sliding" movement of incised tissue.[1] The movement is in one direction, and the flap advances directly over the primary defect. The basic design of an advancement flap is to extend an incision along parallel sides of the defect and then directly advance the tissue over the defect. Wound repair with use of an advancement flap consists of both primary and secondary tissue movement.[2] The primary movement involves the forward pushing, pulling, or sliding action of the incised flap as well as a small amount of stretching of the flap itself. There will usually be secondary movement in the opposite direction of the skin and soft tissue immediately adjacent to the defect, in which case the surrounding skin may move or stretch toward the advancing edge of the flap. This secondary movement either may help in the closure by providing for less wound-closure tension or may at times be detrimental if located near a free margin of a facial structure. Complete undermining of the advancement flap as well as the skin and soft tissue around the flap pedicle is very important. In addition, the skin and soft tissue around the defect opposite the flap can be undermined if secondary movement is desirable. At times it may be preferable to have only movement of the flap, and in this case there should be no undermining of the stationary margins of the defect.

Standing cutaneous deformities are created when advancement flaps are used and usually require excision accomplished by the removal of Burow's triangles. Excision of Burow's triangles may also facilitate movement of the flap. In fact, a variation on the basic advancement flap is a Burow's triangle (or wedge) flap, in which a large triangle or crescent of tissue is removed to allow greater mobility and advancement of the free edge of the flap.[3,4] Not all advancement flaps are pure advancement. For example, the common laterally based cheek advancement flap relies primarily on the sliding of loose cheek tissue from lateral to medial directions but often also involve a lesser amount of inferior to superior rotational movement.[5]

One of the basic advantages of the advancement flap is to allow a change in the position and/or location of a standing cutaneous deformity that might have resulted from a side-to-side closure of a primary defect.[6] A rectangular or geometric advancement flap allows this displacement of the standing cutaneous deformity to an area distant from the defect and thus may allow for better cosmesis. The actual location of where to excise Burow's triangle is best determined after the advancing edge of the flap is secured. The incision lines for Burow's triangles can then be carefully placed into appropriate relaxed skin tension lines (RSTLs) or cosmetic boundary lines when possible. Burow's triangles will not always be the same size or location on both sides of the flap. Occasionally if the flap is sufficiently long, the standing cutaneous deformities might be subdivided into multiple smaller puckers of tissue that need not be excised but merely "sewn out" by sequential suturing of the length of the wound in half (rule of halves).[1,3] This is accomplished by dividing the length of the wound in half by placement of a suture. The two halves are then each divided in half by placement of additional sutures. This process continues until the entire length of the wound is closed.

Advancement flaps can be very useful for reconstruction of surgical defects of the face. It is a truism that certain flaps seem to work best in certain anatomic locations, and this holds true for advancement flaps. Table 7-1 describes some of the facial sites where advancement flaps are particularly useful. The chapter begins with a general discussion of several common advancement flaps—how they work, where they work best, and why they sometimes do not work. All flaps have inherent advantages and disadvantages. At the

Table 7-1   Advancement Flaps

Type	Location
Single and bilateral (U and H-plasty)	Forehead
	Eyebrow
	Helical rim
O-T, A-T (T-plasty)	Forehead
	Lower eyelid
	Lip
	Chin
	Posterior sulcus (ear)
Island pedicle	Upper lip
	Cheek
	Nasal sidewall
Cheek advancement	Medial cheek
Mucosal advancement	Lower lip
Wedge resection with advancement	Lip
	Ear

end of the chapter five case examples will illustrate the use of advancement flaps, which resulted in acceptable cosmesis. As with all flaps it is important to evaluate the adjacent tissue for matching qualities of skin texture, color, consistency, and hair growth. Before use of an advancement flap it is imperative to evaluate the following criteria: (1) the location of the tension vectors of the flap, (2) the location of the incision lines and whether they respect skin tension lines and cosmetic boundary lines, and (3) the location where the standing cutaneous deformity is likely to be and how best it will be removed.[7]

SINGLE-PEDICLE ADVANCEMENT FLAP

The single-pedicle advancement flap, sometimes referred to as U-plasty, is the most basic of the advancement flaps (Fig. 7-1). This advancement flap works well on the forehead by use of horizontal crease lines and in the eyebrow region by hiding a portion of the scar in the hair-bearing region. Although the flap and defect should be visualized as a geometric rectangle or square, in reality most surgical defects are round or oval. The rectangular flap does not always fit precisely into a round defect and may need to be rounded or the defect squared off to allow more precise approximation (Fig. 7-1**B**). However, this should not be performed until the flap has first been elevated and shown to cover the defect completely. The typical ratio of defect length to flap length is 3:1.[1,7]

The following steps should be followed in the use of a single-pedicle advancement flap. First, wide undermining is performed. On the forehead undermining should be performed in the fibrous level just above the outer frontalis muscle fascia. On the scalp the flap

should be incised down through galea and undermining should be carried out in a subgaleal plane. Undermining before incision of the flap helps to accurately determine the incisional depth of the flap. At times, if the flap is long and is stretched excessively in the direction of its long axis, it may seemingly decrease in width, especially at the distal end. For relief of this phenomenon, undermining of the surrounding tissue adjacent to the flap's pedicle is helpful. Undermining also facilitates the wound closure without causing excess wound-closure tension and helps prevent excessive pull on free margins such as an eyebrow or hairline.

Next, parallel incisions are made, preferably in RSTLs such as forehead crease lines. The length of the flap is dependent on several factors, including anatomic location, skin laxity, and defect size. The flap is dissected carefully and elevated to its pedicle base. As with all flaps, careful and meticulous hemostasis is obtained. The mobility of the flap and its ability to close the defect are tested by placing a skin hook at the advancing edge and sliding the flap forward. If sufficient coverage is obtained, the key stitch is placed, which is an absorbable suture (polyglactin [Vicryl], polydiaxanone [PDS]) placed through the subcutis and dermis at the central aspect of the advancing edge of the flap and in the opposite edge of the defect. This key stitch will effectively close the defect. Absorbable sutures are then placed in the deep levels of the wound along the remainder of the primary and secondary defects. Use only enough absorbable sutures to align the skin edges and remove wound-closure tension. Burow's triangles are excised if standing cutaneous deformities remain. Burow's triangles are typically excised near the base of the flap (Fig. 7-1). However, the exact location and size of these triangles will depend on esthetic units, esthetic boundary lines, and RSTLs. The epidermis is then carefully approximated using nonabsorbable sutures. Vertical mattress sutures are often helpful to prevent inversion of wound edges.

BILATERAL ADVANCEMENT FLAPS

Bilateral or H-plasty advancement flaps are typically used when a single-pedicle advancement flap does not provide adequate tissue for closure of the primary defect (Fig. 7-2). The basic principles of tissue movement and closure are identical to those for the single-pedicle advancement flap. Bilateral advancement flaps allow for movement of tissue from both sides of the defect, as shown in Fig. 7-2. In the plan and design of bilateral advancement flaps, it is wise to first incise and elevate a single advancement flap. Occasionally, sufficient movement is achieved with the first flap so that

Figure 7-1   Single-pedicle advancement flap. Primary and secondary skin movement noted.

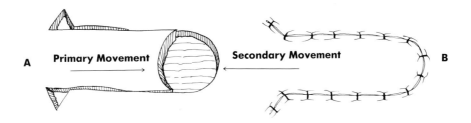

Figure 7-2   Bilateral advancement flaps.

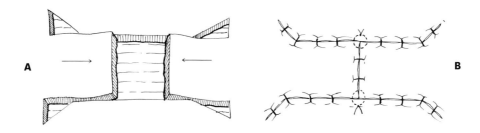

the second flap is not necessary. However, if the single flap is under excessive tension, then the opposite flap is incised, which completes the H-plasty. As with a single advancement flap, bilateral flaps work well on the forehead, eyebrow, and scalp.

Skin hooks may be used to advance the flaps to determine whether they will freely meet in the middle of the defect. The flaps harvested from the two opposite edges of the wound do not necessarily have to be of the same length or demonstrate the same amount of mobility and elasticity. For example, in the temple there is often more movement from the laterally based flap as opposed to a medially based flap. On advancement of the two flaps, if there is excessive tension at the midpoint, it may be necessary to extend the parallel incision lines, thus lengthening the two flaps. It is best not to exceed a 3:1 ratio of flap length to defect length. A 4:1 ratio is possible if the flap is based on a named artery.[7] The key suture to secure the advancement of the two flaps is an absorbable suture placed in the subcutaneous and dermal planes at the center of the two advancing flap edges. Wounds of unequal length are created, which will require removal of Burow's triangles. These triangles may vary in size and location depending on the location of the flaps and the elasticity of the tissues (Fig. 7-3).[1] Fig. 7-3 shows Burow's triangles removed at different locations above and below the two flaps. In theory these locations correspond to areas that result in the best cosmesis. Fig. 7-3**B** shows half-buried mattress sutures at the sites of the Burow's triangle excisions. Inferiorly a four-point corner tip stitch is used. A disadvantage of bilateral

advancement flaps is that it can be an extensive procedure requiring long suture lines.

CHEEK ADVANCEMENT FLAP

Cheek advancement flaps are commonly used and have to their advantage the relative mobility and elasticity of the skin and soft tissue of the cheek (Fig. 7-4).[5,8] A common site for the development of skin cancers is the junction between the nose and cheek along the nasal-facial sulcus. If defects that result from removal of cancers in this area cannot be closed primarily, it is usually best to move cheek skin medially rather than nasal skin laterally because cheek skin is more mobile and generally results in an improved cosmetic result after reconstruction. Medium to large defects in this area can be closed by advancement of lateral cheek skin. Standing cutaneous deformities, which develop with all advancement flaps, are excised superiorly at the natural junction line between the cheek and the lower eyelid and inferiorly along the melolabial fold (Fig. 7-4**B**). For smaller defects of the medial cheek or nasal sidewall, incisions to create the advancement flap may be placed closer together in appropriate RSTLs that parallel the infraorbital and melolabial lines.

For defects of the medial cheek it is important to maintain the integrity and contour of the nasal-facial sulcus, which will avoid blunting or bridging across this concave area. This undesirable tenting can be minimized by the use of a periosteal tacking suture made of absorbable polyglactin (Vicryl) or polydiaxanone (PDS)

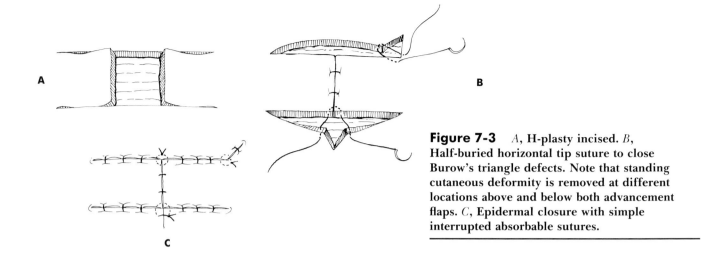

Figure 7-3 *A,* H-plasty incised. *B,* Half-buried horizontal tip suture to close Burow's triangle defects. Note that standing cutaneous deformity is removed at different locations above and below both advancement flaps. *C,* Epidermal closure with simple interrupted absorbable sutures.

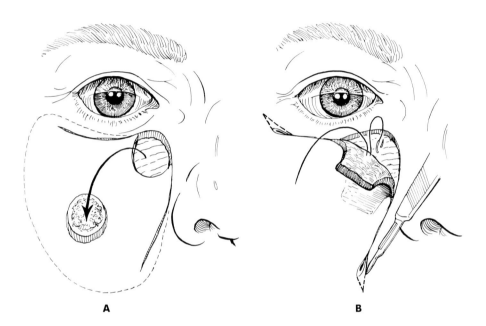

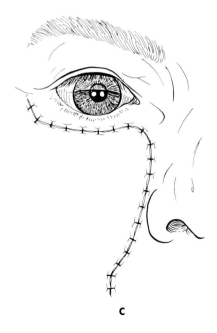

Figure 7-4 *A,* Cheek advancement flap for repair of defect in nasal-facial sulcus. Superior incision is made at infraorbital crease, and inferior incision is made at melolabial sulcus. Dotted line represents degree of skin undermining. *B,* Suspension suture attaching dermis of flap to periosteum of nasal-facial sulcus and excision of Burow's triangles. *C,* Cheek advancement flap sewn into place, with recreation of melolabial sulcus and avoidance of eyelid ectropion.

(Fig. 7-4**B**).[9] This suture is placed in the dermis of the advancing flap several millimeters behind the advancing edge and is sutured deeply to the periosteum of the underlying bone. This technique helps relieve tension on the suture line of the distal flap and concomitantly helps maintain the nasal-facial sulcus. If the defect on the nasal sidewall is large, it may be best to advance the cheek tissue only as far as the nasal-facial sulcus. The remaining defect on the more medial nasal sidewall is allowed to heal by second intention or is repaired by another flap or graft. Standing cutaneous deformities usually form at the base of the flap's pedicle and can be easily removed by extension of the incisions along the same cosmetic junction lines as shown in Fig. 7-4**B.** The excised skin provides an excellent source for grafting of any remaining defect on the sidewall of the nose.

For a defect located near the lower eyelid or medial canthus, advancement of tissue should be based laterally rather than inferiorly to help prevent the development of lower eyelid ectropion. When a defect of the anterior lamella of the lower eyelid is encountered, a horizontal subcilial incision is made along the length of the eyelid approximately 2 mm beneath the lash line.[10] A sliding skin muscle flap of the entire lower eyelid is then developed. To avoid any distortion of the eyelid or fat pads, it is important that the flaps be dissected completely free of any adherence to the underlying orbital septum. It may be necessary to carry this incision well past the lateral canthus to mobilize adequate tissue for advancement. If needed, an inferior incision along the nasal-facial sulcus can also be used to free up additional tissue for the superior movement of cheek skin.

ISLAND ADVANCEMENT FLAP

The island advancement flap uses the basic principles of V-Y advancement and closure (Fig. 7-5). This advancement flap works especially well for repair of medium-sized defects on the upper lip near the alar base.[11] Island advancement flaps involve the isolation of a segment of skin as an island disconnected from the peripheral epidermal-dermal attachments. The only connection with the face, which is left intact, is through the underlying subcutaneous tissue. The geometric shape of the cutaneous island may vary but is usually triangular. As the flap advances toward the recipient site, the donor area is closed in a simple V to Y manner. The vascular supply for this flap is through its connection to the subcutaneous fat.[12]

The size of the flap should be approximately that of the primary defect. Incisions are made to create an island of skin shaped like the defect, which is attached to the underlying muscle by the vascularized subcuta-neous pedicle. Initial incisions around the perimeter of the flap are usually made to the level of the midsubcutaneous plane. After the flap is incised, undermining is gently performed around but *not* underneath the flap. Undermining beneath the flap itself will compromise the vascular supply. With the use of a skin hook, the flap is advanced into the defect (Fig. 7-5**B**). Up to one third of the advancing and trailing edges of the flap may be released from the subcutaneous pedicle depending on the vascular supply to the central portion of the pedicle.[7] This flap is most dependable in areas where the skin has an ample blood supply from the underlying muscle. An example of this is the upper lip, where the skin is adherent to the deep muscle. Undermining around the flap and edges of the defect helps prevent flap fullness or trapdoor deformity. The donor or secondary defect is closed in a V-Y manner, which effectively pushes the island advancement flap into the primary defect. The key suture is at the advancing edge of the flap. It is sometimes necessary to trim the leading edge of the triangular flap to better fit round surgical defects (Fig. 7-5**B**).

The island advancement flap offers several advantages when used to repair skin defects of the lateral upper lip near the base of the nasal ala.[11] The potential for skin color and texture are excellent as the flap originates entirely from the upper lip. If properly designed there should be no distortion of the cosmetic boundaries of the lip. All incision lines are confined to the esthetic unit of the upper lip and most can be well camouflaged by placing them in the boundary lines of the adjacent esthetic units. The advancing edge of the flap is often hidden in the junction of the upper lip and nasal sill. The lateral limb of the flap usually can be placed in the melolabial sulcus. In men this flap permits reconstruction of the mustache; the flap utilizes hair-bearing tissue of like quality with proper orientation of the facial hair. The island advancement flap can also be used for defects on the cheek and the nasal sidewall.[3,12] The major disadvantage of this flap is the potential for pincushioning of the flap but this is usually self-resolving and is minimized by proper undermining around the perimeter of the defect. The flap may be bulky if too much subdermal fat is left in place. It is important to avoid any damage to important anatomic structures during the development of the pedicle such as branches of the facial nerve.

O-T OR A-T FLAP (T-PLASTY)

The O-T or A-T wound repair is so named because it transforms a triangular (A-shaped) or round (O-shaped) defect into a final T-shaped scar. It represents a type of bilateral advancement flap. In essence, a

Figure 7-5   *A*, Incision of triangular subcutaneous island pedicle flap. *B*, Removal of small triangles of tissue to allow better fit of the flap into round defect. Skin hook is used to test advancement of flap. *C*, Secondary defect closed in V-Y fashion. *D*, Circular defect (3 × 3 cm) of upper lip after removal of skin cancer. Island pedicle advancement flap is outlined. The more peripheral marking represents the area undermined. *E*, Defect repaired with V-Y closure. *F*, Appearance 6 months postoperatively. (From Johnson TM, Nelson BR: Aesthetic reconstruction of skin cancer defects using flaps and grafts, *Am J Cosmetic Surg*, 9:256-257, 1992.)

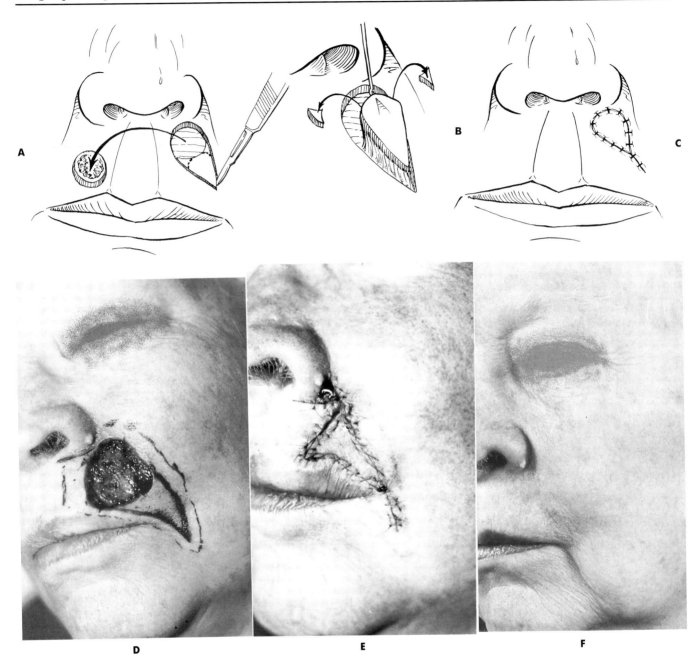

A   B   C

D   E   F

Figure 7-6   *A*, T-plasty designed for circular defect on upper lip near cutaneous vermilion junction. *B*, Final T closure, avoiding incisions onto vermilion. *C*, A 3 × 2.5 cm skin defect of upper lip. Lines mark proposed incisions for bilateral advancement flaps. *D*, Appearance 3 months after repair by T-plasty technique.

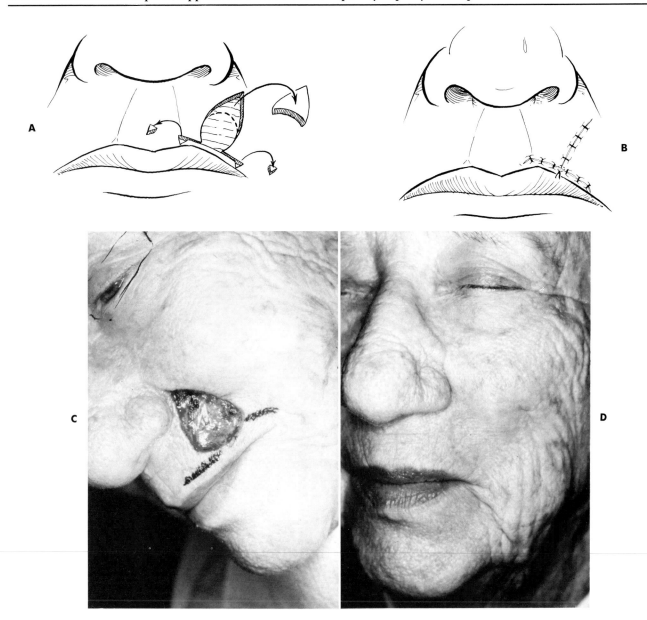

triangular defect is closed by advancing flaps in opposite directions from either side of the triangle (Figs. 7-6 and 7-7). An advantage of this reconstructive technique is the ability to essentially divide the defect in half by the use of two flaps for closure and to concomitantly place most incisions in natural lines, creases, or junctions of esthetic units. The T-plasty works very well on the central forehead when the vertical limb can be placed in the midline. The technique can also be used just above the eyebrow or the temple adjacent to the hairline, where the horizontal component of the T is placed along the eyebrow margin or in the hairline. Other excellent locations are the upper lip adjacent to the vermilion, the chin, and the preauricular and postauricular areas.[13]

The T-plasty is considered a reliable method of wound closure because the pedicles of the two flaps are generally large. A T-plasty can be used in the removal of skin lesions that are asymmetrical with one portion larger than another, thus resulting in a triangular defect. A triangular excision may conserve more tissue than a larger elliptical excision. Since natural crease

Figure 7-7 *A*, Schematic of O-T repair for circular defect above eyebrow. Wedges of tissue are removed from perimeter of circle. Superiorly, M-plasty helps to shorten vertical scar length. Burow's triangles are removed at end of horizontal limb of flaps. *B*, Half-buried horizontal mattress tip sutures. *C*, T closure with M-plasty, avoiding distortion of eyebrow.

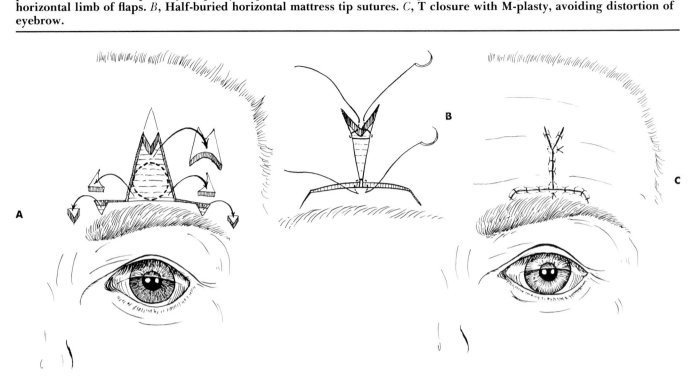

lines are usually used for much of the T-plasty repair, a large portion of the scar is generally imperceptible. However, the vertical limb of the scar, which by necessity is perpendicular to the horizontal component of the repair, can be more noticeable in certain parts of the face.

Figs. 7-6**A** and **B** demonstrate the use of the T-plasty repair for a defect adjacent to the vermilion cutaneous junction. A simple side-to-side closure would result in a large standing cutaneous deformity inferiorly, which would necessitate an incision into the vermilion. The use of a T-plasty repair eliminates this requirement and keeps all incision lines on the cutaneous portion of the upper lip. Incisions are made bilaterally along the vermilion margin at the base of the defect, thus creating the horizontal limbs of the flap. The superior border of the defect is extended in a fusiform manner by removal of a triangle of tissue, which converts the round defect into a triangular defect (Fig. 7-6A). Wide undermining is important to allow closure of the wound with less tension, thus minimizing the risk of distortion of the philtrum. A four-point suture is placed at the central base of the defect to precisely align the edges (Fig. 7-6**B**). Burow's triangles are removed only after the flaps have been advanced and secured. Schematically, small Burow's triangles are removed at the most medial and lateral aspects of the horizontal limbs of the flaps (Fig. 7-6A). At times, due to the

elasticity of the lip tissue, these small Burow's triangles can be efficiently sewn out and not require removal.[13]

Fig. 7-7**A** shows a typical round surgical defect above the left eyebrow, an area where the T-plasty repair works well. First it is helpful to mentally superimpose a triangle over the circular defect. In reality, the circle is converted to a triangle by removal of wedges of tissue at the perimeter of the circle at three points equally separated from each other (Fig. 7-7**A**). In Fig. 7-7**A** note that the superior wedge is in the form of an M-plasty, which helps to minimize the final length of the vertical limb of the scar. Undermining should be sufficient to allow minimal wound-closure tension. Two horizontal incisions are made perpendicular to the vertical limb in order to create the advancement flaps. These incisions may be varied in length and may curve allowing for proper placement in RSTLs, such as the horizontal crease lines of the forehead. The flaps are then elevated and advanced into the primary defect with the key suture being placed at the central advancing edge of the two flaps. It is preferred not to excise Burow's triangles until complete undermining is accomplished and the flaps are advanced into the primary defect. Burow's triangles are usually removed near the base of the flaps but in actuality can be removed from any area along the incision if it hides well into a RSTL (Fig. 7-7**A**). A four-point suture is used to attach the opposing distal tips of the two flaps to each other and to the adjacent skin (Fig. 7-7**B**). The tip of the M-plasty is closed with a similar half-buried horizontal mattress tip suture. Repair is completed by suturing of the flaps together by layered closure (Fig. 7-7**C**).

CASE EXAMPLES

The following case examples illustrate the successful use of advancement flaps.

CASE 1

A 56-year-old man underwent excision of a recurrent infiltrative basal cell carcinoma from the left

postauricular area with a two-stage Mohs micrographic procedure. The resultant defect was 4 × 3 cm and extended to the level of the deep subcutaneous tissue (Fig. 7-8**A**). Adjacent tissue movement was noted to be greatest in the superior and anterior directions. Therefore, a single-pedicle advancement flap was designed with this movement in mind. Parallel incisions were made along the diagrammed lines and extended for a distance of approximately 3 cm (Fig. 7-8**B**). The flap was carefully undermined in a subcutaneous plane and then advanced anteriorly and somewhat superiorly into the posterior sulcus of the ear. Deep closure was achieved by placement of 3-0 absorbable polyglactin (Vicryl) sutures in the subcutaneous tissue and dermis. The key suture was placed at the central aspect of the advancing edge of the flap. Standing cutaneous defor-

Figure 7-8   *A*, Postauricular skin defect measuring 4 × 3 cm. *B*, Diagrammed incision lines and Burow's triangles for single-pedicle advancement flap in postauricular area. *C*, Advancement flap sewn in place. A limited area of posterior aspect of earlobe was sutured to itself. *D*, Appearance 3 weeks postoperatively.

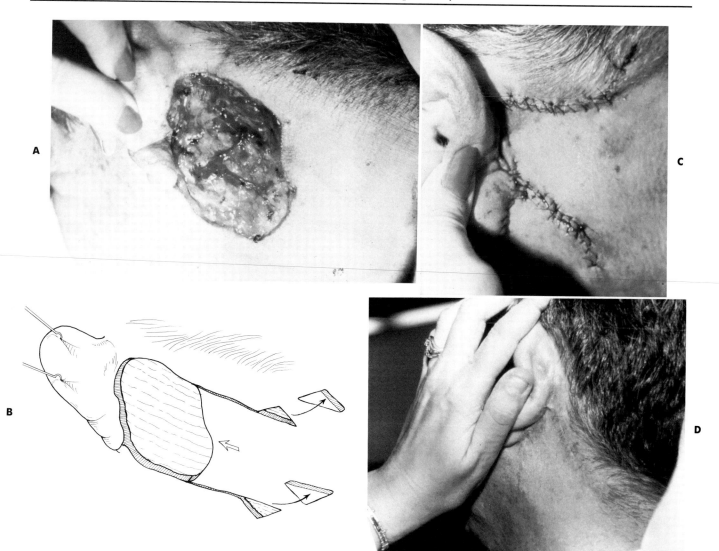

mities were excised at the base of the flap. The epidermis was carefully approximated with a simple running 5-0 polypropylene (Prolene) suture. Fig. 7-8**C** shows completion of the repair, and Fig. 7-8**D** shows follow-up at 3 weeks.

CASE 2

A 48-year-old woman was left with a 2.6 × 2.2 cm defect on the left forehead after Mohs surgery to remove a basal cell carcinoma (Fig. 7-9**A**). Attempts at a primary linear closure resulted in unacceptable wound-closure tension and excessive superior distortion of the eyebrow. It was decided to use bilateral advancement flaps (H-plasty) to prevent eyebrow distortion and maintain most of the scar lines in horizontal skin creases (Fig. 7-9**B**). The length and thus the surface area of the flaps were unequal. In this location there is usually more movement of the laterally based flap compared with the medial flap, and it is wise to first incise and elevate only the more mobile flap to determine if there is sufficient movement for closure before incision of the second flap. However, this patient did not exhibit as much skin laxity as is often found in the forehead skin of older patients, and both flaps were therefore required. Repair of the deep portions of the wound was accomplished with 5-0 absorbable polyglactin (Vicryl) sutures, and the epidermis was closed with simple interrupted 6-0 polypropylene (Prolene) sutures (Fig. 7-9**C**). The inferior incisions were well camouflaged in the upper eyebrow. Small standing cutaneous deformities were removed in

Figure 7-9 *A,* A 2.6 × 2.2 cm circular defect of forehead after removal of skin cancer. *B,* Diagram of H-plasty for forehead defect above left eyebrow. Burow's triangles are removed in superior lateral and inferior central location. *C,* Bilateral advancement flaps sewn in place, with good camouflage of inferior incision lines in eyebrow. *D,* Appearance 3 months postoperatively.

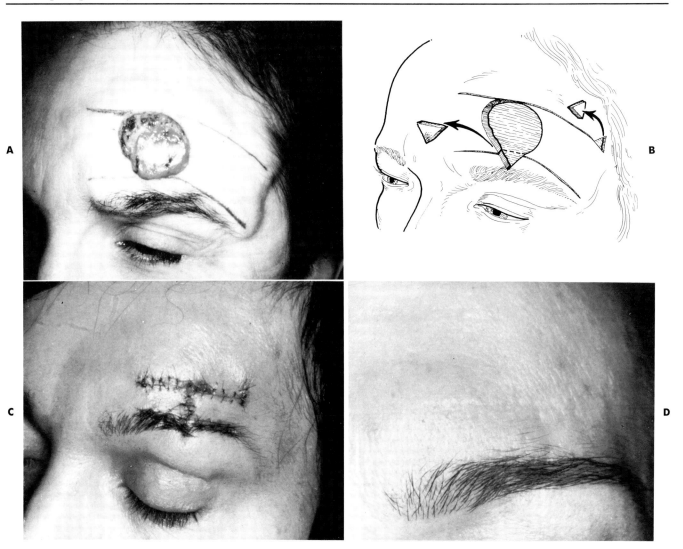

a superior lateral and inferior central location (similar to that in Fig. 7-3). Fig. 7-9 **D** shows excellent cosmesis at 3 months postoperatively. No scar dermabrasion was necessary.

CASE 3

A 65-year-old patient had a history of a recurrent squamous cell carcinoma, which was previously treated with electrodesiccation and curettage. Mohs surgery resulted in a relatively small (1-cm) but deep defect on the midhelical rim (Fig. 7-10**A**). Reconstructive options included an ear wedge or an advancement flap.[14] The latter was chosen because it has the advantage of allowing helical reconstruction without vertical shortening of the ear. Fig. 7-10**A** shows the advancement flap diagrammed with the base of the flap located inferiorly at the level of the earlobe. The incision was made full thickness through skin and cartilage along the helical crease (Fig. 7-10**B**). (A small Burow's triangle can be removed in the earlobe if necessary.) The key suture was placed at the advancing edge of the flap, which was gently held by forceps (Fig. 7-10**C**). Deep closure was achieved with 5-0 polyglactin (Vicryl) sutures placed through cartilage, which give excellent wound strength. Meticulous approximation of the skin of the helical rim was necessary to prevent any helical notching (Fig. 7-10**D**). Vertical mattress sutures of 6-0 polypropylene (Prolene) were used to prevent wound inversion (Fig. 7-10**D**). At suture removal 1 week after surgery, the helix had an excellent contour (Fig. 7-10**E**). There was slight venous engorgement of the distal flap, but this did not influence the final cosmetic result.

Figure 7-10   *A*, A 1-cm helical rim defect and diagrammed helical rim advancement flap. *B*, Helical rim advancement flap elevated to pedicle base at earlobe. *C*, Leading edge of flap advanced. *D*, Helical advancement flap sewn in place with 6-0 polypropylene (Prolene) sutures. Advancing edge approximation with vertical mattress sutures. *E*, Appearance 1 week postoperatively, after removal of sutures.

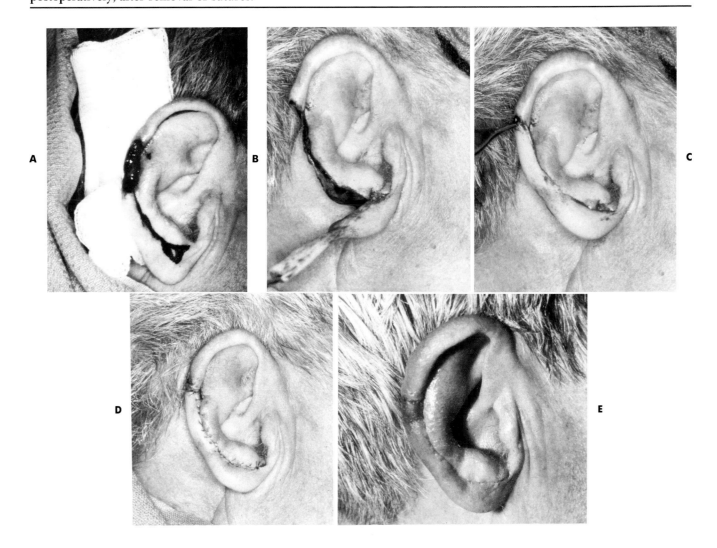

CASE 4

A 78-year-old woman with a twice-recurrent basal cell carcinoma underwent excision with the Mohs surgical technique, which resulted in a 3 × 2 cm defect that extended to the level of the periosteum. An H-plasty was considered but would involve more incisions and resultant scar lines than would a T-plasty. A T-plasty was selected because the vertical limb heals almost imperceptibly in the midline region of elderly individuals and the horizontal limbs are camouflaged nicely in the forehead horizontal crease lines. The horizontal limbs of the flaps were located superiorly, with the base of the flaps located laterally and inferiorly. The O-shaped surgical defect was converted to an A-shaped defect by removal of a wedge of tissue inferiorly, with the use of a W-plasty placed in the glabellar area (Figs. 7-11**A** and **B**). Incisions were made superiorly in a horizontal direction away from the defect, and the flap was carefully dissected to the pedicle base. Initially, wide undermining (1 to 2 cm) was performed to minimize tension on the repair. Undermining was performed just above the periosteum because the defect extended to the periosteum and was located centrally. Contraction of the flaps after this dissection will make the defect appear larger. Deep closure was achieved with placement of subcutaneous and dermal 4-0 absorbable polyglactin (Vicryl) sutures. Burow's triangles were excised laterally to remove standing cutaneous deformities. Epidermal approximation was with simple and vertical mattress 6-0 polypropylene (Prolene) sutures (Fig. 7-11**C**). Fig. 7-11**D** shows the forehead 1 month after reconstruction.

Figure 7-11   *A*, A 3 × 2 cm midforehead circular skin defect and diagrammed O-T repair with inferior vertical limb W-plasty. *B*, Diagram showing advancement flaps. Both flaps are based laterally. Burow's triangles are excised at base of both flaps. *C*, Closure of T-plasty, with removal of Burow's triangles laterally. *D*, Appearance 1 month postoperatively.

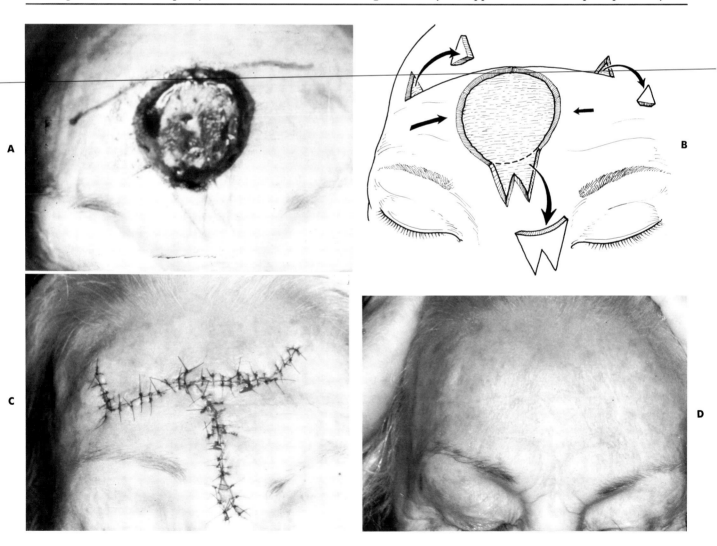

CASE 5

A 67-year-old woman had a 3 × 2 cm skin defect of the central forehead that was similar in size to that in case 4 (Fig. 7-12**A**). However, the defect was located at a more superior location in the central forehead. As in case 4, the defect was repaired with a T-plasty technique (Fig. 7-12**B**). Standing cutaneous deformities were removed laterally (Figs. 7-12**B** and **C**). Fig. 7-12**D** shows the results of reconstructive surgery 3 months later.

Figure 7-12   *A*, A 3 × 2 cm circular defect of central forehead. *B*, Diagram of T-plasty closure showing location of Burow's triangle excisions. *C*, Defect closed in two layers. Skin closure is achieved with simple running cutaneous suture. *D*, Appearance 3 months postoperatively.

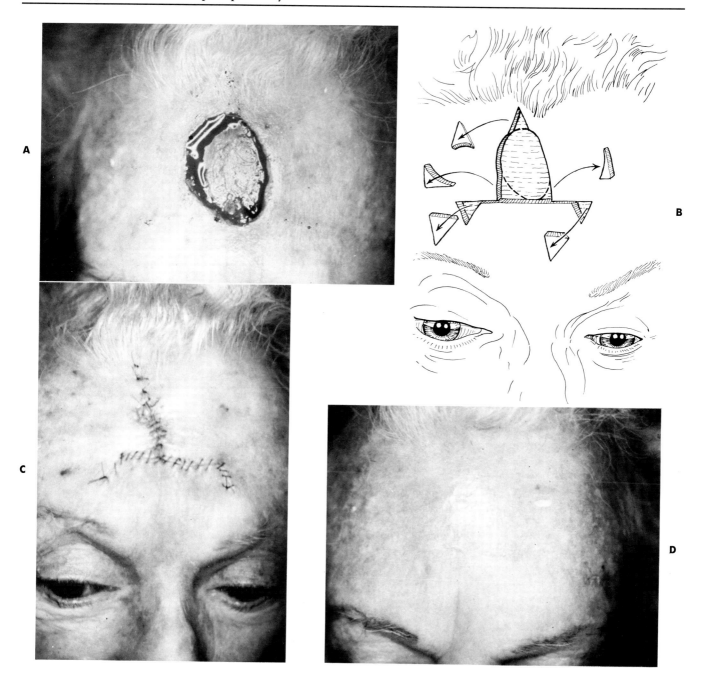

CASE 6

An 80-year-old woman had a poorly differentiated squamous cell carcinoma excised from the right cheek, with a resultant 3 × 2 cm defect. This defect, located on the medial cheek, was ideally suited for a cheek advancement flap. Fortunately, the defect did not extend onto the nasal sidewall, thus avoiding the risk of tenting as the flap crosses esthetic boundary lines (nasal-facial sulcus). In this elderly patient there was significant tissue laxity in the lateral cheek to allow for easy advancement of tissue with minimal wound-closure tension. Undermining was accomplished in a subcutaneous plane at the level of the defect. Incisions were then placed superiorly near the infraorbital crease and inferiorly parallel to the melolabial crease (Fig. 7-13**A**). Tissue movement was both medial and superior. It was important to prevent any tension on the eyelid, which could possibly result in an ectropion. Deep-wound closure was achieved with subcutaneous and dermal placement of 4-0 polyglactin (Vicryl) sutures (5-0 also can be used), and epidermal closure was completed with a simple running 6-0 polypropylene (Prolene) suture (Fig. 7-13**B**). Sutures were removed in 5 days. Fig. 7-13**C** shows good cosmesis at 1 month postoperatively.

SUMMARY

Advancement flaps are useful for repair of many types of cutaneous defects in various locations of the head and neck. Salient features concerning the use of advancement flaps are as follows:

1. An advancement flap is composed of a pushing, pulling, or sliding movement of incised tissue. A component of rotational movement often accompanies flap advancement.

2. A wound repair with an advancement flap consists of both primary and secondary tissue movement.

3. Complete undermining is important for both the advancement flap and surrounding tissue to allow adequate movement.

4. Excision of Burow's triangles allows for removal of standing cutaneous deformities as well as for facilitation of flap movement. Burow's triangles are best removed after the flap is secured over the primary defect.

5. The necessary length of an advancement flap depends on location and size of the defect and skin laxity. A 3 : 1 ratio of length to width is a common design.

Figure 7-13 *A*, A 3 × 2 cm medial cheek skin defect and diagrammed cheek advancement flap. *B*, Cheek flap sewn in place. *C*, Appearance 1 month postoperatively.

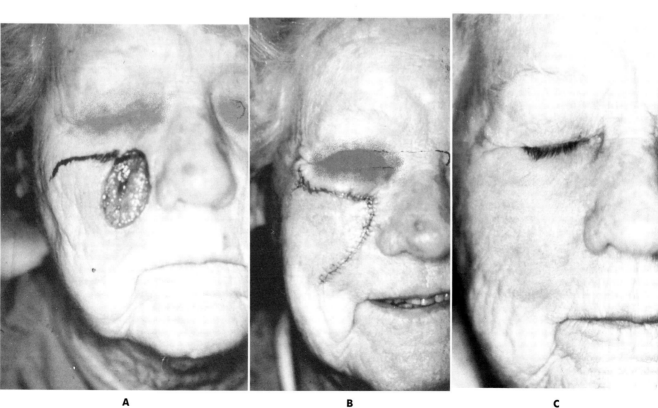

A   B   C

6. The key suture for wound repair is usually an absorbable suture placed through the dermis and subcutaneous tissue at the central aspect of the advancing edge of the flap.

REFERENCES

1. Swanson NA: *Atlas of cutaneous surgery*, Boston, 1987, Little Brown.

2. Tromovitch TA, Stegman SJ, Glogau RG: *Flaps and grafts in dermatologic surgery*, St. Louis, 1989, Mosby–Year Book.

3. Dzubow LM: Flap dynamics, *J Dermatol Surg Oncol* 17:116, 1991.

4. Mellette JR, Harington AC: Applications of the crescent advancement flap, *J Dermatol Surg Oncol* 17:447, 1991.

5. Juri J, Juri C: Cheek reconstruction with advancement-rotation flaps, *Clin Plast Surg* 8:223, 1981.

6. Dzubow LM: *Facial flaps: biomechanics and regional application*, Norwalk, Conn, 1990, Appleton & Lange.

7. Johnson TM, Nelson BR: Aesthetic reconstruction of skin cancer defects using flaps and grafts, *Am J Cosmetic Surg* 9:253, 1992.

8. Bennett, RG: Local skin flaps on the cheeks, *J Dermatol Surg Oncol* 17:161, 1991.

9. Salache SJ, Jarchow R, Feldman BD et al: The suspension suture, *J Dermatol Surg Oncol* 13:973, 1978.

10. Khan JA: Subcilial sliding skin muscle flap repair of anterior lamella lower eyelid defects, *J Dermatol Surg Oncol* 17:167, 1991.

11. Skouge JW: Upper lip repair: the subcutaneous island pedicle flap, *J Dermatol Surg Oncol* 16:63, 1990.

12. Tomich JM, Wentzell JM, Grande DJ: Subcutaneous island pedicle flaps, *Arch Dermatol* 123:514, 1987.

13. Salache SJ, Grabski WJ: *Flaps for the central face*, New York, 1990, Churchill Livingstone.

14. Antia NH, Buch VI: Chondrocutaneous advancement flaps for the marginal defect of the ear, *Plast Reconstr Surg* 39:472, 1967.

EDITORIAL COMMENTS

Shan R. Baker

Most local flaps used in the head and neck have some component of advancement during movement of the flap to the recipient site. An example is the median or perimedian forehead interpolation flap. Although they are pivotal flaps, frequently it is necessary to undermine the pedicle in the brow area to gain additional mobility and length for the flaps. Thus, the pedicle is advanced inferiorly below the bony orbital rim, adding some advancement to the main pivotal movement of the flaps. The rhombic flap is another example where both pivotal movement and advancement are important in transposition of the flap to the recipient site. Most rotation flaps are also facilitated by advancement of their point of pivot.

The T-plasty, discussed in this chapter, involves advancement of two flaps in opposite directions toward each other. The standing cutaneous deformity that occurs to some degree with all advancement flaps is excised at the vertical limb of the T. If the horizontal limbs of the T-plasty are curved, flap movement is not solely advancement but a combination of rotation (pivotal movement) and advancement. Advancement flaps are pure advancement flaps when they move in the direction of a single straight vector and have no pivotal movement. Primary wound closure is the simplest form of advancement in that skin is advanced toward the wound, but no additional incisions are made in the skin.

The author of this chapter discusses different uses and designs of advancement flaps for facial reconstruction. An important type that was not discussed is the V-Y advancement flap. This is a unique flap in that the V-shaped flap is not stretched toward the recipient site but achieves its advancement by recoil in that the flap is allowed to move into the recipient site without any wound-closure tension placed on the flap. The secondary triangular donor defect is then repaired with wound-closure tension by advancement of the two edges of the wound toward each other. In so doing, the wound-closure suture line assumes a Y configuration, and the vertical component of the Y represents the suture line that results from closure of the secondary defect.

V-Y advancement is useful in situations when a structure or region requires lengthening or release from a contracted state. The technique is particularly effective in lengthening the columella in the repair of cleft lip nasal deformities in which a portion or all of the columella is underdeveloped. A V-Y advancement flap is elevated by recruiting skin from the midportion of the lip between the filtral ridges. The length of the columella is augmented by advancement of the flap upward into the base of the columella (Fig. 7-14). The secondary donor defect is approximated by advancement of the remaining lip skin together in the midline. V-Y advancement is helpful in releasing contracted scars, which are distorting adjacent structures such as the eyelid or vermilion. An example is the correction of an ectropion of the vermilion caused by scarring. The segment of distorted vermilion is incorporated into the

Figure 7-14   V-Y advancement using central lip skin to augment vertical length of columella.

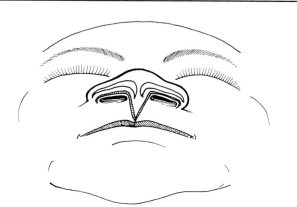

A

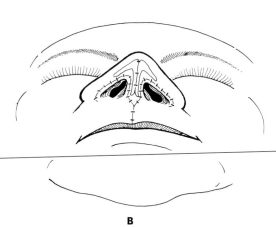

B

Figure 7-15   V-Y advancement to release ectropion of upper vermilion.

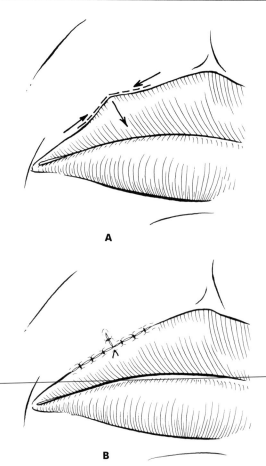

A

B

V-shaped flap and advanced toward the lip to restore the natural topography of the cutaneous vermilion junction. The lip skin adjacent to the secondary defect

is then advanced toward each other and sutured. This suture line becomes the vertical component of the Y configuration (Fig. 7-15).

EDITORIAL COMMENTS

Neil A. Swanson

The advancement flap is the most basic of the sliding flaps. As the author correctly indicates, there are relatively few pure advancement flaps, and many encompass both rotation and advancement in a sliding fashion.

Dr. Brown gives a lucid explanation of primary and secondary motion and its importance with an advancement flap. The secondary defect created by advancing (sliding) tissue to cover a primary defect is a wound of unequal lengths. This is surgically closed, usually by removal of a triangle of tissue, shortening the long arc

of wounds of unequal length created by the advancement of tissue. As Dr. Brown indicates, this is often removed as a displaced standing cutaneous cone. It can be removed anywhere on the long arc of the flap and can be visualized by means of displacement of a cutaneous cone from one position to another. The art in creation of these sliding flaps is learning how and where to place the Burow's triangle.

The author gives an excellent basic discussion of the criteria for performing an advancement flap. He discusses tension factors, placement of incisional lines, and where the secondary defect is created.

In advancement flaps, technically the key suture closes

the primary defect, as he aptly demonstrates. I prefer to square the edges of a defect to meet squared edges of an advancing flap instead of rounding the flap to meet the rounded edges of a circular defect. This results in better cosmetic result and less chance of "pooching" tissue. This is true with the advancement flap, better designed (Fig. 7-1**B**) as a squared-off suture line, and the island pedicle advancement flap, better designed as a squared-off advancing edge.

The discussion of the cheek advancement flap is particularly good. The concept of a tacking suture to remove tension and the gravitational impact of this flap is important. Equally important is the placement of the incision under the eyelid in the subciliary line.

The island pedicle advancement flap is another particularly useful flap. One technical point that I've found useful is that, after perpendicularly incising the skin into fatty tissue, the scalpel blade is angled outward (away from the pedicle) as I cut more deeply. This allows for a wider subcutaneous pedicle.

This chapter gives an excellent summary of different types of advancement (sliding) flaps, many of which are discussed during reconstruction of regional defects.

8

TRANSPOSITION FLAPS

David J. Leffell

INTRODUCTION

Transposition flaps provide a number of versatile reconstructive options. These flaps of tissue are harvested at one site and transferred to a site immediately adjacent to the base of the flap. This transfer is accomplished by moving the flap through an arc of rotation on a pivotal point located at the base of the flap's pedicle. Although transposition and rotation flaps are both pivotal flaps, they differ in that the axis of the transposition flap is linear whereas the axis of a rotation flap is curvilinear. This difference enables transposition flaps to be oriented so that wound-closure tension is reduced and the most favorable orientation of the scar results.[1] In effect, excess tissue is transposed from an area where it is abundant to an area where it is required for resurfacing purposes. The tension of wound closure resulting from the use of transposition flaps depends on the regional laxity of adjacent tissue.

A common variant of the transposition flap is the rhombic flap. Although the primary movement of the rhombic flap is transposition about a pivotal point, the flap also is advanced toward the defect that it is resurfacing. Other varied transposition flaps frequently used in the reconstruction of facial defects include the banner,[2] bilobed flap,[3] bilateral rhomboid flap,[4] and 30° modification of the rhombic flap.[5]

The geometry of the transposition flap is important to understand, but precise angle measurement is not critical to success. Too much intrinsic variation in movement of adjacent secondary tissue exists to predicate flap design on a strict interpretation of flap angles or the absolute geometry of the defect to be repaired by the flap. Regional differences in tissue mobility have greater impact on flap design than does geometry. For example, it may not be possible to design the perfect rhombic flap on the temple near the hairline, where tissue mobility is not great, despite the proper geometric design. In fact, the most important element in the design of transposition flaps is establishment of the location of the pivot point.[6] The flap must be designed in such a way that, when transposed into the defect, there is minimal tension across the flap, so that strangulation does not occur and the defect is repaired without excess wound-closure tension or distortion of adjacent structures.

ADVANTAGES

An important advantage of transposition flaps is the ability to design the flap in the appropriate orientation so that wound-closure tension and the resulting scars provide maximum preservation of function and cosmesis.[7] An example is the design of a rhombic flap in the periorbital region, which, if done properly, will minimize the risk of developing an ectropion that might have resulted from another type of adjacent tissue transfer. Another advantage of transposition flaps is the ability to repair large defects by the use of multiple flaps. An example is the use of several rhombic flaps to correct a defect of the central scalp.[8] The surface area of the defect can be divided by the number of flaps harvested, with each flap contributing to the closure of the defect. Likewise the surface area of the secondary donor defect is divided by the number of flaps transferred. Due to the inelasticity of the scalp, it is technically easier to repair several smaller defects of the donor site than to close a single large secondary defect.

DISADVANTAGES

Disadvantages of transposition flaps include risk of necrosis and the development of a trapdoor deformity.[9] In general, flap necrosis in the head and neck region is not a serious complication. It results from poor design of the flap in which an inadequate base has been provided; injury to the base of the flap during flap elevation; or factors related to the patient, such as impaired skin vascularity because of smoking or diabetes. Flaps smaller than 5 cm^2, such as the kind one would construct on the nose, rarely suffer necrosis of more than the peripheral tip. The earliest sign of this is pallor or even duskiness in the first 24 hours after surgery. The patient should be advised of this evolving complication and told that it is not serious. I tell patients that they might develop a small scab, which they should leave alone (debriding is contraindicated), and that the wound will heal from beneath the scab. The final appearance of the reconstructed area, usually apparent by 2 months, varies from excellent in patients with a ruddy complexion whose adjacent blood supply has probably salvaged some of the vascular compromised tip, to poor in patients with thick sebaceous skin of the nose. When poor results do occur, dermabrasion is helpful to improve the final result.

Trapdoor deformity is a complication that can be observed with transposition flaps.[8,9] The deformity is one in which the flap appears bulky, protruding from the surrounding skin and giving the appearance of a pincushion. This complication tends to occur a few weeks following transfer. It may develop because adjacent tissue surrounding the recipient site is not sufficiently undermined at the time of flap transposition. The "plate" of scar tissue, which forms between the undersurface of the flap and the floor of the defect, contracts relative to the flap itself. Contraction of this scar beneath the flap causes the flap to bulge upward. In addition, loss of contact inhibition during scar production may promote excessive scar tissue. Suturing of the flap to the base of the defect in a way that does not compromise the vascularity of the flap may minimize trapdoor deformity. Fortunately trapdoor deformity usually resolves with time. Resolution also is assisted by the use of intralesional triamcinolone (Kenalog), 40 mg/ml, injected in small amounts (0.1 ml) every 4 to 6 weeks. Similarly, if after 8 months the deformity has not resolved, a frequently successful solution is scar revision—achieved by entry through a portion of the present scar to debulk the flap and free surrounding tissue.

Transposition flaps are so versatile that there is virtually no situation in which they would not be a reconstructive option. However, the location and size of a defect dictate the preferred repair. That is, for a defect of a given size, a transposition flap may be preferable to primary closure or the use of other types of flaps. Defects of the glabellar area are especially amenable to repair by transposition flaps. Although defects in this region often can be closed primarily, primary closure may result in the loss of the glabellar crease, distortion of the medial brow, or the development of a depression over the nasion, thus warranting the use of a transposition flap. A banner or transposi-

tion flap harvested from the centrally located forehead skin will permit closure with the donor site scar camouflaged in natural vertical forehead furrows. However, it is important to be aware of the potential mismatch of the thick sebaceous forehead skin and the thinner skin of the glabella, upper nose, and medial canthi.

Another common location where transposition flaps are especially helpful in repair of facial defects is the temple region. In this anatomic subunit a linear closure, although technically possible, might result in distortion of the lateral brow or webbing of the lateral canthus. Transposition flaps are especially helpful in reconstruction of the lower third of the nose. Options in designing such flaps range from melolabial flaps, which work well for reconstruction of the ala, to transposition flaps (of various designs) harvested from other locations on the medial cheek. Skin of the nasal tip is difficult to match by grafting or by flap repair with the use of cheek skin. The problem in the reconstruction of nasal tip defects can often be resolved with a bilobe transposition flap. This flap takes advantage of the laxity of the skin on the superior lateral aspect of the nose and in effect permits movement of this relatively more relaxed skin into the nasal tip defect.

SURGICAL TECHNIQUE

It is important to discuss the various reconstructive options with the patient. Smokers, for example, have a greater risk of flap failure because of vascular compromise and should be advised of this. In the selection of a reconstructive flap, it is important to think of alternative approaches should the preferred flap not be possible because of the quality or quantity of tissue available. Maintain an open mind. Success in reconstruction depends on creativity. If, after you prepare the site for reconstruction, your original plan proves inadequate, proceed to the next option.

The patient should be seated during evaluation, especially if the repair is to occur near the eye. With the patient facing forward and the head placed in the Frankfort plane, ask the patient to show his or her teeth or to smile so that relaxed skin tension lines (RSTLs) can be determined. Observe the natural tendency of the wound to close and what effect movement of adjacent tissues has on the borders of the wound. Next diagram the intended flap with the use of an indelible felt marker (which is more convenient than marking dyes, which can sometimes spill). If a rhombic flap is being considered for repair of a circular wound, use a dashed line to denote the skin adjacent to the wound, which will require excision to accommodate the geometric form of the flap. This does not mandate excision before elevation of the rhombic flap, but the markings do maintain landmarks after some distortion following infiltration of the local anesthetic.

The patient is prepared and draped for surgery in the usual fashion. When possible, do not prepare with the antimicrobial skin cleanser Hibiclens and certainly not in the periorbital region because Hibiclens can cause keratitis if it comes in contact with the eye.[10] The skin cleanser pHisoDerm is a safe, excellent alternative. Most facial transposition flaps can be completed within 45 minutes. For this reason, lidocaine is sufficient for anesthesia. A balance must be achieved between the benefit of hemostasis due to the use of epinephrine and the disadvantage of postoperative bleeding, which occasionally occurs once the effect of the epinephrine wears off. This compounds the bleeding that occasionally can occur when a vessel, even in the absence of epinephrine, emerges from spasm. I prefer to use epinephrine and believe the benefits outweigh the disadvantages. Bleeding due to loss of the vasoconstrictive effect of epinephrine, in my experience, occurs primarily in the region of the lateral cheek when dissection has occurred in the high subcutis. Lacerated blood vessels perforating through the fat can often be missed in this area during development of the flap. Control of bleeding is best accomplished by following the simple rule of "visualize and cauterize." There is no alternative to meticulous hemostasis.

I prefer to undermine the flap and surrounding skin with the use of blunt (Mayo) scissors and handle the wound edges exclusively with single pronged hooks. This minimizes trauma to the wound edges, upon which the cosmetic result ultimately depends. In most cases, undermining should be performed just beneath the dermis, in the high subcutis. The danger zones of the temple must be respected. During dissection in the region of the zygomatic arch, it is important to remember that the temporal and eye branches of the facial nerve are superficial and thus prone to injury.[11]

In the temple region, flap undermining often results in an encounter with branches of the temporal artery. Anticipate this and have hemostats ready. Any transected vessel larger than 2 mm in diameter should be tied using 3-0 polyglactin (Vicryl) sutures because electrocautery of larger vessels often leads to delayed bleeding when clots dislodge. After the wound has been undermined to allow the desired tissue movement and before the flap is incised, simulate the tension that will be imposed on the donor site with the use of skin hooks. Evaluate whether there may be unexpected distortion of adjacent tissue structures such as eyelids. Mentally recapitulate what tissue is to be transposed and make a rough assessment of whether a smaller or shorter flap will suffice. If so, redesign the flap, but remember that a flap designed too long can always be

shortened after transposition. In general the length of the flap should be no longer than three times the width of the base. This ratio may vary depending on skin type, location of the flap, and depth of undermining. When developing a flap from sebaceous nasal skin, where the dermis is very thick and thus requires increased blood supply, use the broadest based flap possible. In contrast, flaps developed on the cheek or on the temple, where there is excellent skin vascularity, may exceed the standard 3:1 ratio of length to width.

After the flap has been incised, the secondary donor defect should be approximated with 4-0 or 5-0 polyglactin (Vicryl) sutures placed in the deeper layers of the wound. The approximation should be sufficient so that epidermal sutures are not necessarily required. Next transpose the flap into the defect, being certain to handle it as little as possible and then only with skin hooks. Careless handling of the flap after elevation may lead to necrosis by violating the blood supply at the base, on which the flap is solely dependent. The flap should then be positioned and secured with buried dermal sutures. Only the minimum number of sutures to secure the flap should be used. The possibility of tissue strangulation from the use of an excessive number of sutures should be a concern. The epidermal surface of the flap can be sutured with 5-0 or 6-0 nylon or other monofilament synthetic suture material such as polypropylene (Prolene). Unless perfect approximation of the edges of the epidermis is possible, a running suture should not be used. Interrupted sutures, especially when flaps located in the region of the nose and melolabial fold are sutured, are able to even wound edges that might not have been accomplished with deep sutures.

The blood supply to most transposition flaps of the face is random, which means the more distal portions of the flap are nourished by the dermal and subdermal plexuses. Historically there has been a hesitancy to trim transposition flaps of subcutaneous fat for fear that the blood supply to the flap would be compromised. Although there is some validity to this concern, it is usually safe to eliminate excessive fat with a scissors. Observe the wound edge for dermal bleeding. Remember that if epinephrine was used with the local anesthesia it may be several hours before the true vascularity of the flap can be assessed. After transposition of the flap, the tip may well look white and even be cool to touch when compared with the surrounding tissue. These ominous changes are usually due to the vasoconstrictive effects of epinephrine and the vasoconstrictive shock that results from flap elevation itself.

After reconstruction the flap is cleaned with peroxide, and a thin film of antibiotic salve is applied. A nonadherent (for example, Telfa) dressing is covered by gauze and secured with plastic tape to provide maximal compression of the repair during the first 24 hours. If the flap is on the forehead, the compression dressing may be reinforced with elasticized compression bandage or an easy-to-obtain custom, elastic bandage. This minimizes postoperative edema and the risk of bleeding and protects the flap from inadvertent trauma. Elastic compression dressings should not be applied too tightly over a bony prominence because the vascularity of the skin may be compromised. For flaps on the nose a temporary nasal plug that consists of cotton coated with petrolatum will provide some intranasal compression, although this is uncomfortable to most patients.

The patient should return in 24 hours for bandage change if needed, evaluation for the possibility of hematoma, assessment of the condition of the flap, and review of instructions for wound care. On the face, sutures are removed no later than 5 days unless the patient schedule does not permit. I have observed no suture marks when sutures remain in place 7 days except on the lip, where they occasionally occur even if sutures are removed after 3 days. This may occur because of the constant tension on the wound produced by movement of the lip.

CASE EXAMPLES

CASE 1: 30° TRANSPOSITION FLAP

A 67-year-old man had a 1 × 1.1 cm skin defect on the tip of the nose after Mohs surgical excision of a basal cell carcinoma (Fig. 8-1**A**). The skin was sebaceous, and almost any adjacent tissue transfer in this area was at risk for distorting the nasal tip. However, careful evaluation of the nasal tip and adjacent alar esthetic units indicated that the broad nasal tip and ala might allow for lateral movement of skin. This suggested that a transposition flap from the skin of the lateral nasal tip might be sufficient to close the wound. By creating an acute angle to the flap it is possible, assuming enough lateral skin laxity, to close the defect without much vertical distortion of the nasal tip. The 30° angle transposition flap was designed with its base located at the left lateral aspect of the wound just inferior to the midpoint (Fig. 8-1**B**). The base of the flap was narrower than that used in a conventional rhombic flap, thus placing flap survival somewhat at risk. The standing cutaneous deformity, which was anticipated at the inferior pole of the defect, was excised in a triangular fashion, extending the excision under the nasal tip, where the resulting scar was less visible (Fig. 8-1**C**). (It is extremely important to undermine widely on the nose to avoid a trapdoor deformity.

Of special concern is when broad undermining extends into the region of the angular arteries. These vessels can bleed profusely, and under the thick immobile skin of the nose they may be difficult to identify to obtain hemostasis if injured.)

In Fig. 8-1**C** and **D**, the flap has been sutured in place with 4-0 deep dermal polyglactin (Vicryl) sutures and 5-0 polypropylene (Prolene) simple sutures. Note that the direction of wound-closure tension is upward from the left nostril (Fig. 8-1**D**). However, because of the thickness of the nasal skin in this patient, the ala was minimally elevated. The nasal tip maintained its contour. (A three-point tip suture may be used at the superior aspect of the flap.)

Owing to the sebaceous nature of the skin of the nasal tip, the wound healed well but with a noticeable scar line (Fig. 8-1**E**). There was no trapdoor deformity, but a depressed scar was visible. Excellent camouflage of the scar was accomplished by a single dermabrasion 2 months after flap transfer. (Dermabrasion can be performed as early as 4 to 6 weeks postoperatively and repeated 4 weeks later. Dermabrasion of sebaceous skin must be performed with a refrigerant such as Frigiderm, and hemostasis after dermabrasion is accomplished with the use of aluminum chloride or ferric chloride. The resulting wound is cleaned daily and covered with polysporin B-bacitracin [Polysporin] ointment and a nonadherent [Telfa] dressing for 5 to 7 days.) Fig. 8-1 **F** shows the patient's nose 3 months after initial reconstruction.

Figure 8-1 *A*, **A 67-year-old man with 1 × 1.3 cm skin defect of tip of nose after Mohs surgical excision of basal cell carcinoma.**

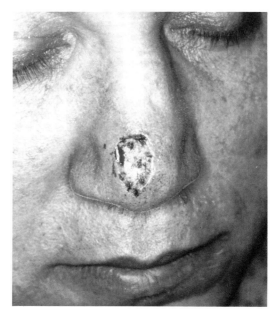

A

Figure 8-1, cont'd.   *B*, A 30° transposition flap is selected because broad nasal tip provides sufficient skin laterally for reconstruction. Inferior pedicle of flap assists lymphatic drainage. Standing cutaneous deformity is excised inferiorly. *C*, Flap sutured in place after wide undermining, which is important when the surgeon works with sebaceous skin to help reduce the risk for a trapdoor deformity. *D*, Drawing highlights slight elevation of left nasal alar rim, which resulted from flap transposition. This elevation, also noted in Fig. 8-1C, rapidly resolves, but patients should be advised of possible temporary nasal deformity. *E*, Repair is shown 6 weeks postoperatively. Uneven scar is noted, and there is even a suggestion of puckering seen in early trapdoor deformity. Scar dermabrasion was performed at this time. *F*, Results of reconstruction 3 months postoperatively demonstrating beneficial effect of dermabrasion with resolution of uneven scar line.

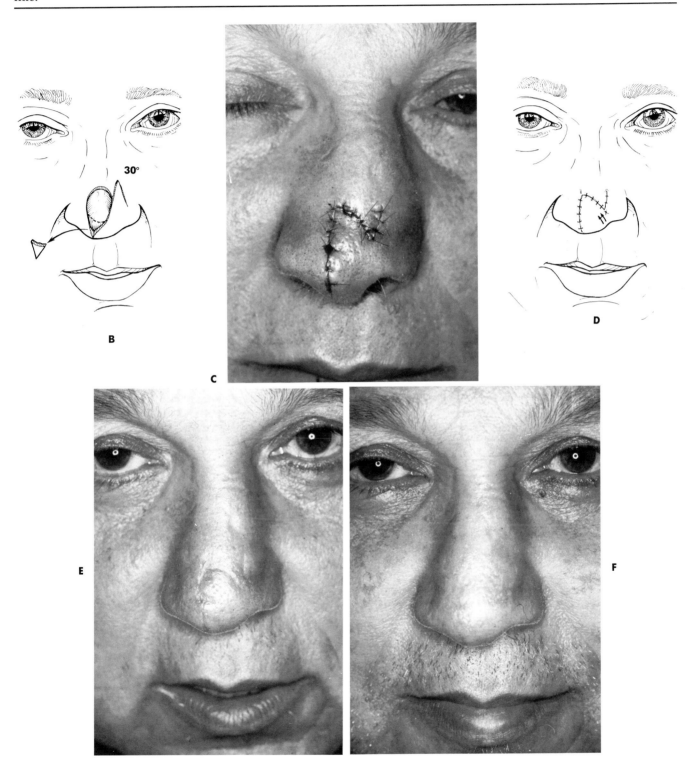

CASE 2: MODIFIED RHOMBIC FLAP

A 73-year-old man presented with a 1.8 × 1.5 cm skin defect of the medial cheek after Mohs surgery for removal of a keratotic basal cell carcinoma (Fig. 8-2A). Options that were considered for repair of this defect included a cheek advancement flap, which would have resulted in a relatively linear scar extending from below the medial canthus into the melolabial fold adjacent to the lip; a rotation flap from the lateral cheek; a rhombic transposition flap; or a variant of a rhombic flap. A modified rhombic flap was selected because of the location of the defect (on the border of three esthetic subunits: the lateral nasal wall, ala, and cheek) and concern about causing eyelid retraction in a patient who already had senile laxity of the lower lid (Fig. 8-2B). The shape of the defect, after undermining, indicated that it could be modified to accommodate a variant of a rhombic flap.

By designing the flap such that the anterior border was located in the melolabial groove and by excising minimal additional skin at the lateral and medial edges of the defect to accommodate the configuration of the flap (Fig. 8-2C), it was possible to keep the length of the final scar short, hide most of the scar deep in the melolabial sulcus, and minimize risk of distortion of the eyelid. A similar flap designed on the contralateral aspect of the defect would have resulted in downward pull on the eye and the possible development of an ectropion. As initially designed, wound-closure tension was directed horizontally from the lateral cheek across the alar-facial sulcus (Fig. 8-2C).

After flap transposition (Fig. 8-2D and E), a standing cutaneous deformity was removed laterally. No distortion of the eyelid was noted. Conversely a cheek advancement flap in this area might have put undue tension, although lateral, on the lower eyelid, and the resulting lymphedema may have resulted in protracted swelling.

Minor hypertrophic scarring was noted at the lateral aspect of the flap but resolved within 3 months (Fig. 8-2F). (Massage and occasionally triamcinolone (Kenalog) injections are helpful in hastening resolution of such scarring.)

Figure 8-2 *A,* A 73-year-old man with 1.1 × 1.3 cm skin defect of right cheek. *B,* Inferior transposition flap is designed, and surrounding tissue is undermined at level of subcutis. Angular artery is located medially, and care should be taken not to lacerate it. *C,* Modified rhombic flap is designed, taking advantage of the proximity of defect to melolabial fold. Inferior aspect of flap is then positioned in defect so that it parallels lateral border of nasal esthetic unit. Transposition of flap is facilitated by excision of tissue adjacent to defect medially and laterally to better approximate rhombic shape of flap. Dotted line indicates area of skin undermining; *arrows,* wound-closure tension vectors. *D,* Flap sutured in place. Lower suture line is concealed along alar base and superior aspect curves along superior border of ala itself. *E,* Standing cutaneous deformity is removed at lateral aspect of repair. Note use of Gilles tip suture at medial aspect of flap. *F,* Result is shown 3 months postoperatively. Melolabial fold is not blunted, as might have been the case with more broadly based cheek advancement flap. Scar is well camouflaged in the alar-facial sulcus.

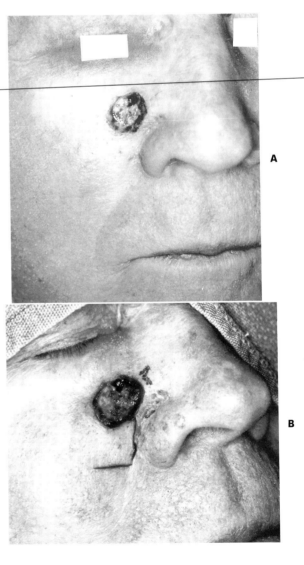

Figure 8-2, cont'd. For legend see opposite page.

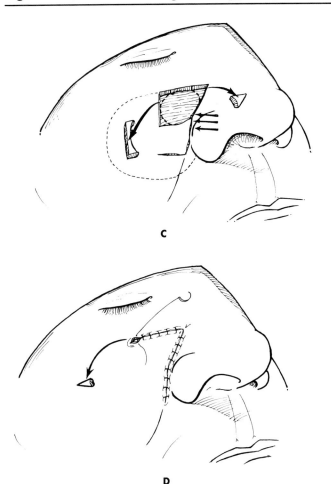

C

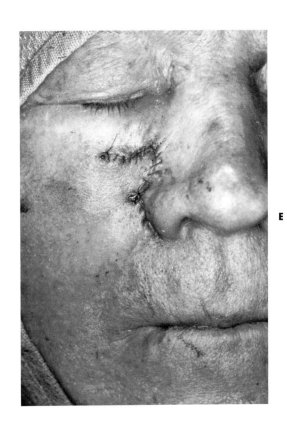

E

D

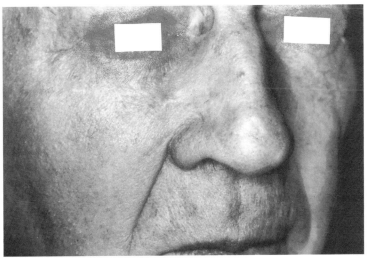

F

CASE 3: BILATERAL TRANSPOSITION FLAPS

A 70-year-old man had a 2 × 3 cm defect of the central nasal skin after excision of a basal cell carcinoma (Fig. 8-3**A**). A full-thickness skin graft, although functional, would not have been cosmetically acceptable because it would have been a poor match with the patient's severely sun-damaged nasal skin. A forehead flap was another option considered but would not repair the defect with skin of similar color and texture to that which was removed. Although a forehead flap is excellent for large defects of the nose in which a substantial amount of nasal tissue has been removed, in this defect only minimal subcutis was resected. A large unilateral melolabial transposition or interpolation flap was another reconstructive option, but transfer of the flap would be technically difficult because of the central location of the defect. As a consequence of these considerations, 30° transposition flaps were selected for reconstruction because of the relative abundance and mobility of lateral nasal skin and the superior color and texture match this skin would provide.

The two flaps were designed to extend superiorly up onto the lateral aspects of the nose and still remain within a single esthetic unit (Fig. 8-3**B** and **C**). Wide undermining of nasal skin was essential before the flaps were transposed. As is best in such cases, the secondary defects were first closed with 4-0 deep dermal polyglactin (Vicryl) sutures. Next the superior flap tips were sutured in place with a deep Vicryl suture passed through the dermis of both the flap tip and the superior edge of the defect (Gilles flap tip suture, Fig. 8-3**B**). (This is a horizontal mattress skin suture that passes through the dermis of the tip of the flap and exits through the skin of the recipient site.) The remainder of the wound was then closed in layers with 4-0 Vicryl sutures for the dermal layer and 5-0 polypropylene (Prolene) sutures for the epidermal layer (Fig. 8-3**C** and **D**). (If adequate approximation of the epidermis is obtained with dermal sutures, sterile bandages (Steristrips) can be used without the need for the Prolene sutures.) After suturing of the flaps, residual redundant skin at the base of the flaps was excised (Fig. 8-3**C**). Note how the central suture line extends under the tip of the nose for additional scar camouflage (Fig. 8-3**E**).

Fig. 8-3**F** shows the wound-closure tension vectors directed primarily from the lateral cheek and to a lesser degree from the superior edge of the nostril. The elevation that resulted from the latter forces temporarily created a bulging appearance to the nostril. However, this resolved with time, largely because of the persistent downward forces exerted by the cartilaginous structures within the nose which directly underlie the region of the flap. The results of reconstruction 6 months postoperatively are shown in Fig. 8-3**G** and **H**. (The success of this approach relies primarily on the laxity of the lateral nasal skin frequently observed in elderly patients. A similarly sized skin defect in a younger patient will prove to be more difficult to repair using this approach without untoward secondary deformity.)

Figure 8-3 *A*, **A 70-year-old man with 2 × 2.4 cm nasal skin defect encompassing most of lower dorsum of nose that resulted from resection of nodular basal cell carcinoma. Thorough evaluation of wound indicated only a deficiency of epidermis, dermis, and a small amount of subcutis.** *B*, **Bilateral transposition flaps are designed to take advantage of relaxed skin on lateral aspects of nose.** *C*, **Following wide undermining both flaps are approximated with three-point tip suture. Inferiorly triangle of skin is excised in anticipation of a standing cutaneous deformity. Gilles tip sutures permit even approximation of all flap tips.** *D*, **Simple interrupted sutures are used to evenly distribute wound-closure tension along edges of wound. Blanching of superior tips of flaps is related to vasoconstrictive effect of epinephrine and is not a sign of permanent vascular compromise.** *E*, **Constriction of lower part of nose from reconstruction creates a slight supratip depression and elevation of the alar margins (on profile view). These deformities are temporary and will resolve in time due to forces exerted by cartilaginous structures, natural tissue creep, and effects of gravity.** *F*, **Drawing highlights lateral vectors of force exerted on nasal tip and distortion of alar margin.** *G* and *H*, **Result of reconstruction at 6 months postoperatively. Alar margins and nasal tip once again have normal contour. Ridging of nasal bridge in area of rhinion is due to patient wearing glasses. Success of this approach relies primarily on the profound laxity of skin frequently observed in elderly patients.**

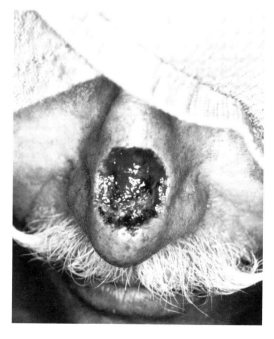

A

Figure 8-3, cont'd.   For legend see opposite page.

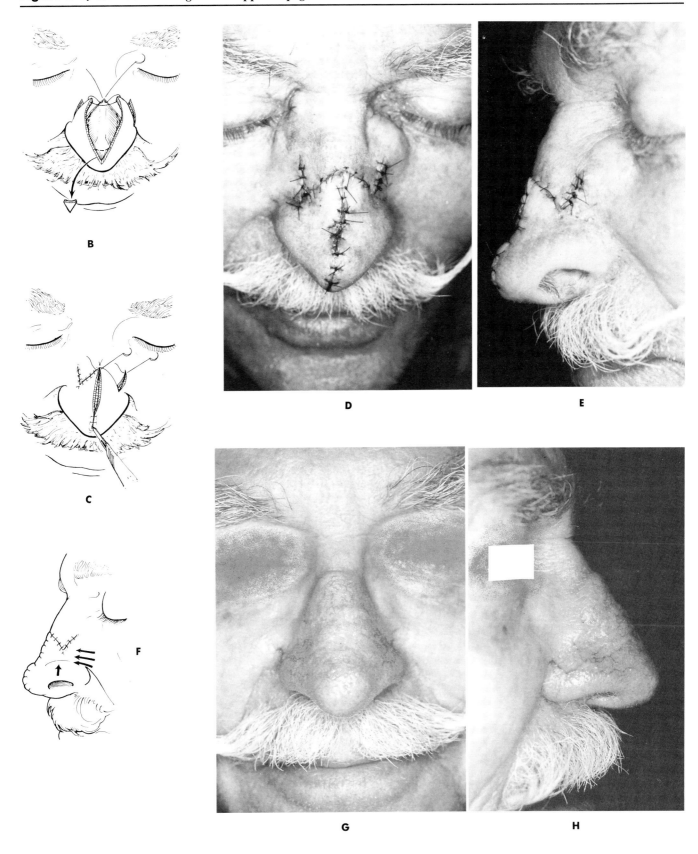

B

C

F

D

E

G

H

CASE 4: BILATERAL RHOMBIC FLAPS

A 45-year-old woman had a 3 × 3 cm skin defect of the chin after excision of a deeply invasive microcystic adnexal carcinoma (Fig. 8-4**A**). A full-thickness skin graft was considered to resurface the defect, but it has the disadvantage of a poor color and texture match with the adjacent cheek skin. In addition, wrinkling of the graft can be a problem from constant movement of the chin from speech and chewing. Hypertrophic scarring on the chin was also a concern because of this movement, and there is a greater risk of this occurring with use of a skin graft. Other reconstructive options included bilateral rotation flaps; submental advancement flap, which would involve extensive dissection of anterior neck skin; or bilateral rhombic flaps. The latter option was selected because it permitted less skin undermining than the use of an advancement flap and promised to maintain the architecture of the mental sulcus. In addition, because the forces of wound-closure tension after repair are lateral, there is less risk of distortion of the lip.

Unlike the bilateral 30° transposition flaps used in case 3, conventional 60° rhombic flaps were designed so as not to interfere with the patient's natural mental sulcus (Fig. 8-4**B**). (Wide undermining of the skin, with meticulous attention to hemostasis, is necessary on the chin. Undermining is accomplished at the level of the muscular fascia, and any branches of the labial arteries must be identified and cauterized if transected during dissection.)

After transposition, the flaps were secured with a 4-0 polyglactin (Vicryl) three-point tip suture at the superior and inferior aspects of the flaps (Fig. 8-4**C** and **D**). Note that the design of these flaps permitted removal of the standing cutaneous deformity at the inferior aspect of the defect in the midline without narrowing the base of either flap.

Final wound closure usually is accomplished with single interrupted cutaneous 5-0 or 6-0 polypropylene (Prolene) sutures. Alternatively, provided that approximation with deep dermal Vicryl sutures was excellent (Fig. 8-4**E**), sterile bandages (Steri-strips) alone are sufficient (Fig. 8-4**F**). (These bandages have the advantage of minimizing the chance of permanent skin suture marks.) Fig. 8-4**G** shows the early postoperative results 3 weeks after repair.

Figure 8-4   *A,* A 45-year-old woman with 3 × 3 cm skin defect of chin following Mohs surgical excision of microcystic adnexal carcinoma. *B,* Bilateral rhombic flaps are designed on either side of defect so that each flap will resurface approximately half of wound. *C,* Flaps have been incised and transposed, and adjacent tissue is undermined widely. *D,* Flaps are approximated with deep dermal polyglactin (Vicryl) sutures. Similar sutures can be used to secure tips of flaps. *E,* Wound is completely closed with deep sutures. Where there is considerable skin movement, as on the chin, risk of skin suture marks is greater; therefore, use of only deep sutures is likely to yield improved results. *F,* Sterile bandages (Steri-Strips) are placed to secure incision lines. Patient is instructed to remove them in 5 days. In perioral region when Steri-strips are allowed to remain in place too long, the possibility of moisture collecting along suture line may result in *Candida albicans* skin infection. *G,* Photograph of chin 3 weeks postoperatively. Extrusion of deep suture is seen. Massage of wound beginning 3 to 4 weeks postoperatively may be helpful in retarding or preventing development of hypertrophic scarring, which can be problematic with chin incisions.

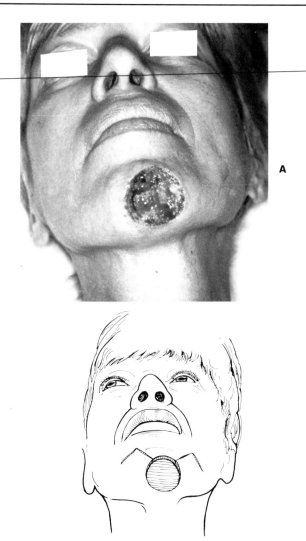

A

B

Figure 8-4, cont'd.   For legend see opposite page.

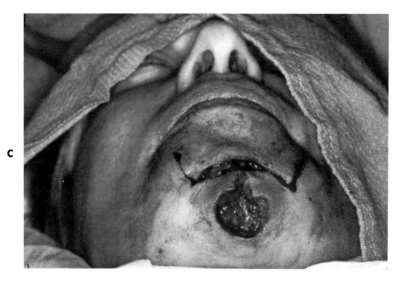

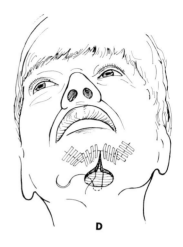

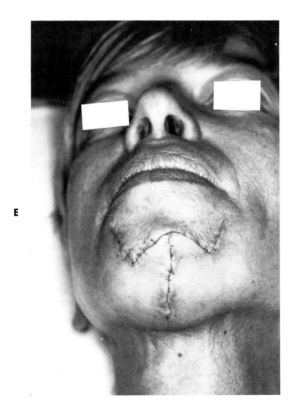

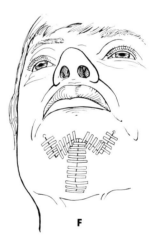

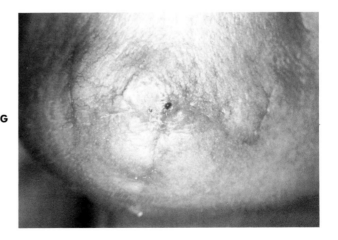

CASE 5: COMBINATION TRANSPOSITION FLAPS

An 85-year-old mentally compromised patient at a nursing home had a 3.5 × 1.8 cm skin defect involving the alar margin, nasal tip, and part of the cheek after resection of a neglected basal cell carcinoma with morpheaform features (Fig. 8-5**A**). The defect involved two nasal esthetic subunits (Fig. 8-5**B**). Although this patient's defect could have been adequately resurfaced with a full-thickness skin graft, adjacent tissue transfer requires less postoperative wound care and provides greater structural support to the nostril. Two transposition flaps were selected for reconstruction of this defect.

A bilobe flap was planned for the central nasal defect (Fig. 8-5**C**). The flap was designed so that the secondary lobe of the flap would transpose through only a 90° pivot. The secondary lobe of the flap was assisted by an adjacent melolabial transposition flap in repair of the remaining nasal and cheek defect (Fig. 8-5**D**). A free cartilage graft was positioned along the inferior alar margin to prevent upward contraction. The melolabial flap was designed so that it was sufficiently long to reach the lateral aspect of the bilobe flap (Fig. 8-5**E**). After transposition the flaps were draped in place in a fashion that minimized wound-closure tension, and the excess skin of the secondary lobe of the bilobe flap was trimmed (Fig. 8-5**F** and **G**). Wound tension from primary closure of the donor site of the melolabial flap was amply accommodated by the laxity of the patient's cheek skin. (Although the base of the melolabial flap may appear narrow relative to the length of the flap, the flap is well vascularized.)

The two flaps were secured in place with deep polyglactin (Vicryl) dermal and interrupted epidermal polypropylene (Prolene) sutures (Fig. 8-5**G**). A cosmetic disadvantage of this combined dual flap approach is the obliteration of the alar-facial sulcus and loss of some of the melolabial sulcus. Melolabial transposition flaps tend to obscure the alar-facial sulcus unless the base of the flap is above it. However, in this case the reconstructed alar margin was minimally distorted, and the overall results of the reconstruction were functional and continued to improve in appearance (Fig. 8-5**H** and **I**).

Figure 8-5 *A,* **An 85-year-old patient with large skin defect (3.5 × 1.8 cm) after excision of basal cell carcinoma.** *B,* **Three esthetic nasal subunits are violated by skin defect: sidewall, ala, and nasal tip.** *C,* **Bilobe transposition flap is selected to repair nasal tip defect. It is anticipated that secondary lobe of flap will assist in repairing superior aspect of ala.** *D,* **Melolabial flap is designed to repair lateral nasal and medial cheek defect. An auricular cartilage graft is used to support alar margin.** *E,* **Both flaps are draped in place. Slight amount of excess skin at distal end of secondary lobe of bilobe flap is trimmed.** *F* **and** *G,* **Both flaps are sutured in place with deep dermal polyglactin (Vicryl) and running epidermal polypropylene (Prolene) sutures. No substantial wound-closure tension is present.** *H,* **Frontal view of repair 6 weeks postoperatively demonstrating preservation of contour of alar rim.** *I,* **Lateral view of nose skin 6 weeks postoperatively. There is no marked elevation of alar margin.**

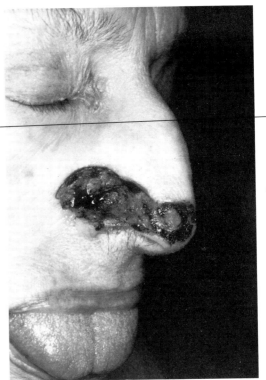

A

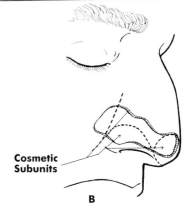

Cosmetic Subunits

B

Figure 8-5, cont'd.   For legend see opposite page.

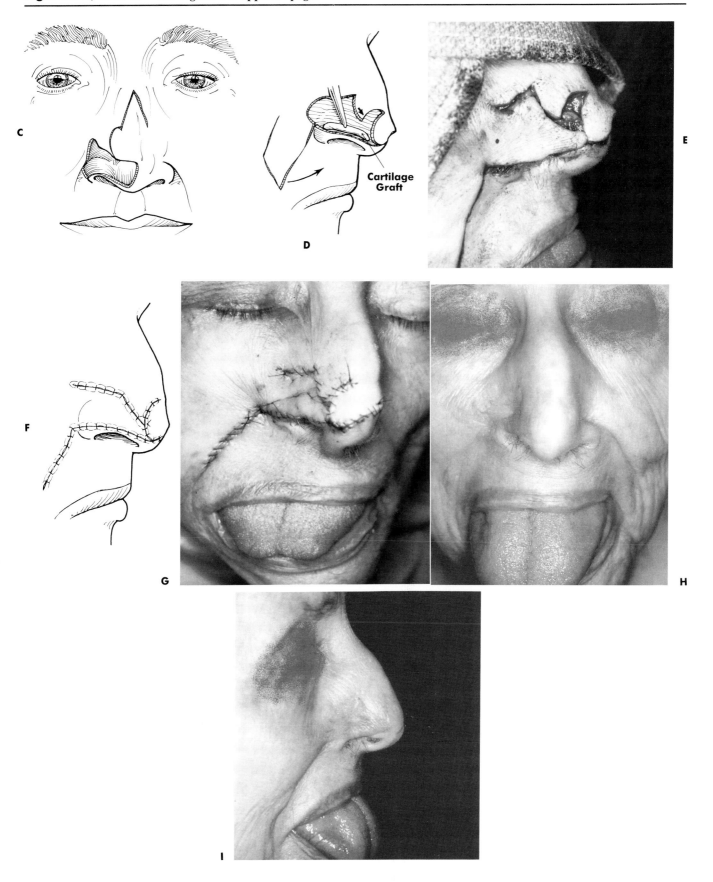

CASE 6: RHOMBIC FLAP

A 60-year-old woman had a 1.8 × 1.9 cm skin defect of the cheek and upper lip after excision of a basal cell carcinoma (Fig. 8-6**A**). The defect was similar to that in case 2, except that it was more inferior and traversed the upper lip and cheek cosmetic junction zone. Traditionally one does not like to violate cosmetic boundaries in the process of reconstructing a facial defect. However, like most rules in a creative pursuit such as reconstructive surgery, there are exceptions. Many repair options present a significant risk of distorting the upper lip. In this case the defect is viewed as a rhombus, and a rhombic flap is designed superiorly in a way that most of the scar from repair is hidden in the melolabial sulcus. Maintenance of the alar-facial sulcus was facilitated by deepithelialization of the beveled flap margin and by tucking this portion of the flap under the alar margin (Fig. 8-6**B**). In addition, the cheek skin was approximated to the nasal skin at a slightly deeper plane by placement of deep dermal and epidermal sutures at a lower depth on the nasal side compared with the cheek side of the wound (Fig. 8-6**C** and **D**). (If this adjustment is not made, partial obliteration of the alar-facial sulcus may occur.)

After incision and undermining, the flap was transposed. The secondary defect was then closed to assist in maintaining the melolabial sulcus after repair of the donor site. The skin edges were approximated at slightly different levels so as to create a "step-down" between the skin of the cheek and lip. This was accomplished by insertion of the needle at a lower depth in the lateral skin edges during placement of deep dermal and epidermal sutures (Fig. 8-6**D**). (This will create a slight unevenness of the epidermis of the suture line, which when healed will help accentuate the melolabial sulcus.) The standing cutaneous deformity created by the movement of the flap should be removed in such a way that the scar lies within the melolabial sulcus (Fig. 8-6**D**). However, the excision was positioned too laterally (X$_1$, Fig. 8-6**D**) and caused the resulting scar to lie beyond the sulcus (Fig. 8-6**E**). A more medially located excision would have placed the scar directly in the sulcus (X$_2$, Fig. 8-6**D**). Fig. 8-6**F** shows the postoperative result 2 months after reconstruction.

Figure 8-6 *A*, A 60-year-old woman with 1.8 × 1.9 cm skin defect of left cheek extending onto left upper lip after excision of basal cell carcinoma. *B*, Rhombic flap is designed to conceal much of resulting scar along alar-facial sulcus. This figure demonstrates important principles of mobilizing and transferring transposition flaps in this region; wide skin undermining *(dotted line)*; excision of standing cutaneous deformities; and beveling margin of flap where it joins nasal ala. Maintenance of alar-facial sulcus is facilitated by deepithelialization of beveled flap margin and tucking this portion of flap under alar margin. *C*, Standing cutaneous deformity is excised. *D*, In region of melolabial sulcus it is important to maintain appearance of a "step-down" between skin of cheek and lip. This is accomplished by approximation of skin edges at slightly different levels. Lateral edge is placed higher than medial edge by insertion of needle at lower depth in lateral edge when deep dermal or epidermal sutures are placed. This creates slight unevenness of epidermis along suture line, which when healed will help accentuate melolabial sulcus. In contrast, to help maintain alar-facial sulcus, lateral cheek skin is approximated to nasal skin at slightly lower level with use of deep dermal and epidermal sutures. *E*, Flap is secured with 5-0 polypropylene (Prolene) cutaneous sutures. *F*, Postoperative result 2 months after reconstruction. There is minimal trapdoor deformity or distortion of melolabial sulcus.

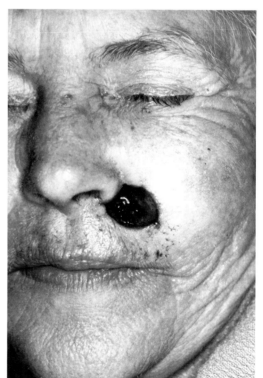

A

Figure 8-6, cont'd.   For legend see opposite page.

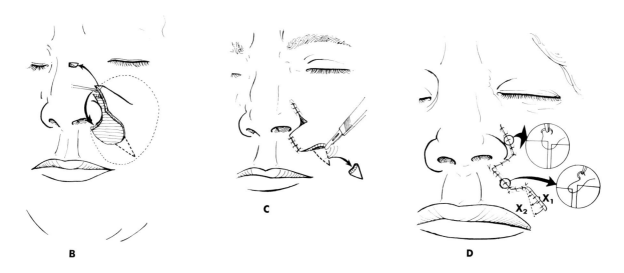

B   C   D

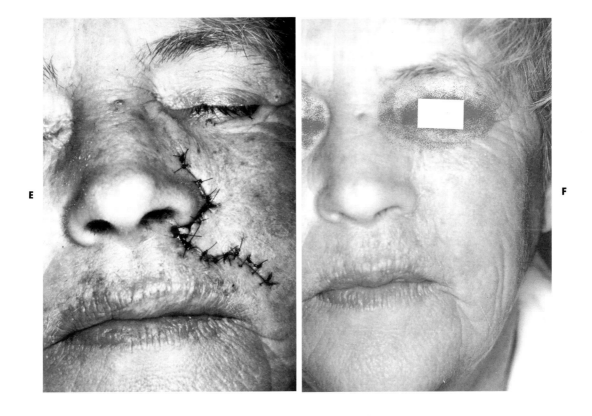

E   F

CASE 7

A 63-year-old man had a large skin defect (3 × 1.9 cm) of the melolabial sulcus (Fig. 8-7**A**) after Mohs surgical excision of a recurrent basal cell carcinoma. A V-Y advancement flap from the region of the lateral oral commissure was one reconstructive option considered. This approach, however, may blunt the melolabial sulcus. A 30° transposition flap, as demonstrated in Fig. 8-7**B** and **C,** traverses both esthetic units (cheek and upper lip) and causes upward distortion of the vermilion (Fig. 8-7**D**). However, in anticipation of the downward pull from the constant movement of the orbicularis oris muscle, it is reasonable to predict that in time the vermilion will return to its anatomic position (Fig. 8-7**E**). Fig. 8-7**B** demonstrates trimming of fat from the flap, which is essential when transposing fatty cheek skin to the lip. (This maneuver does not compromise vascularity of the flap. Use of a skin hook to minimize trauma is demonstrated.) The standing cutaneous deformity was excised at the inferior aspect of the wound (Fig. 8-7**C**).

A useful technique to make the surface of the melolabial flap even is depicted in Fig. 8-7**C.** (If deep sutures have misaligned the two wound edges, so that one is higher than the other, epidermal polypropylene [Prolene] sutures placed properly can adjust this misalignment. This adjustment is accomplished by insertion of the needle in a more superficial plane on the high side of the suture line compared with the low side. The effect will be to even the two epithelial edges when the suture is tied. This variable discrepancy in placement of sutures at different tissue depths can also be used to intentionally create misalignment. For example, to create a "step-down" in the lower melolabial region, exit the lateral wound low and enter the medial edge high so that the lateral side of the wound heals, a fraction of a millimeter higher.)

Fig. 8-7**F** demonstrates the result 4 months after reconstruction. During the first 3 postoperative months, some trapdoor deformity was noted (Fig. 8-7**E**), which resolved spontaneously. Note that there is no distortion of the lip or nostril.

Figure 8-7 *A,* A 63-year-old man with 3 × 1.9 cm skin defect involving melolabial sulcus after excision of recurrent basal cell carcinoma. *B,* A 30° transposition flap is designed so that inferior border of flap will assist in restoration of melolabial sulcus. Excess fat is trimmed from flap to minimize flap bulkiness. *C,* After transposition, flap is sutured with Gilles tip sutures and running sutures. Suturing skin margins together with discrepancy in the level of the medial and lateral edges helps simulate melolabial sulcus. *D,* Flap is sutured in place. Minimal lip distortion observed will resolve. *E,* Six weeks postoperatively some trapdoor deformity is seen, but treatment is not necessary. *F,* Twelve weeks postoperatively trapdoor deformity has resolved. Note how two superior scars are positioned mostly in RSTLs and inferior scar is well situated in melolabial sulcus.

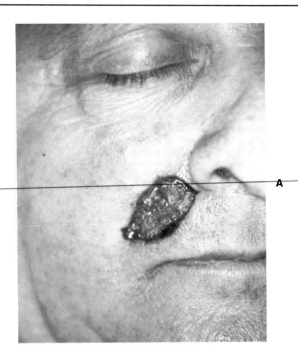

A

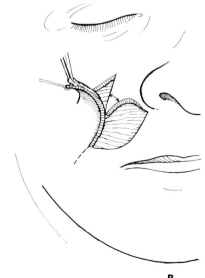

B

Figure 8-7, cont'd.   For legend see opposite page.

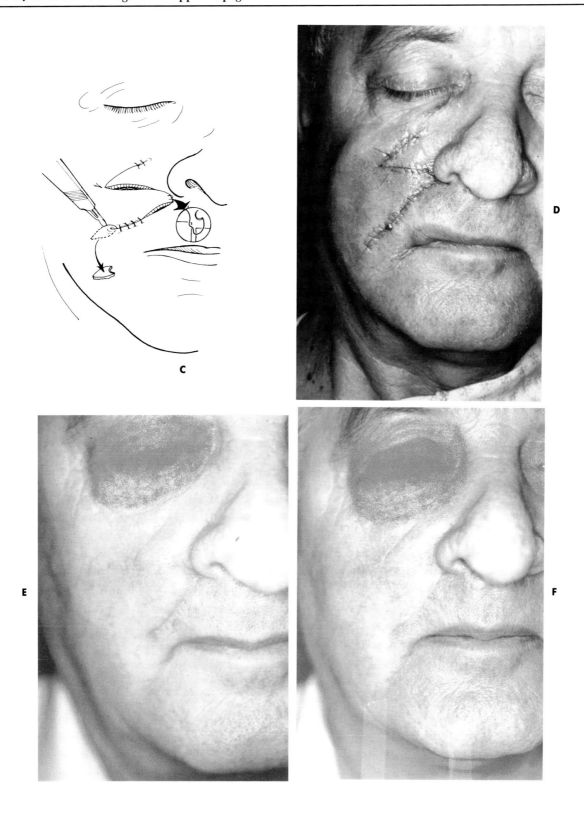

CASE 8: LARGE DEFECTS

A 70-year-old man underwent Mohs surgical excision of a recurrent basal cell carcinoma. The large facial skin defect (5 × 5.5 cm) that resulted is shown in Fig. 8-8**A**. The defect was rhombic and occurred in the region of the zygomaticotemporal branch of the facial nerve, which was spared. A large transposition flap was designed in a somewhat nontraditional way. A measurement was made from the superior pole of the defect to the inferior pole, and an incision of the same length was made in the cheek skin beneath the defect from a point centered along the inferior border of the defect (Fig. 8-8**A**). A traditionally designed rhombic flap would have more appropriately positioned this incision closer to the ear, but such a design would result in undue pulling and distortion of the earlobe.

After incision and hemostasis, the flap was transposed into the defect and secured with deep polyglactin (Vicryl) sutures (Fig. 8-8**B** and **C**). A large area of redundant skin, which resulted from the standing cutaneous deformity that developed after transposition, was removed in the preauricular area and was preserved (Fig. 8-8**C**). The limited availability of lax skin in the neck and the surprising tautness of the skin over the temple prevented the complete repair of the defect with the flap alone. The preserved skin was trimmed of fat, and the deep one third of the dermis was used to cover the remaining defect (Fig. 8-8**D**). (It is important to save all skin during a reconstructive procedure because a small Burow's graft may prove helpful in situations when the flap used for reconstruction is found to provide insufficient skin for repair of the defect.) Fig. 8-8**E** shows the results of the reconstruction 3 months postoperatively.

SUMMARY

Transposition is one of the most versatile methods of transfer of flaps because it permits realignment of skin tension lines. In addition, because of the broad range of flaps available in this category, reconstruction with matching tissue is a major benefit. However, the successful use of transposition flaps depends on a thorough appreciation of tissue movement. It is critical to have an understanding of the concept of the pivot point and the relation of flap movement about this pivotal point and secondary tissue movement of adjacent skin. Because the basic movement of a transposition flap is around a fixed pivotal point, the flap will not reach the most distant portion of the defect unless the surgeon has adjusted the design of the flap. The effective length of the flap should be reduced as the flap moves around the pivotal point or unless there has

Figure 8-8 *A*, A 70-year-old patient with 5 × 5.5 cm skin defect of cheek and temple following excision of basal cell carcinoma. Rhombic transposition flap is designed to take advantage of skin laxity of cheek and upper part of neck. *B*, Flap transposed. *C*, Flap sutured in place with deep dermal polyglactin (Vicryl) sutures and epidermal polypropylene (Prolene) sutures. Standing cutaneous deformity is excised and preserved for use as full-thickness skin graft. *D*, An inability to sufficiently mobilize flap prevented complete resurfacing of defect with flap alone. Previously excised skin is used as full-thickness skin graft (Burow's graft) to complete closure of defect superiorly. *E*, Results of reconstruction 3 months postoperatively. Portion of full-thickness skin graft did not survive, and healing in that area was by second intention. This did not impair final cosmetic result.

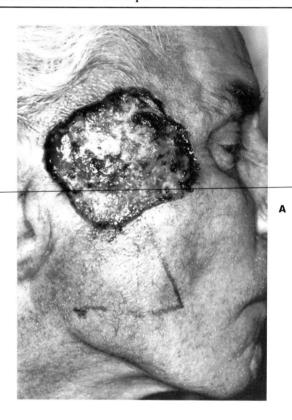

A

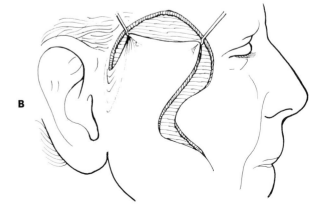

B

Figure 8–8, cont'd   For legend see opposite page.

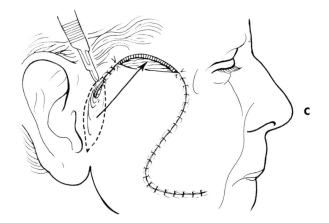

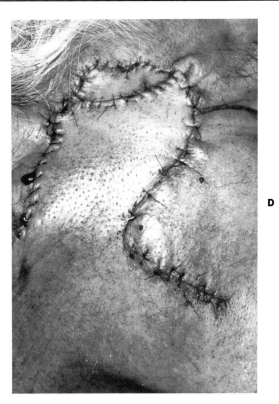

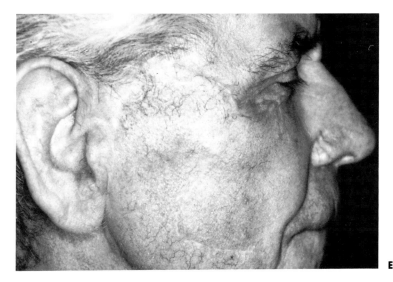

been secondary movement of recipient tissue toward the flap. It is important to be aware of surrounding facial structures that might be distorted.

It is axiomatic that a flap based on a random blood supply requires a sufficiently broad base to support all the tissues encompassed within the flap. In general, random-pattern transposition flaps should not have a longer linear axis than three times the width of the flap, but this rule is influenced by the facial region. For instance, the skin of the temple appears to have more vascularity than the thicker, more sebaceous skin of the nose, and thus relatively more narrow flaps can be used in this area.

Transposition flaps should be designed so that closure of the donor site occurs in favorable RSTLs. Careful attention to flap design will permit the versatile application of the whole range of transposition flaps.

REFERENCES

1. Dzubow LM: Facial flaps: *Biomechanics and regional application*, Norwalk, Conn, 1990, Appleton & Lange.

2. Masson JK, Mendelson BC: The banner flap, *Am J Surg* 1977; 134:419-423.

3. McGregor JC, Soutar DS: A critical assessment of the bilobed flap, *Br J Plast Surg* 34:197, 1981.

4. Cuono CB: Double Z-plasty repair of large and small rhombic defects: the double-Z rhomboid, *Plast Reconstr Surg* 71:658, 1983.

5. Webster RC, Davidson TM, Smith RC: The thirty degree transposition flap, *Laryngoscope* 88:85, 1978.

6. Dzubow LM: The dynamics of flap movements: the effect of pivotal restraint on flap rotation and transposition, *J Dermatol Surg Oncol* 13:1348, 1987.

7. Fee WE Jr, Gunter JP, Carder HM: Rhomboid flap

principles and common variations, *Laryngoscope*
86:1706, 1976.

8. Koranda FC, Webster RC: Trapdoor effect in
nasolabial flaps, *Arch Otolaryngol* 111:421, 1985.

9. Webster RC, Benjamin RJ, Smith RC: Treatment of
"trapdoor deformity," *Laryngoscope* 88:707, 1978.

10. Hamed LM et al: Hibiclens keratitis, *Am J Ophthalmol*
104:50, 1987.

11. Salasche SJ, Bernstein G, Senkarik M: *Surgical anatomy
of the skin,* Norwalk, Conn, 1988, Appleton & Lange.

12. Katoh H, Nakajima T, Yoshimura Y: The double-Z
rhomboid plasty: an important in design, *Plast Reconstr
Surg* 74:817, 1984.

EDITORIAL COMMENTS

Shan R. Baker

In contrast to rotation flaps that have a curvilinear configuration, transposition flaps have a straight linear axis. Both flaps move around a pivotal point, with their effective length decreasing as they pivot. Rotation flaps must be designed in such a way that one border of the flap is also a border of the defect for which it is intended to repair. Like rotation flaps, transposition flaps can be designed so that a border of the flap is also a border of the defect; they also may be designed with borders that are removed from the defect with only the base of the flap contiguous with the defect. The ability to construct a flap at some distance from the defect with an axis that is independent of the linear axis of the defect is one of the greatest advantages of transposition flaps. This fact enables the surgeon to recruit skin at variable distances from the defect, selecting areas where there is skin elasticity or redundancy. In addition, the ability to select a specific site to harvest a flap ensures that the scar at the donor site will be best camouflaged by its location and orientation.

Transposition is the most common method to move local flaps into skin defects of the head and neck. They are elevated in a multitude of sizes, shapes, and orientations and are usually random cutaneous flaps but may occasionally be axial (that is, glabellar, transposition flaps) or compound. A transposition flap as a reconstructive option is applicable to almost any conceivable configuration or location of small to medium-sized defects, thus making this the most useful of local flaps in head and neck reconstruction. Although the author of this chapter observes that random cutaneous transposition flaps generally should not exceed a 3:1 length-to-width ratio, this rule is not applicable to such flaps designed on the face and scalp. More important

than such a ratio are the location and orientation of transposition flaps. The abundant vascularity of the skin of the face and scalp often enables the development of flaps that exceed the 3:1 ratio. An example of this is the inferiorly based melolabial transposition flap, which can be successfully transferred with a length considerably longer than three times the width of the flap's base. This is due to the fact that the linear axis of the flap is directly above and parallel to the linear axis of the angular artery. Although the flap is rarely elevated as a true axial flap incorporating the angular artery, many small peripheral branches of the artery are probably included in the base of the melolabial flap. This accounts for its dependable viability when designed even as a lengthy flap.

I would like to comment on two additional points discussed in this chapter. The modified rhombic flap that the author shows in Fig. 8-8**A,** in my opinion, could have been better designed by recruitment of the relatively lax skin of the central cheek. A rhombic flap based medially instead of laterally would provide for greater flap mobility and probably would allow repair of the defect without the use of a skin graft. The author also emphasizes the importance of creation of a discrepancy of the skin levels during repair of wounds in the area of the alar-facial and melolabial sulcus. I do not advocate this technique because I believe it may create a scar that is more apparent than may otherwise occur. Instead, I prefer reconstruction of the sulcus by aggressive defatting of the flap in the appropriate locations. In addition, with time, there is a natural return of the melolabial sulcus to greater or lesser degrees depending on how much the remaining cheek skin relaxes during the ensuing months and years. This gradual return is also partly related to the constant movement of the cheek and lip from continued activity of the facial musculature.

EDITORIAL COMMENTS

Neil A. Swanson

Transposition is the second basic tissue movement. It is based on a lifting and repositioning of the flap from one point to another about a fixed pivotal point. Therefore, as Dr. Leffell clearly states, the mechanics of this flap and an understanding of the movement about a fixed pivotal point are critical to its design. The flap must always be designed longer than the height of the defect because the real height extends from the pivotal point to the side of the defect instead of from one side to the other. The most common error in transposition flaps of any kind is to cut the flap too short because of a poor understanding of this concept.

This chapter nicely introduces several of the individual flaps that will be discussed in detail in other chapters. Transposition flaps in general are some of the most versatile flaps used in reconstructive surgery, and an understanding of their principles is paramount.

Some general technique principles that hold true for all transposition flaps include the following: (1) Design the flap with enough length or tissue volume to fill the defect. It is always easier to excise excess flap length than it is to try and harvest it later. (2) Suture the secondary defect first. This allows the properly designed transposition flap to drape into place with very little tension. (3) Defat the flap before suturing it in place. This can often prevent the need to go back as a secondary procedure and remove the fibrofatty tissue that is redundant.

The concept of a trapdoor with transposition flaps is real. It can be minimized or prevented by the following: (1) Widely undermine the primary defect. (2) Defat the flap during transposition. (3) Suture with buried as well as meticulous cutaneous sutures. (4) In sebaceous skin maintain the bevel of the defect resulting from Mohs surgery (or create one) and counterbevel the edge of the flap. This results in a tongue and groove fit and allows for a better suture line and a flattening of the flap surface. (5) Create lines and angles rather than curvilinear lines during the final suturing of the flap. (6) If it looks as if a trapdoor is forming, at approximately 4 weeks begin to inject triamcinolone, 5 to 10 mg/ml, into the base of the flap and repeat at approximately 4-week intervals.

If a secondary procedure such as dermabrasion and/or defatting a disk of fibrofatty is necessary, the optimum time for dermabrasion is under debate. I usually dermabrade at 6 to 8 weeks and dermabrade the entire esthetic unit, not just the suture line. I disagree with Dr. Leffell about the use of ferric chloride as a hemostatic agent after dermabrasion. I never use this agent because it has resulted in documented instances of iron tattooing, which can be very difficult to treat.

9

Z-PLASTY

John L. Frodel

Tom D. Wang

INTRODUCTION

The Z-plasty principle is one of the most versatile concepts in reconstructive surgery. The dynamics of tissue movement involved in this technique work particularly well in the area of scar revision. A clear understanding of the underlying principles of Z-plasty will allow the reconstructive surgeon to apply this versatile technique to a wide array of clinical situations.

The history of the Z-plasty has been well reviewed by Borges[1] and Davis and Renner.[2] Classically this technique involves three limbs of equal length that form two equally triangulated flaps. Although the initial description of such equilateral transposition flaps was by Berger[3] in 1904, numerous other descriptions have been noted. In the 1800s Fricke,[4] Horner,[5] Serre,[6] and Denonvilliers[7] described the transposition of cheek and temporal skin to correct eyelid ectropion and regional defects. In these case descriptions, however, the tissue transposed consisted of neither symmetric angles nor limbs of equal length. In the late 1920s Limberg elucidated the geometric principles involved in Z-plasty.[8] He also noted that Z-plasties, as well as the related Limberg or rhombic flap, are best described as having both pivotal and advancement components. Whereas the classic Z-plasty follows very specific geometric guidelines, this historical perspective demonstrates the flexibility of the underlying principles. It is this flexibility that allows the wide-ranging applications and significant variations from the classic description of this versatile technique.

The Z-plasty is designed to accomplish three things: change scar direction, interrupt scar linearity, and lengthen scar contracture. In application, the Z-plasty should be considered when it is optimal to change the direction of a scar such that it is concealed either within a relaxed skin tension line (RSTL) or in a natural junction between facial esthetic units. Similarly a long straight scar may be broken into smaller segments to allow better camouflage. Finally, scars that cause distortion of facial features secondary to contracture may be lengthened with the Z-plasty techniques.

Although the principle function of Z-plasty remains this change of scar direction and scar lengthening, its main advantage over other techniques, such as W-plasty, is that usually no further skin needs to be removed. Additionally, a properly planned Z-plasty results in minimal distortion of surrounding structures. As with many techniques that interrupt a straight scar, the Z-plasty scar will counter forces of scar contracture. This is particularly important in contracted or webbed scars as well as with scars that distort anatomic landmarks.

Proper planning is critical to the success of this technique. As will be seen when geometric planning is discussed, projected scar locations are in the ideal theoretical situation and do not take into account the surrounding skin tensile properties. Accordingly it is not always possible to place the limbs of the Z-plasty exactly as planned. As noted by Borges,[1] a Z-plasty that requires a relatively long segmental scar can lead to an occasional bowstring effect in the central limb. This may result in irregularity of scar contour. Although scar contracture lengthening may be optimal for contracted scars, in other situations the lengthening caused by Z-plasty may also distort adjacent facial structures.

Mastery of the principles of Z-plasty allows its myriad applications in the head and neck. Any contracted or webbed scar in concavities is amenable to correction by Z-plasty. This includes vertical scars along the concave neckline, radial contractures that traverse the concavities of the auricle, and scar bands that cross the concave medial canthal region. Conversely, depressed contracted scars may occur in convex regions with limited structural support, such as in the nasal ala. Eyelid scars are often best corrected with Z-plasty because of contracture in the vertical direction, leading to lid ectropions. Similarly, lip scars are often contracted and require Z-plasty both to lengthen the scarred segment and to prevent recurrence of the contracture. Scars that cross the melolabial sulcus represent a classic application for Z-plasty. The central limb of the Z-plasty not only is camouflaged by the sulcus but also is incorporated into its reconstruction. Wide or confluent scars treated with excision and primary closure often lead to significant wound tension. The use of Z-plasties along the wound edges allows interdigitation to break scar linearity and disperse wound tension. Short (less than 2 cm) scars that oppose RSTLs are often best managed by Z-plasty. It should be made clear that this listing of indications is far from inclusive. It is important to note that for optimal results many situations require a combination of reconstructive techniques, such as W-plasty or geometric broken-line closure, in addition to Z-plasty.

GEOMETRY AND DESIGN

In the classic description, Z-plasty consists of one central limb and two peripheral limbs in the shape of a Z such that two triangular flaps of equal size are created. All three limbs are of identical length, and the central limb consists of the scar that is to be lengthened and realigned. In the classic 60° Z-plasty (Fig. 9-1) a protractor may be used to measure the angles. However, a more practical means for estimation of this angle is to mark out a 90° angle and divide it into thirds. Similarly, a caliper or ruler is useful in the design of limbs of equal lengths. Transposition of these triangular flaps (angles ABC and BCD in Fig. 9-1) brings about the following changes: the central limb is rotated 90°, from a vertical to a horizontal direction; the distance between B and C of the original vertical limb is increased; and the final scar is "broken" from a straight line to a nonlinear Z configuration.

Although a 60° Z-plasty is perhaps the most common design, angles between 30° and 90° are possible. Changing the angle of the flaps will cause a change in the length gained in the dimension of the original central limb (B-C) (Fig. 9-2). Theoretically the percentage gain in length increases with larger angles (Table 9-1). The amount of lengthening noted in actual practice, however, is usually less.

A range in the amount of directional change of the resultant central limb (B-C) is also noted. In the 60° Z-plasty the central limb is changed 90° from its initial position. In the 45° Z-plasty the resultant central limb lies in a more oblique position, approximately 60° from the initial position. In the 30° Z-plasty the direction of change is even less, approximately 45° from the initial position of the central limb (Fig. 9-2). This characteristic is extremely important during planning of the final limb locations after flap transposition.

The initial length of the central limb affects the final outcome as well. As the central limb is increased in length, so is the linear length gained with the Z-plasty (Fig. 9-3).[9] Unfortunately, as the three limbs of the Z-plasty become longer, there is also a greater likelihood of a more apparent scar. The multiple Z-plasty was developed to circumvent this problem (Fig. 9-4). In the classic sense a single long scar is divided into several smaller Z-plasties, usually with 60° angles.[10] A single large 60° Z-plasty provides more gain in length than multiple small 60° Z-plasties along the same central limb.[11] However, the esthetic ramifications and tissue availability will often preclude the use of the single, large Z-plasty. On the face the limb length is usually limited to 1 cm or less. On the neck the limb length should not exceed 2 cm.

Another variation is the four-flap compound Z-plasty. These will increase the length gained by increasing the initial angles of the flaps and by increasing the number of limbs. In the 90° compound Z-plasty each 90° angle is bisected into 45° triangular

Figure 9-1 Design of 60° Z-plasty.

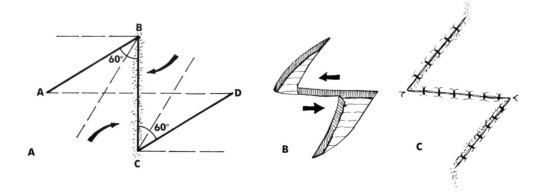

Figure 9-2   Changes in scar contracture length gained relative to Z-plasty angle. Also demonstrated is variation in central limb direction.

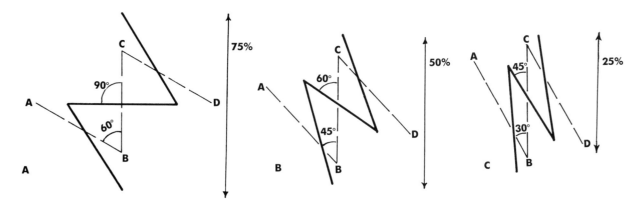

Table 9-1   Theoretical Increases in Length of B-C Dimension*

Angles (degrees)	Gain in Length (percent)
30-30	25
45-45	50
60-60	75
75-75	100
90-90	125

*See Fig. 9-2.

Figure 9-3   Increase in overall scar length with increasing limb length. There is eventual loss of effect of scar camouflage.

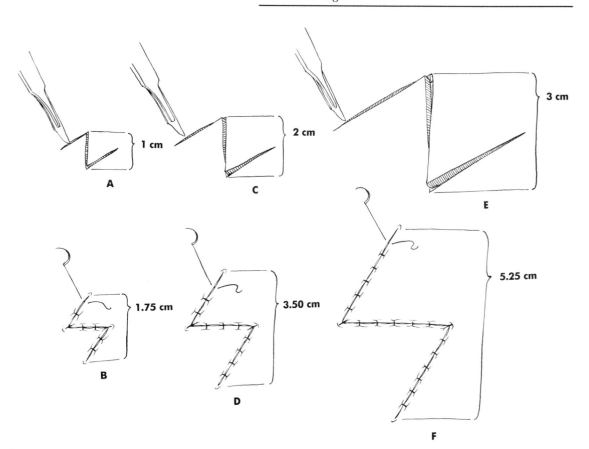

Figure 9-4   Multiple Z-plasty. Limbs are limited to less than 1 cm on face.

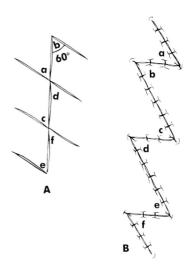

Figure 9-5   Four-flap compound Z-plasty at 45°.

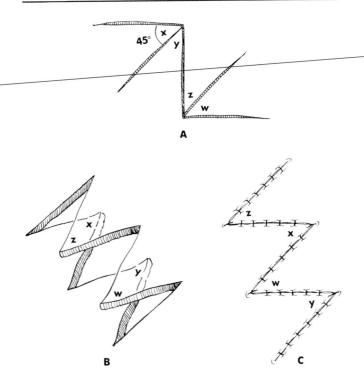

Figure 9-6   Four-flap compound Z-plasty at 60°.

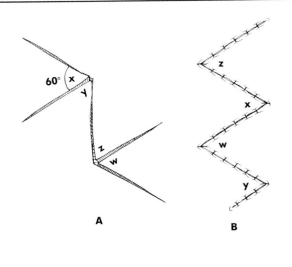

Figure 9-7   Unequal-angle Z-plasty.

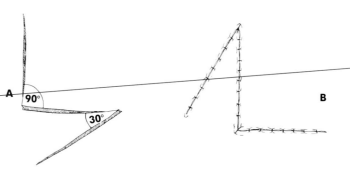

flaps which are then transposed (Fig. 9-5). Even further length can be obtained by starting with 120° angles, which subsequently are bisected into four 60° flaps (Fig. 9-6). Variations on this theme are plentiful, such as the six-flap Z-plasty and other multiple compound flaps. However, due to the extreme degree of standing cutaneous deformity on final closure, these designs are of minimal usefulness in the head and neck region.

Finally, while the classic Z-plasty consists of triangles with equal angles, these angles may vary considerably. In such situations the flap with the smaller triangle (more acute angles) will be transposed considerably more than that of the larger triangle (Fig. 9-7). Minimal gain in length will occur with unequal-angle Z-plasties, because the main purpose is to transpose the smaller flap over the larger flap.[2]

SURGICAL APPLICATION AND TECHNIQUE

The discussion to this point has involved theoretical concerns regarding classical geometry of the Z-plasty. It must be made extremely clear that much of what has been reviewed is theoretical. An understanding of the classic design is critical, but practical clinical considerations are even more important. Before a discussion of specific clinical uses of the Z-plasty, these theoretical considerations should be addressed from a practical perspective.

Figure 9-8   Acutely angled Z-plasty with curving of limbs to maximize blood supply to tip.

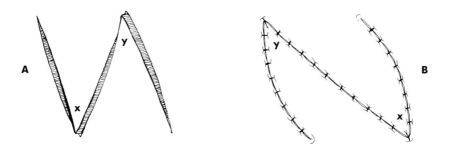

Figure 9-9   Release of underlying scar tissue to allow adequate transposition.

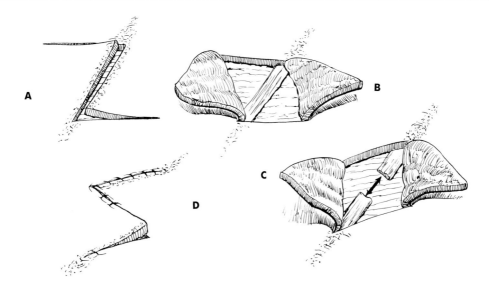

Whereas length in the direction of the central limb is indeed gained, it is usually not increased to the degree calculated.[9] Various studies have shown the increase to be considerably less in practice.[11] Similarly there is a limit to the angle of the triangular flap that may be used. Angles below 30° generally should not be used because of concern for tip vascularity. In the design of such acutely angulated flaps, the width of the flap may be broadened by curving the limbs of the flap (Fig. 9-8). This is important in skin with a reduced blood supply, such as in a contracture associated with a burn or radiation. Conversely, angles greater than 60° to 75° will commonly produce standing cutaneous deformities and should be avoided.

Complete evaluation of the surrounding skin and structures is necessary before design of a Z-plasty. The laxity at the base of each transposed flap must be adequate to allow movement into the new position. If the tissue is contracted perpendicular to the central limb, transposition may not be possible. Likewise, if an important anatomic structure such as the eyelid, oral commissure, lip, or nasal ala is near the flap base,

transposition may lead to distortion. Finally, if the scar tissue of the central limb is not released adequately, resistance to transposition will occur (Fig. 9-9).

As was demonstrated in Fig. 9-2, although a 60° Z-plasty will tend to reposition the central limb at a right angle, more acute Z-plasties will place the central limb at more acute angles. An understanding of these changes will assist in proper positioning of Z-plasty limbs in relation to RSTLs. To maximally camouflage scars in or near RSTLs, the Z-plasty angles should be calculated accordingly. With scars located approximately 90° to the RSTL, a 60° Z-plasty is required to relocate the central limb parallel to the RSTL. As the angle of the scar to the RSTLs becomes more acute, the Z-plasty angles should become more acute to position the central limb and the two peripheral limb scars more parallel to the RSTLs (Table 9-2).[2] For scars less than 30° to the RSTL, Z-plasty may not be necessary for realignment. For each particular scar there are always two choices for the alignment of the peripheral limbs, these being mirror images of one another. Both options should always be considered. One usually will

Table 9-2   Limb Direction and Scar Revision*

Variance to RSTL (degrees)	Z-Plasty Design
90	60° Z
60-90	60° Z (try to follow RSTL as much as possible)
30-60	Parallel to RSTL
30	Fusiform excision best

From Davis WE, Renner GJ: Z-plasty. In Thomas JR, editor: Scar revision, St. Louis, 1989, Mosby–Year Book.

be a better choice for scar camouflage due to better placement of the lateral limbs (Fig. 9-10).

The example of a wide scar perpendicular to the melolabial sulcus will be used to illustrate the specific surgical technique (Fig. 9-11). This scar is clearly noticeable due to its width and perpendicular orientation to the RSTL. Correction of these two factors will improve scar camouflage and with this in mind, a plan is made for a Z-plasty to translocate the scar or central limb into a RSTL, (in this case the melolabial sulcus). Since the scar is aligned 90° from the RSTL, a 60° Z-plasty is planned. This will reposition the resultant

Figure 9-10   Two options (A to B and C to D) for limb positioning. Choose one that will provide maximal scar camouflage in RSTLs.

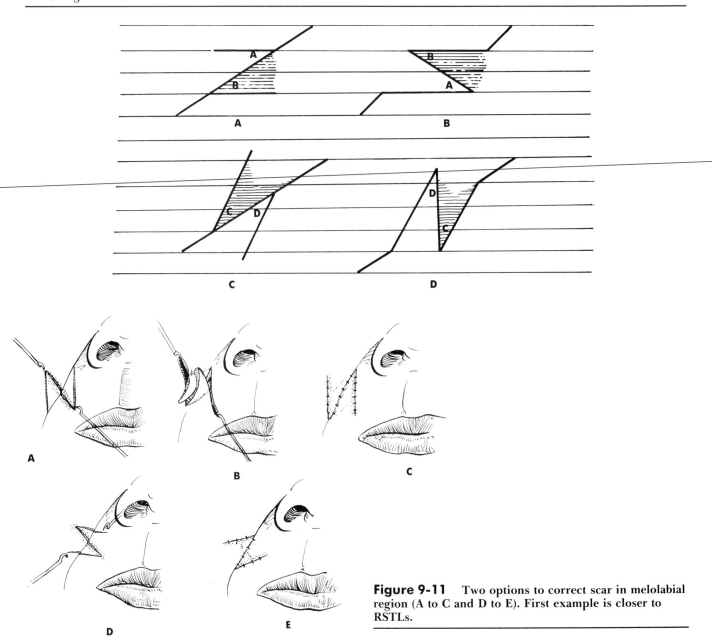

Figure 9-11   Two options to correct scar in melolabial region (A to C and D to E). First example is closer to RSTLs.

central limb at right angles to the original central limb. Note that two options exist for 60° Z-plasty design (Fig. 9-11**A** to **C** and **D** to **E**). As with any scar revision or local flap procedure, the design should be marked before the injection of local anesthetic to avoid distortion of the skin. Proper limb length is precisely measured by a caliper. Fig. 9-11**A** illustrates the preferred option. After transposition of the flaps, the central limb lies within a RSTL, in the melolabial sulcus, and the two lateral limbs approximate the RSTL of the lateral upper lip and medial cheek (Fig. 9-11**C**). Conversely, even though the mirror image (Fig. 9-11**D**) also realigns the central limb appropriately, the resultant lateral limbs cross the RSTL of the lip and cheek in an undesirable perpendicular fashion. Accordingly the first option is optimal, and the skin is marked with this Z-plasty.

A sterile solution is used to prepare the skin, followed by injection with a local anesthetic. Note that significant undermining of the skin surrounding the flaps is necessary to allow for the planned transposition without distortion of the lip, commissure, and alar base. Therefore, local anesthetic is injected to the extent of anticipated undermining. After a 7- to 10-minute wait for maximal vasoconstrictive effect, the scar is excised. In cases in which the scar is quite wide, it is occasionally useful to quickly suture the central limb of the wound closed at this time to confirm the design of the lateral limbs. Incision of the lateral limb follows and is best accomplished with skin fixation and incision from the flap base to the apex. Due to skin contraction after release of the central limb scar, there is a tendency to incise the tip of the Z-plasty such that it becomes overly narrowed. This tendency can be countered by slightly rounding and widening the incision as the lateral limb approximates the central limb. Elevation of the flaps is then undertaken beginning at the flap tip. This tip is delicately retracted with a skin hook and meticulous sharp dissection performed in a plane just within the subdermal fat. As mentioned, dissection continues well beyond the flap bases. After

appropriate undermining, the flaps are easily transposed by retraction of the ends of the central limb with skin hooks (Fig. 9-11**B**). Occasionally, tension prohibits adequate transposition and necessitates further undermining and extension of the incision at the base of one or both of the flaps.

The flaps are then sutured in place beginning with placement of several antitension subcutaneous sutures made of an absorbable material. The number of sutures should be limited, however, so as to not compromise the vascularity of the flap. Finally, the skin is closed using a fine suture material and a meticulous, atraumatic, wound-everting technique. These sutures are removed at 3 to 5 days postoperatively.

This case of a melolabial fold scar illustrates the classic use of a Z-plasty to change the direction of a scar so that it is located in a more esthetic position. It demonstrates that while the scar has been lengthened by the addition of two lateral limbs, the central portion of the scar is located directly within a RSTL, the melolabial sulcus in this case. To demonstrate the other principles of Z-plasty, several other situations will be illustrated.

Lengthening of contracted areas is often necessary, particularly if there is distortion of an anatomic structure or interference with function. An example of upper lip notching and retraction, which may occur from a deep laceration of the upper lip or after cleft lip repair, is shown in Fig. 9-12. Since additional length is required along the direction of the scar, a Z-plasty is designed with the lateral limbs along the malpositioned vermilion-cutaneous junction. The flaps are transposed, resulting in increased lip length in the scarred region and realignment of the vermilion border.

A more extreme example of the requirement for scar lengthening is in the contracted scar on the neck (Fig. 9-13). A long, webbed scar on the neck can ideally be approached with a Z-plasty. This will not only lengthen the scar and correct the webbing but will also approximate the new scars in better relationship to the obliquely positioned RSTLs. However, whereas a sin-

Figure 9-12   **Z-plasty in upper lip vermilion-cutaneous notching.**

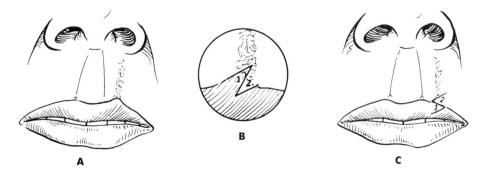

Figure 9-13   Z-plasty in webbed neck scar. A and B, single Z-plasty. C and D, multiple Z-plasty.

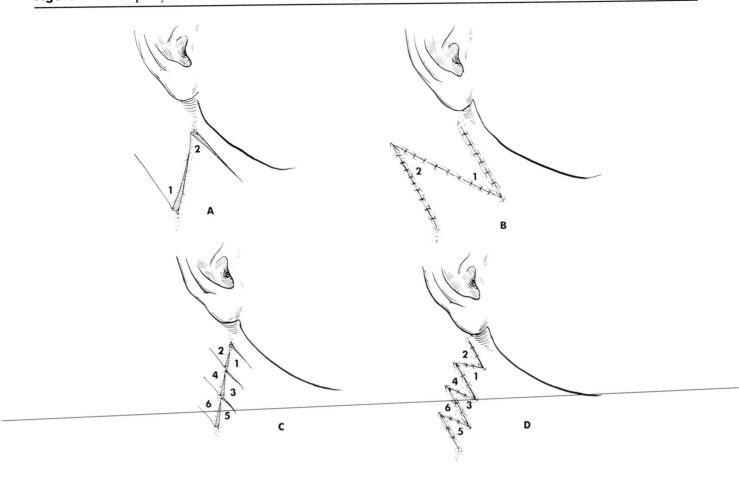

Figure 9-14   Multiple Z-plasty for vertical forehead scar and contracted lower eyelid and cheek scar, corrected using compound Z-plasty.

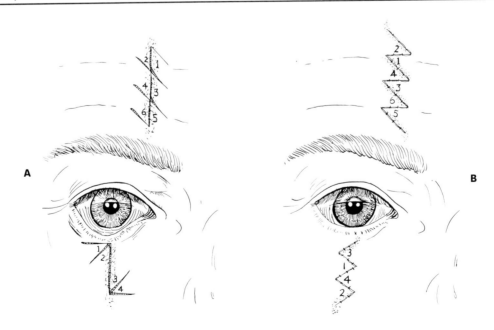

Figure 9-15   Multiple Z-plasties in rounded scar.

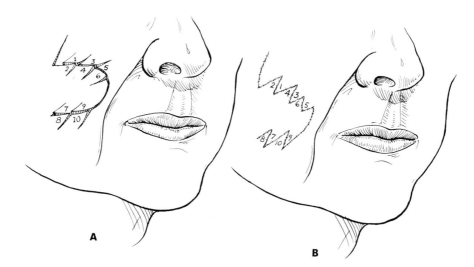

Figure 9-16   Z-plasty for correction of contracted oral commissure.

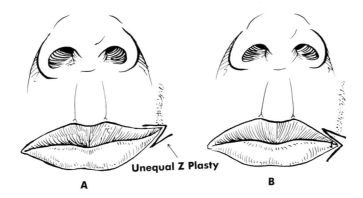

gle Z-plasty might provide maximum lengthening, it will tend to be more noticeable because of the long and uninterrupted nature of the resulting limbs. Accordingly a multiple Z-plasty will better circumvent this problem (Fig. 9-13**C** and **D**).

The multiple Z-plasty may also be of value in forehead scars; a repositioned central limb may be placed within a forehead crease (Fig. 9-14). While the complex four-flap Z-plasty has few indications in the head and neck, it might be considered for correction of a lower eyelid ectropion (Fig. 9-14). Finally, a multiple Z-plasty is sometimes useful to improve contour on round flaps, which have resulted in pincushion or trapdoor deformities, such as might occur with a cheek transposition flap (Fig. 9-15). Such deformities essentially represent a form of scar contracture, and a scar lengthening procedure such as Z-plasty is appropriate.

In a Z-plasty with unequal angles, the more acutely angulated flap will transpose a greater distance than the less acute flap. This simply represents a transposition flap of the more acute angled flap. Variations on such unequal Z-plasties can be used in situations of asymmetry, such as in a scar contracture of the oral commissure (Fig. 9-16). In such cases, the larger flap, that is, the commissure, is not undermined and the smaller flap is transposed. This allows for repositioning of the oral commissure.

CASE EXAMPLES

The following case examples demonstrate the Z-plasty technique.

CASE 1

Fig. 9-17**A** shows a patient with an oblique forehead scar extending under the right eyebrow and onto the right upper eyelid. Revision surgery to improve scar camouflage of the forehead component of this scar required excision of the existing widened erythematous scar tissue and realignment of the oblique portions more parallel to the horizontal RSTLs of the forehead. Fig. 9-17**B** demonstrates the proposed excision of the forehead scar, with two Z-plasties designed. The diagram of the patient's right forehead shows the anticipated outcome.

Fig. 9-17**C** demonstrates the immediate postoperative appearance of the procedure. The outcome 1 year postoperatively showed an improvement of scar camouflage (Fig. 9-17**D**).

Figure 9-17 *A*, Oblique forehead scar extending to the upper eyelid. *B*, **Double Z-plasty combined with scar revision. Markings on the patient's right side indicate the anticipated outcome.** *C*, **Wound repaired.** *D*, **One-year postoperative.**

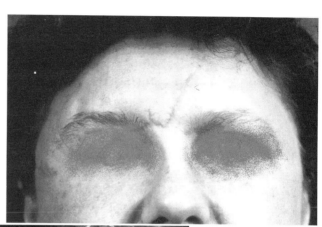

A

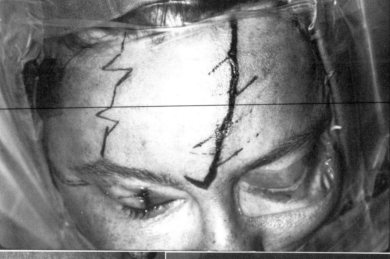

B

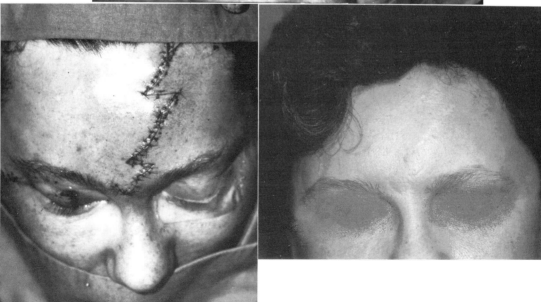

C

D

CASE 2

A patient had a contracted scar across the concavity of the scapha (Fig. 9-18**A**). Z-plasty was an ideal solution for this problem in that both the contracture and the misalignment of the central limb could be corrected. Fig. 9-18**B** shows the planned Z-plasty incision. Note the orientation of the side limbs, which conform with the surrounding anatomy. The mirror image of this planned Z-plasty would be less desirable because the side limbs will conform less well with the surrounding structures.

Shown in Fig. 9-18**C** is the transposition of equilateral triangles. Final closure of the wound was accomplished with 5-0 polyglactin (Vicryl) subcutaneous sutures and 6-0 fast-absorbing gut skin sutures (Fig. 9-18**D**).

One year after Z-plasty there was restoration of the normal auricular architecture and scapha (Fig. 9-18**E**).

Figure 9-18   *A*, Scar of the scapha. *B*, **Z-plasty marked.** *C*, **Flaps transposed.** *D*, **Completion of Z-plasty. Note release of the scar contracture.** *E*, **One-year postoperative.**

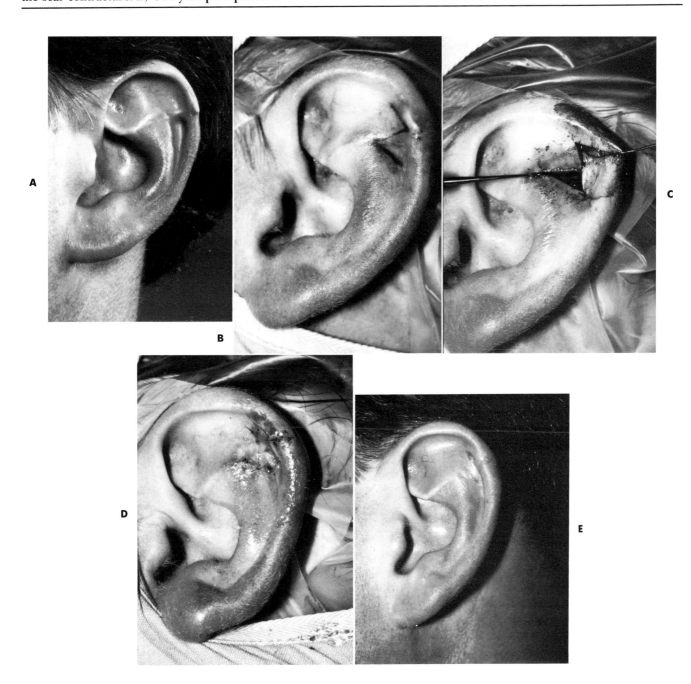

CASE 3

Fig. 9-19**A** demonstrates a frontal view of a small alar notch and the effects of scar contracture along an orifice. It was believed that simple excision of the notch would not correct the contracture. A small Z-plasty was performed, which redirected the central limb to be parallel with the alar margin and allowed the transposed flaps to reestablish the smooth nostril contour. Fig. 9-19**B** demonstrates the postoperative frontal view after correction of the alar notching.

Figure 9-19   **Correction of notching accomplished with Z-plasty.**

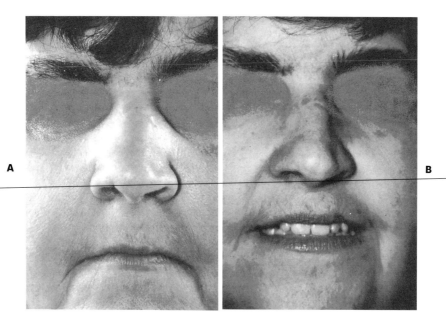

CASE 4

A patient had a unilateral cleft lip deformity with nasal alar tissue loss secondary to an unrelated injury that resulted in alar foreshortening and contracture (Fig. 9-20**A**). Two Z-plasties were required for correction of the contracted ala and were performed approximately 6 months apart. Fig. 9-20**B** shows the orientation for the first Z-plasty to release the horizontal contracture along the central limb as marked. Fig. 9-20**C** shows the second Z-plasty, demonstrating placement of the central limb along the contracted alar notch.

A preoperative oblique view of the ala (Fig. 9-20**D**) is compared with a 1-year postoperative result showing correction of the shortened ala and the notching (Fig. 9-20**E**).

Figure 9-20 *A*, **Alar notching secondary to tissue loss.** *B*, **Z-plasty designed to release horizontal scar contracture.** *C*, **Second Z-plasty (performed subsequently) designed to correct alar notching.** *D*, **Preoperative oblique view of alar deformity.** *E*, **One year postoperative showing correction of shortened and notched alar.**

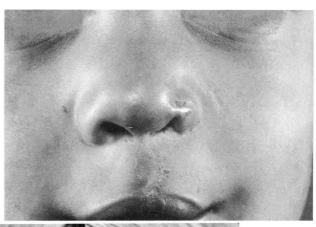

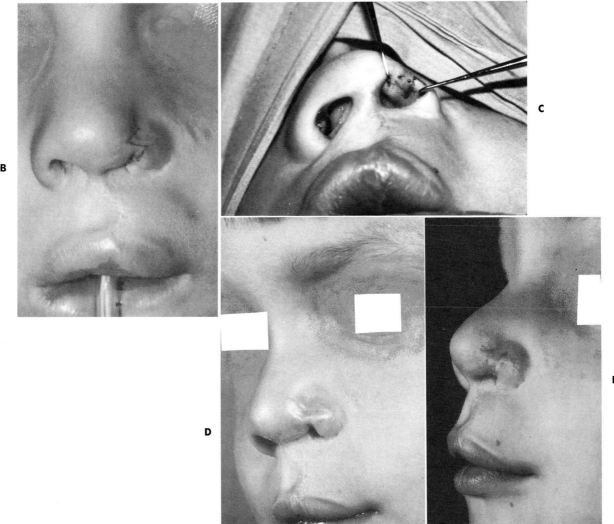

CASE 5

A patient had a contracted postauricular scar after a face lift procedure (Fig. 9-21**A**). This horizontal band interfered with the patient's ability to wear eyeglasses and was an ideal situation for Z-plasty correction. Fig. 9-21**B** shows the flaps after incision and undermining. Distraction along the central limb demonstrates the transposition of the two flaps.

Shown in Fig. 9-21**C,** after final closure, is correction of the contracture and lengthening of the original scar.

Figure 9-21   *A,* **Contracted postauricular scar.** *B,* **Transposed flaps following incision of Z-plasty.** *C,* **Release of scar contracture following completion of Z-plasty.**

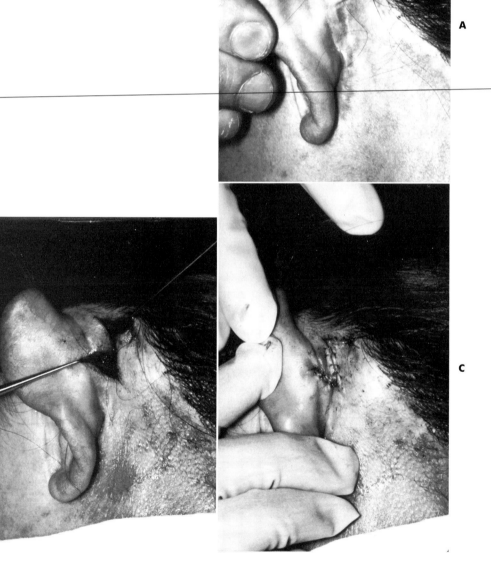

CASE 6

A young girl had a vertical hypertrophic widened neck scar in the anterior concavity of the neck (Fig. 9-22**A**).

Fig. 9-22**B** shows the immediate postoperative appearance after scar excision and multiple Z-plasties. Although the Z-plasty was successful in transposing a portion of the scar into a more parallel relationship with the horizontal RSTLs of the neck, a large portion of the scar was still aligned in the vertical dimension.

Fig. 9-22**C** demonstrates the 1-year outcome showing good camouflage of the portions of the scar that were aligned with the horizontal RSTLs but recurrent hypertrophy of the vertical portions of the neck scar. Further Z-plasties are required to improve the scar alignment of the remaining hypertrophic portions. This case demonstrates the importance of appropriate scar alignment in scar camouflage.

Figure 9-22   *A*, Vertically oriented hypertrophic neck scar. *B*, **Following scar excision and multiple z-plasties.** *C*, **One year postoperatively vertical components of the scar have become hypertrophic.**

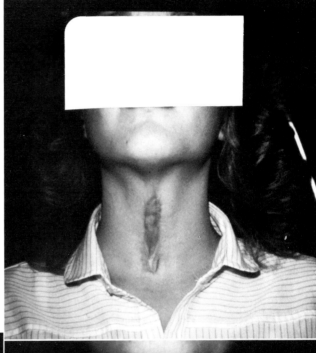

A

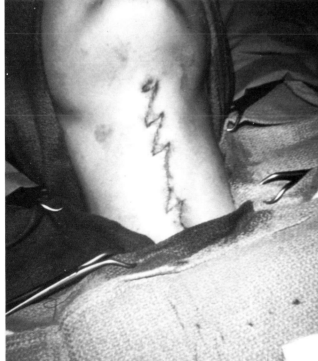

B

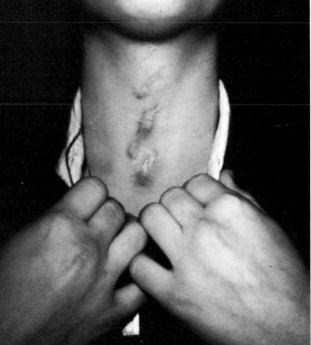

C

CASE 7

After trauma a patient had substantial soft-tissue loss with foreshortened upper lip contracture and tethering of the lower lip due to scarring across the inferior labial sulcus and absence of lateral commissure (Fig. 9-23**A**). Fig. 9-23**B** demonstrates the procedures planned: rotation advancement correction of the upper lip to achieve lengthening along with Z-plasty incorporated in the superior portion of the rotation advancement procedure. A commissuroplasty was planned as was a Z-plasty to release the lower lip and correct the notched vermilion border. Fig. 9-23**C** demonstrates the immediate postoperative outcome.

The proposed second-stage revision included further rotation advancement of the upper lip plus Z-plasty interdigitation to lengthen the upper lip scar, Z-plasty at the vermilion-cutaneous junction of the upper lip for better alignment, and Z-plasty in the mental region to create greater length for the lower lip and release the vertical scar contracture (Fig. 9-23**D**). The final outcome 1 year postoperatively showed improved positioning and alignment of the upper and lower lips (Fig. 9-23**E**).

Figure 9-23 *A*, Traumatic deformation of upper and lower lip. *B*, Rotation advancement flap facilitated by z-plasty is designed to lengthen upper lip. Z-plasty to release distorted lower vermillion as well as a commissuroplasty is also designed. *C*, Following completion of surgery. *D*, Six months following first scar revisions, Z-plasties of upper and lower lip scars are planned. *E*, One year postoperative.

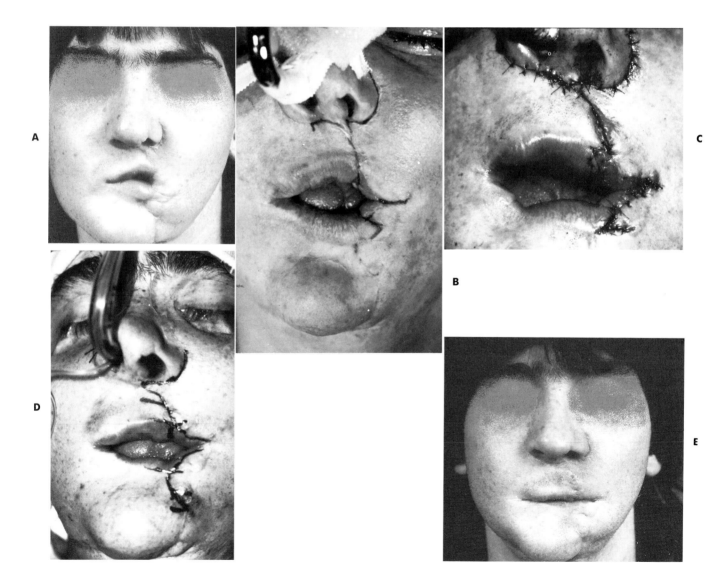

CASE 8

A patient had an oral cutaneous fistula after composite resection for squamous cell carcinoma of the mandible (Fig. 9-24**A**). An unequal Z-plasty was planned, involving transposition of the cheek flap for external lining of the fistula.

Fig. 9-24**B** demonstrates closure of the donor site before insetting of the flap. Wound repair with 4-0 polyglactin (Vicryl) subcutaneous sutures and 6-0 fast-absorbing gut skin sutures (Fig. 9-24**C**).

Fig. 9-24**D** shows the patient 2 years after surgery. This case illustrates the versatility of the Z-plasty and its application in this type of tissue transposition.

Figure 9-24   *A,* **Unequal Z-plasty designed to repair oral cutaneous fistula.** *B,* **Flaps transposed.** *C,* **Wound repair completed.** *D,* **Two years postoperative.**

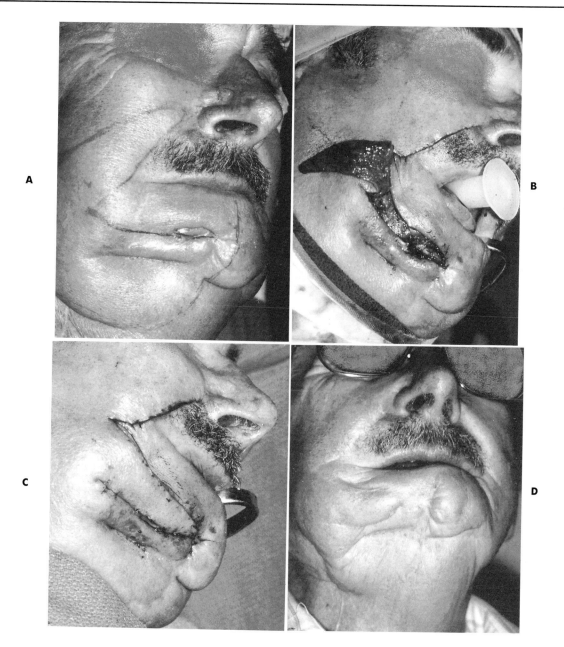

SUMMARY

The Z-plasty, one of the oldest concepts in plastic surgery, remains a prevalent and important technique. An encompassing understanding of its geometric and basic principles is critical to successful application. As a form of transposition flaps, the Z-plasty is useful to lengthen a contracted scar, change the direction of a scar for better alignment with RSTLs, and interrupt a straight scar to better camouflage it. It is also helpful in the closure of some defects and to realign malpositioned anatomic landmarks. Classic indications exist, such as correction of a contracted and webbed scar of the neck or realignment of a scar that crosses RSTLs or a facial esthetic junction such as the melolabial sulcus. However, knowledge of the principles involved allows the surgeon to adapt the Z-plasty to other more complex situations. These might include correction of a malpositioned oral commissure or an ectropion, correction of a congenital or posttraumatic epicanthal fold,[12,13] or even use in the functional repair of a primary cleft palate.[14] It is impossible to list all of the reported uses for the Z-plasty as described in the literature. Suffice it to say that with a thorough understanding of its principles, the Z-plasty is an extremely powerful tool in the reconstructive surgeon's armamentarium.

REFERENCES

1. Borges AF: Z-plasty. In Borge AF, editor: *Elective incisions and scar revision*, Boston, 1973, Little Brown.
2. Davis WE, Renner GJ: Z-plasty. In Thomas JR, editor: *Scar revision*, St Louis, 1989, Mosby–Year Book.
3. Berger P: Autoplastic par dedoublement de la palmure et echange de la lambeaux. In Berger P, Banzat S, editors: *Chivurgie orthopdique*, Paris, 1904, G Steinheil.
4. Fricke JC: Bildung nerur Augenlider nach Zerstörung und dadurch hervorgebrachter Auswartswendung derselben. Hamburg, 1829, Perthes & Basse.
5. Horner WE: Clinical report on the surgical department of the Philadelphia. *Am J Med Sci* 21:99, 1837.
6. Serre M: Traite sus l'art de restaurer les déformités de la face, selon la methode par deplacement, ou methode française. Montpellier, France, 1842, L Castel.
7. Denonvilliers CP: Blepharoplasie. *Bull Soc Chir* 7:213, 1856.
8. McCarthy JG: Introduction to plastic surgery. In McCarthy JG, editor: *Plastic surgery, vol 1, General principles*, Philadelphia, 1990, WB Saunders.
9. Limberg AA: Design of local flaps. In Gibson T, editor: *Modern trends in plastic surgery*, London, 1966, Butterworth.
10. Jankauskas A, Cohen IK, Grabb WC: Basic technique of plastic surgery. In Grabb WC, Aston SJ, editors: *Plastic surgery*, Boston, 1991, Little Brown.
11. Davis JS, Kitlowsky EA: The theory and practical use of the Z-incision for the relief of scar constriction. *Ann Surg* 109:1001, 1939.
12. Furnas DW, Fischer GW: The Z-plasty: biomechanics and mathematics. *Br J Plast Surg* 24:144, 1971.
13. Converse JM, Smith B: Naso-orbital fractures and traumatic deformities of the medial canthus. *Plast Reconstr Surg* 38:156, 1966.

EDITORIAL COMMENTS

Shan R. Baker

The authors have nicely explained Z-plasty in geometric terms. They have provided examples and have listed common indications for this technique. Perhaps a few comments concerning the dynamics of tissue movement occurring during Z-plasty is also in order. The Z-plasty procedure consists of a dual transposition of triangular flaps, each with independent points of pivot. One flap is transposed about its pivotal point in a clockwise direction and the other in a counterclockwise direction. In addition to pivoting, the flaps are advanced into their triangular recipient sites. Thus, to achieve proper flap movement, it is necessary to undermine widely at the base of each flap.

When Z-plasty is used for scar revision, it changes the direction of the old scar and relieves scar contracture at the expense of increasing the final length of the scar that results from revision. Another way of saying this is that a scar modified by Z-plasty results in the "lengthening" or release of the segment of adjacent skin that is distorted by contraction by creating two triangular flaps, which require additional skin incisions and thus an increase in the length of the final scar. The advancement, not the pivotal movement of the Z-plasty flaps, accounts for the lengthening in the axis of scar contracture, because in essence skin adjacent to the scar is recruited through the mechanism of advancement to augment the contracted area. The larger the triangular flaps used in Z-plasty, both in terms of angles and length of limbs, the greater the amount of skin advancement toward the contracted site and the greater the lengthening of the contracted segment. However, the greater the angles of the triangular flaps, the greater the resulting standing cutaneous deformity and the longer the limbs, the greater will be the length of the final revised scar. Used appropriately, the Z-plasty technique is a highly effective method of improving the appearance of scars, relieving tension during wound closure, and correcting distorted facial structures that result from scar contraction.

EDITORIAL COMMENTS

Neil A. Swanson

The Z-plasty is a superb tool for the reconstructive surgeon. An understanding of the concepts, geometry, and complexity of the Z-plasty can be challenging. This chapter explains these concepts in practical terms better than any I have read. I have few comments, other than to encourage the reader to spend time learning the practical points, which are clearly elucidated by the authors.

Tables 9-1 and 9-2 are particularly good summaries. The four-flap compound Z-plasty, illustrated in Fig. 9-5, is a particularly useful variant of the standard Z-plasty. One of the keys with this, as well as the standard Z-plasty, is to make sure that once the flaps are cut, they are actually transposed and interchanged. I have seen more than one training fellow proudly show me the results of a Z-plasty, when actually they sewed the cut flaps back in place without transposition. Therefore, when starting this procedure, one should find a way of inking the tips of the triangles to be transposed to ensure that transposition occurs.

Last, a small but realistic point is illustrated in Fig. 9-9. In the use of Z-plasty for scar revision (contrary to Z-plasty designed into the reconstructive effort primarily) it is important to realize that underlying scar tissue can be quite fibrotic and deep. If the Z-plasty is elevated above the linear fibrous band of the scar, that fibrous band must be released to maximize the gain in length or change in direction of that particular Z-plasty.

10

RHOMBIC FLAPS

David A. Bray

INTRODUCTION

The rhombic flap, although one of the most popular transposition flaps used today, has always been surrounded by problems with nomenclature (also called rhomboid flap) and even more so by problems of design. A rhombus is an equilateral parallelogram, whereas a rhomboid is a parallelogram in which the angles are oblique and adjacent sides are unequal. In any event, the transposition flap most often associated with the name Limberg flap is not the rhombus. Rather, the surgical defect to be corrected by the flap is the true rhombus.

The Limberg flap, on which all future variations of the rhombic flap were developed, was first described by Alexander A. Limberg[1] in 1963. The credit for the development and mathematical analysis of the first rhombic flap belongs to Limberg. It also should be noted, for the student of soft-tissue surgery, that his work was all done on paper models. Paper, of course, lacks the distensibility characteristics of human or even pig skin. Thus the uniqueness of his work should be duly noted. For example, the development of transposition "puckers" and "dog-ears" (standing cutaneous deformities) are far more impressive and demanding in paper models in which Limberg coined the terms *lying* and *standing cones*. It is the desire to eliminate these cones that in essence drives the surgeon to continually attempt to improve on the original Limberg model.

In the ensuing years since Limberg's work, multiple variations of the rhombic flap have appeared as well as multiple articles that report a broad range of surgical use. Unlike many soft-tissue closure procedures, the Limberg flap and all of its variations require a vigorous understanding of the geometry involved. Because this flap was designed on paper models, the geometry is exacting and becomes even more exacting with newer variations on the theme, such as the Dufourmental,

Webster, and Becker modifications.[2-5] Therefore, a thorough understanding of the Limberg flap must be accomplished before any derivatives or surgical indications can be discussed.

The Limberg rhombus defect consists of two equilateral triangles placed base to base to form a rhombus with opposing angles of 60° and 120°. In simplistic fashion, if one simply rounds off 60° and 120° angles, the rhombus becomes a 60° tip-to-tip ellipse (Fig. 10-1). This straight-line ellipse is the basis of the most common and simple linear advancement closure; however, when the opposing sides are simply too far apart for closure without undue tension, a flap should be created and hence the rhombic flap. The design of the 60° to 120° defect has often been incorrectly taught. Although often causing a great deal of confusion, the actual design is quite simple. The major problem in the technique seems to be with which angles correspond to each other from defect to flap.

In the Limberg flap, all of the sides of the defect and the flap are equal in length and they are, in turn, equal to the short diagonal of the rhombus defect. Thus the ever-present question of which angles correspond to each other is a moot point, and one needs only to remember that all sides and the short diagonal of the defect must be equal in a 60° to 120° rhombus defect and flap. Once the 60° to 120° rhombus defect has been drawn with all sides equal, by definition, the short diagonal is directly extended. This creates the first side of the flap and should be extended a distance equal to all other sides. The second side of the flap, again equal to all other sides, is drawn parallel to one of the attached sides of the defect[6] (Fig. 10-1).

As mentioned above, the Limberg flap represents the transposition of equilateral triangles and can be thought of as a modified Z-plasty.[1,6,7] This concept eventually leads to the Dufourmental modification using isosceles triangles and the various Z-plasty closure techniques originally described by Becker.[5]

Figure 10-1 *Left,* A 60° ellipse and 60° straight-line ellipse. *Right,* Classic Limberg flap in which all sides of defect, short diagonal of defect, and flap are equal. Flap is designed by extension of short diagonal (B-D) one length equal to itself (D-E) and then cutting back of a similar length (E-F) parallel to nearest side of defect. (From Bray DA: Clinical applications of the rhomboid flap, *Arch Otolaryngol* 109:37-42, 1983. Copyright 1983, American Medical Association.)

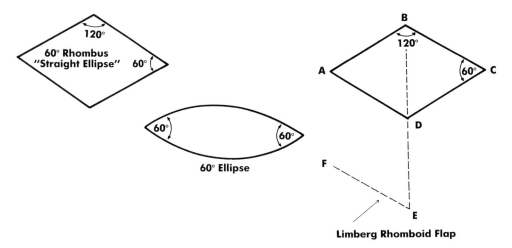

Another important feature to note is that the flap itself only closes one half of the defect, and the other 60° angle is closed upon itself. Thus, even with undermining and use of a transposition flap, one is at the base of the defect, still closing an ellipse under tension. Therefore the subject of flap dynamics and flap tension needs to be discussed.

The majority of the tension is at the closure point of the donor flap site. Wide undermining of the surrounding tissue does not change the relative tension distribution.[7] The resultant total tension vector has been calculated to be 20° to the short diagonal of the rhombus defect (Fig. 10-2).[8] Thus, skin mobility or extensibility is important in appropriate flap design, but an understanding of the resultant tension vector is critical to avoid distortion of surrounding structures. The lines of maximal extensibility (LME), or the direction of the most skin laxness, lie perpendicular to the facial crease lines.[9,10] If significant facial wrinkles do not exist, then the surgeon can determine the LME by simply picking up the skin with his or her fingers. This is an important concept because every rhombus defect may have four potential flaps for closure. In placement of the lines of the rhombus defect, two parallel sides should be drawn on lines of maximal extensibility. Two more parallel lines need to be drawn to create a 60° to 120° rhombus defect. The appropriate two flaps are created by direct extension of the short diagonal and a cutback line that would intersect the theoretical extension of the defect sides that lie on the LME (Fig. 10-2).[6,11]

In the perfect Limberg flap procedure, the transposed flap equals the size of the defect; however, as the rhombus defect approaches a 90° or square defect, the

resultant flap is reduced to 40% of the defect.[12] There may be times when the defect location does not allow a 60° to 120° rhombus, or the skin available for closure is less than full defect size.

Once the basics of the Limberg 60° to 120° flap are understood—that is, all sides are equal to the short diagonal and also to the flap sides—the placement factors depend on the following. Two parallel sides should be on the LME, the cutback line of the flap is parallel to one of the defect sides and would intersect a theoretical extension of the LME defect side, and the resultant tension vector is 20° from the short diagonal. (Fig. 10-2). Fortunately for the surgeon, skin is very distensible, and slight errors are easily tolerated.

COMMON VARIATIONS

The first variation and one that often develops inadvertently in the 60° to 120° defect is as the defect is altered by frozen-section margin adjustments, a gradual change toward a 90° or square defect develops. For a well-detailed analysis of the effect, the reader is referred to the article by Koss and Bullock.[12]

Perhaps the best known modification of the Limberg flap is the Dufourmental flap that was designed to close rhombus defects with any acute angle, rather than just 60° to 120° defects.[2,13] The design of this flap is more complex than that of the Limberg flap and as a consequence may be more difficult for some surgeons to use. The peripheral sides of the defect are equal in length, but the short diagonal will vary with the acuteness of the angles employed. Thus the defect from the Dufourmental procedure should be thought of as two isosceles triangles placed base to base. The

Figure 10-2   *Top*, Limberg rhombus defect and flap with resultant lines of tension before and after closure. *Bottom*, Placement of proper line of four flaps to take advantage of LME of facial skin. Either side of defect (B-C or A-D) is placed on LME. Short diagonal is extended equal to its length and cutback line G-H or E-F is drawn parallel to closest defect side and thus theoretical lines H-B and D-F complete equilateral triangle with base on LME. (From Bray DA: Clinical applications of the rhomboid flap, *Arch Otolaryngol* 109:37-42, 1983. Copyright 1983, American Medical Association.)

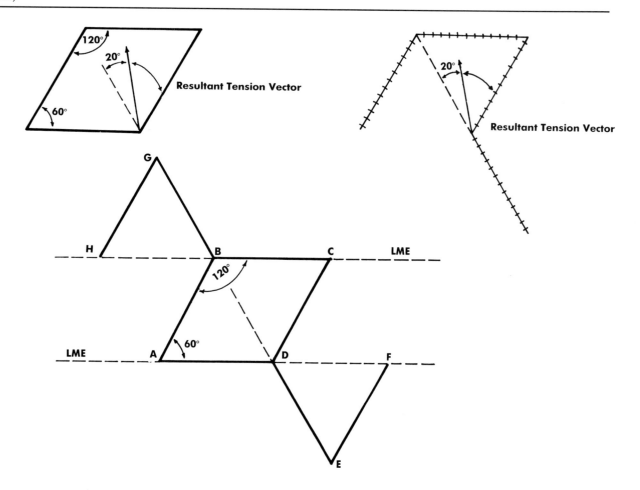

actual design of the flap is accomplished by extending the short diagonal and an adjacent side from the same point. These two lines are then bisected to create the first side of the flap. The cutback or second side of the flap is formed by a line parallel to the long diagonal. The flap sides are equal in length to the defect sides (Fig. 10-3). The placement of the Dufourmental flap is based on the fact that as the defect varies from a 60° acute angle up to a 90° or square defect, the short diagonal of the flap changes only 4° from an angle of 150° (Fig. 10-3). Thus placement of the short diagonal of the defect can be placed at 150° from the LME to obtain the most tension-free transfer.

The Webster 30° flap deserves discussion because it is obvious that the smaller the angles of closure are, the easier the closure is. This is true of a single elliptical closure, in which many soft-tissue surgeons prefer 30° angles to 60° angles to avoid standing cutaneous deformities. As was pointed out earlier in the 60° to

120° Limberg flap, the bottom half of the defect is closed directly. Therefore, if this portion of the defect could be extended to create a 30° angle, the closure would be easier and there would be less tendency for a standing cutaneous deformity to develop. To do this, a great deal more tissue must be sacrificed and a long straight line must be created. Webster et al[4] solved this problem by simply dividing the aforementioned 60° angle with an M-plasty to create two 30° angles, thus preserving tissue and breaking up the line of closure (Fig. 10-4). Webster et al further modified the Limberg flap by designing a 30° flap for transposition. Angle C in Fig. 10-4 must be 110° or greater to prevent the distance C-E from becoming so short that flap viability is compromised. The above-mentioned flaps are shown side by side for comparison (Fig. 10-4).

Two additional modifications or extensions of the Limberg flap need to be discussed because they really create an extended-use situation, as opposed to a

Figure 10-3 Dufourmental flap design in relation to LME of facial skin. Since all sides of defect and flap are equal, entire design may be started by drawing imaginary line C-F on LME. Line A-C may then be drawn at 150° from line C-F. Short diagonal length is not known until all four sides of defect are drawn and acute angles of rhombus are varied from 60° to accommodate anatomy. All sides of defect and flap are equal but are not equal to short diagonal of defect. Once rhombic defect is drawn, short diagonal A-C is directly extended, as is side D-C. Angle thus created is bisected to form first side of flap (C-E). Second side (E-F) is created parallel to long axis of defect (B-D). (From Bray DA: Clinical applications of the rhomboid defect, *Arch Otolaryngol* 109:37-42, 1983. Copyright 1983, American Medical Association.)

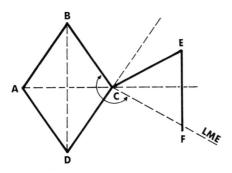

Figure 10-4 Limberg (*bottom*), Dufourmental (*center*), and Webster 30° flap (*top*). See text (Common Variations) for details. (From Bray DA: Clinical applications of the rhomboid flap, *Arch Otolaryngol* 109:37-42, 1983. Copyright 1983, American Medical Association.)

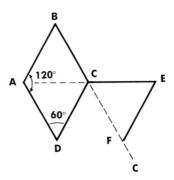

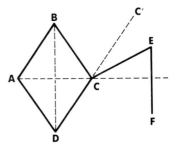

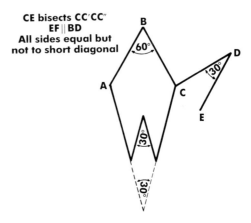

CE bisects CC′CC″
EF∥BD
All sides equal but not to short diagonal

modification only. The first is the double Z-plasty technique, described by Cuono[13] and revised by Katoh et al,[11] which extends the use of excision of a rhombic defect to larger areas. The technique is as follows. Two parallel lines are drawn perpendicular to the LME along the relaxed skin tension lines (RSTLs). Two more parallel lines are drawn to create the 60° to 120° all-sides-equal defect of Limberg. Then with use of an extension of the first parallel lines as a central limb, two 60° Z-plasties are formed with all sides equal. The Z-plasties are transposed for closure. This procedure allows tissue to be taken from two areas instead of one for closure (Fig. 10-5). Thus, larger defects can be closed while reducing undue tension that would be created by a single Limberg, Dufourmental, or Webster flap.

The last modification of the Limberg flap to be discussed was originally described by Limberg[1] and again by Lister and Gibson.[10] This modification or extension really represents the use of multiple rhombic flaps. As one thinks of a rhombus defect as an ellipse with straight sides, one can also imagine a hexagon as a squared-off circle. Thus three rhombic flaps can be used to close a single defect (Fig. 10-6). The sides of the hexagon are equal to the radius, and the flaps are drawn at every other corner so as not to share common sides. Again, all sides are equal and in turn are equal to the radius, the extension of which is the first line of the flap. The cutback parallels the appropriate side. The

flaps are then elevated and transposed into position for closure.

SURGICAL TECHNIQUE

The surgical procedure of the rhombic flap requires extreme accuracy and faultless soft-tissue handling (Fig. 10-7**A** to **H**). The initial lesion seen in the figure is bordered by three landmarks: the ear, beard line,

Figure 10-5   Double Z rhomboid begins with two parallel lines drawn on LME. Another set of parallel lines that creates 60° angles is then drawn. With extensions of first parallel lines as central limb, a 60° angle is created to generate cutback line parallel to one side of defect. Only one pair of Z-plasties can be made. All sides are equal.

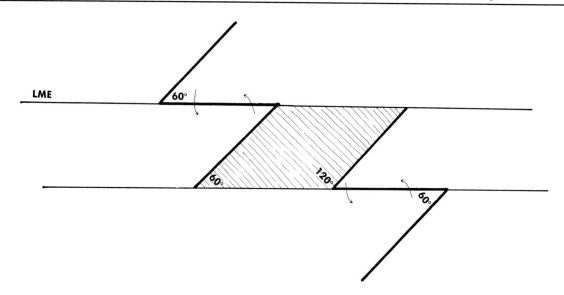

Figure 10-6   Sides of hexagon are equal to radius of circle. First side of flaps are created by direct extensions of radius at alternate corners to prevent sharing of common sides. Second side is created parallel to appropriate side of hexagon.

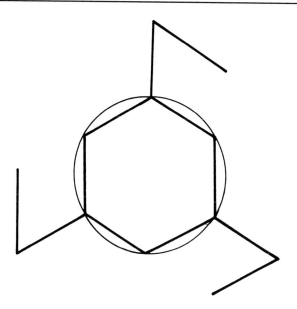

Figure 10-7   *A-H,* Sequence of intraoperative photographs demonstrate technique employed in Limberg flap. See text (Surgical Technique) for details. *I,* Results of healing 4 months postoperatively.

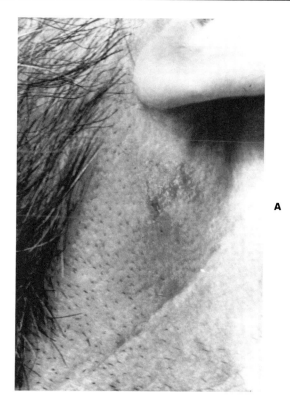

and an old discolored scar (Fig. 10-7**A**). In this case, as in many, the flap was designed to accommodate structures, whereas some compromise was made in the LME. The inexperienced surgeon needs only calipers to outline the rhombus defect of Limberg (Fig. 10-7**B**). Once the anticipated defect is drawn, the

Continued.

Figure 10-7, cont'd.   For legend see p. 155.

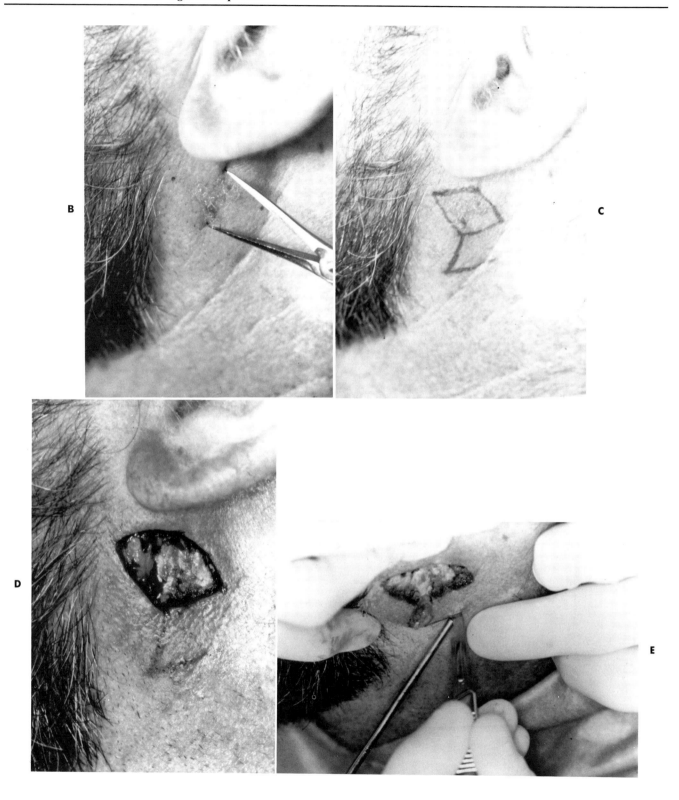

Figure 10-7, cont'd.   For legend see p. 155.

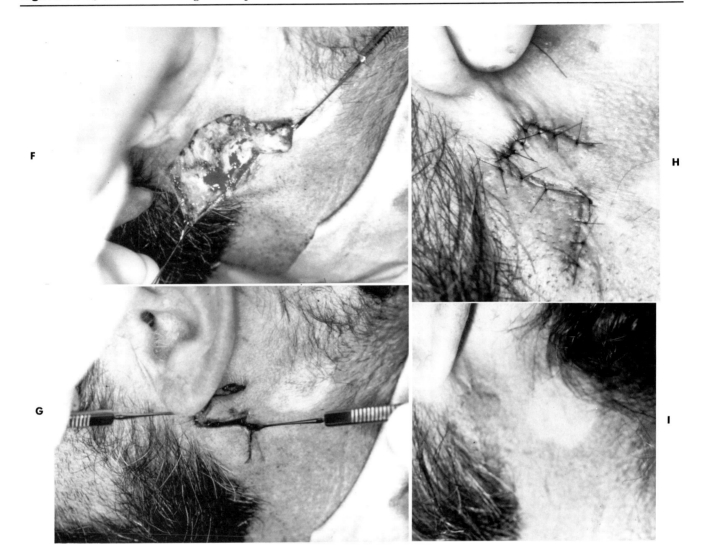

proposed flap with dependent drainage is also drawn (Fig. 10-7**C**). After the tissue specimen is removed, note how the length-to-length relationships of the sides of the defect seem to change (Fig. 10-7**D**). However, one must respect the original drawing, unless the defect is altered by the need to resect additional tissue for tumor-free margins. The creation of the defect and the flap may be performed with a No. 15 or No. 11 surgical blade (Fig. 10-7**E**). However, for precise margin cuts, any additional margin resections should be accomplished with a No. 11 blade and cut along an entire side for accuracy. Because of the elasticity of skin, one or two repeated margin resections can be tolerated without the need to redesign the entire flap, depending, of course, on the amount of tissue removed. Both donor and recipient sites are widely undermined (Fig. 10-7**F**). Although this does not change the basic tension vectors, it does facilitate a

good everted tissue closure.[7] The flap is now easily transposed into the defect site (Fig. 10-7**G**). The wound is repaired by deep and superficial everting tip sutures (Fig. 10-7**H**).

Fig. 10-8**A** to **G** demonstrates additional technical aspects of the rhombic flap. In this case, the key anatomic structures are the hairline, eyebrow, and eyelid (Fig. 10-8**A**). Distortion of the latter two must not occur. With the lesion removed, the flap is cut with use of skin hooks and constant suction to keep visualization optimal (Fig. 10-8**B**). The flap should be easily transposed without undue tension (Fig. 10-8**C**). Note how the donor defect is automatically filled as the flap is transferred. However, the donor site is the point of greatest tension. In practice, either this point or the most distant tip of the transposition flap should be closed first with a permanent or nearly permanent suture such as 4-0 clear monofilament nylon or 4-0

Figure 10-8 *A-G,* Sequence of surgical technique for Limberg flap. See text (Surgical Technique) for details. *H,* Appearance 4 months postoperatively.

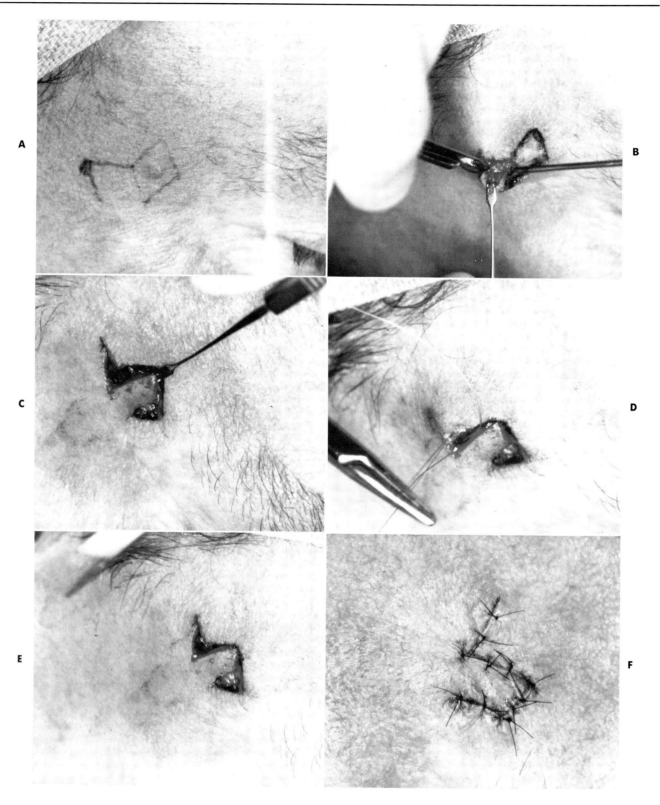

Figure 10-8, cont'd.   For legend see p. 158.

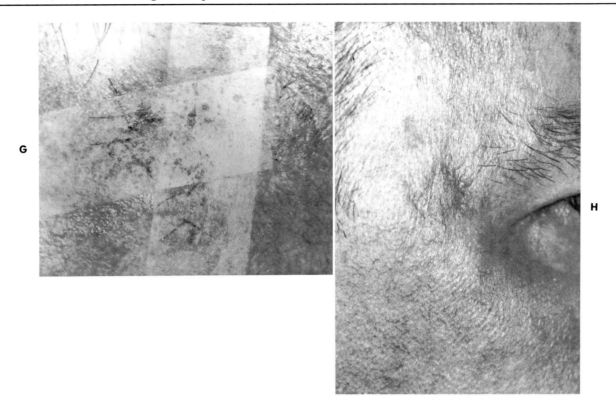

CASE EXAMPLES

clear polyglactin (Vicryl) (Fig. 10-8**D**). One cannot overemphasize the importance of a good subcutaneous closure. Chromic sutures are usually unsatisfactory (Fig. 10-8**E**). Final skin sutures should be placed so as to obtain skin eversion. Despite the undermining inherent with the use of a transposition flap, skin tension will always exist, as can be seen by the stress on the repaired wound (Fig. 10-8**F**). The final dressing need only be plain paper tape placed so as to give an occlusion effect and allow total debridement of all scabs and debris when removed 24 hours after surgery (Fig. 10-8**G**).

The postoperative care of rhombic flaps is routine and simple, assuming that the procedure is performed with the correct geometry, minimal wound tension, and good soft-tissue techniques. Failure to properly design the defect or flap may lead to a standing cutaneous deformity or anatomic distortion of adjacent structures, while excessive wound tension may cause a depressed scar, especially at the distal tips of the flap. Flap edema poses no more problem than in any other flap, but the risk is higher when the distal end of the flap is brought downward into a dependent position. Very rarely are defatting or postsurgical dermabrasion necessary.

The examples selected to describe the surgical technique are ideal situations for the use of classic Limberg flaps. The surgical defects are relatively small and in areas where straight lines are common. This is easily demonstrated by examination of the results of healing at 4 months postoperatively in the two cases already mentioned (Figs. 10-7**I**, 10-8**H**).

CASE 1

An example of the Dufourmental modification of the Limberg flap is shown in Fig. 10-9**A** and **B.** Note how nicely the resulting wound-closure lines fall into facial and lip creases if appropriately planned. The flap was designed to have the resultant scar fall into the preexisting lines as possible. In this case, or whenever possible, the flap is inferiorly based. The advantage to this is to prevent tip edema that occurs with superiorly based flaps. However, if the weight of the flap causes stress or distortion of the structures above, a superiorly based or laterally based flap may be used.

Figure 10-9 Dufourmental flap demonstrating adaptation to melolabial sulcus and vertical lip lines. Note lack of distortion of free border of lip.

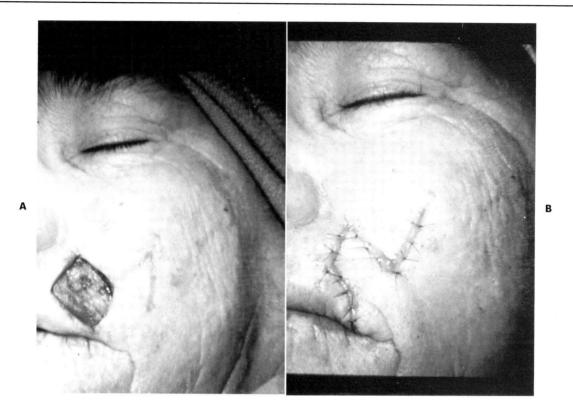

CASE 2

An example of the Dufourmental procedure on the nose is shown in Fig. 10-10. The glabellar skin offers an excellent source of tissue for nasal repairs. Almost any flap, for example, a bilobe flap, will succeed in this area. The rhombic flap, however, results in a series of straight lines blending well with the typical nasal crease lines. The defect of about 1.5 cm is easily closed, using the glabellar skin. Unfortunately, the nasal skin stiffens and adheres to bone and cartilage in the lower caudal extent of the nose. Large rhombic flaps in this area become much more difficult to close without tension, producing distortion to the tip of the nose. The final cosmetic result in this case is seen at 1 year after surgery (Fig. 10-10**D**).

Figure 10-10 *A to C,* **Dufourmental flap procedure is shown on nose.** *D,* **Appearance at 1 year postoperatively.**

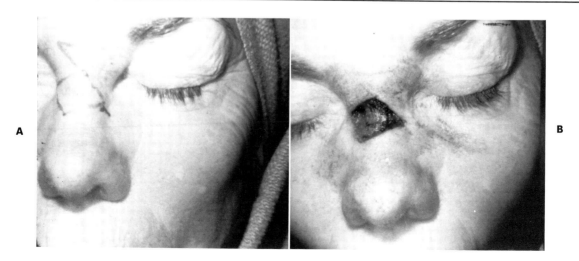

Figure 10-10, cont'd.   For legend see p. 160.

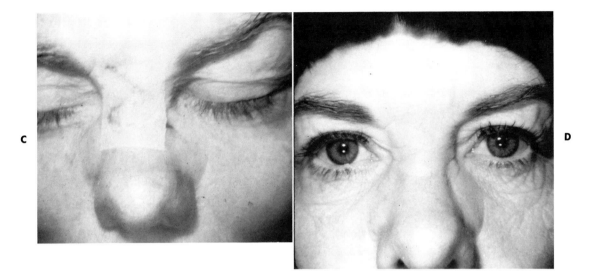

CASE 3

A rhombic flap was used for reconstruction of a defect in the temple area. A large (greater than 2 cm) lesion had been removed, resulting in a defect that measured approximately 2 × 2.5 cm. No undue tension was created in the eyebrow, and the hairline remained undisturbed. Nonetheless, the patient must be prepared to live with a scar shaped like a bucket handle (Fig. 10-11). Approximately one half of the scar length is not parallel with the natural skin creases.

LIMITATIONS VERSUS INDICATIONS

The decision as to when to use a rhombic flap is based on several factors. Perhaps the most critical factor is not to overdo the procedure; that is, do not use such a flap when simple elliptical excision and closure will do. Also do not remain committed to a rhombic flap when a flap of a different design can better accomplish the goals of reconstruction. An example is a defect of the nasal tip that would be best repaired with a dorsal nasal flap.[14] There are also certain areas of the face that lend themselves to straight-line closures and other areas where rhombic flaps do not work well.[15] A good example is the forehead, which is not an ideal location for use of a rhombic flap, because even though the closure is a series of straight lines resembling a bucket with handles, the multiple directions of the scar resulting from wound closure fail to complement the horizontal forehead creases. The scalp is also not a good location for rhomboid excisions when hair is present. The transposition of the flap reorients the hair

Figure 10-11   Two-year result of a rhombic flap used to reconstruct a 2 × 2 cm defect in the temple area. This case clearly avoided structure distortion; however, the patient must be prepared to live with the scar.

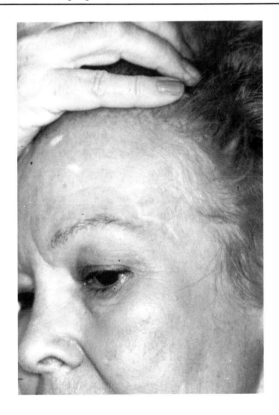

follicles into an unnatural position. However, when non–hair-bearing scalp is being removed in scalp reduction procedures, a multiple rhombic flap procedure can be quite useful to avoid significant wound closure tension.[16]

The use of the rhombic flap is by no means confined to the face. It is of note that large rhombic flaps or multiple rhombic flaps have been used for various genitourinary procedures.[17-19] Myelomeningoceles also lend themselves to rhombic flap repair,[20] the most innovative of which has been the creation of a Limberg-latissimus dorsi myocutaneous flap.[21] Large trunk lesions such as decubitus ulcers, partial mastectomy defects, and defects created by removing melanomas have all been treated with the Limberg flap or its modifications.[22-24]

SUMMARY

The rhombic flap possesses many qualities. The first and foremost is that it works with great reliability. The geometry allows precise incisions and wound closure that result in a predictable set of straight-line scars. The rhomboid-shaped specimen is a pathologist's dream, as all the sides are straight and easy to cut for frozen-section margins.

The disadvantages of the rhombic flap usually occur as a result of poor surgical judgment. Examples are inappropriate use, when simpler closures could have been used, and/or attempts to stretch the flap too far, with resultant standing cutaneous deformities and undue tension lines. The initial rigors of the geometry are easily mastered, and skin extensibility covers many small errors. This can even be carried to the extreme where little rigorous geometry is applied to the closure.[25] As in all soft-tissue repairs, surgical judgment and case selection are critical to success. If these are exercised correctly, the rhombic flap and its variations and extensions will prove highly successful.

As an addendum, I would like to mention my pleasant meeting with Dr. Alexander A. Limberg's daughter, Anna K. Limberg, in Leningrad in 1988. The Russians are still as excited about his work as we are and pleased to see its extensive use in the United States.

REFERENCES

1. Limberg AA: *Design of the local flaps.* In Gibson T, editor: *Modern trends in plastic surgery,* Sevenoaks, England, 1966, Butterworth.

2. Dufourmental C: *An L-shaped flap for lozenge-shaped defects.* In Transactions of the Third International Congress of Plastic Surgery, Amsterdam, 1964, Excerpta Medica.

3. Dufourmental C: Le formeture des pertes de substance cutanée limitées le lambeau de rotation en losange, *Ann Chir Plast* 7:61, 1962.

4. Webster RC, Davidson TM, Smith RC: The 30° transposition flap, *Laryngoscope* 88:85, 1978.

5. Becker H: The rhomboid-to-W flap, *Ann Plast Surg* 11:123, 1983.

6. Bray DA: Clinical applications of the rhomboid flap, *Arch Otolaryngol* 109:37, 1983.

7. Larrabee WF Jr, Trachy R, Sutton D et al: Rhomboid flap dynamics, *Arch Otolaryngol* 107:755, 1981.

8. Fee WE, Gunter JP: Rhomboid flap principles and common variations, *Laryngoscope* 86:1706, 1976.

9. Gibson T, Stark H, Evans JH: Directional variation in extensibility of human skin in vivo, *J Biomech* 2:201, 1969.

10. Lister GD, Gibson T: Closure of rhomboid skin defects: the flaps of Limberg and Dufourmental, *Br J Plast Surg* 25:300, 1972.

11. Katoh H, Nakajima, Yoshimura Y: The double-Z rhomboid plasty: an improvement in design, *Plast Reconstr Surg* 76:817, 1984.

12. Koss N, Bullock JD: A mathematical analysis of the rhomboid flap, *Surg Gynecol Obstet* 141:439, 1975.

13. Cuono CB: Double Z-plasty repair of large and small rhombic defects: the double-Z rhomboid. *Plast Reconstr Surg* 71:658, 1982.

14. Bray DA, Eichel BS, Kaplan HJ: The dorsal nasal flap. *Arch Otolaryngol* 107:765, 1981.

15. Bray DA: Preferred placement of facial incisions. In *Transactions of the fourth international symposium on facial plastic and reconstructive surgery,* St Louis, 1984, CV Mosby.

16. Stough DB, Stough DB: *Triple rhomboid flap for crown alopecia correction, J Dermatol Surg Oncol* 16:543, 1990.

17. Barnhill DR, Hoskins WJ, Metz P: Use of the rhomboid flap after partial vulvectomy, *Obstet Gynecol* 62:444, 1983.

18. Kramer SA, Jackson IT: Bilateral rhomboid flaps for reconstruction of the external genitalia in epispadias-exstrophy, *Plast Reconstr Surg* 77:621, 1985.

19. Romero CJ, Alcade M, Martin F et al: Treatment of pilonidal sinus by excision and rhomboid flap, *Int J Colorect Dis* 5:200, 1990.

20. Cruz NI, Ariyan S, Duncan CC et al: Repair of lumbosacral myelomeningoceles with double Z-rhomboid flaps, *J Neurosurg* 59:714, 1983.

21. Munro IR, Bernd RN, Humphreys RP et al: Limberg-latissimus dorsi myocutaneous flap for closure of myelomeningocele, *Child Brain* 10:381, 1983.

22. Cuono CB, Ariyan S: Versatility and safety of flap coverage for wide excision of cutaneous melanomas. *Plast Reconstr Surg* 76:281, 1985.

23. Gwynn BR, Williams CR: Use of the Limberg flap to close breast wounds after partial mastectomy, *Ann R Coll Surg Engl* 67:245, 1985.

24. Luscher NJ, Kuhn W, Zach GA: Rhomboid flaps in surgery for decubital ulcers: indications and results, *Ann Plast Surg* 16:415, 1986.

25. Quaba AA, Sommerland BC: "A square peg into a round hole": a modified rhomboid flap and its clinical application, *Br J Plast Surg* 40:163, 1987.

EDITORIAL COMMENTS

Shan R. Baker

The author has described the geometry of the rhombus defect, its common variations and his surgical technique for harvesting rhombic flaps. The flap is mainly a transposition flap that moves about a pivot but is also an advancement flap in which the flap's pivotal point is advanced toward the defect in an attempt to close the donor site. A standing cutaneous deformity always develops at the pivotal point of the flap. The greatest wound tension is located along a vector extending from the pivotal point 20° to the short diagonal of the rhombic defect. Reconstruction with a rhombic flap often makes use of secondary tissue movement, thus care must be exercised in design of the flap so that secondary movement will not distort important facial structures such as the vermilion, eyelid, or margin of the nasal ala.

Design of the rhombic flap is more complex than most other facial skin flaps because of the geometry and the option of placing the flap in four separate locations about a rhombus defect. I do not use the rhombic flap frequently in my practice, primarily because approximately half of the entire length of the scar that results from such repair is not parallel with or does not fall within the natural skin creases of the face. This disadvantage is more important in the area of the forehead and temple, where skin creases are more prominent; it is less important in the cheek, where creases are not as prominent, the skin is thinner, and the resulting scar tends to blend better with the adjacent skin.

EDITORIAL COMMENTS

Neil A. Swanson

The rhombus flap and its variations are perhaps the most useful reconstructive options for the surgeon. They also can be the most difficult to visualize. This chapter begins with an excellent review of the history and pertinent geometry of the rhombic flap. Also helpful is a review of the semantics of a rhombus, rhomboid, and rhombic flap.

The geometry of this flap is important. It is one of the few flaps in which I actually measure limbs. Each side of the parallelogram as well as each side of the flap to be transposed should be equal in length. The only case in which this does not hold true is when one is attempting to place a larger flap into a smaller defect. This is done along functional areas, such as an eyelid or lip, where one wishes to make sure that the free margin is not distorted by secondary tissue motion. I have begun to think of this flap in terms of tissue volume. In the sense of the pure rhombus (Limberg) flap, the angles in the parallelogram as well as the flap to be transposed are 60°. This means that the volume of tissue being transposed will be approximately equal to the volume of the defect. Once the secondary defect is closed, the flap should lie in place and basically fill the entire defect without tension. There will be very little secondary motion. As Dr. Bray states, this flap in its purest sense is seldom used. One usually varies the

angle that the initial arm of the rhombic flap exits the defect as well as the angle of the flap itself depending on several factors. For me, these factors include (1) where I wish to place the flap in relation to RSTLs, (2) the degree of secondary motion that is possible to assist closure of the primary defect, (3) the degree of tissue movement that allows closure of the secondary defect, and (4) blood supply.

If one refers to Fig. 10-4 *(left)* in Dr. Bray's chapter, on transposition of tissue into the defect the side of the flap, B-A-D, will collapse. This is the secondary motion. The degree of this collapse will depend on the take-off angle of line C-E as well as the absolute angle C-E-F. With a pure rhombus flap, there is very little collapse or secondary motion. With a Dufourmental (45° angle), there is some collapse and with the 30° angle flap there is collapse of approximately half of the volume of the defect. Therefore, one must understand the principle of secondary tissue motion when deciding the appropriate option of the rhombic flap. It is also sometimes difficult to visualize what the final suture line will be. I like to teach resident physicians to cover lines C-D and E-F (Fig. 10-4) with their finger, obliterating them. The remaining lines E-C-B-A-D, are the approximate lines of closure. This has been useful in getting beginners to visualize what the final scar will be with this flap.

By geometric definition, there will always be a standing cutaneous deformity with rhombic flaps. Unless one enlarges the defect to make a 30° angle, as does Webster, or uses a 30° flap, any angle other than this will usually leave a standing cutaneous deformity. The placement of this deformity can become very important in the design of the flap. During removal of the deformity, remember to widen the base of the flap.

As a Mohs reconstructive surgeon, I often place a rhombic flap into a circle. The beginning Mohs surgeon may wish to make the circle into a parallelogram. However, with experience one can pick the exit point from the circle, visualizing the circle as a parallelogram, and transpose the flap. When I started to use rhombic flaps several years ago, I would cut the flap to fit into the circle, producing rounded lines. With more experience, I will now make sure the flap is cut with a generous volume and, once the secondary defect is closed, will enlarge the circular defect to fit the angular transposition flap. This results in straight lines in the closure and lessens the chance of "pooching" of the flap itself.

Last, I'd like to comment on case 1, the lip example (Fig. 10-9). Whenever possible, I like to stay within the esthetic unit of the lip during lip reconstruction. Occasionally one needs to move cheek tissue into the lip. The design of the flap shown results in the suture line from closure of the secondary defect going against RSTLs. Although a portion of the flap fits within the melolabial sulcus, the sulcus itself will be blunted compared with the opposite side. This will often recover over time. There are times when this flap or an inferiorly based melolabial flap is necessary to close a large esthetic unit defect of the lip. However, I try hard to stay within the lip's esthetic unit during reconstruction of the lip itself.

11

BILOBE FLAPS

John A. Zitelli

Shan Ray Baker

INTRODUCTION

The bilobe flap is a workhorse flap for facial reconstruction and historically has been underused. With modifications from its original design, it is the flap of choice for reconstruction of certain defects on the lower third of the nose.

The bilobe flap is a double transposition flap. The primary flap is used to repair the surgical defect and a secondary flap is elevated to repair the original flap donor site. The secondary flap donor site is then closed primarily.

The original design of the bilobe flap is attributed to Esser,[1] who described its use in 1918 for reconstruction of nasal tip defects. Ziminy[2] and others later described an expanded use for the flap for defects on the trunk and soles. However, most authors now share the opinion that this flap is most useful for facial reconstruction, particularly the nose.

Esser's original design required that the angle of tissue transfer be 90° between each lobe of the flap, for a total transposition over 180° (Fig. 11-1). An example of this design for a nasal tip defect would be a primary donor flap from the nasal sidewall and a secondary flap from the glabella. This design of a 180° transfer maximizes the distance that skin can be moved, but the wide angles also maximize standing cutaneous deformities and the likelihood of pincushioning of both primary and secondary flaps. These are common complications of the original design that limit the use of this flap for facial reconstruction.

McGregor and Soutar[3] later altered this design and noted that the angle of tissue transfer could be varied greatly from the original 90° between each flap. In 1989 Zitelli[4] published his experience using the bilobe flap for nasal reconstruction. He emphasized the use of narrow angles of transfer: 45° between each lobe, so that the total transposition occurs over no more than 90° to 110° (Fig. 11-2). Complications of trapdoor deformities and pincushioning were thus avoided. Burget[5] confirmed excellent results using this flap on the nose. Other surgeons also advocated a similar design using narrow transposition angles and achieved better results than when using 180° transposition bilobe flaps on the cheek, chin, and lips.[6]

BIOMECHANICS

At first glance the bilobe flap would appear to be a modified rotation flap with some component of transposition. However, during movement of tissue, there is a greater release of tension on the primary donor flap than might be predicted by rotation alone. This increased movement of the primary flap and release of tension is accomplished by the transposion of skin. The mechanical release of tension is identical to that of a Z-plasty (Fig. 11-3). Assuming that the primary flap (without the creation of the second lobe) would be transposed into the defect under tension, the addition of a Z-plasty releases tension and enhances transposition about a pivotal point.

Bilobe flaps expand the use of the transposition flap. Defects that cannot be covered with a single transposition flap because the tension of wound closure causes distortion of important cosmetic structures may now be repaired with less wound closure tension by the addition of the second tension-releasing lobe. Furthermore, these flaps transfer the tension of wound closure through a 90° arc, which is more than the usual 45° to 60° pivot of a single transposition flap. This greater movement about a pivotal point also helps to minimize distortion of the primary defect.

One apparent disadvantage of this flap is the use of multiple small curved lines that do not follow preexisting skin folds or wrinkles. An alternative modification using a bilobe double rhombic flap can be used to eliminate the curves. The design is similar but the circular lobes of the flaps are replaced by rhombic flaps. This modification still requires the use of multiple short lines in various directions. Fortunately, with accurate suturing techniques and postoperative dermabrasion, the scars resulting from both types of flaps may be barely noticeable.

Figure 11-1 Standard design of bilobe flap. Design results in prominent standing cutaneous deformity at base of two flaps.

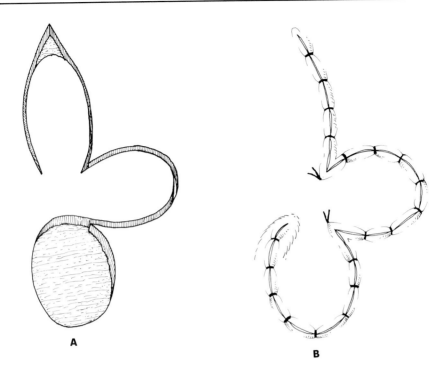

A

B

Figure 11-2 Improved design minimizes standing cutaneous deformities and reduces chance of trapdoor deformation.

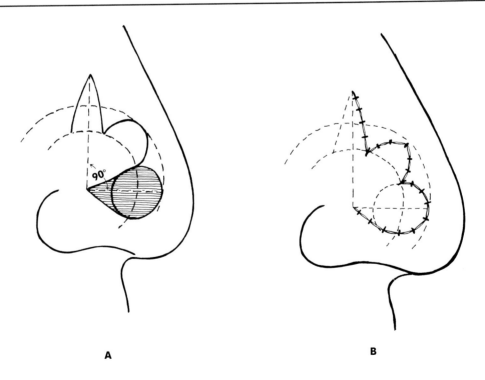

A

B

Figure 11-3   Use of Z-plasty transposition to improve tissue movement. If line A represents line of maximum tension, then Z-plasty as drawn will lengthen line A. This in turn will improve movement and reduce tension on primary flap.

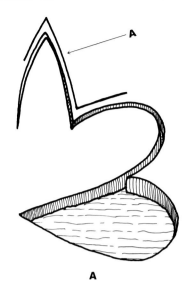

A

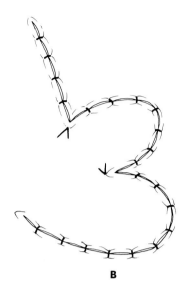

B

CLINICAL APPLICATIONS

Many surgeons with experience using bilobe flaps report that it is best suited for use on the lower third of the nose. In one review of 400 nasal reconstructions the bilobe flap was the most commonly used flap.[4]

The nose has unique characteristics that a surgeon must consider when choosing a local flap for reconstruction. The topography is complex, with multiple adjacent convex and concave surfaces. The free margins of the alar rims are mobile and easily elevated or displaced. The skin over the lower third of the nose has limited mobility and cannot be recruited for local flaps. The texture is unique so that only nearby skin will provide an adequate match.

The bilobe flap is well suited for the nose. With little wound closure tension on the primary flap, there is little or no distortion when the flap is used for repair of defects located near the alar rim. The use of skin adjacent to the defect allows for excellent color and texture match. The donor site of the secondary flap is closed primarily because the secondary flap lies in the lax skin of the upper dorsum and nasal sidewall, where easy side-to-side closure can occur. The base of the bilobe flap is usually positioned laterally, and the nasalis muscle is included in the substance of the flap, enhancing an excellent blood supply with little risk of necrosis. Even medially based flaps do well, although the vascular supply is not as rich without a musculocutaneous component.

As mentioned, this flap works best for defects on the lower third of the nose. The upper limit in size of such defects is approximately 1.5 cm. Repair of these defects uses skin from the upper dorsum and sidewall, where the generous lax skin allows easy transposition of the secondary lobe. However, for defects higher on the nose the recruitment of skin for the secondary flap must occur nearer to the medial canthus, where the skin is immobile. Thus defects on the upper half of the nose are not well suited for reconstruction with use of this flap.

The bilobe flap has limited usefulness on the ear because of the lack of lax skin to recruit for construction of the flap. The flap may be used for some helical rim defects in which skin is recruited from the medial surface of the auricle and the postauricular sulcus. Even in these cases free grafts, helical rim advancement flaps, or pedicle flaps are more useful for reconstruction than the bilobe flap.

On the cheek the bilobe flap can be useful when simple rotation flaps will not provide enough tissue. This occurs when the defect is large and located in the midcheek away from the central part of the face. In this situation the amount of remaining cheek skin available for reconstruction may not fill a large cheek defect and still enable closure of the donor site. Instead, the bilobe flap designed to recruit infraauricular (cervical) skin can be useful. Obviously lines of closure do not fall in wrinkle lines on the cheek, but the advantage of lack of wound closure tension and subsequent distortion outweigh the disadvantages of the final curvilinear scar.

SURGICAL TECHNIQUE

The ideal choice for the bilobe flap is a small defect (less than 1.5 cm) located on the lateral nasal tip or sidewall. This flap is usually small, and therefore the use of local anesthesia consisting of lidocaine and epinephrine is adequate for elevation of the flap. The flap has a geometrically important design. Initially a Burow's triangle is designed with its apex pointing laterally and one side parallel to the alar crease. The base of this triangle is approximately one half to two thirds the diameter of the defect. The apex serves as a focal point for the rest of the design. Each donor lobe is designed around one arc through the center of the defect and another arc through the distal end of the defect (Fig. 11-2). Each flap's center radius is positioned at approximately 45° from each other and 45° from the radius of the defect. After outlining the flap, local anesthesia is infiltrated. The flap is incised and elevated.

The level of undermining during elevation is important. In general, undermining occurs just above perichondrium and periosteum. In most cases nasalis muscle is included in the base of the flap but not in the tip of the flap. The thickness at the tip of the primary donor flap can vary. If it is recruited from thick skin and placed into a shallow defect, the distal most portion of the flap can be thinned to dermis. In this situation it is important that the recipient defect is as deep as possible (to cartilage) before thinning the flap. If fat is present on the donor flap, it can easily be thinned so no more than 1 mm of fat is included at the distal edges. Ideally the donor flap should be just slightly thinner than the depth of the defect. In this way elevation during the healing phase results in a flat, level flap.

After elevation of the flap, wide peripheral undermining is important. This helps not only to reduce wound tension on the closure and facilitate flap movement but also to reduce the chance of development of a trapdoor deformity. Although the true pathogenesis of trapdoor deformity of flaps is unknown, it is my opinion that when no peripheral undermining is done around the recipient site of a flap, the contraction phase of wound healing is limited to the base of the flap. This contraction reduces the base area of the flap but not its volume, and therefore the flap elevates. On the other hand, when wide undermining is done around the defect, the platelike scar that is continuous beneath both the flap and its adjacent skin edge will contract uniformly, stabilizing the entire surgical site and preventing the trapdoor deformity.

After elevation of the flap and undermining the edges of the recipient site, hemostasis is obtained. On the nose, bleeding is often profuse especially at the flap's base and superficial skin edges. Hemostasis must be precise so that a dry field is obtained without excess char from electrocautery. Destruction of tissue by excess electrocoagulation and/or a hematoma from inadequate hemostasis will result in vigorous wound contraction and an increased likelihood of a trapdoor deformation.

The primary flap is transposed into the defect and the secondary flap is transposed into the donor site of the primary flap. As with most transposition flaps, closure begins with the donor site of the secondary flap. Next, the primary flap is sutured into place and finally, the secondary flap is trimmed to fit the remaining defect before it is sutured.

The type of suture technique used is important in determination of the final cosmetic result. Most important, the flap's wound edges (deep aspect) need to be sutured together just as do the more superficial skin edges. When the flap is first elevated, the elastic deep dermal tissue retracts more than the inelastic superficial skin edges. If the superficial edges alone are sutured, the retracted dermis leaves a dead space that heals by contraction, leaving a depressed scar. The deep dermal component of the flap and wound edges are approximated by buried vertical mattress sutures which will also provide prolonged eversion of the wound until healing is complete.[7] The final skin closure must be meticulous so that the edges are even, minimizing the visible scar resulting from wound healing.

On the nose the cosmetic results are best when the bilobe flap is used in patients with thin lax skin in contrast to thick inelastic skin. Patients with thick sebaceous or rhinophymatous skin have a higher risk of flap necrosis and infection. These patients are best managed with prophylactic antibiotics administered preoperatively or intraoperatively. Attention to details such as aspirin intake and avoidance of smoking will help to minimize complications in nearly all patients.

The complication rate is low with a properly designed and executed bilobe flap. The risk of wound infection is less than 1%. Although slight epidermal sloughing of the flap may occur in as many as 10% of the cases, full-thickness necrosis is much less common. When flap necrosis does occur, it is managed by occlusive dressings as the wound heals. Rarely is any surgical debridement necessary. Trapdoor deformities are extremely rare and quickly respond to treatment with less than 1 ml of intralesional triamcinolone 40 mg/ml.

Dermabrasion is often useful after nasal reconstruction with use of a bilobe flap. This is best accomplished at 6 weeks after surgery when the scar is young.[8] It is most often necessary in cases with thick sebaceous nasal skin and rarely necessary with thin skin if there has been meticulous attention to suturing techniques.

CASE EXAMPLES

CASE 1

A 54-year-old woman was referred for treatment of a 1.5-cm ulcerated basal cell carcinoma on the right lower sidewall and tip of the nose. It was excised with Mohs surgery, leaving the surgical defect shown in Fig. 11-4**A.** The location of this defect on the lower sidewall and tip presented a classical choice for a bilobe flap. It was too low on the nose and too large for a single transposition flap (rhombic or Banner) but was well suited for borrowing of skin from the nasal sidewall in the form of a bilobe flap. The planned incision lines were marked with the Burow's triangle that already was excised. At this stage the closure of the defect resulting from the secondary flap will be by horizontal skin movement and will result in a vertical line. Note in Fig. 11-4**A** how narrow the base of the flap may be and still remain viable.

In Fig. 11-4**B** the flap has been undermined, transposed, and sutured. There is no distortion of the ala. If alar distortion occurs with this flap, it is more likely caused by tight closure of the secondary donor site, although suturing of the primary flap occasionally pulls slightly on the nasal tip. Fig. 11-4**C** shows the cosmetic results 6 months after reconstruction without dermabrasion.

CASE 2

A 47-year-old woman with a basal cell carcinoma on the right lower nasal sidewall and tip resulted in a 1 × 1 cm defect of the lower sidewall of the nose after Mohs surgery (Fig. 11-5**A**). This was repaired with a bilobe flap similar to that in case 1 (Fig. 11-5**B**). (The Burow's triangle should be kept above the alar crease when possible; this design keeps all incisions within a single esthetic unit.) If this defect had been more lateral, a single transposition flap based inferiorly at the junction of the nose and cheek would have been a good reconstruction option. However, the more medial location of the defect made a single transposition flap difficult and likely to distort the ala and nasal tip as well as violate the alar-facial sulcus, which is an important esthetic junction zone between the cheek and sidewall of the nose. The flap was sutured so that it was level or slightly below the surrounding nasal skin (Fig. 11-5**C**). The second lobe of the flap was trimmed appropriately to accommodate the shape of the donor site resulting from harvesting of the primary lobe. The result 1 year after reconstruction without dermabrasion of the scar is seen in Fig. 11-5**D.**

Figure 11-4   *A,* A 2.5 × 1 cm nasal defect ideally located for repair with bilobe flap. Bilobe flap is designed with narrow base and will pivot through arc of 90°. *B,* Transposed flap. *C,* Appearance 6 months postoperatively.

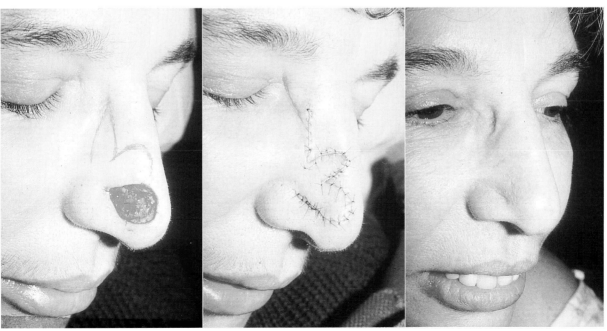

A   B   C

Figure 11-5   *A*, 1 × 1 cm skin defect after removal of nasal skin cancer. *B*, Bilobe flap designed. Standing cutaneous deformity is excised in alar-nasal crease for maximum scar camouflage. *C*, Flap transposed. *D*, Appearance 1 year postoperatively.

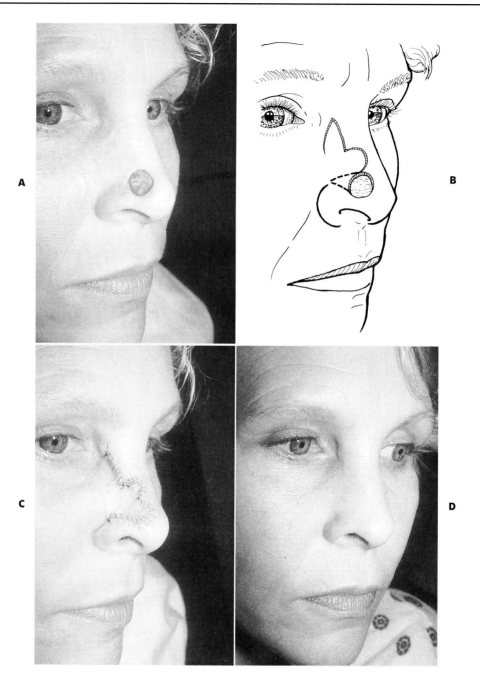

CASE 3

A 72-year-old woman had a recurrent basal cell carcinoma on the lower midnasal dorsum in the supratip area. The lesion was excised by Mohs surgery and resulted in a circular surgical defect with a diameter that measured 1.6 cm (Fig. 11-6**A**). The skin surrounding the defect was thick and would have been difficult to match with a free skin graft other than one harvested from the immediate adjacent nasal dorsum. Use of a bilobe flap was believed to be a good method

of repair because it was more likely to provide a perfect color and texture match and less likely to necrose than a free graft or more peripherally located flap.

After transposition and suturing of the flap, there was a slight upward pull on the patient's right nasal tip and ala (Fig. 11-6**B**). This pull is almost always a temporary deformation unless the distortion is extreme (more than 3 mm). The alar distortion resolved spontaneously by 6 months postoperatively (Fig. 11-6**C** and **D**). A very light dermabrasion was performed 6 weeks postoperatively.

Figure 11-6   *A*, **Supratip nasal defect 1.6 cm in diameter. Bilobe flap is designed to recruit skin from remaining lower nasal dorsum and lateral nose.** *B*, **Flap transposed. Standing cutaneous deformity has been excised in supratip area.** *C* **and** *D*, **Appearance 6 months postoperatively. Dermabrasion of scar was performed 6 weeks after flap transfer.**

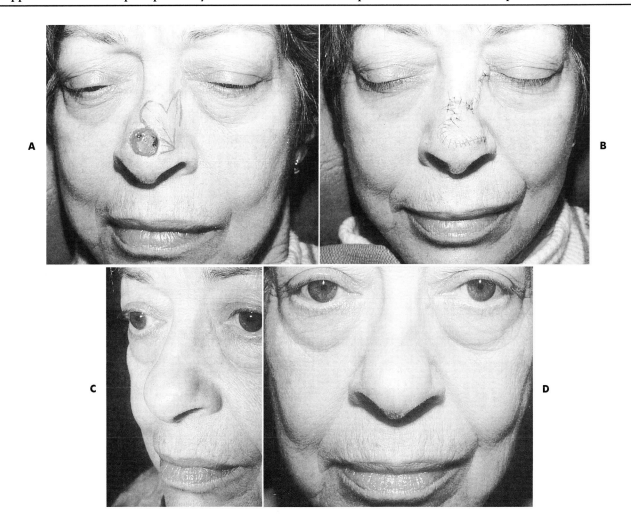

CASE 4

A 41-year-old man had a 1 × 1 cm skin defect on the left lateral nasal tip after excision of a basal cell carcinoma by Mohs surgery (Fig. 11-7**A**). Although the location of this defect was common, reconstruction was difficult because the patient's skin was thick and sebaceous. A skin graft would have poorly matched the thickness of adjacent nasal skin. Furthermore, his taunt nasal skin made a scar more noticeable and more difficult to camouflage than would be the case in thin loose nasal skin of an older patient who may have other skin blemishes to help camouflage the scar. A bilobe flap provided the means to use well-matched nearby skin. (The surgeon must take care with this type of skin to incise the full thickness of the skin to the plane above the perichondrium, because in patients with thicker skin there is a tendency to undermine too superficially, which increases the risk of flap necrosis.) The flap was designed and transposed with use of the methods discussed in the Surgical Technique section (Fig. 11-7**B** and **C**). Fig. 11-7**D** and **E** shows the result of reconstruction 6 months after wound repair without dermabrasion of the scars.

Figure 11-7 *A*, 1 × 1 cm lateral nasal tip defect located in thick sebaceous skin. *B*, **Bilobe flap designed. Standing cutaneous deformity is removed from lateral tip area.** *C*, **Flap transposed.** *D* and *E*, **Appearance 6 months postoperatively.**

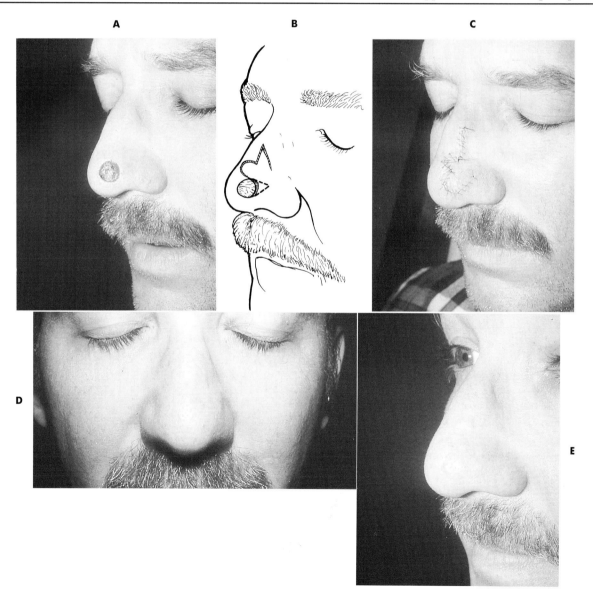

CASE 5

A 63-year-old woman was referred for treatment of a primary basal cell carcinoma on the nose. It was excised by Mohs surgery and resulted in a circular surgical defect on the right lateral nasal tip and lower sidewall that measured 1.5 cm in diameter. This case presented a reconstructive challenge not only because of the location of the defect but also because of the thick skin surrounding the defect (Fig. 11-8**A** and **B**). The bilobe flap was best based medially to prevent alar distortion. If based laterally, as in the previous cases, excision of the standing cutaneous deformity would be located on the surface of the ala and could distort it after repair of the defect. Furthermore, the base of the flap would be positioned in the alar-nasal crease, which may not provide an adequate blood supply for the flap and at best would distort the crease. There are significant disadvantages to a medially based bilobe nasal flap. First, the potential standing cutaneous deformity occurs toward the midline and may accentuate a prominent nasal tip; the blood supply to the flap's base is not as great as if it were based laterally. There is not as much skin laxity and motion compared with the laterally based flap. However, in this case the advantages outweighed the disadvantages.

After transposition and suturing of the flap, there was a slight upward pull on the medial alar rim (Fig. 11-8**C**). This mild distortion of the alar margin completely resolved by 6 months postoperatively (Fig. 11-8**D**).

Figure 11-8   *A,* **Defect of lateral nasal tip measuring 1.5 cm in diameter. Defect is surrounded by thick sebaceous skin.** *B,* **Medially based bilobe flap designed. Standing cutaneous deformity will be excised in supratip region.** *C,* **Flap transposed. There is mild distortion of alar margin.** *D,* **Six months postoperatively alar margin distortion is no longer apparent.**

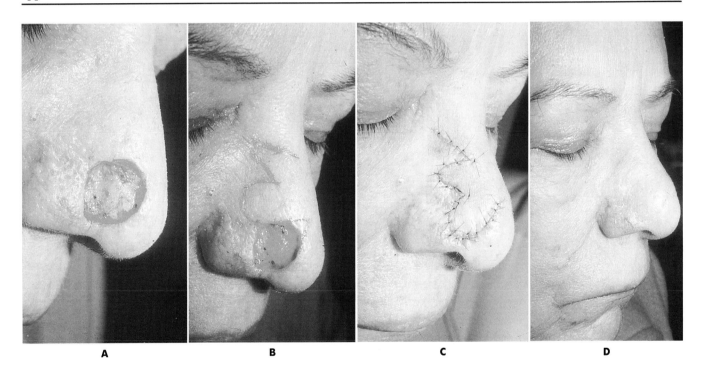

A   B   C   D

CASE 6

An 80-year-old man presented with a 1.8 × 1.5 cm defect on the right alar lobule after Mohs surgery for a basal cell carcinoma (Fig. 11-9**A**). A medially based bilobe nasal flap was used for reconstruction (Fig. 11-9**B**). Other reconstructive options included a melolabial transposition flap or a full-thickness skin graft. A conchal bowl full-thickness skin graft might have provided adequate thickness, good texture, and mini-

mal contraction. Instead a bilobe flap was utilized based medially.

For reduction of wound closure tension, the flap was widely undermined over much of the nose before transposition and suturing (Fig. 11-9**C**). Fig. 11-9**D** and **E** shows the results 2 years postoperatively. Note the pull on the patient's left alar rim, which may have resulted from excessive wound closure tension after repair of the secondary donor site.

Figure 11-9   *A*, 1.8 × 1.5 cm right alar lobule defect after Mohs surgery for basal cell carcinoma. *B*, **Medially based bilobe flap designed.** *C*, **Flap transposed. Standing cutaneous deformity is partly excised in alar-nasal crease.** *D* and *E*, **Two years postoperatively some distortion of alar margin is noted.**

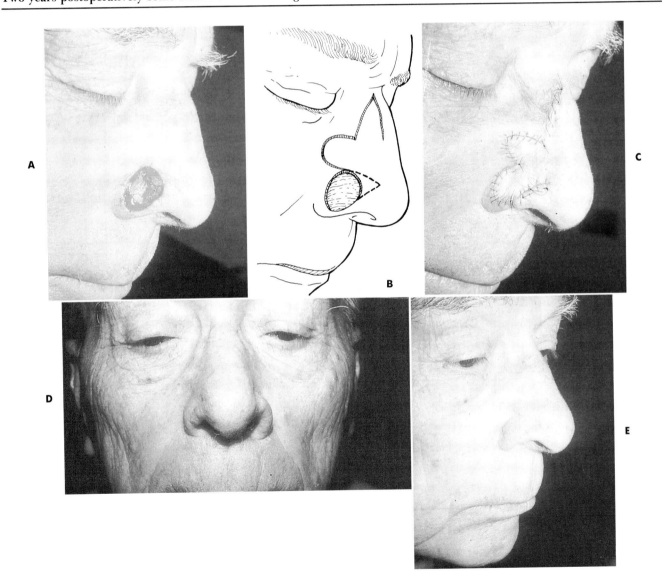

CASE 7

A 79-year-old woman was treated for a recurrent basal cell carcinoma on the lower nasal dorsum above the supratip area. It resulted in a circular full-thickness skin defect with a diameter of 9 mm (Fig. 11-10**A**). This case demonstrated a variation of the classical curvilinear bilobe flap: a bilobe rhombic flap (Fig. 11-10**B**). This flap uses short straight lines, which may provide better scar camouflage compared with the curved lines of the traditional bilobe flap. It is not commonly used, however, because it requires enlargement of the typical circular defect into a rhombic defect and uses the tips of the flaps for wound closure (Fig. 11-10**C**). The most peripheral tips of the flap were the portions that are most susceptible to necrosis. The rhombic modification of the bilobe flap is most useful for small rectangular defects. For larger defects the movement of the surrounding skin after transposition of the primary flap and closure of the site of the secondary flap results in a change in the shape of the donor site of the primary flap. For a small flap this change is minor and the precut rhombic flap fits nicely. But for larger defects, the secondary flap must be trimmed to fit the altered shape of the donor site of the primary flap. Fig. 11-10**D** shows the reconstructed area 6 months postoperatively. The scar was dermabraded.

Figure 11-10   *A*, Circular defect after Mohs surgery for recurrent basal cell carcinoma. *B*, Bilobe flap modified to have rhombic flaps is planned for reconstruction. Circular defect must be converted to rhombic defect. *C*, Flap transposed. *D*, Six months postoperatively. Scar has been dermabraded.

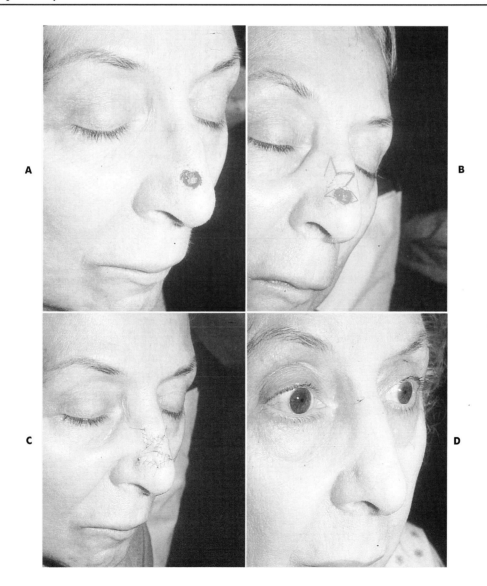

CASE 8

This 63-year-old man had a recurrent amelanotic lentigo maligna on the right cheek after multiple treatments with destructive techniques (Fig. 11-11*A*). The area was excised with the use of Mohs surgery, resulting in a large defect that measured 5 × 7 cm (Fig. 11-11*B*). The patient's ruddy skin provided a challenge for a match of any skin used for reconstruction. The defect was too large and too near the ear for a single inferiorly based rotation cheek flap and would other-wise require a much larger cervicofacial flap. A bilobe flap was designed using the skin in the preauricular, infraauricular, and upper cervical areas (Fig. 11-11*C*).

The extra motion allowed during transposition of the second flap, as discussed earlier, provided coverage without the need for a larger cervicofacial rotation advancement flap. This flap was completed with the patient under local anesthesia (Fig. 11-11*D*). To minimize tension on the wound edge in the area of the lateral canthus, the flap was suspended from the periosteum of the zygoma with periosteal sutures. The

Figure 11-11 *A*, Recurrent amelanotic lentigo maligna in 63-year-old man. *B*, After resection 5 × 7 cm defect of facial skin is present in central area of cheek. *C*, Design of bilobe flap uses skin in preauricular, infraauricular, and upper cervical areas. *D*, Flap transposed. Large standing cutaneous deformity is excised near melolabial fold. *E* and *F*, Appearance 6 months postoperatively.

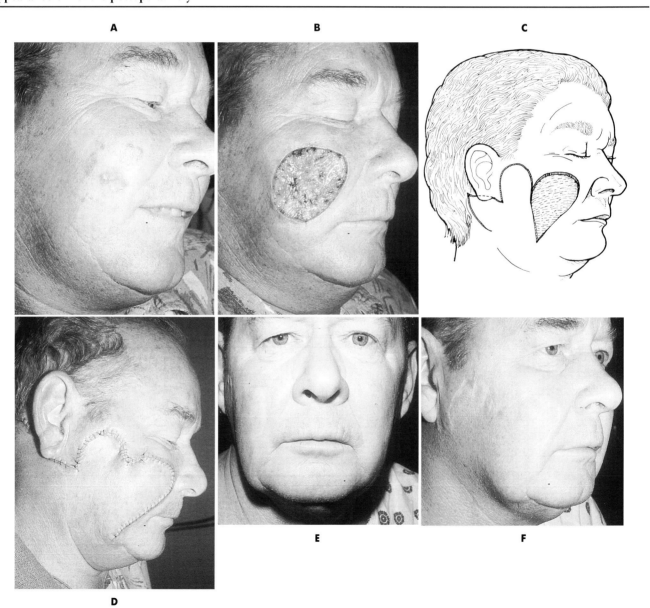

usual Burow's triangle was excised in the jowl area. Additional redundant skin in the jowl area was later excised again for a better cosmetic result. The patient's ruddy complexion and some necrosis of the secondary flap accentuated the scar line, which is observed in Fig.

11-11**E** and **F** 6 months after initial reconstruction.

Fig. 11-11**G** through **L** shows a similar case in which a bilobe flap was used to reconstruct an even larger central cheek defect.

Figure 11-11, cont'd. *G,* Lentigo maligna in a 74-year-old man. *H,* Proposed border of resection margin with large bilobe flap designed. *I,* Primary lobe of bilobe flap is remaining preauricular skin. Source for secondary lobe is from postauricular and upper posterior cervical skin. *J,* Oval surgical defect measures 14 × 7 cm. *K,* Bilobe flap transposed. *L,* Four months postoperatively small persistent standing cutaneous deformity is noted at junction of base of primary and secondary flaps. (Courtesy Ted Cook, M.D.)

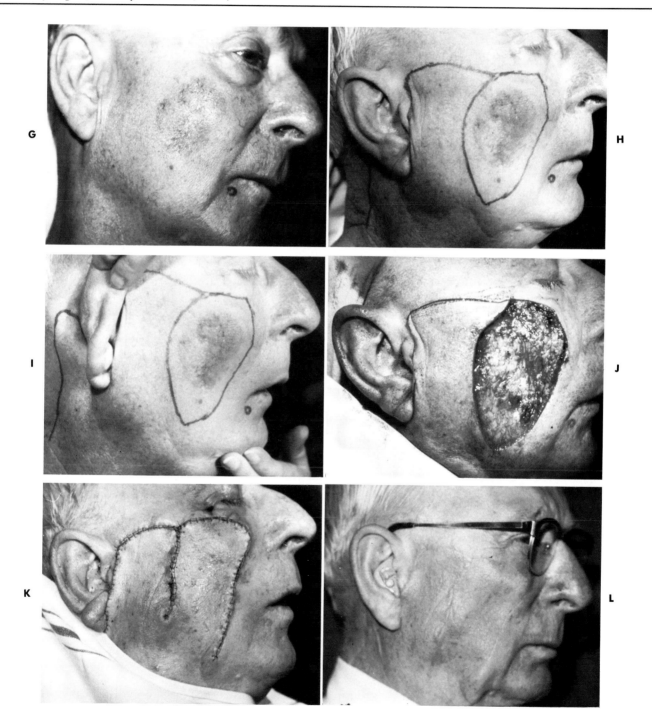

CASE 9

A 60-year-old patient had a primary basal cell carcinoma on the posterior surface of the right helix. The tumor was excised by Mohs surgery and resulted in an extensive loss of skin and cartilage and a surgical defect measuring 1.3 × 2.5 cm (Fig. 11-12**A**). If cartilage and perichondrium had been spared, a skin graft would have been a good option for reconstruction. If a smaller amount of cartilage and skin had been missing, helical rim advancement flaps would have been a good choice and would have reduced the vertical height of the ear slightly. Alternatively a cartilage graft and two-stage pedicle flap could have

Figure 11-12 *A*, Skin and cartilage defect of helix measuring 1.3 × 2.5 cm. Bilobe flap is designed in anticipation of reconstruction. *B*, Appearance of ear immediately after flap transposition. *C* and *D*, One month postoperatively notching of helix resulted from lack of replacement of missing cartilage with free cartilage graft and from use of flap insufficient in size to provide adequate soft-tissue replacement.

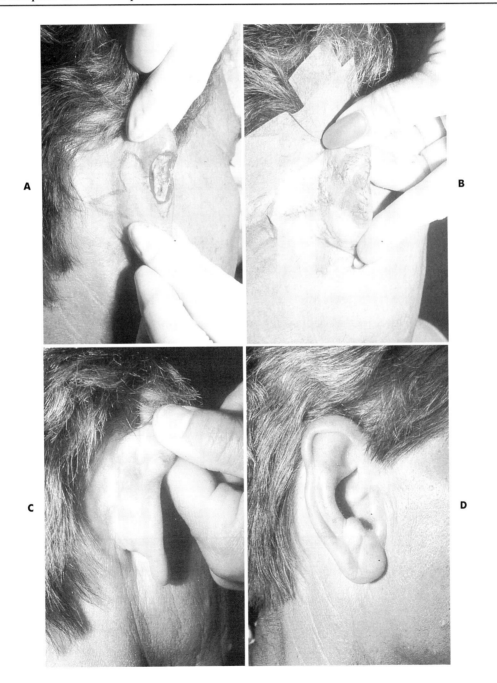

been used to repair the defect. However, a single-stage procedure with use of a bilobe flap was chosen to provide the soft-tissue coverage.

The bilobe flap was designed to use the postauricular skin (Fig. 11-12**A**). Wide peripheral undermining was performed before transposition and suturing of the flap (Fig. 11-12**B**). Fig. 12**C** and **D** shows the results 1 month postoperatively. Note the notching of the helix. This was accentuated because the cartilage deficit was not replaced. The deformity also reflects the tension on the bilobe flap when used on the ear compared with the greater laxity possible with bilobe flaps on the nose. This notch might have been prevented by use of a wider flap. A wider primary lobe was not employed because the larger convex surface of the helical rim was not accounted for during measurement of the defect. The defect was, in error, measured in a flat plane from side to side.

SUMMARY

The bilobe flap is a useful flap for surgical reconstruction. This chapter described a few variations in design that improve its usefulness, including the following: (1) the use of a Burow's triangle at the base,(2) transposition of each flap over 45° instead of 90° for a total of only 90° for both flaps, and (3) the need for wide peripheral undermining of the skin surrounding the defect as well as the flap and its donor sites. With these modifications the bilobe flap is unique in its ability to mobilize skin from nearby donor sites without causing distortion of the skin near the defect. The biomechanics of this skin motion are similar to the release of tension provided by the Z-plasty transposition flap.

The bilobe flap is best suited for reconstruction of circular defects on the lower third of the nose. In this location reconstruction with other types of flaps is difficult. The bilobe nasal flap allows movement of well-matched nearby skin without causing nasal distortion. The cosmetic result is excellent and easily surpasses the commonly used skin graft. As a consequence

the bilobe flap is a preferred flap for reconstruction of the distal lateral aspect of the nose.

Variations of this flap are useful. The flap can be based medially on the nose, although it works best and is most often used with a lateral base. Its lobes may be designed in rhombic shapes for smaller defects. A bilobe flap may be used for large defects located on the cheek in lieu of larger cervicofacial rotation advancement flaps. It also may be useful for transfer of skin from the postauricular area to cover helical rim defects that might otherwise require more difficult reconstructive techniques.

The bilobe flap is a true workhorse flap that should be in the armamentarium of every reconstructive surgeon. With the modifications described herein, it is a flap of choice for reconstruction of defects on the lower one third of the nose.

REFERENCES

1. Esser JFS: Gestielte lokale Nasenplastik mit Zweizipfligem lappen Deckung des Sekundaren Detektes vom ersten Zipfel durch den Zweiten, *Dtsch Z Chirurgie* 143:385, 1918.

2. Zimany A: The bilobed flap, *Plast Reconstr Surg* 11:424, 1953.

3. McGregor JC, Soutar DS: A critical assessment of the bilobed flap, *Br J Plast Surg* 34:197, 1981.

4. Zitelli JA: The bilobed flap for nasal reconstruction, *Arch Dermatol* 125:957, 1989.

5. Burget G: Creating a nasal form with flaps and grafts. In Bardach J, editor: *Local flaps and free skin grafts*, Philadelphia, 1992, Mosby-Year Book.

6. Marschall MA: Bilobed flap in head and neck reconstruction. In Bardach J, editor: *Local flaps and free skin grafts*, Philadelphia, 1992, Mosby-Year Book.

7. Zitelli JA, Moy RL: The buried vertical mattress suture, *J Dermatol Surg Oncol* 15:17, 1989.

8. Yarborough JM: Ablation of facial scars by programmed dermabrasion, *J Dermatol Surg Oncol* 14:292, 1988.

EDITORIAL COMMENTS

Shan R. Baker

Bilobe flaps are double transposition flaps that share a single base. Similar to a single transposition flap, bilobe flaps move around a pivotal point located at the base of the flap and develop standing cutaneous deformities as they pivot. The greater the arc of rotation about the pivotal point, the greater the standing cutaneous deformity. To minimize this deformity, it is wise to limit the degree of movement through the arc by

design of both flaps within 90° of the axis of the defect. However, the primary factor in determination of the location of the primary and secondary flaps of the bilobe flap is the location of the defect and the availability of donor skin for construction of the two flaps. The primary and secondary flaps are designed in areas of greatest skin laxity and/or in areas where scar camouflage will be maximized. This may on occasion necessitate design of the secondary flap along an axis that is 180° to the axis of the defect.

The great advantage of bilobe flaps is the ability to use lax skin, which may be located at some distance from the defect and which would be difficult to transfer to the defect by other surgical approaches. In general, bilobe flaps are designed in such a way that the primary flap is immediately adjacent to the defect and has a surface area that is less than the surface area of the defect. Thus, part of the closure of the defect is achieved by secondary movement of surrounding skin through direct advancement. The degree of reduction in surface area of the primary flap compared with the surface area of the defect depends on the location of the defect and the elasticity of surrounding skin. On the lower nose the primary flap must nearly approximate the size of the defect because of the inelasticity of nasal tip skin. In the cheek area, however, the primary flap may be designed considerably smaller than the size of the defect (up to 25% less in surface area) because of the elasticity of the skin of the cheek.

The secondary flap of a bilobe flap is usually designed so that its surface area is less than the surface area of the defect left by harvesting of the primary flap. Again, advancement of adjacent skin assists the secondary flap in repair of the donor site of the primary flap. The defect left by the secondary flap is closed primarily by direct advancement of surrounding skin. Thus, for the bilobe flap to work, there must be considerable skin laxity in the vicinity of the primary and secondary flap to achieve wound closure without excessive wound-closure tension.

In my opinion, the primary disadvantage of the bilobe flap is that most of the incision necessary to elevate and transfer the flap produces scars that do not parallel relaxed skin tension lines. The resulting scar is also lengthy due to the need to elevate two flaps.

EDITORIAL COMMENTS

Neil A. Swanson

Dr. Zitelli proves again why he's one of the most respected and talented teachers and surgeons of the local flap. He has mastered the bilobe flap and presents in a clear concise form his well-conceived technique. I agree completely that the best results with this flap occur when both lobes are transposed in less than a 180° arc. Whenever possible this flap should be designed as such. When one is forced to design the flap in the traditional 180° arc, the biggest mistake is to make the second flap of the bilobe too short. The longer the arc (180°), the longer the transposition reach of the second lobe of the bilobe. This also needs to extend well into the glabella to be long enough to fill the length of the defect created by transposition of the first lobe of the flap.

Again, this is a flap with a rounded edge. When this happens, "pooching" or trapdoor deformities can occur. I personally think that this can be prevented by the following: (1) extensive undermining of the surgical defect; (2) defatting, especially centrally, of the flap

to be transposed; and (3) meticulous suture technique with buried and cutaneous sutures. Again, I often maintain the Mohs surgical bevel and counterbevel the edge of the flap to form a tongue and groove type of fit for an improved suture line.

One point on which Dr. Zatelli and I disagree is when to remove the triangle which is, in essence, the redundant standing cutaneous deformity. He proposes to remove the triangle during the flap design before the tissue is moved. I remove this redundant tissue after I have transposed the flap. In doing so, often less tissue is removed than if preexcised and in a slightly different location than if the triangle of tissue were removed early. When this is done, one must always widen the base of the flap during removal of the triangle of redundant tissue.

As the author mentions, the suture lines of this flap can often be improved by dermabrasion. I agree that early dermabrasion in 7 to 8 weeks is certainly of benefit. I favor dermabrasion of the entire esthetic unit and not just the scar. I think that this leaves a superior result.

12

MELOLABIAL FLAPS

Ferdinand F. Becker

Robert E. Adham

INTRODUCTION

The nose is the most prominent feature on the face. As such, the nose is highly exposed to the sun and is the area that most frequently experiences the development of neoplastic skin lesions. In fact, cancer of the skin of the nose is the most common cancer in humans. Occasionally, congenital abnormalities, vascular abnormalities, and infectious processes (and the surgery used to eradicate these processes) leave significant nasal or perinasal skin deficits. Esthetic reconstruction of nasal and perinasal soft-tissue deficits must satisfy several goals: reproduction of the gentle and complex folds and margins of the nose without unnecessary bulk, good color and texture match, and maintenance of structural support to ensure an adequately patent nasal airway.

The melolabial cheek fold adjacent to the nose and lips contains abundant skin with many of the attributes required for excellent nasal and perinasal reconstruction. The color match and texture is good, the skin is usually free of hair, and the skin has an excellent blood supply from branches of the facial artery.

Perinasal skin has been used for nasal reconstruction since the earliest descriptions of flaps.[1,2] During the late 19th and early 20th centuries, many varieties of melolabial flaps were reported,[3] and since then multiple variations have been described. These flaps have been called nasolabial flaps for years, but the term *melolabial* is more accurate and descriptive.

It is important to understand that superficial defects that do not extend to or through the nasal cartilages or bony skeleton are sometimes better left to heal by second intention (secondary scar tissue contracture) or may best be treated by skin grafting with suitable skin taken from the preauricular, cervical, supraclavicular, or infraclavicular donor areas. The decision whether to use primary closure, secondary intention healing, skin grafting, or a flap procedure is a matter of surgical judgment. In this chapter we discuss only melolabial flap procedures. Most of the wounds chosen for flap reconstruction will be too large or deep or unfavorably located so as to preclude secondary healing or skin grafting.

ANATOMIC CONSIDERATIONS

The melolabial sulcus is formed by the junction of the upper lip and lower nose with the cheek. It is created by the insertion of several of the mimetic facial muscles into the skin of the lip at this juncture. The forces of muscle contraction and gravity with time create an outpouching or mound of skin lateral to this crease in the medial area of the cheek, which is called the melolabial cheek fold. The cheek skin in this region has an extensive and excellent blood supply from perforating branches of the facial artery and is drained by the facial and angular veins. Because of this rich blood supply, melolabial flaps may be based superiorly or inferiorly and, if properly designed and executed, will rarely fail in a suitable host. Abundant tissue is usually available in the melolabial area, and the size of the flap is limited only by the amount of cheek tissue that can be used in the flap and still effect a primary closure of the donor site in the melolabial sulcus. Because the melolabial sulcus is a prominent facial landmark, the donor site closure is usually easily hidden in this area.

COMMON TYPES

Superiorly Based Melolabial Flaps

The superiorly based melolabial flap is most useful for deep central and lateral nasal dorsal defects and defects of the nasal ala and tip. Superficial defects are frequently better left to heal by secondary intention or closed with a skin graft. The area of the nose where this flap is not as useful is the superior portion of the nose. If the flap is carried too far superiorly, it can result in a medial lower eyelid ectropion when the donor site is closed. The most cephalad portion of the nose lends itself better to coverage from the glabella and forehead area if flaps are chosen for closure.

Like all melolabial flaps, the superiorly based flap can usually be performed on an outpatient basis with use of local anesthesia or monitored anesthesia care in a treatment-room setting. General anesthesia in an operating room may be required for unhealthy or particularly sensitive patients or patients with a very large or deep defect.

Potential disadvantages of the superiorly based melolabial flap include the trapdoor or pincushion effect caused by scar contracture, blunting of the nasofacial sulcus, and asymmetry of the melolabial sulcus. These problems, however, can largely be eliminated or corrected with careful execution of the flap or with minor secondary procedures.

Inferiorly Based Melolabial Flaps

The inferiorly based melolabial flap is most useful for defects of the upper and lower lip, floor of the nose, and columella. This flap is ideal for lateral upper lip defects that involve only skin and muscle and do not involve the vermilion of the lip.

Potential disadvantages include scarring across the alar-facial groove and trapdoor deformity of the upper lip. Almost invariably when this flap is used, there is obliteration of the melolabial sulcus from the alar-facial sulcus to the level of the lateral commissure of the mouth. This problem can be corrected with a secondary procedure to recreate the melolabial fold. The pivotal point of the flap will often leave some bulkiness of the upper lip on the involved side, and this, too, can be corrected with a secondary procedure if necessary.

Advancement Melolabial Flaps

The sliding advancement melolabial flap is most useful for defects of the most lateral aspect of the nasal dorsum, lateral nasal alar defects which do not involve the alar rim, and defects which extend onto the cheek. It is particularly useful in closure of defects that are narrow and long. One of the major advantages of this flap is the fact that the closure lines of the donor and recipient areas fall in natural creases and natural shadows. The most superior line is usually along the junction of the nasal dorsal and sidewall esthetic subunits. The horizontal portion of the closure on the

nose is usually located somewhere near the nasal alar sulcus, and the donor site closure line is usually along the melolabial sulcus.

The main disadvantage of the advancement melolabial flap is distortion and loss of definition of the nasofacial sulcus.

SURGICAL TECHNIQUE

Preoperative planning begins with careful assessment of the depth, location, and extent of the defect. Photographs of the defect help the surgeon to plan and to mentally perform the reconstruction before entering the operative arena. All satisfactory alternatives for reconstruction of the nasal defect should be considered, from the simplest to the most complex. Healing by second intention (secondary scar tissue contracture), primary closure, full-thickness skin graft closure, and other local and regional flaps must be considered. Involvement of donor skin by scarring, actinic changes, or radiation effects must be considered and may preclude the use of a melolabial flap. The surgeon must also decide if creation of a larger defect to encompass an entire or several esthetic subunits would lend a more favorable final esthetic result.

Superiorly Based Melolabial Flap

Local anesthesia, sometimes supplemented with monitored anesthesia care, is usually possible during creation of a superiorly based melolabial flap. Infraorbital nerve block will anesthetize most of the area but should be reinforced with judicious local infiltration of local anesthetic. We almost invariably use 1% lidocaine with epinephrine, and have had no problems with flap necrosis attributed to vasoconstriction caused by the anesthetic agent.

In design of the flap, several points must be kept in mind. In general, melolabial flaps with a ratio of up to 4:1 in length to width can be used without the need for delay. The maximum width of the flap is limited by the amount of donor tissue available that can be elevated and still allow closure of the primary donor site. In general, defects greater than 2.5 to 3 cm in width are difficult to close with a melolabial flap. The medial incision for the flap should be planned to lie in the melolabial sulcus (Fig. 12-1**A**). The lateral incision should be kept as short as possible superiorly and can always be lengthened as the procedure continues. Generally this incision should be no higher on the cheek than the most inferior part of the nasal defect that is being reconstructed. If the lateral limb is made too high, it will narrow the base and could compromise the blood supply of the flap.

Figure 12-1 Design *(A)* and transposition *(B)* of superiorly based melolabial flap.

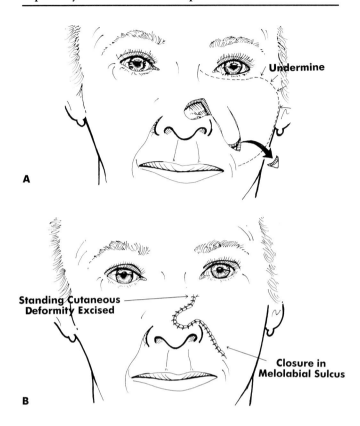

It is also important to design the flap so that the width of the flap is as wide as the height of the defect. The flap should fit the defect to allow little or no wound tension on closure (Fig. 12-1**B**). On the other hand, the flap should not be so large as to require crowding it into the defect. This would create a bulky, unnatural-looking repair.

In general, flaps should be kept thin and should consist only of skin and a thin layer of subdermal fat, maintaining the dermal-subdermal plexus. The subcutaneous layer can be thinned to approximately 2 mm proximally and 1 mm at the distal end of the flap. If bulk is required to fill a deep defect, fat should be trimmed to keep the surface of the flap slightly beneath the level of the surrounding skin. The reason for this is that excess fat will contract and could contribute to a significant trapdoor deformity. Before transposition of the flap into the defect and to allow closure of the donor site, wide undermining of the cheek skin lateral to the donor site must be performed in the midsubcutaneous plane (Fig. 12-1**A**). Frequently, undermining must be extended to the periorbital area, where the skin is very thin. In this area a small layer of orbicularis muscle may be lifted with the flap to ensure viability. Closure of the donor defect before closure of the primary defect brings the base of the flap closer to the nose, thereby facilitating subsequent closure of the primary defect with minimal wound closure tension. During transposition of the flap, there is an occasional tendency for blunting of the nasofacial sulcus. The normal concavity of the nasofacial sulcus can be reestablished with the use of an absorbable suspension suture placed between the undersurface of the dermis of the flap and the periosteum of the nasal bone or maxilla.

Some surgeons believe that the nasal skin around the primary defect should be undermined before closure to minimize the chance of trapdoor deformities.[5] Other surgeons condemn undermining of the primary defect, because they believe that undermining will blunt the natural subtle depressions around the nose, such as the nasofacial sulcus. Our feeling is that judicious undermining is prudent, as long as the surgeon is aware of the risk of subtle changes to the nasal contour.

It is often necessary to remove a standing cutaneous cone deformity (dog-ear) at the inferior limit of the donor site. If the flap has been incised in a pointed fashion, such as in a fusiform excision, this step will be unnecessary (Fig. 12-1**A**). In addition, there is usually a standing cutaneous deformity at the pivotal point of the flap. The excision of this redundant tissue should always be carried out away from the base of the flap so as not to narrow the base, which carries the vascular supply of the flap. If there is any question about the viability of the flap, the redundant tissue can be left in place. The patient is then informed that a secondary procedure to remove this redundant tissue will be carried out approximately 3 weeks after the primary procedure. If the defect on the nose directly abuts the flap, reconstruction can be accomplished in a single stage or a small skin bridge can be excised, resulting in a one-stage procedure. If the skin bridge is large between the defect and the flap, and it is impractical to excise, an interpolation flap may be necessary. In such cases a second stage to detach the flap is required 10 to 21 days after the primary procedure.

Postoperatively the wound is left uncovered or is covered with a light dressing to absorb any blood that may ooze from the suture line, with no significant compression applied on the flap or its base. The wound edges are cleaned with peroxide and covered with antibiotic ointment once or twice daily. Sutures are removed from 5 to 7 days postoperatively.

If troublesome hairs grow from the transposed skin, epilation may be performed after 1 month.

Inferiorly Based Melolabial Flap

The inferiorly based flap is designed by marking the medial incision of the flap along the melolabial sulcus and nasofacial sulcus as far as is necessary to allow

Figure 12-2   Design *(A)* and transposition *(B)* of inferiorly based melolabial flap.

Figure 12-3   Design *(A)* and transfer *(B)* of advancement melolabial flap.

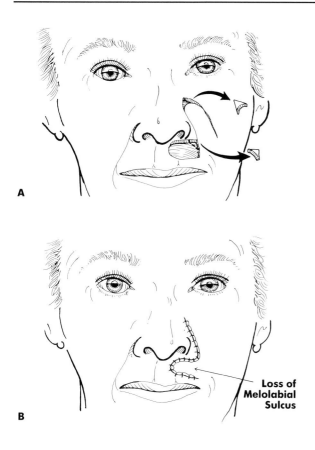

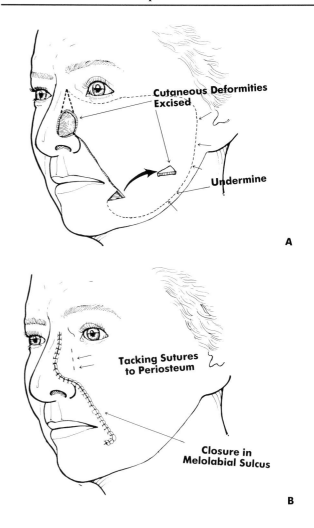

closure of the primary defect (Fig. 12-2**A**). This flap is frequently used to reconstruct upper and lower lip defects. The width of the flap is determined by the height of the defect. It is imperative that the flap be as wide as or slightly wider than the height of the defect to ensure that the lip is not shortened. The superior tip of the flap is tapered to a point to allow closure without a standing cutaneous deformity (Fig. 12-2**A**).

The use of local anesthesia, dissection of the flap and the surrounding cheek, and undermining of the skin adjacent to the recipient site is performed as described for the superiorly based flap. The donor site is closed in the natural melolabial sulcus and nasofacial sulcus. The pivotal point of the inferiorly based flap is located adjacent to the angle of the mouth (Fig. 12-2**B**). Since this area is not a fixed point, it is usually capable of being repositioned without distortion of the symmetry of the mouth. If this area is distorted, a secondary procedure can be carried out to improve the appearance. It is often necessary to perform a secondary procedure to recreate a melolabial sulcus, which is often obliterated by the inferiorly based melolabial flap (see case 8 in the Case Examples).

Advancement Melolabial Flap

The advancement melolabial flap is the easiest flap to design but requires considerable care in execution. The inferior limb of the flap is marked in the melolabial sulcus and is continued superiorly into the nasofacial sulcus and into the inferior aspect of the nasal defect. One usually needs to excise a triangle of skin at the superior aspect of lateral nasal defects reconstructed with this flap because this is the location for one of two standing cutaneous deformities that occur. The other cutaneous deformity develops at the inferior aspect of the flap near the oral commissure and also requires resection (Fig. 12-3**A**).

To prevent unnecessary blunting of the nasofacial sulcus, excess subcutaneous fat and muscle tissue is excised from the nasofacial sulcus, and 4-0 polyglycolic acid sutures are used to tack the flap to the underlying periosteum at the nasofacial sulcus (Fig. 12-3**B**).

Secondary Esthetic Refinement Procedures

There are generally three types of refinement procedures that may be required after facial reconstruction with the use of melolabial flaps: (1) deepening of the nasofacial sulcus, (2) release of a contracture of the alar-facial sulcus with the use of a Z-plasty, and (3) deepening of the nasoalar crease. These refinement procedures are described in the Case Examples.

CASE EXAMPLES

CASE 1

This case demonstrates the use of a superiorly based melolabial flap for repair of a lateral nasal defect. Fig. 12-4**A** shows a 2-cm lateral nasal defect located superior to the alar rim and the proposed flap design. The medial aspect of the designed flap lay in the melolabial sulcus. The lateral border of the flap was designed such that the height of the defect was equal to the width of the flap. The tip of the flap was pointed to allow closure of the secondary defect without a standing cutaneous

deformity. Fig. 12-4**B** shows the wide undermining on the cheek and nose. The skin of the upper lip medial to the melolabial fold was not undermined, thereby preventing lateral migration of the fold. (It often is necessary to carry the dissection up to the orbital rim, exposing the orbicularis oculi muscles. One may dissect the skin above or deep to this muscle.) Fat and soft tissue were excised down to periosteum in the area of the melolabial fold to recreate a deep melolabial sulcus (Fig. 12-4**C**). Once the flap was incised and the surrounding cheek skin was widely undermined, the flap was transposed into the defect, with no closure tension on the wound edges. The flap was then trimmed to fit the defect (Fig. 12-4**D**). The standing cutaneous cone deformity at the pivotal point of the flap was then excised (Fig. 12-4**E**). (Note that the excision should not narrow the base of the flap.)

The wound was closed with interrupted subcuticular 4-0 polyglactin sutures and a running 6-0 polypropylene skin sutures (Fig. 12-4**F**). The sutures were removed in 5 to 7 days. Fig. 12-4**G** shows the 3-month postoperative result.

Figure 12-4   Superiorly based melolabial flap. *A*, Design. *B*, Extent of undermining. *C*, Subcutaneous tissues excised from melolabial fold. *D*, Trimming of the flap. *E*, Excision of standing cutaneous deformity at pivotal point. *F*, Closure of wound. *G*, Postoperative result.

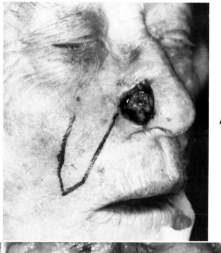

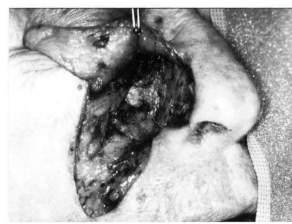

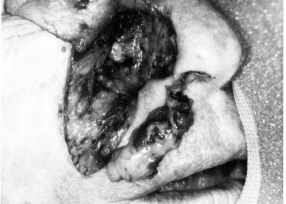

Figure 12-4—cont'd   For legend see p 185.

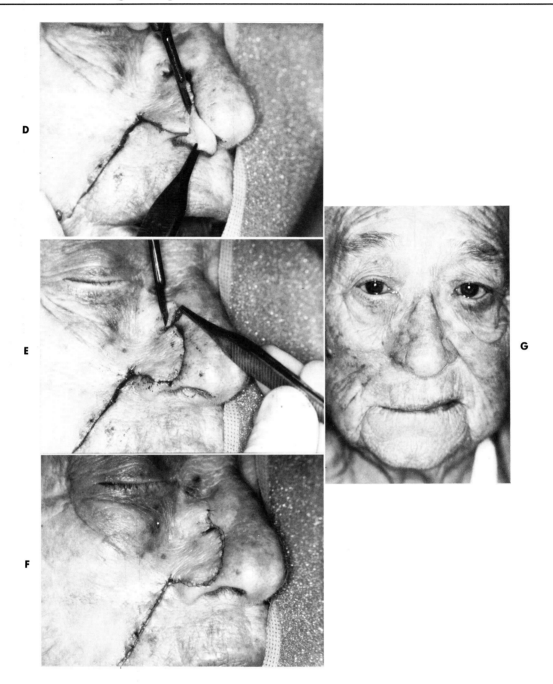

CASE 2

This case demonstrates the technique of using of a superiorly based melolabial flap for reconstruction of a 2.5 × 2 cm dorsal nasal defect. In design of the flap (Fig. 12-5**A**) the apex of the flap was not pointed, requiring excision of a standing cutaneous deformity during closure of the secondary wound. Fig. 12-5**B** shows elevation of the flap in the proper plane, which was in the subcutaneous plane in the cheek and just superficial to the perichondrium and periosteum over the cartilage and bone of the nose. After transposition of the flap, it was necessary to excise a standing cutaneous deformity at the pivotal point of the flap (Fig. 12-5**C**). The base of the flap was not narrowed by excision of the deformity (Fig. 12-5**D**). It is also necessary to excise a standing cutaneous deformity at the inferior aspect of the donor site, as shown in Fig. 12-5**E.**

The primary and secondary wounds were closed in layers. The skin was closed with a running locking 6-0 nylon suture (Fig. 12-5**F**). Fig. 12-5**G** shows the patient 3 months after reconstruction.

Figure 12-5   Superiorly based melolabial flap. *A*, **Design.** *B*, **Flap raised.** *C* and *D*, **Excision of standing cutaneous deformity at pivotal point.** *E*, **Excision of inferior standing cutaneous deformity.** *F*, **Closure of wound.** *G*, **Six-month postoperative result.**

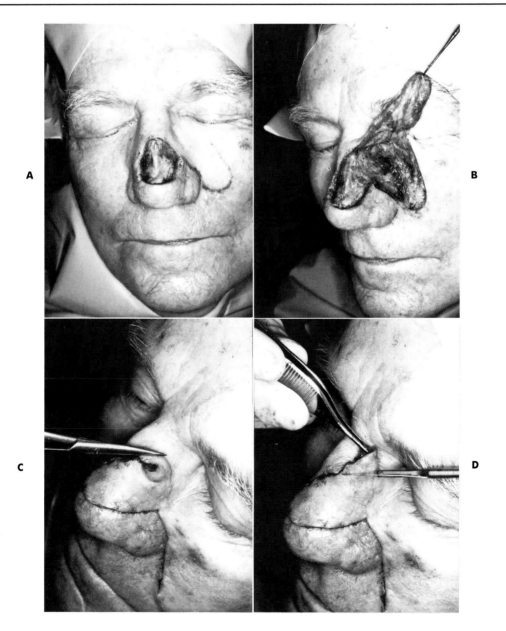

Figure 12-5—cont'd   For legend see p 187.

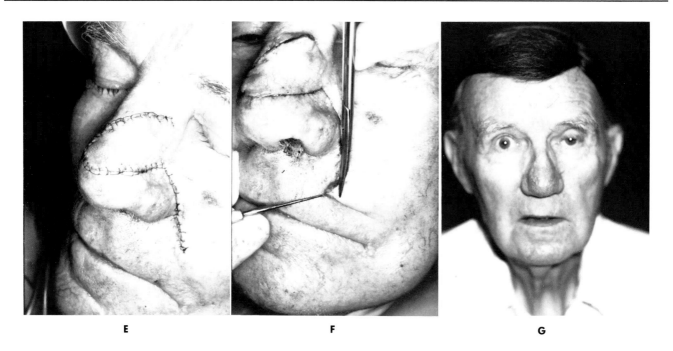

E   F   G

CASE 3

This case (Fig. 12-6**A** to **C**) demonstrates the use of bilateral melolabial flaps for closure of a large (3.5 × 3 cm) midline dorsal nasal defect. This technique may be used in patients who are at high risk for recurrence of their skin cancer, to save the forehead for possible future use for reconstructive procedures, or in patients with considerable redundancy of their medial cheek skin. This method of reconstruction is also particularly useful in patients with large nasal defects who have previously undergone nasal reconstruction with one or more paramedian forehead flaps. The postoperative result is shown 3 months after reconstruction (Fig. 12-6**D**).

Figure 12-6   Bilateral superiorly based melolabial flaps. *A,* Design. *B,* Flaps raised. *C,* Closure of wound. *D,* Six-month postoperative result.

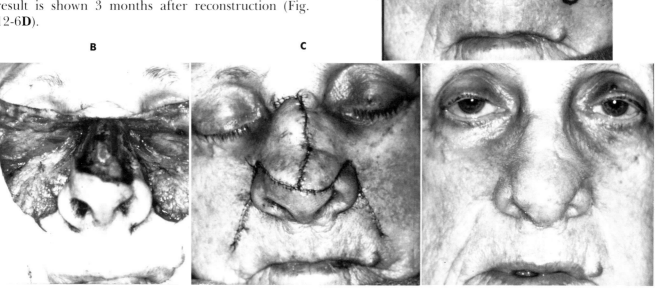

B   C

A

D

CASE 4

This case demonstrates the use of conchal cartilage for alar support in combination with a superiorly based melolabial flap for repair of a full-thickness defect of the nasal dome after Mohs surgery for an extensive nasal skin cancer. The defect measured 1.5 × 2 cm and included loss of the entire lateral crus of the lower lateral cartilage and the skin and soft tissue of the alar rim (Fig. 12-7**A**). The internal lining defect of the nasal vestibule was repaired by mobilization of adjacent skin. A conchal cartilage graft was used to replace the missing alar cartilage and to support the alar rim (Fig. 12-7**B**). The conchal cartilage was placed very close to the alar rim and was not positioned in a manner that attempted to duplicate the anatomy of the lateral crus of the lower lateral cartilage. This inferior placement of the graft helped prevent upward migration and notching of the reconstructed alar margin. The cartilage graft was sutured to adjacent fibrous connective tissue in the alar base and to the remaining medial crus in the dome area. The melolabial flap was then elevated (Fig. 12-7**C**) and transposed (Fig. 12-7**D**) using the skin of the flap to reconstruct the alar margin.

Fig. 12-7**E** shows the result 2 months after reconstruction. The patient had some notching of the alar rim. This is probably due to not placing the cartilage graft sufficiently low enough to prevent scar contraction upward. Repair of the internal lining primarily without the use of additional tissue may also have contributed to the notching.

Figure 12-7   Superiorly based flap with conchal cartilage graft. *A*, 1.5 × 2cm defect. *B*, Conchal cartilage support in place. *C*, Flap raised. *D*, Flap transposed. *E*, Two-month postoperative result.

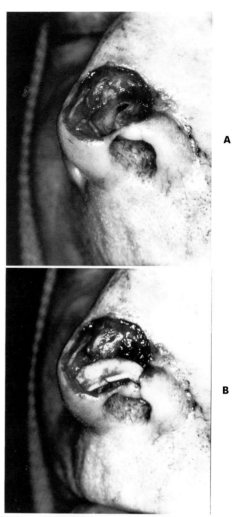

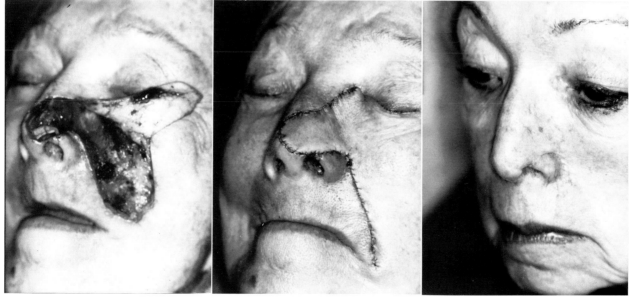

CASE 5

This case demonstrates the use of a superiorly based interpolation melolabial flap for reconstruction of the nasal tip (Fig. 12-8**A** to **C**). The defect, which measured 2.5 × 2.5 cm, could instead have been closed with a forehead flap. The interpolation melolabial flap is useful when the edge of the defect does not abut the nasofacial sulcus. In such cases the interpolation flap has the advantage of not disturbing the alar-cheek or nasofacial sulcus. The flap is usually inset 3 to 4 weeks after the primary reconstruction, (as shown in Fig. 12-8**D**).

Fig. 12-8**E** shows the patient 6 months postoperatively. There is some trapdoor deformity of the flap, which is a common problem encountered with interpolation flaps. This undesirable quality can be minimized by undermining of the tissues surrounding the primary defect and by creation of a uniformly thick flap.

Figure 12-8   Interpolation melolabial flap. *A*, 2.5 × 2.5 cm defect. *B*, Design. *C*, Flap transposed. *D*, Second stage of closure (flap inset). *E*, Six-month postoperative result.

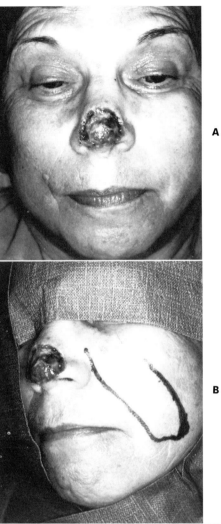

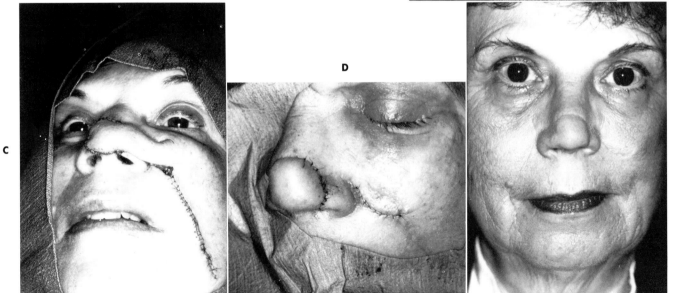

CASE 6

This case demonstrates the use of an inferiorly based melolabial flap for reconstruction of the upper lip (Fig. 12-9**A**). The defect that resulted after removal of a basal cell carcinoma measured 2.5 × 3 cm and was reconstructed with a 2.5-cm-wide flap (Fig. 12-9**B**). The medial incision was placed in the nasofacial sulcus. The width of the flap was equal to the height of the defect to prevent secondary movement of the vermilion upward (Fig. 12-9**C**).

The patient is seen 4 months postoperatively in Fig.

12-9**D**. No distortion of the vermilion or oral commisure was observed at that time.

The use of melolabial flaps for reconstruction of the lip necessitates closure of the secondary wound by advancement of adjacent cheek skin. This can sometimes cause excessive wound closure tension in the area of the alar-facial sulcus, causing the alar base to migrate laterally. This distortion of the alar base can be lessened by anchoring of the leading edge of the advanced cheek skin to the periosteum of the pyriform aperture with permanent deep sutures.

Figure 12-9   Inferiorly based melolabial flap. *A*, **Design.** *B*, **Flap raised.** *C*, **Closure of wound.** *D*, **Four-month postoperative result.**

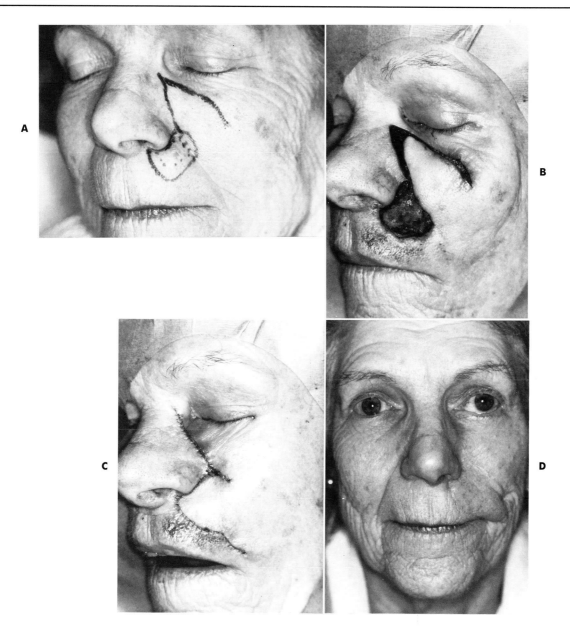

CASE 7

This case demonstrates the use of an advancement melolabial flap for repair of a 2.5 × 2.5 cm lateral nasal defect (Fig. 12-10**A** to **D**). (For larger defects a horizontal incision may be made in the infraorbital or subciliary area to allow more medial advancement of the flap.) In this case, as with virtually all melolabial advancement flaps, it was necessary to remove standing cutaneous deformities superiorly and inferiorly (Fig. 12-10**B**). A Burow's triangle, which was designed to fall in a relaxed skin tension line, facilitated the excision of the inferior redundant skin. Fig. 12-10**E** shows the postoperative result 10 months after reconstruction.

The major disadvantage of advancement flaps to close defects of the lateral aspect of the nose is that blunting of the nasofacial sulcus may occur. This can be minimized by suturing of the subcuticular soft tissue of the underside of the flap to the periosteum of the maxilla at the nasofacial sulcus.

Figure 12-10   Advancement melolabial flap. *A*, 2.5 × 2.5 cm defect. *B*, Flap incised, with excision of Burow's triangle. *C*, Flap raised. *D*, Closure of wound. *E*, Ten-month postoperative result. There is blunting of the alar-facial sulcus.

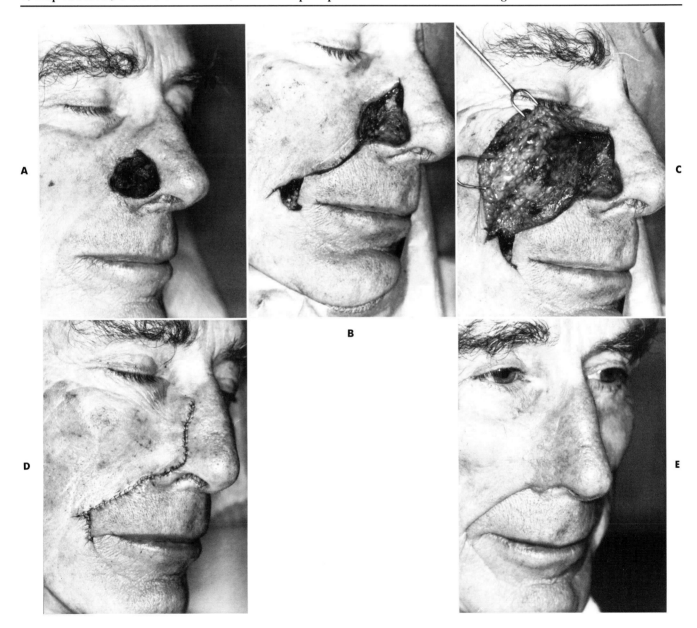

CASE 8

One of the major disadvantages of melolabial flaps for facial reconstruction is the resulting loss of definition of the normal melolabial sulcus and melolabial cheek fold. Case 8 demonstrates the technique of sculpting of the deep soft tissues in the area of the melolabial fold to better define the fold in a patient who previously had undergone an inferiorly based melolabial flap (Fig. 12-11**A**). This technique can be performed as a secondary revision surgery or at the time of primary reconstruction. The subcutaneous fat in the area of the intended melolabial sulcus was exposed by making an incision along the linear scar that resulted from the closure of the donor site of the melolabial flap (Fig. 12-11**B**). Fat was then excised along the intended melolabial sulcus (Fig. 12-11**C**). (The excised fat could conceivably be developed as a flap of tissue in a hinged-door fashion and turned laterally to create or enhance the new melolabial cheek fold.)

The wound was closed in layers (Fig. 12-11**D**). Fig. 12-11**E** shows the postoperative result 3 months after surgery.

Figure 12-11   Defatting and redefinition of melolabial sulcus. *A*, Preoperative photograph. *B*, Skin incised. *C*, Soft tissue excised. *D*, Closure of wound. *E*, Three-month postoperative result.

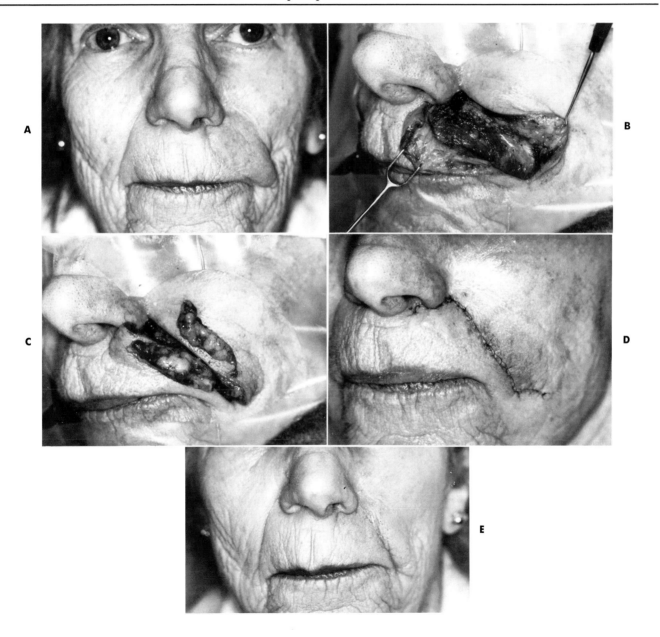

CASE 9

Similar to the disadvantage of loss of definition of the melolabial sulcus and fold when melolabial flaps are used to reconstruct the lip, loss of definition of the alar-facial sulcus often occurs when the flap is used to reconstruct nasal alar defects unless the flap is transposed as an interpolation flap. Case 9 demonstrates the use of a Z-plasty to refine a blunted alar-facial sulcus and the use of excision of subcutaneous of soft tissue to recreate a more defined nasal-alar sulcus.

The patient had previously undergone a superiorly based melolabial flap to reconstruct a lateral alar defect. The alar-facial web and poorly defined sulcus were sequelae of the nasal reconstruction (Fig. 12-12A). The design of the Z-plasty should be planned with the central limb centered along the linear axis of the web and one limb located in the alar-facial sulcus (Fig. 12-12B). The triangular flaps were widely undermined, and the fibrofatty tissue was excised to better define the sulcus (Fig. 12-12C). The triangular flaps were then transposed, and the wound was repaired with fine sutures (Fig. 12-12D). Fig. 12-12E shows the 3-month postoperative result.

Figure 12-12 Secondary refinement of alar-facial sulcus. *A*, Preoperative photograph. *B*, Design of Z-plasty. *C*, Excision of soft tissue. *D*, Closure of wound. *E*, Three-month postoperative result.

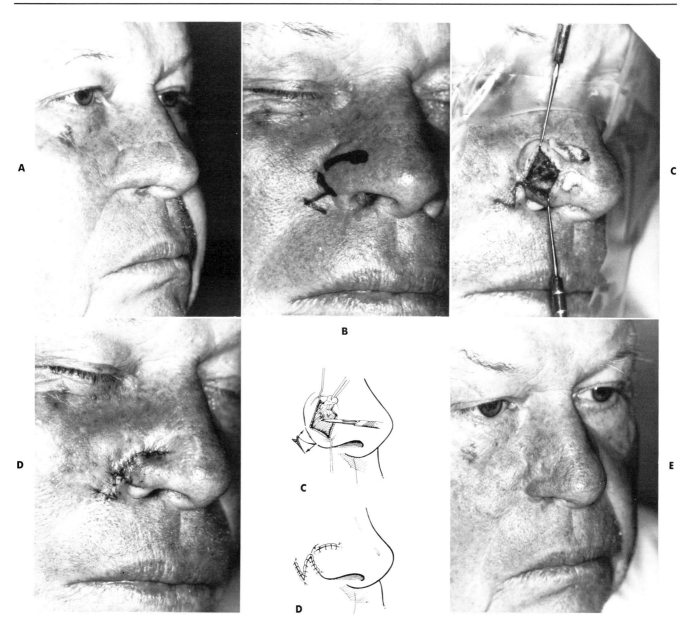

SUMMARY

Melolabial flaps are very useful in the repair of small to medium-sized defects of the lower two thirds of the nose, the immediate perinasal area, and the nonvermilion upper lip. They are frequently used to repair partial-thickness nasal and perinasal defects that are too large or deep for repair by primary closure, healing by second intention, or skin grafting. These flaps are limited primarily by the size of the donor defect, which should be closed primarily. Melolabial flaps are reliable and useful for esthetic reconstruction of nasal and perinasal skin defects.

REFERENCES

1. Cameron RR, Latham WD, Dowling JA: Reconstructions of the nose and upper lip with nasolabial flaps, *Plast Reconstr Surg* 52:145, 1973.

2. Pers M: Cheek flaps in partial rhinoplasty. *Scand J Plast Reconstr Surg* 1:37, 1967.

3. Cameron RR: Nasal reconstruction with nasolabial cheek flaps. In Grabb WC, Myers MB, editors: *Skin flaps*, Boston, 1975, Little Brown.

4. Zitelli JA: The nasolabial flap as a single-stage procedure, *Arch Dermatol* 126:1445, 1990.

5. Larrabee WF: Personal communication, May 1992.

EDITORIAL COMMENTS

Shan R. Baker

Melolabial flaps are perhaps the most frequently used facial skin flap. This is due to the fact that the nose is the most common site of skin cancer and the melolabial flap is extremely useful in reconstruction of partial and full-thickness defects of the distal third of the nose following surgical management of skin cancer. Although the flap could be dissected as an axial flap by inclusion of the angular artery and vein in its pedicle, these vessels lie too deep to easily incorporate. Thus the flap is dissected as a random skin flap. However, it has ample vascular supply through the dermal and subdermal plexus to allow the flap to be designed as a superiorly or inferiorly based flap and to be dissected as a very thin flap consisting of skin and only a minimal amount of subcutaneous fat.

I prefer design of an inferiorly based melolabial flap when I reconstruct portions of the upper or lower lip. It is an excellent flap for repair of defects of the lip. The thickness of the flap can be adjusted to match the depth of the lip defect by inclusion of more or less subcutaneous fat. Full-thickness melolabial flaps that consist of skin, subcutaneous fat, muscle, and mucosa can be transferred to reconstruct full-thickness loss of the upper or lower lip. If the vermilion is also missing, the mucosa on the deep side of the flap can be advanced over the edge of the flap to reconstruct this portion of the lip.

In reconstruction of the nose the melolabial flap is best suited for repair of defects involving the columella, nasal sill, nasal ala, and the lateral portion of the caudal one third of the nose. In the case of the columella and sill, I prefer a superiorly based flap. For reconstruction of the entire columella, bilateral flaps are most effec-

tive. Defects of the ala and lateral wall of the nose that do not extend to the nasal-facial or alar-facial sulcus are, in my opinion, best reconstructed with an interpolation melolabial flap that does not violate these important esthetic junction zones. This is then a two-stage reconstruction, in contrast to a one-stage reconstruction that designs the melolabial flap as a transposition flap; however, the maintained natural alar-facial and nasal-facial sulcus are far superior in appearance compared with any attempt to restore them with revision surgery.

Advancement melolabial flaps used to repair lateral nasal defects almost always blunt the nasal-facial sulcus and in my opinion, should be confined to defects that are centered within the sulcus. I prefer tie over bolster sutures along the entire length of the nasal facial sulcus in attempts to maintain the sulcus integrity rather than deep sutures placed between the dermis of the advancement flap and the underlying periosteum of the sulcus. The bolster sutures are placed so that the suture extends through the flap into the underlying periosteum and soft tissues of the sulcus; these sutures are left in place for 7 to 10 days.

The authors have discussed a method to restore or maintain the melolabial sulcus following harvest of a melolabial flap by removal of an ample amount of cheek fat in the area of the sulcus. Although this appears to have worked well in case 8, the technique may not be as effective in individuals with minimal soft tissue, including subcutaneous fat. In such cases excision of skin in the contralateral melolabial sulcus will provide facial symmetry and often enhance the youthful appearance of the central area of the cheek. However, this excision is at the expense of a second facial scar, albeit with good camouflaging of the scar in the melolabial sulcus.

EDITORIAL COMMENTS

Neil A. Swanson

The melolabial flap is incredibly useful. It has obtained a bad reputation in some plastic surgery literature. Dr. Becker and I believe that this "bad rap" is because of a poor understanding of the mechanics and performance of this flap. I perform these flaps with some differences from the authors and will try to elucidate these.

With the superior based melolabial flap, the initial design is important. Remember that with transposition flaps the movement of tissue around the pivotal point makes the measurement of the length of the flap critical. It must be measured from the pivotal point rather than using the diameter of the defect itself. I always add to that length a triangle of tissue that would be removed as the redundant standing cutaneous deformity. Therefore, if I have mismeasured the length of the flap, I have this extra tissue to use instead of having it discarded. I agree with the placement of the medial incision; however, I bring my lateral incision much higher than do the authors. I have not found this to be a problem with restriction of blood flow, and it allows me to drape the flap more than rotate it. I think this leads to a better esthetic result, less of a trapdoor deformity, and an ability to close the secondary defect directly in the cheek-nasal esthetic junction. During draping of the flap, the width is more a tangential measurement than the height of the flap. Undermining of the cheek occurs as described, and in someone with fatty or protuberant cheeks the level of undermining should be carefully uniform and curved. The temptation is to undermine in a straight line, giving a more fatty edge to the advancement flap and with less fat on the remainder of the flap. By undermining all in one plane, some of the blunting effect of the mesolabial sulcus can be prevented. As the authors mention, the flap can then be dramatically thinned and can maintain its rich blood supply. I also will often thin or defat at the nasal-facial sulcus in an attempt to assist in the reestablishment of that line. The secondary defect is closed first, allowing the flap to drape over the primary defect. I agree with the authors that judicial undermining around the primary defect assists in closure and prevention, to a degree, of trapdoor deformities. The flap is then tacked in place within the primary defect. I then remove the resulting standing cutaneous deformity, as do the authors, by curving away from the base of the flap, thus widening the base and providing additional blood supply. The flap is then finally positioned and sutured using a two-layered closure. Once this has occurred, the excess tissue in length (the standing cutaneous deformity, if you will) is trimmed to fit the defect. The final suturing then continues. As the authors state, the flap itself should be slightly thinner and lower than the surrounding tissue. The use of a suspension suture as described can be useful at times. Their discussion of the use of this flap as an interpolation flap that bridges alar tissue is also pertinent.

Regarding the inferiorly based melolabial flap, the key again is measurement. I will always design this flap to be oversized, remembering the concept of turning about a transposition point, effectively shortening the length of the flap when transposition occurs. Because this flap is usually used to correct lip defects, it is imperative that the flap be large enough to fill the defect and not to pull up on the lip. It's easier to trim the flap than it is to secondarily repair the snarl effect. When this flap is used for lip reconstruction, a blunting of the melolabial sulcus occurs as described. This must be discussed with the patient preoperatively.

The advancement melolabial flap is a good choice for lateral nasal defects. In elderly patients with very elastic skin, it can even be stretched to reach further up the nasal sidewall. I will usually delay removal of the inferior and superior redundant standing cutaneous deformities until after the flap has been carefully sutured in place. One is often surprised as to the amount (or lack) of standing cutaneous deformity that is left, and I find it very difficult to prejudge that cutaneous deformity.

The authors show several excellent examples of the versatility of this flap. When the flap is used for repair of a deep defect, a defect in which cartilage has been lost and needs replacement to maintain the nasal valve, or a through-and-through defect in which a cartilage-composite skin graft has been inverted and used for lining and cartilaginous support covered by a melolabial flap, I use a compression dressing and nasal pack. The nasal pack can wrap around a cut straw, so that the patient maintains nasal patency and the ability to breathe. The compression dressing uses a dental roll, to assist in remolding that structure during the early phases of wound healing.

13

MIDFOREHEAD FLAPS

Eugene L. Alford

Shan R. Baker

Kevin A. Shumrick

INTRODUCTION

The art of facial plastic and reconstructive surgery is said to have begun more than 2000 years ago in India with the use of the midforehead flap or Indian rhinoplasty for reconstruction of the nose. Midforehead flaps were first described in the Indian medical treatise, the *Sushruta Samita*, in approximately 700 BC.[1-6] The operation was performed by members of a caste of potters known as the Koomas. The need for this operation arose from the common Indian practice of amputation of the tip of the nose as punishment for various crimes ranging from robbery to adultery.[7,8]

The first reported use of the midforehead flap outside of India was by Antonio Branca of Italy. Based on an Arabic translation of the *Sushruta Samita*, Branca performed a nasal reconstruction using the midforehead flap in the 15th century.[4,9] In the 16th and early 17th centuries, little advancement was seen in the use of the midforehead flap because plastic and reconstructive surgery fell into disrepute.[7-9]

The midforehead flap saw a revival in 1794 after Carpue read an editorial letter in *Gentlemen's Magazine* of London that described the use of the midforehead flap for nasal reconstruction.[5,10-12] Initially Carpue practiced the midforehead flap operation on cadavers. Twenty years passed before he actually performed the operation on two patients and reported his successful results in a monograph entitled, "An Account of Two Successful Operations for Restoring a Lost Nose From the Integuments of the Forehead."[13] His monograph was widely circulated throughout Europe and served to popularize the operation.[4,11,13,14] In the 1830s Ernst Blausius, chief of ophthalmologic surgery of Berlin; Johann Friedereich Diffenbach, chief of surgery at Munich Hospital; and Natale Petrali of Milan simultaneously reported on uses and variations of the midforehead flap for reconstruction of the face and nose.

Based on their influence as respected surgeons at large European teaching hospitals, the practice and popularity of the midforehead flap grew.[4] In the late 1830s use of the midforehead flap for nasal and facial reconstruction crossed the Atlantic when Warren first performed the operation in America.[7,15]

Reconstructive rhinoplasty and use of the midforehead flap progressed in the early 1900s to reconstruct losses of the nose secondary to battle, scrofula, syphilis, and cancer. Many great American surgeons such as Pancoast, Mutter, Buck, Davis, and Fomon wrote about the use of the midforehead flap in nasal reconstruction.[4] Little modification in design, use, harvest, or donor site closure of the midforehead flap occurred until articles by Kazanjian appeared in the plastic surgery literature in the 1930s. This pioneering plastic surgeon was the first to delineate that the primary blood supply of the flap came from the supratrochlear and supraorbital arteries. Kazanjian[16] described a precise midline forehead flap with primary closure of the donor site, which minimized the major morbidity of the operation, forehead donor site scarring. His technique was a major advance in the use of the midforehead flap, as before this time, the donor site had either been skin grafted or left open to close secondarily by granulation and contraction. This practice frequently left the patient more scarred and disfigured than before reconstructive surgery.[16]

In the 1960s Millard[15,17] followed Kazanjian's lead by designing larger modified midforehead flaps, such as the "seagull" flap. This median forehead flap allowed lateral extensions that could be used to recreate the nasal ala. Additionally, the incision for this flap extended below the orbital rim to gain extra flap length and rotation. Millard also described donor site closure techniques to recreate nasal support, all of which improved the outcome when midforehead flaps were used for nasal reconstruction.[15,17-19]

Figure 13-1 Forehead divided into vascular territories according to primary vascular supply. *A,* **Dorsal nasal artery.** *B,* **Supratrochlear artery.** *C,* **Supraorbital artery.** *D,* **Anterior branch of superficial temporal artery.**

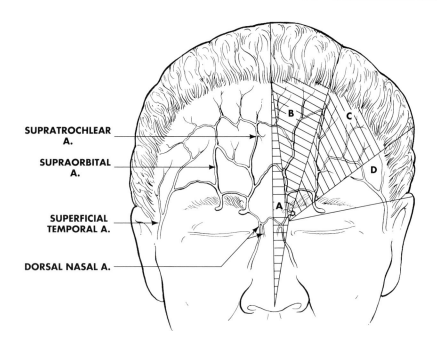

SUPRATROCHLEAR A.

SUPRAORBITAL A.

SUPERFICIAL TEMPORAL A.

DORSAL NASAL A.

In the 1970s and 1980s, Burget[20,21] and Menick[22] found that by extending incisions below the orbital rim, one did not need to curve the flap or extend it superiorly into the hairline to reach the nasal tip. They also determined that the end arterioles of the supratrochlear artery travel just under the dermis, superficial to the frontalis muscle. Thus the frontalis muscle could be removed from the flap, allowing for better flap contouring to meet the three-dimensional tissue requirements of the defect.[1] Menick[9] also described the paramedian forehead flap based on a single supratrochlear artery. This vertical forehead flap has a much narrower base than a median forehead flap, and thus has much greater freedom of rotation, yielding a flap with greater effective length.[9]

More recent anatomic studies by surgeons such as Mangold and co-workers,[23] McCarthy et al,[24] and Shumrick and Smith[5] better defined the vascular anatomy of the forehead region. In 1980 Mangold et al[23] determined that the major blood vessels of the forehead—the dorsal nasal artery (or angular artery), supratrochlear artery, supraorbital artery, and superficial temporal artery—had numerous interconnecting anastomoses, and each was the primary blood supply to a particular region of the forehead. Their injection studies and dissections of cadavers implied subdivision of the forehead into regions based on its primary vascular supply (Fig. 13-1).[23] Relying on these principles of vascular subdivision of the forehead, Mangold and co-workers[23] determined that median and parame-

dian vertical forehead flaps are nourished primarily by the supratrochlear artery and secondarily by the dorsal nasal artery (angular artery) and supraorbital artery. In cases in which the supratrochlear artery is absent, the paramedian or median vertical forehead flap may still survive based on the dorsal nasal artery.

McCarthy, working alone and with others,[24,25] confirmed the work of Mangold's group in clinical experiences with patients. McCarthy[24,25] noted that injection of the facial artery after ligation of the supraorbital and supratrochlear arteries yielded sufficient filling of forehead vessels to supply the vertically oriented flaps in the region of the central forehead.

In 1992, Shumrick and Smith[5] performed detailed anatomic studies of the forehead using techniques of latex injection, radiography, and microdissection to determine the precise vascular anatomy of the midforehead flap. Examination of the radiographic data confirmed a clinically apparent fact—that the forehead region contained an intricate system of anastomosing vessels between the angular, supratrochlear, supraorbital, and superficial temporal arteries (Fig. 13-2A). The paired supratrochlear arteries anastomosed with each other via several horizontal unnamed arteries that crossed the midline. Moreover, the supratrochlear artery consistently anastomosed with the angular artery and supraorbital artery in the medial canthal region. Microdissection of the forehead vasculature confirmed these radiographic findings. The supratrochlear artery was consistently found to exit the

Figure 13-2   A, Radiograph showing forehead skin vasculature after injection of contrast medium. Note intricate system of anastomosing vessels. *A,* Dorsal nasal artery. *B,* Supratrochlear artery. *C,* Supraorbital artery. *D,* Superficial temporal artery. **B,** Contrast study similar to that of Fig. 13-2**A** with wire markers to delineate supraorbital rim, and medial aspect of brow. (From Shumrick KA, Smith TL: The anatomic basis for the design of forehead flaps in nasal reconstruction, *Arch Otolaryngol Head Neck Surg* 118:373-379, 1992; Copyright 1992, American Medical Association.)

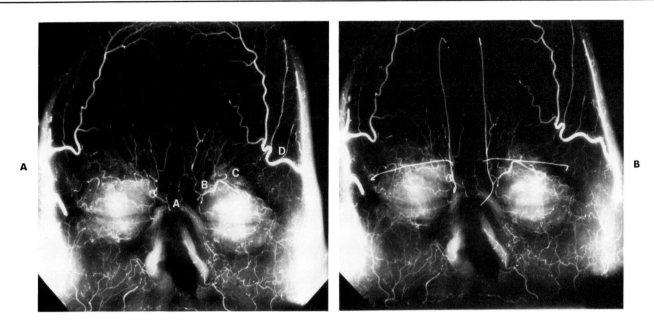

superior medial orbit approximately 1.7 to 2.2 cm lateral to the midline, and it continued its course vertically in a paramedian position approximately 2 cm lateral to the midline. This paramedian position closely corresponded to the location of the medial portion of the eyebrow (Fig. 13-2**B**). The supratrochlear artery was seen to exit the orbit by piercing the orbital septum and passing under the orbicularis oculi muscle and over the corrugator supercilii muscle (Fig. 13-3).[5] At approximately the level of the eyebrow, the supratrochlear artery passed through the orbicularis and frontalis muscles and continues upward in the superficial subcutaneous tissue.[5]

Further confirmation of the change in anatomic levels of the supratrochlear artery was obtained by histologic examination of cross sections of the forehead skin at various levels.[5] These cross sections clearly showed the supratrochlear artery passing external to the corrugator supercilii muscle but deep to the orbicularis oculi muscle and then piercing the frontalis muscle to enter into the superficial subcutaneous tissues external to the frontalis muscle. Doppler examination and localization studies in healthy volunteers confirmed these cadaver findings.[5]

These studies of the vascular anatomy of the forehead have confirmed that the supratrochlear artery is the primary axial blood supply of midforehead flaps, which by our definition include median and paramed-

Figure 13-3   Anatomic relationship of supratrochlear artery and adjacent musculature.

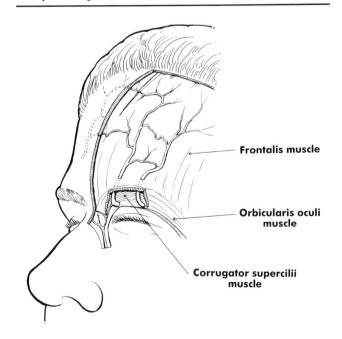

Frontalis muscle

Orbicularis oculi muscle

Corrugator supercilii muscle

ian vertically oriented flaps. Additionally, these studies have shown that a rich anastomotic network exists in the medial canthal region between the supratrochlear, supraorbital, and angular arteries. Identification of this vascular network and the surgical techniques of flap harvest that preserve this regional blood flow have allowed surgeons to harvest paramedian forehead flaps based on pedicles narrower than those used for median forehead flaps. The narrower pedicle gives the flap more freedom of rotation about its pivot point and therefore provides a more effective length. This pedicle, which can be as narrow as 1.2 cm, reduces donor site deformity in the glabellar area that results from transposition of the flap.[9,26]

The midforehead flaps, which include the median and paramedian flaps and their many variations, have withstood the test of time and have proved to be a workhorse flap for midfacial reconstruction.[2,3,27-31] Their high success rate, reliability, and popularity are primarily the result of the dependable axial blood supply. Based on the supratrochlear artery and its anastomoses to surrounding vessels, the midforehead flap is an axial pivotal interpolation flap with an outstanding blood supply that provides a dependable flap, which can be transferred without delay. This highly vascular flap also allows primary incorporation of cartilage or tissue grafts, which can then act as support structures or lining tissue when needed.[1,15,27,32] Correct removal of the muscle and subcutaneous fat from the distal portion of the flap makes it thin, pliable, and easily contoured to fit any defect of the midface. Including the frontalis muscle and fascia in the flap is useful when more stiffness and bulk is required to better fill defects with irregular thicknesses.[33]

Appropriate contouring and thinning of the flap is essential for an acceptable esthetic result. It can be accomplished without concern for compromise of the flap vasculature due to the fact that the supratrochlear artery travels superiorly in the subcutaneous-subdermal plane from a point 1 cm above the level of the eyebrow.[5] This allows for three-dimensional sculpturing of the flap by removal of the fascia and frontalis muscle and, if necessary, a portion of the subcutaneous tissue from the distal portion of the flap. The ability to create a flap of the correct thickness that exactly matches and fills the defect greatly enhances the cosmetic and functional results of vertical midforehead flaps. Excellent reliability, ease of flap harvest and contouring, and an abundant vascular supply are the major advantages of midforehead flaps. The close proximity of forehead skin to the midface provides a source of skin with an excellent color and texture match to that of the central face. Additionally, midforehead flaps do not transfer hair-bearing skin to the face,

have no effect on the mimetic musculature of the face, and do not undergo a great deal of wound contracture.[7,33] These characteristics of the flap combine to lessen the need for later revision surgery. Depending on the characteristics of individual patients' forehead skin laxity, primary donor site closure can be achieved with flaps as wide as 4.5 cm. Combined with its long pedicle and ability to reach almost any point on the midface, the midforehead flap is a versatile method of midfacial reconstruction.

Midforehead flaps are often used as interpolation flaps. When this is the case, a second operation is required to separate the pedicle of the flap.[34] The pedicle can safely be detached as early as 10 to 14 days after transfer, but an interval of 3 weeks is preferred. At three weeks the distal portion of the flap has developed sufficient collateral blood supply from the nose to allow thinning and sculpturing of the more proximal portion of the flap left attached to the recipient site. This portion of the flap is not usually sculptured at the time of initial transposition.

Disadvantages of the midforehead flap are few but notable. The major disadvantage is the forehead scar. Care must be taken to correctly approximate the donor site, which will minimize wound tension. This is facilitated by wide undermining bilaterally to the anterior border of the temporalis muscle and the use of three or four vertical fasciotomies on either side of the incision site. These maneuvers often provide an extra 1 cm of skin laxity to assist in wound closure and reduction of wound tension.[35] Primary closure of the donor site is preferred; however, inability to close the donor site is not in itself a contraindication to use of the midforehead flap. Excellent donor site healing can result, even when areas up to 2 cm^2 have been allowed to granulate and heal by second intention and wound contracture.[7,9,26,36] In general, midforehead flaps wider than 4.5 cm are too large to allow primary closure of the donor site. In such circumstances the donor site must, in part, be left to heal by second intention.

Another disadvantage of the midforehead flap is its limited length. In patients with a low forehead hairline or a widow's peak, a midforehead flap may not have adequate pedicle length for the desired reconstruction. Modifications such as the oblique forehead flap, tissue expansion, or extension of the flap into the hair-bearing scalp may be considered.[35,37-39,45] When midforehead flaps are designed to include hair-bearing scalp, the surgeon must markedly thin the distal flap and meticulously remove all hair follicles at the time of transfer or pedicle division.[39]

Finally, in the case of interpolation flaps, the requirement of a second operation to divide the pedicle is widely seen as the major drawback to the use of midforehead flaps. It is important to counsel the patient preoperatively concerning the deformity caused by the flap during the interval between flap transfer and pedicle division.

Historically, the midforehead flap has been used primarily for the reconstruction of larger defects of the nose or nasal tip. It is the method of choice for the closure of nasal defects too large or too deep to close with full-thickness skin grafts, composite auricular grafts, or adjacent tissue flaps such as the melolabial flap.[7,8,16] In general, nasal defects larger than 2.5 cm in length along the horizontal transverse plane are best closed with a midforehead flap.[16] Additionally, nasal defects with exposed bone and cartilage deficient of periosteum or perichondrium, or cases in which the central face has been irradiated, are best served by a midforehead flap repair.[8,16,40]

Modern use of the midforehead flap has expanded beyond nasal reconstruction to include any soft-tissue defect of the midface that the flap can be designed to reach. Defects of the medial canthal region, upper or lower eyelids, medial cheek, melolabial region, or upper lip may be reconstructed with midforehead flaps.[8,34] Midforehead flaps may also be used in combination with other larger flaps for reconstruction of complex facial defects.[3,8,39,41] A classic example of this is the use of a midforehead flap in combination with a scalping flap for total nasal reconstruction.[2,8,27] Use of midforehead flaps in facial reconstruction is limited only by the length and width of the flap and the ingenuity of the surgeon.

Reconstruction of facial defects with midforehead flaps requires precise planning and preoperative preparation. Preoperative assessment of the patient should include measurement of the defect and contemplation of the required length and width of the flap. Attention should be given to the height of the hairline and the degree of forehead skin laxity. When an interpolation flap is planned, patients should be counseled concerning their appearance between the first- and second-stage operations. Wound care of the pedicle, donor site, and recipient areas should be discussed as well as information regarding realistic expectations and goals of the reconstructive procedure.

SURGICAL TECHNIQUE

The following discussion of surgical techniques applies to the use of the midforehead flap for nasal reconstruction. Midforehead flaps are usually harvested and transferred with the patient under general anesthesia; however, long-acting local anesthetics such as bupivacaine (Marcaine) combined with intravenous sedation may be adequate for some patients. Thirty minutes before skin incision, a broad-spectrum prophylactic

intravenous antibiotic of the surgeon's choice is administered. The patient is placed on the operating room table in the supine position in 20° to 30° of reverse Trendelenburg. This position decreases venous pooling, causing less intraoperative blood loss during flap harvest and transfer. After general endotracheal anesthesia is induced, the patient's eyes are protected by suturing of the upper and lower eyelids together with a horizontal mattress suture. The full face and scalp, from midvertex to submentum, is prepared with a sterilizing solution of the surgeon's choice. A sterile head drape is placed, and full-body draping is completed in the usual sterile fashion.

The flap is often designed with the assistance of a Doppler probe to localize the supratrochlear, supraorbital, and angular or dorsal nasal arteries.[5,9] The base of the pedicle is placed in the glabellar region, either in the midline in the case of a median flap, or centered over the supratrochlear artery on the same side as the majority of the defect in the case of a paramedian flap. Flaring of the base of a median flap may include both supratrochlear arteries, but this restricts rotation of the flap about its pivotal point. Limitation of the vascular input of the pedicle to a single supratrochlear artery will allow considerable narrowing of the pedicle base and facilitate transposition. A three-dimensional template exactly mimicking the surface defect to be reconstructed is fashioned from foil or foam rubber. The template is then used to outline the flap design on the forehead skin (Figs. 13-4 and 13-5).

In the case of a paramedian flap, the center of the template should be located approximately 2 cm lateral to the midline of the forehead. This will approximate the location of the supratrochlear artery based on the anatomic and clinical studies of Shumrick and Smith.[5] The length of the flap is then determined by measurement using a length of suture from the distal tip of the positioned template to the base of the pedicle. With the suture held at the base of the pedicle, the suture is then rotated 180° in the coronal plane to the distal recipient site on the face. If the suture does not reach this point, the template and measurement must be repositioned higher on the forehead, or the pedicle base must be lowered by extending it below the level of the eyebrow. It may be necessary to repeat this step of relocation of the template several times until adequate length has been incorporated into the flap design. The flap is then precisely outlined on the forehead with a surgical marker, following the exact shape of the template.

Lidocaine (0.5%) with a 1:100,000 concentration of epinephrine is then injected subcutaneously circumferentially about the surgical defect and the forehead flap design, except near the pedicle base. The defect is sharply debrided of any nonviable tissue, the margins

Figures 13-4, 13-5   Template is used to outline midforehead flap. Template should reflect exact surface defect to be reconstructed.

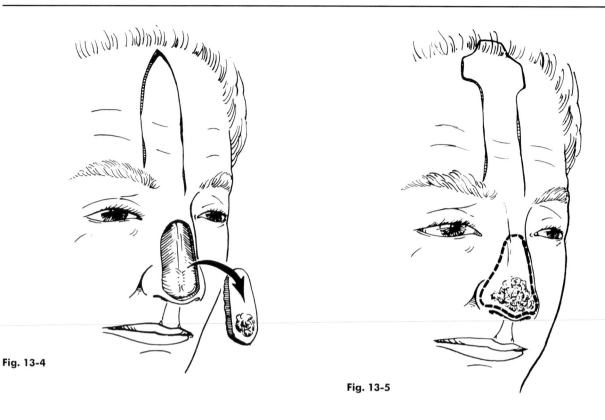

Fig. 13-4

Fig. 13-5

are freshened with a scalpel, and all its edges are undermined completely. Incisions for flap elevation should be made through the skin, subcutaneous tissue, muscle, and fascia. The flap is elevated in the subfascial plane, just superficial to the periosteum of the frontal bone, from the superior to inferior direction (Fig. 13-6). Careful attention must be paid to flap dissection once elevation reaches the region 1 to 2 cm above the eyebrow. To avoid injury or inadvertent cutting of the arterial pedicle, blunt dissection with a dissecting hemostat or cotton-tipped applicator is used to separate slips of corrugator supercilii muscle, which are then cut with a scalpel. If incisions are necessary at or below the brow level, they are made using a scalpel through skin only. Blunt dissection by spread of tissue with a hemostat is then used to mobilize the pedicle away from the medial bony orbit. The supratrochlear artery can usually be identified visually or with the aid of a Doppler probe from superiorly to inferiorly on the deep surface of the frontalis muscle, just as it exits over the corrugator supercilii muscle and before it passes deep to the orbicularis oculi muscle to enter the orbit. Adequate flap mobilization usually requires complete sectioning of the corrugator supercilii muscle to achieve free movement of the flap. Once the supratrochlear artery is identified and preserved, blunt and sharp dissections are used to continue flap eleva-

Figure 13-6   Midforehead flap is elevated in subfascial plane.

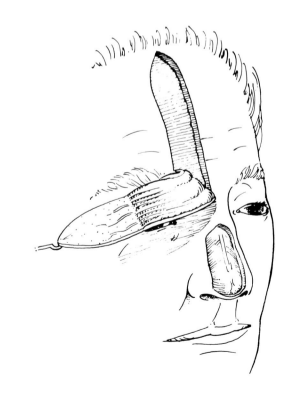

Figure 13-7   Flap is thinned in subcutaneous plane.

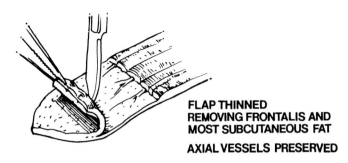

FLAP THINNED
REMOVING FRONTALIS AND
MOST SUBCUTANEOUS FAT

AXIAL VESSELS PRESERVED

Figure 13-8   All hair follicles are removed from flap.

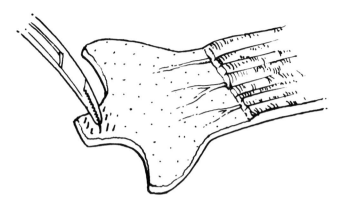

Figure 13-9   Beveled edge of flap. Cutting back deep dermis along edge of flap provides better thickness match with that of adjacent nasal skin.

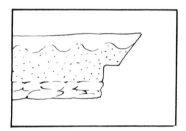

SKIN EDGE BEVELED

RETICULAR DERMIS
CUT-BACK

SUBDERMAL FAT
PRESERVED

Figure 13-10   Extensive undermining of remaining forehead skin and fasciotomies facilitate closure of donor site.

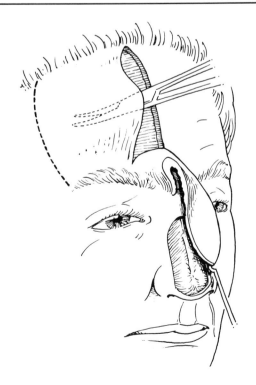

tion down onto the root of the nose, or until adequate pedicle length and mobility has been attained.

Hemostasis in the superior portion of the flap may be accomplished by Bovie electrocautery. Precise, bipolar electrocautery or fine 4-0 silk sutures should be used for hemostasis at the base of the flap.

Once adequate flap mobilization has been accomplished, the flap is rotated about its pivot point in the coronal plane to the defect. The flap is then sculptured and contoured to fit the depth, breadth, and height of the defect by removal of all or some of the muscle and subcutaneous tissue from the distal portion of the flap (Fig. 13-7). When necessary, all but 1 mm of the fat beneath the dermis may be removed. Muscle removal may be accomplished beginning 1 cm above the point at which the supratrochlear artery pierces the frontalis muscle. Any hair follicles transferred with the flap should be meticulously removed (Fig. 13-8). Only the distal three fourths of the flap required for reconstruction is sculptured; the proximal one fourth is left thick and is debulked at the time of pedicle detachment. Forehead skin is often thicker than nasal skin. To compensate for this discrepancy, it is often helpful to bevel the edge of the forehead flap. It may also be helpful to split the dermis along the edge of the flap, removing the deep portion (Fig. 13-9).

Donor site closure is accomplished by extensive undermining of the forehead in the subfascial plane, from the anterior border of one temporalis muscle to the other (Fig. 13-10).[42] Several parallel vertical fasciotomies, 2 to 3 cm apart, are made just to the level of the subcutaneous fat with Bovie electrocautery. This maneuver will provide additional skin laxity to assist in wound closure. The muscle and fascia are closed as a single layer with 3-0 absorbable sutures, and the skin is closed with 5-0 polypropylene (Prolene) vertical mattress sutures (Fig. 13-11). No drain is employed.

The extreme cephalic border of the defect under the flap pedicle is not closed. This portion of the surgical defect and the exposed raw surface area of the pedicle are wrapped in petrolatum gauze, and antibiotic oint-

Figure 13-11 Skin is approximated with vertical mattress sutures. Muscle and fascia are approximated as single layer.

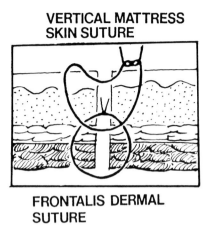

VERTICAL MATTRESS
SKIN SUTURE

FRONTALIS DERMAL
SUTURE

Figure 13-12 Vertical mattress sutures are used to suture midforehead flap. Distal excess flap tissue is excised.

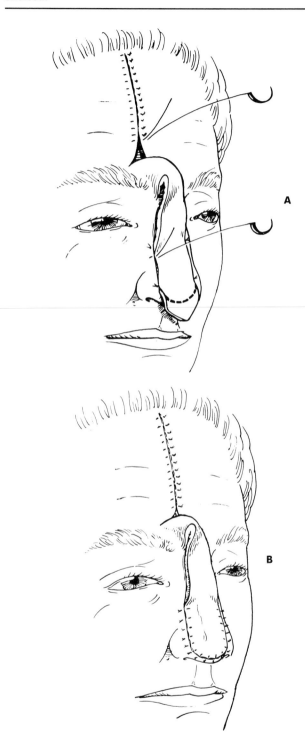

ment is applied to the suture lines. Flap inset is accomplished with 4-0 absorbable sutures in the deep layers of wound closure, and skin closure is performed with 5-0 or 6-0 polypropylene sutures placed in vertical mattress fashion (Fig. 13-12).

Patients may be discharged home the day of surgery or admitted for overnight observation and wound care at the surgeon's discretion. Prescriptions to give the patient at discharge usually include a broad-spectrum oral antibiotic; a mild pain reliever, such as acetaminophen (Tylenol) with codeine; an antiemetic, such as promethazine (Phenergan) or trimethobenzamide (Tigan) suppositories; and a topical antibacterial ointment, such as bacitracin or mupirocin (Bactroban). Postoperative wound care consists of twice-daily cleansing of the suture lines with hydrogen peroxide and application of the antibacterial ointment. The xeroform gauze around the pedicle remains in place for 24 hours and is then removed.

On the fifth to seventh postoperative day, sutures are removed and benzoin and adhesive strips (Steri-Strips) are applied to the forehead wound. These remain in place for an additional 10 days. The wound is carefully checked for flap viability, healing, or signs of infection. If all appears well and the wound is healing as expected, the patient is then scheduled for pedicle separation approximately 3 weeks from the date of initial flap transfer. Some surgeons prefer to separate the pedicle 2 weeks after flap transfer; however, this earlier detachment may limit the ability to debulk and sculpture the proximal flap remaining at the recipient site. Other surgeons advocate leaving pedicle attached throughout the sculpting and revision procedures, which allows for more aggressive debulking due to the flap's enhanced blood supply.

Pedicle separation is accomplished with the patient

under local anesthesia. One percent lidocaine with epinephrine is injected into the base of the pedicle and circumferentially around the recipient site after the usual sterile preparation and draping has been completed. The pedicle is separated with a scalpel exactly at the superior margin of the defect. The skin superiorly surrounding the defect is undermined for approximately 1 cm. The portion of the skin flap left attached to the recipient site and not thinned at the time of transposition is now thinned appropriately. In the case of reconstruction of skin-only nasal defects that extend to the rhinion, the flap must be aggressively thinned to the level of the dermis. All subcutaneous fat must be removed so that the thin skin of the rhinion will be replicated. Deep-layer closure is not necessary, since the wound should not be under any tension. The skin is closed with 5-0 or 6-0 polypropylene sutures in a vertical mattress fashion.

The base of the pedicle is now returned to its donor site in such a way as to recreate the normal intereyebrow distance. It is often necessary to debulk early scar deposition in the donor area to enable the pedicle to lie flat between the brow. Any excess pedicle should not be returned to the forehead above the brow but should be resected and discarded. The deep layers of the pedicle wound are closed with 4-0 absorbable sutures, and the skin is closed with 5-0 or 6-0 polypropylene sutures in a vertical mattress fashion. The patient may return to work and normal daily activities within 5 days after pedicle separation.

Postoperative care after pedicle detachment consists of local wound cleansing with hydrogen peroxide solution and application of an antibacterial ointment twice daily for 5 days. The sutures are removed 5 to 7 days postoperatively. The patient is advised to avoid sunlight to the forehead and face for 3 months to prevent darkening or pigmentation of the scars. Additionally the patient is warned that extremes of heat or cold may cause reversible temporary color changes in the flap skin at the recipient site for several months. Revision surgery such as thinning of the flap should be delayed 3 to 6 months to allow complete wound healing, contracture, and beginning of scar maturation. Revision surgery is accomplished with the use of local anesthesia. Revisions are occasionally necessary.

CASE EXAMPLES

CASE 1

Fig. 13-13 shows a 60-year-old woman who presented with a tumor of the right nasal lobule and supralobular area that measured 2.8 × 1.8 cm. A biopsy specimen of the lesion demonstrated a basal cell carcinoma with an aggressive growth pattern. Several

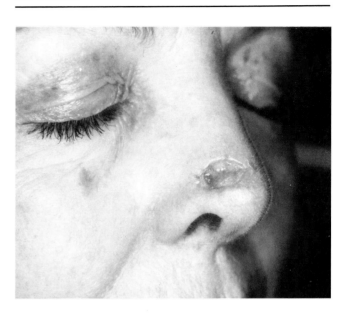

Figure 13-13 **Basal cell carcinoma of nose in 60-year-old woman.**

years earlier the patient had undergone removal of a basal cell carcinoma from her forehead and repair of the subsequent defect with a split-thickness skin graft. The nasal tumor was removed in a three-stage, seven-section Mohs surgical procedure. The final defect was 3.4 × 2.8 cm and involved a full-thickness loss of the entire right nasal lobule and portions of skin of the left lobule and left ala. The right medial alar rim and sublobular soft triangle was also missing (Fig. 13-14).

A 3 × 4 cm wide paramedian forehead flap, based on the right supratrochlear artery and vein, was designed tangential to the skin graft of the forehead and was transposed to the nose (Fig. 13-15**A**). The distal flap was thinned and folded on itself to create an alar rim and to provide for internal lining of the nasal vestibule (Fig. 13-15**B**). The internal portion of the flap was sutured to the nasal mucosa surrounding the nasal defect. The skin margins of the external flap were approximated with interrupted 5-0 nylon vertical mattress sutures. The donor site was closed primarily after adequate mobilization, with the muscular and skin layers closed separately. Aggressive thinning of the distal forehead flap enabled folding of the flap without creation of excessive bulkiness to the reconstructed ala. Three weeks after flap transposition, the proximal pedicle was detached and amputated. Only the very most proximal portion of the pedicle was preserved to ensure medial brow symmetry. The distally attached flap was debulked of any residual frontalis muscle and excess subcutaneous fat (Fig. 13-15**C**).

Ten months after reconstruction, the patient underwent refinement. An incision was made along the inferior edge of the reconstructed ala, and that portion

Figure 13-14 Full-thickness defect of entire right nasal lobule and portions of left lobule and ala after Mohs surgical excision.

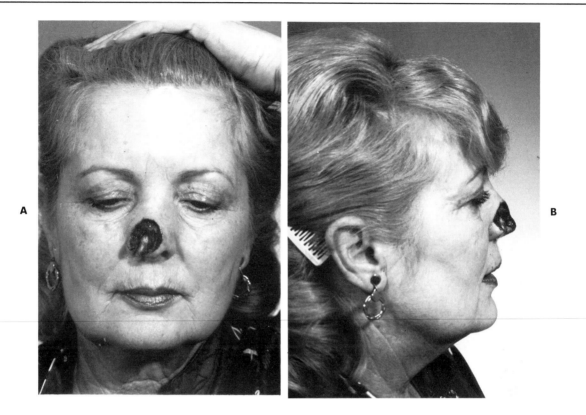

Figure 13-15 *A,* Tangential paramedian forehead flap. *B,* Distal portion of flap folded inward to provide alar margin and internal lining of right nasal vestibule. *C,* Detachment of pedicle.

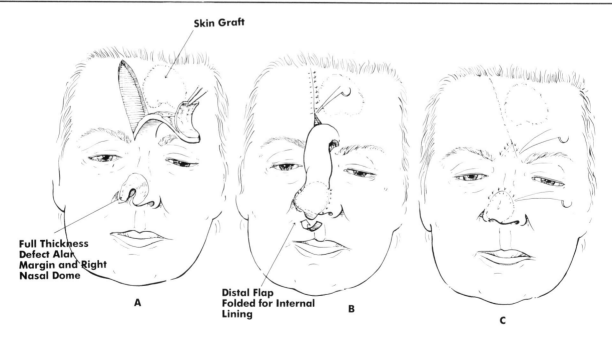

Figure 13-16 Appearance 2.5 years after reconstruction.

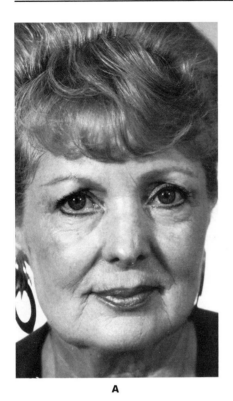 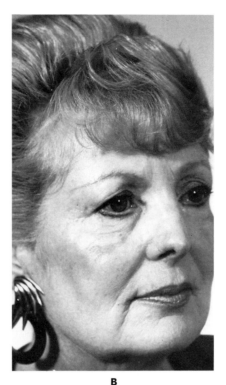 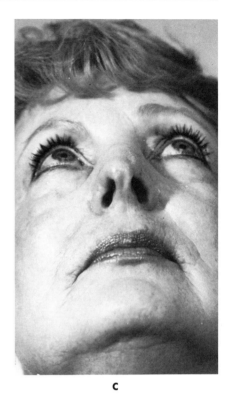

A   B   C

of the flap lining the nasal vestibule was undermined. Fibrofatty scar tissue was removed from the interior of the folded flap to thin the nasal ala and create a more acute angle between the lateral and medial crura. A cartilage graft was also placed between the medial crural cartilages as a cartilagenous strut to provide for support of the nasal tip. The cartilage was placed through a skin incision on the membranous septum. For improvement of the patient's profile, an intercartilaginous incision was made, and the cartilaginous dorsum at the anterior septal angle was trimmed.

Fig. 13-16**A** and **B** shows the patient 2.5 years after reconstruction. The size of the skin graft on the forehead was reduced by partial excision at the time of primary closure of the donor site. The patient had slight distortion of the nostril shape on basal view, but no alar retraction or notching was present (Fig. 13-16**C**). The patient has not had any airway compromise. If cartilage grafts had been used at the time of the initial reconstruction, this may have prevented the need for subsequent revision surgery.

CASE 2

Fig. 13-17[10] shows a 59-year-old woman with recurrent basal cell carcinoma of the nasal tip. Ten years earlier the patient had undergone removal of a similar

tumor from the nasal tip and repair with a skin graft followed by postoperative irradiation. She smoked a pack of cigarettes a day and reported occasional angina pectoris. Mohs surgery was used to resect the tumor, leaving a 5 × 3.5 cm defect of the nasal dorsum. There was full-thickness loss of both nasal lobules, with loss of the medial dome portion of both lower lateral cartilages and the sublobule soft-tissue triangles. There was also loss of the medial alar margins, more so on the right side (Fig. 13-18).[10] A 3.5 cm median forehead flap was used for reconstruction. Appropriately sized skin grafts were used for inner lining of the nasal dome and vestibule areas bilaterally. The skin grafts were quilted to the underside of the thinned forehead flap, and the flap was sutured in place as described for case 1 (Fig. 13-19). This was facilitated by development of, from either side of the dorsal cartilaginous septum, small superiorly based septal mucosal flaps hinged along the length of the upper nasal septum. Each of the mucosal flaps was sutured to the medial edge of its corresponding skin grafts. Fig. 13-20 shows the forehead flap transposed to the nose. The donor site was closed primarily in a fashion described in the Surgical Technique section.

Fig. 13-21 shows the patient 1 week after detachment of the pedicle. The proximal pedicle was trimmed and inset between the brows. The most

Figure 13-17 Recurrent basal cell carcinoma of nasal tip in 59-year-old woman. (From Baker SR: Regional flaps in facial reconstruction, *Otolaryngol Clin North Am* 23:924-945, 1990.)

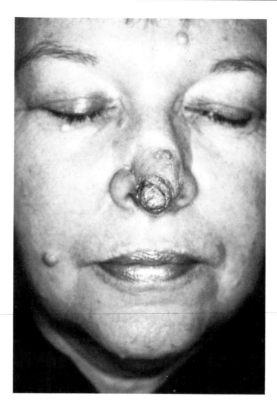

Figure 13-18 Full-thickness defect of nasal dome bilaterally and right alar margin after Mohs surgical excision. (*A* from *Otolaryngol Clin North Am* 23:924-945, 1990.)

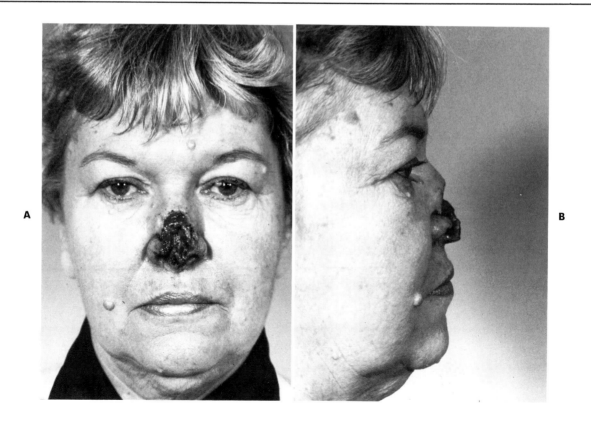

Figure 13-19   Two split-thickness skin grafts placed on underside of thinned forehead flap provide internal lining of nasal vestibules.

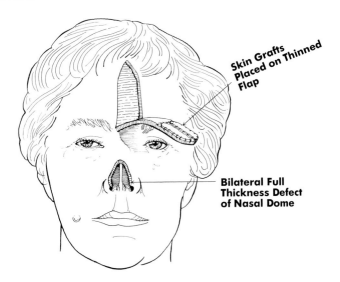

Figure 13-20   Forehead flap is transposed.

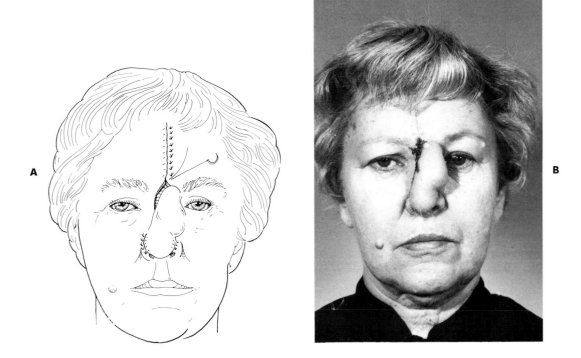

Figure 13-21   Appearance 1 week after detachment of flap pedicle. Only most proximal portion of pedicle is used to restore normal anatomic relationship of eyebrows.

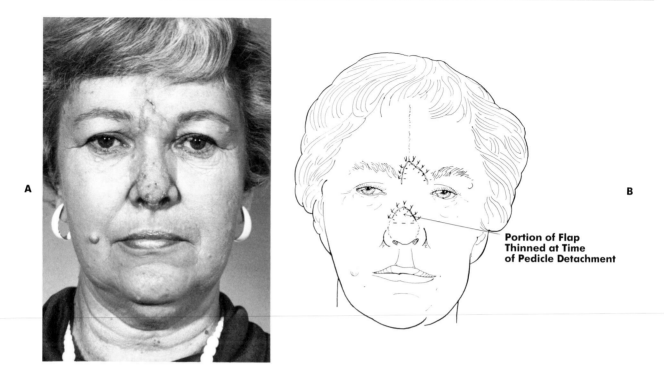

Figure 13-22   Appearance 8 months after reconstruction. (*A* from Baker SR: Regional flaps in facial reconstruction, *Otolaryngol Clin North Am* 23:924-945, 1990.)

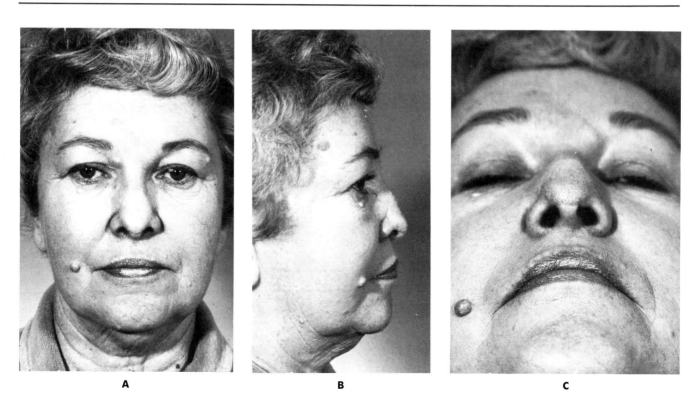

proximal portion of the distal flap left attached to the nose, which was not debulked during the initial transposition, was thinned by removal of the remaining frontalis muscle and all but a very thin layer of subdermal fat.

In attempts to reconstruct an entire esthetic unit, some surgeons advocate removal of the remaining dorsal nasal skin. It is our opinion that such a concept should not be applied to the upper dorsum of the nose when a forehead flap is used for reconstruction. This is because the skin of the rhinion is thin and is not well duplicated by the thick forehead skin. When skin of the rhinion is replaced with forehead skin, it often produces a pseudohump appearance to the profile because of the thickness of the skin.

Fig. 13-22[10] shows the patient 8 months after detachment of the flap pedicle. No revision surgery was performed, and the patient did not complain of nasal obstruction. Although skin grafts can be used for internal lining of full-thickness nasal defects, one of the authors (S.R.B.) prefers to use turn-in skin flaps or intranasal pedicled, mucosal flaps. Mucosal flaps are better vascularized than turn-in skin flaps and can be combined with concurrent cartilage grafts to provide structural support to the nose. Skin grafts tend to contract, often causing distortion of the alar rim and impairment of the airway by compromise of the nasal valve area or the size of the nasal vestibule.

CASE 3

An 11-year-old boy had a history of a progressively enlarging mass of the nasal dorsum at the rhinion. He had fractured his nose 1 year earlier and had noticed the appearance of the mass soon thereafter. The mass had been removed 4 months earlier through an external rhinoplasty approach, but the tumor recurred. Pathologic examination of the tumor revealed an atypical fibrous histiocytoma. The recurrent tumor was diffuse and measured 2×2 cm (Fig. 13-23). Due to the recurrent nature of the lesion, it was resected by Mohs surgical technique. Three stages were necessary to obtain tumor-free margins. This left a full-thickness nasal dorsal defect that measured 4×3 cm. The defect was confined to the dorsum above the lower lateral cartilages and involved loss of portions of the septal cartilage and the medial aspect of both upper lateral nasal cartilages. The defect extended through the mucosa into each nasal passage (Fig. 13-24).

A 4-cm-wide median forehead flap was transposed to provide external reconstruction of the defect (Fig. 13-25). The internal defect was repaired by elevation of bilateral inferiorly based nasal septal mucosal flaps and suturing of the flaps to the edge of the nasal mucosa laterally (Fig. 13-26). The donor defect was closed primarily after wide undermining of the remaining forehead skin (Fig. 13-27). Vertical mattress 5-0 nylon

Figure 13-23   Recurrent atypical fibrous histiocytoma of midnose in 11-year-old boy.

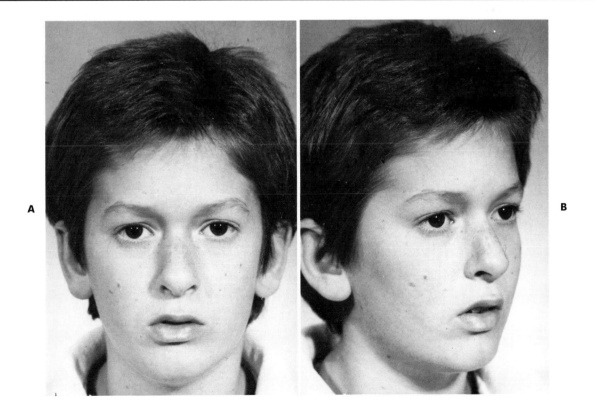

Figure 13-24 Full-thickness defect of cartilaginous dorsum and skin defect of bony dorsum after Mohs surgical excision.

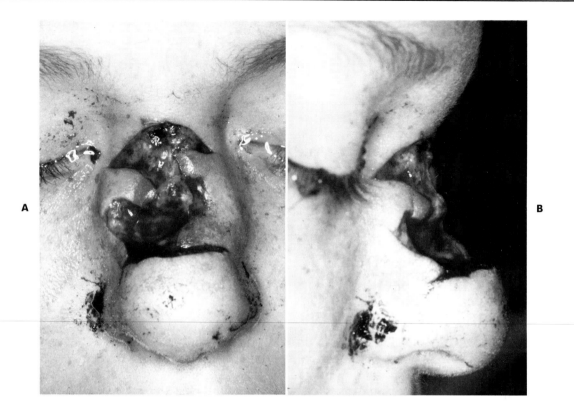

A   B

Figure 13-25 Median forehead flap is transposed to provide external resurfacing of nasal dorsum.

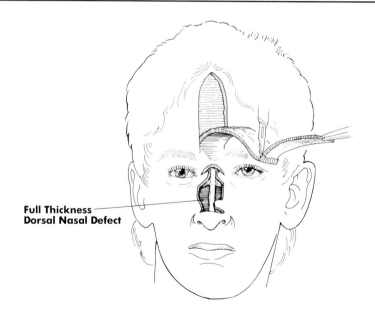

Full Thickness Dorsal Nasal Defect

Figure 13-26   Bilateral nasal septal mucosal flaps provide internal lining.

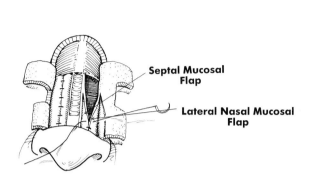

Septal Mucosal
Flap

Lateral Nasal Mucosal
Flap

Figure 13-27   Closure of forehead donor site.

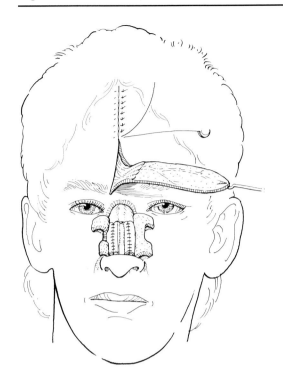

Figure 13-28   Vertical mattress sutures are used to approximate flap to surrounding nasal skin.

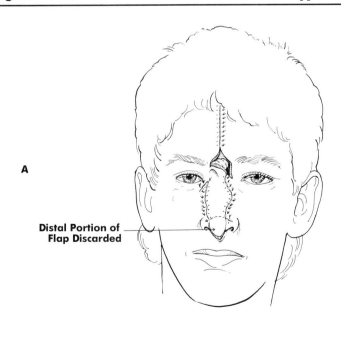

A

Distal Portion of
Flap Discarded

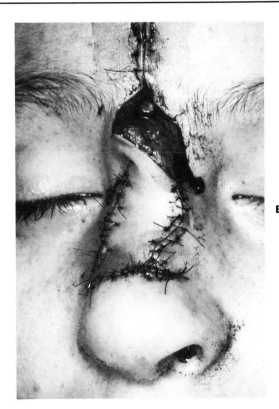

B

sutures were used to approximate the flap to the remaining nasal skin (Fig. 13-28). The pedicle of the flap was separated 3 weeks after flap transfer. At the time of pedicle severance, a cartilage graft was inserted beneath the skin to replace the missing cartilaginous dorsum (Fig. 13-29). Three years after reconstruction, the patient underwent scar revision of the forehead and dermabrasion of the nose (Fig. 13-30).

Figure 13-29 Cartilage graft provides dorsal support to nasal bridge.

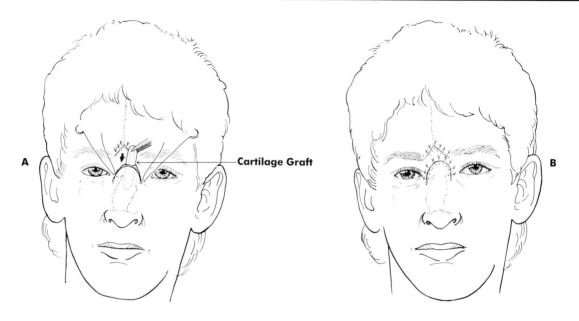

Figure 13-30 Appearance 3 years after reconstruction.

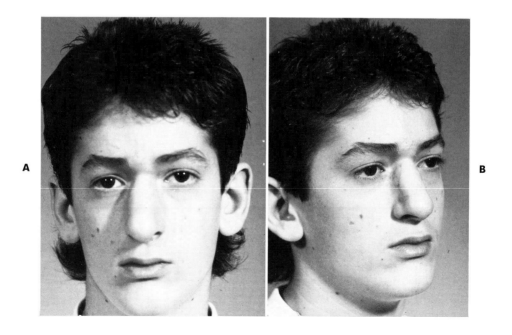

Figure 13-31   Malignant fibrous histiocytoma of right lateral aspect of nose in 37-year-old man.

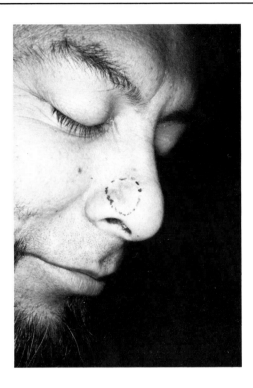

CASE 4

A 37-year-old man had a 1.5 cm × 1.5 cm area of induration over the right lateral aspect of the nose that had been present for 6 months (Fig. 13-31). A biopsy specimen obtained from the area demonstrated a malignant fibrous histiocytoma. The tumor was removed by Mohs surgery in three stages. The final defect after complete resection of the tumor measured 3.5 × 3 cm. The defect consisted of a full-thickness loss of the right nasal vestibule, dome, and lateral crura of the right lower lateral cartilage. The caudal one half of the right upper lateral cartilage was resected, and portions of the cartilaginous dorsum were also absent (Fig. 13-32). The missing portion of the upper and lower lateral cartilages were replaced by a superiorly based full-thickness composite septal flap that consisted of septal cartilage covered on both sides by mucosa transposed in a hinged-door fashion (Fig. 13-33). The mucosa on the right side of the septal flap was turned over as a second hinged flap to provide lining to the nasal dome and lower vestibule, and the mucosa on the deep side of the septal flap provided internal lining to the remaining nasal vestibule (Fig. 13-34). A median forehead flap provided external coverage of the nose (Fig. 13-35). A Bolster suture placed through the forehead flap and the underlying septal flap eliminated potential dead space (Fig. 13-36).

Figure 13-32   Full-thickness defect of right nasal vestibule in addition to loss of portions of cartilaginous dorsum.

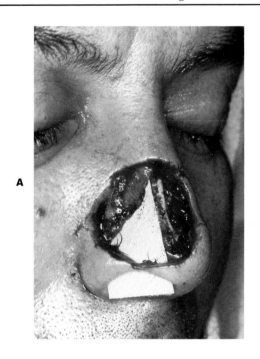

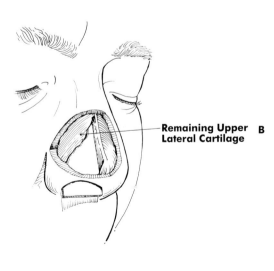

Remaining Upper Lateral Cartilage   B

Figure 13-33 Design of full-thickness hinged-door septal flap.

Figure 13-34 Cartilage from septal flap provides structural replacement of missing upper and lower lateral cartilage. Mucosa on superior aspect of flap provides lining for lower nasal vestibule.

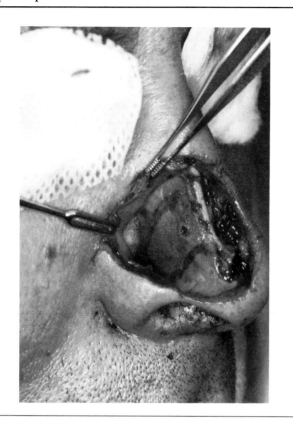

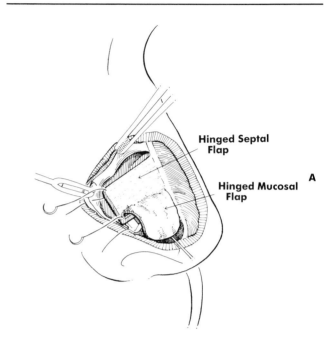

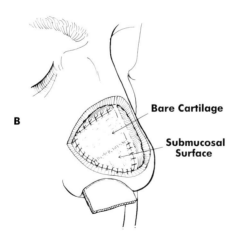

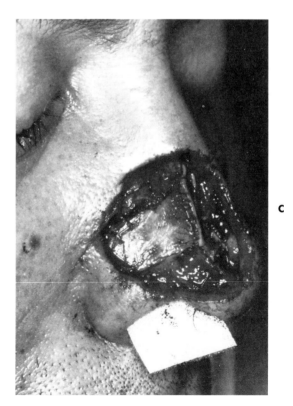

Figure 13-35   Median forehead flap provides external coverage of nose.

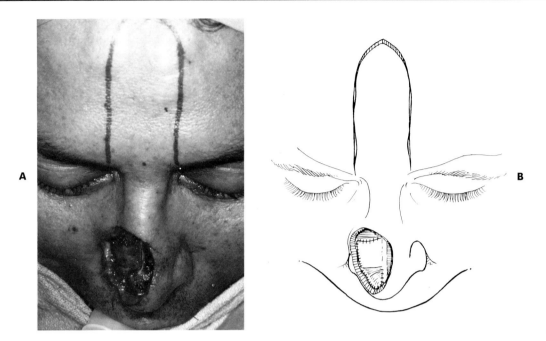

Figure 13-36   Bolster dressing eliminates potential dead space between septal flap and forehead flap.

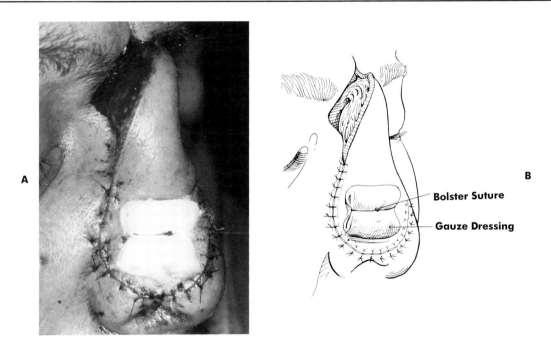

Figure 13-37 Appearance 3 years after reconstruction.

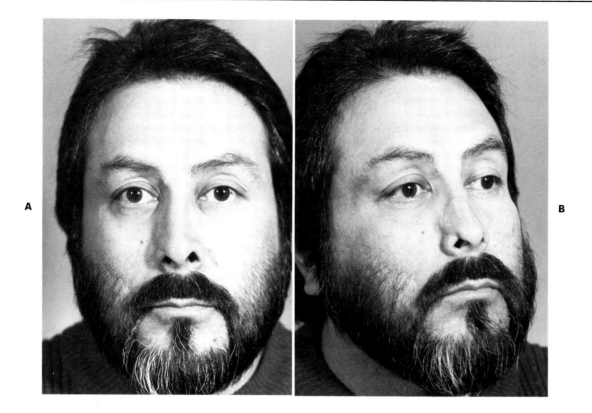

A   B

Fig. 13-37 shows the patient 3 years after reconstruction. No revision surgery was performed. The patient had some notching of the right alar margin as a result of wound contracture. An additional cartilage graft placed in the area of the alar margin below the hinged septal cartilage flap would likely have prevented this upper migration of the alar margin.

CASE 5

A 70-year-old woman presented with a recurrent basal cell carcinoma of the nose measuring 2.5 × 2 cm (Fig. 13-38).[43] The tumor had been treated with surgical resection four times during the preceding 4 years, and on two occasions the patient had skin grafts applied. The patient underwent a five-stage, 19-section Mohs surgical procedure to completely excise the tumor. The resulting defect measured 4 × 4 cm and involved loss of the entire nasal tip and columella. There was loss of all but the lateral portions of both lower lateral cartilages. The entire membraneous septum was missing, and portions of the cartilaginous nasal dorsum and the medial aspect of the right upper lateral cartilage were also absent (Fig. 13-39).[43]

The nose was reconstructed with a paramedian oblique forehead flap. An oblique design was used because of the relatively low hairline and the necessity for the distal end of the flap to reach the upper lip (Fig.

Figure 13-38 Recurrent basal cell carcinoma of nose in 70-year-old woman. (From Baker SR, Swanson NA: Regional and distant skin flaps in nasal reconstruction, *Facial Plast Surg* 2:33-44, 1984.)

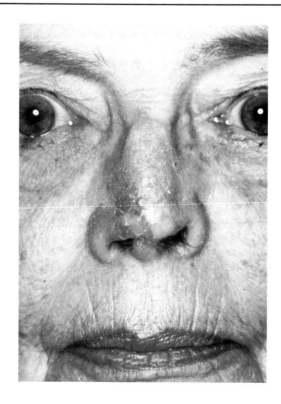

Figure 13-39   Full-thickness defect of nasal tip columella and membranous septum. (From Baker SR, Swanson NA: Regional and distant skin flaps in nasal reconstruction, *Facial Plast Surg* 2:33-44, 1984.)

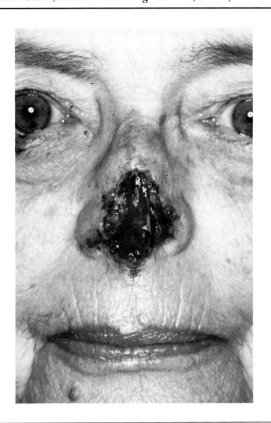

Figure 13-40   Oblique paramedian forehead flap used to reconstruct entire nasal defect. (*A* from Baker SR, Swanson NA: Regional and distant skin flaps in nasal reconstruction, *Facial Plast Surg* 2:33-44, 1984.)

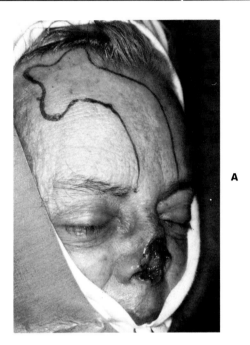

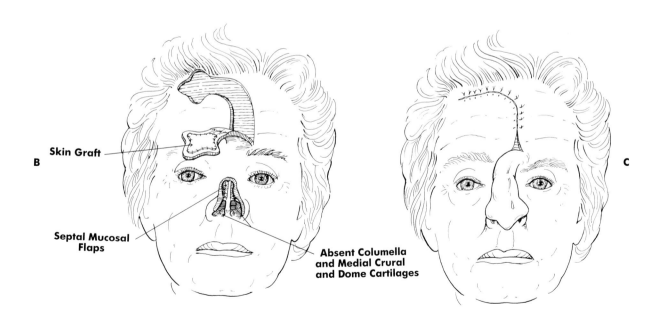

Skin Graft

Septal Mucosal Flaps

Absent Columella and Medial Crural and Dome Cartilages

Figure 13-41   Portions of donor site left to heal by second intention. (From Baker SR, Swanson NA: Regional and distant skin flaps in nasal reconstruction, *Facial Plast Surg* 2:33-44, 1984.)

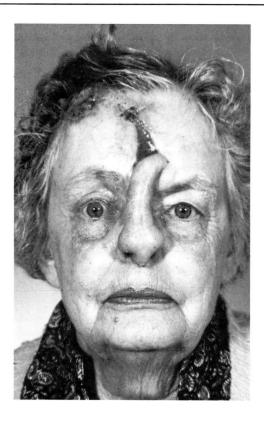

Figure 13-42   Detachment of oblique forehead flap.

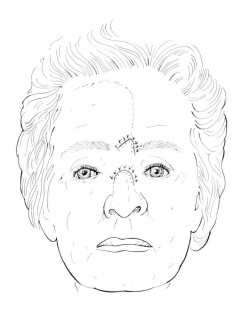

Figure 13-43   Appearance 1 year postoperatively. (From Baker SR, Swanson NA: Regional and distant skin flaps in nasal reconstruction, *Facial Plast Surg* 2:33-44, 1984.)

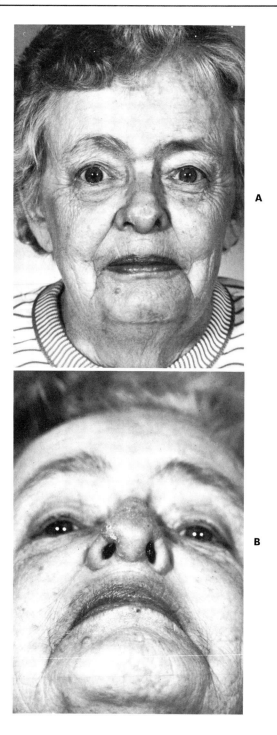

13-40).[43] The internal lining of the missing nasal vestibule was provided by a split-thickness skin graft placed on the deep surface of the distal thinned forehead flap. More posteriorly in the nasal passage, lining was provided by reflecting mucosal flaps from the nasal septum and suturing them to lateral nasal mucosa. No cartilage grafts were used. The distal end of the flap was 5 cm wide, and it was not possible to achieve primary closure of the donor site (Fig. 13-41).[43] The flap was detached 3 weeks after the initial flap transfer (Fig. 13-42).

Fig. 13-43[43] shows the patient 1 year postoperatively. She had one revision of the reconstructed nose 3 months after detachment of the pedicle, which consisted of minor debulking of the flap along the nasal bridge. Despite loss of most of the lower lateral cartilages without replacement, the patient has not had compromise of the nasal airway. This is probably related to the remaining high nasal septum that provides support to the reconstructed tip. As in this case, enough fibrosis may occur between the midforehead flap and the internal skin graft to give the reconstructed areas sufficient rigidity that a cartilaginous framework is not necessary. In general, however, a preferred technique would be to replace missing cartilage with cartilage grafts at the time of initial reconstruction. Although portions of the donor site were allowed to heal by second intention, the final scar was acceptable.

From an esthetic standpoint primary closure of the forehead is not as important as some of the other donor sites about the face, such as the cheek. This is presumably because the forehead is a convex, relatively immobile area of the face and secondary wound healing produces favorable scars. When it is likely that closure of the forehead will not be possible after transfer of a midforehead flap, secondary healing may be facilitated by leaving the frontalis muscle on the forehead and harvesting a skin-only forehead flap in the distal three fourths of the flap. Dissection in the area of the proximal one fourth of the flap extends below the frontalis muscle near the base of the flap to preserve the pedicle's vasculature. The preserved frontalis muscle left attached to the forehead will provide a source of granulation tissue for rapid secondary healing and may help prevent a depressed scar.

SUMMARY

The vertically oriented midforehead flaps are truly the workhorse local rotation flap for nasal and midface reconstruction. When used appropriately by skilled surgeons, large disfiguring nasal and midface defects can be completely reconstructed and camouflaged to the patient's satisfaction. Understanding of flap anatomy and the concepts of lining, support, and covering as outlined by Millard and Burget, as well as a willingness to perform revision surgery as necessary, make this a wildly successful local, regional flap for nasal reconstruction.

REFERENCES

1. Burget GC, Menick FJ: Nasal support and lining: the marriage of beauty and blood supply, *Plast Reconstr Surg* 84:189, 1989.
2. Conley JJ, Price JC: Midline vertical forehead flap, *Otolaryngol Head Neck Surg* 89:38, 1981.
3. Jackson IT: *Local flaps in head and neck reconstruction*, St Louis, 1985, CV Mosby.
4. Mazzola RF, Marcus S: History of total nasal reconstruction with particular emphasis on the folded forehead flap technique, *Plast Reconstruct Surg* 72:408, 1983.
5. Shumrick KA, Smith TL: The anatomic basis for the design of forehead flaps in nasal reconstruction, *Arch Otolaryngol Head Neck Surg* 118:373, 1992.
6. *Sushruta samhita*, Calcutta, 1916, Base (translated by KK Bhishagronta).
7. Deformities of the nose. In Converse JA, editor: *Reconstructive plastic surgery*, Philadelphia, 1964, WB Saunders.
8. Deformities of the nose. In Converse JA, editor: *Reconstructive plastic surgery*, ed 2, Philadelphia, 1977, WB Saunders.
9. Menick FJ: Aesthetic refinements in use of the forehead flap for nasal reconstruction: the paramedian forehead flap, *Clin Plast Surg* 17:607, 1990.
10. Baker SR: Regional flaps in facial reconstruction, *Otolaryngol Clin North Am* 23:925, 1990.
11. McDowell F, Valone JA, Bronn JB: Bibliography and historical note on plastic surgery of the nose, *Plast Reconstruct Surg* 10:149, 1952.
12. BL: Letter to the editor, *Gentleman's Magazine*, London, Oct 1794, p 891. Reprinted in *Plast Reconstruct Surg* 44:67, 1969.
13. Carpue JC: An account of two successful operations for restoring a lost nose from the integuments of the forehead, London, 1816, Longman. Reprinted in *Plast Reconstruct Surg* 44:175, 1969.
14. Cormack GC, Lamberth BG: *The arterial anatomy of skin flaps*, New York, 1986, Churchill Livingstone.
15. Millard DR: Total reconstructive rhinoplasty and a missing link, *Plast Reconstruct Surg* 37:167, 1966.
16. Kazanjian VH: The repair of nasal defects with the median forehead flap: primary closure of the forehead wound, *Surg Gynecol Obstet* 83:37, 1946.

17. Millard DR: Hemi-rhinoplasty, *Plast Reconstruct Surg* 40:440, 1967.

18. Millard DR: Reconstructive rhinoplasty for the lower two-thirds of the nose, *Plast Reconstruct Surg* 57:722, 1976.

19. Millard DR: Reconstructive rhinoplasty for the lower half of the nose, *Plast Reconstruct Surg* 53:133, 1974.

20. Burget GC, Menick FJ: The subunit principle in nasal reconstruction, *Plast Reconstruct Surg* 76:239, 1985.

21. Burget GC: Aesthetic reconstruction of the nose, *Clin Plast Surg* 12:463, 1985.

22. Burget GC, Menick FJ: Nasal reconstruction: seeking a fourth dimension, *Plast Reconstruct Surg* 78:145, 1986.

23. Mangold V, Lierse W, Pfeifer G: The arteries of the forehead as the basis of nasal reconstruction with forehead flaps, *Acta Anat* 107:18, 1980.

24. McCarthy JG, Lorenc ZP, Cuting L et al: The median forehead flap revisited: the blood supply. *Plast Reconstruct Surg* 76:866, 1985.

25. Acquired deformities of the nose. In McCarthy JG, editor: *Plastic surgery*, ed 3, Philadelphia, 1990, WB Saunders.

26. Burget GC: Surgical restoration of the nose, In , editor: *Current therapy in plastic and reconstructive surgery*. New York, 1989, BC Decker.

27. Barton FE: Aesthetic aspects of nasal reconstruction, *Clin Plast Surg* 15:155, 1988.

28. Meyer R, Kesserling VK: Reconstructive surgery of the nose, *Clin Plast Surg* 8:435, 1981.

29. Nichter LS, Morgan RF, Nichter MD: The impact of Indian methods for total nasal reconstruction, *Clin Plast Surg* 10:635, 1983.

30. Taroy ME, Sykes J, Kron T: The precise midline forehead flap in reconstruction of the nose, *Clin Plast Surg* 12:481, 1985.

31. Thomas JR, Griner N, Look T: Precise midline forehead flap as a musculocutaneous flap, *Arch Otolaryngol* 114:79, 1988.

32. Baker SR, Swanson NA: Rapid intraoperative tissue expansion in reconstruction of the head and neck, *Arch Otolaryngol Head Neck Surg* 116:1431, 1990.

33. Hart NB, Goldin JM: The importance of symmetry in forehead flap rhinoplasty, *Br J Plast Surg* 37:477, 1984.

34. Converse JM, Wood-Smith D: Experiences with the forehead island flap with a subcutaneous pedicle, *Plast Reconstruct Surg* 31:521, 1963.

35. Hoffman HT, Baker SR: Nasal reconstruction with the rapidly expanded forehead flap, *Laryngoscope* 99:1096, 1989.

36. Salasche SJ, Brabaski WJ, Mulvaney MJ: Delayed grafting of midline forehead flap donor defects: utilization of residual flap tissue, *J Dermatol Surg Oncol* 16:633, 1990.

37. Baker SR, Swanson NA, Grekin RC: Mohs surgical treatment and reconstruction of cutaneous malignancies of the nose, *Facial Plast Surg* 5:29, 1987.

38. Adamson JE: Nasal reconstruction with the expanded forehead flap, *Plast Reconstr Surg* 81:12, 1987.

39. Zhou LY, Hu QY: Median forehead island skin flap for the correction of severely collapsed nose, *Ann Plast Surg* 22:516, 1989.

40. Mosconda AR, Hirshowitz B: Combined forehead and bilateral cheek flaps for resurfacing a large dorsal nasal defect, *Ann Plast Surg* 7:75, 1981.

41. Gaze NR: Reconstructing the nasal tip with a midline forehead flap, *Br J Plast Surg* 33:122, 1980.

42. Baker SR, Swanson NA: Regional and distant skin flaps in nasal reconstruction, *Facial Plast Surg* 2:33, 1984.

43. Baker SR, Swanson NA: Oblique forehead flap for total reconstruction of the nasal tip and columella, *Arch Otolaryngol Head Neck Surg* 111:425, 1989.

44. Kroll SS: Forehead flap nasal reconstruction with tissue expansion and delayed pedicle separation, *Laryngoscope* 99:448, 1989.

EDITORIAL COMMENTS

Neil A. Swanson

I had the privilege of working with Shan Baker during my tenure at the University of Michigan during the 1980s. Together we shared many patients who had large central nasal and other defects that required reconstruction with the forehead flap. My observation of the evolution of Shan's technique in performing this flap and my participation with Dr. Burget in panel discussions led me to appreciate versatility of this flap when it is performed by talented surgeons who understand the concepts.

This chapter has a very inclusive and well-written background concerning the history of the forehead flap and the anatomy that allows both its use and refinements. Study of the supratrochlear artery has allowed thinning of the distal flap with impunity and narrowing of the pedicle, which facilitates flap transfer.

As a dermatologic surgeon who performs most of my reconstruction surgeries with the use of local anesthesia with or without mild sedation, I believe that the forehead flap can be easily and adequately performed with use of local anesthesia. However, some surgeons may be more comfortable with use of general anesthesia. The design of the flap is well detailed by the authors, as are the techniques of flap interpolation. I would parrot the usefulness of galeotomies and fasciotomies and the importance of the deep galea suture in relief of tension on the skin edge and prevention of "stretch back" in the closure of the secondary defect on the forehead. I also agree that vertical mattress sutures in the forehead are an excellent way to obtain fine tissue eversion.

The authors describe the use of benzolin during placement of Steri-strips. I prefer the use of Masatsol. It is colorless and relatively odorless and does not stain or produce a contact dermatitis.

For surgeons who do not understand this flap and who improperly thin the distant flap, a large, bulky, sausagelike result occurs. The other poor results are due to an improper understanding of flap detachment at 3 weeks. Also, it is critical to not extend the replacement of tissue above the eyebrow line. Sausage-shaped tissue extending onto the forehead does not prove esthetically pleasing. The authors very nicely review in detail the method of flap detachment.

The authors also hint at the concept of enlargement of the defect to fill an esthetic unit with some warning about the inferior part of the defect. Although it can be difficult to deal with the concept of removal of carefully preserved tissue during Mohs surgery, this concept can result in improved esthetic results.

The case examples carefully illustrate several tips on secondary procedures, procedures for lining full-thickness defects, replacement of cartilage, and fine-tuning the final result.

This chapter shows the versatility of this important flap in facial reconstructive surgery.

14

DORSAL NASAL FLAPS

Leonard M. Dzubow

INTRODUCTION

The dorsal nasal flap is a rotation flap that uses all or part of the nasal skin to repair small to moderately sized partial-thickness defects. The use of rotation flaps of the nose for local reconstruction was first described by Elliot.[1] However, the flaps he detailed were the banner and bilobe flaps. Although these flaps employ rotational movement, they transpose over a peninsula of intervening tissue and are currently classified as interpolation flaps. Rieger[2] was the first individual to describe a true rotation flap with the use of the entire dorsal nasal skin to repair a tip defect. He used the technique to repair lower nasal wounds that did not exceed 2 cm in diameter. The flap was designed to pivot around a random-pattern vascular pedicle that extended from the medial canthus and down the nose-cheek junction. The flap was cut from the superior aspect of the defect, up the nose-cheek junction, into the glabella, and back down to the medial canthus. The glabellar incisions essentially provided a back-cut for the rotation flap. Rieger closed the upper end of the flap with a Z-plasty. Of importance, he noted limitation in movement of the flap, which resulted in elevation of the nasal tip.

Further refinements of the dorsal nasal flap were offered by Rigg.[3] He introduced the concept of occasional use of only part rather than all of the nasal skin for the flap. These heminasal flaps could be created by running the free edge of the flap directly down the midline of the nose with a lateral base or down the melonasal junction with a medial base. If the entire nasal dorsum was to be incorporated in the flap, the incision ran across the vasoalar crease to the lateral nasal wall, up through the opposite medial canthus to the glabella, and back down across the glabella to the ipsilateral inner canthus. Rigg also noted the problem of tethering of the flap at the inner canthal pivotal point and suggested further back-cutting into this edge. In fact, one of his postoperative photographs demonstrates alar elevation due to such restraint. He suggested treatment of the redundant glabellar triangle by either amputation or Z-plasty.

Several authors subsequently commented on the utility of this flap alone or in combination with cheek advancement flaps for larger nasal defects.[4-8] However, many of the cases, which were presented photographically, demonstrated mild to extreme alar elevation due to pivotal movement limitation. Cronin[9] described in detail the technique of using only part of the nasal skin for the rotation flap.[9] This heminasal laterally based flap was designated by him as a V-Y rotation flap. He used this for defects up to 2.5 cm in diameter located in the lower or middle third of the nose. Of interest is that Cronin extended his glabellar back-cut through and past the medial canthus. The resulting pedicle was narrower than the classic design and resulted in less apparent alar elevation. Although the pedicle was of a random vascular pattern, ischemia was not noted as a difficulty.

The most recent refinement of the dorsal nasal flap was introduced in 1970 by Marchac[10] but not published in the English literature until 1985.[11] His modification defined an axial pedicle for the flap based on vessels that emerge near the inner canthus. He designated this as the axial frontonasal flap. Extreme narrowing of the pedicle could now be safely accomplished, permitting better rotational movement without restraint. The vascular pedicle was presented as incorporating a constant branch of the angular artery. The flap uses the total nasal surface, such as in the traditional design. However, Marchac's flap permits a longer descent of the glabellar back-cut just up to the location of the medial canthal ligament. Distortion of free alar margins was not noted.

The effectiveness of any rotation flap relies on the transformation and relocation of the primary defect to a secondary wound. As the original wound is partially or totally closed by the movement of the flap, a new secondary defect is created along the curvilinear sweep of the elevated flap edge. This new defect has the same surface area as the original. It is, however, crescentic and hopefully located in a site of available tissue laxity to permit easy closure. Of greatest importance, the longer the sweep of the flap, the narrower will be the secondary defect. The narrower the defect, the easier it will be to close. Therefore, if rotation flaps are to effectively reduce the tension of closure, they must be large relative to the size of the primary wound. This is clearly the greatest source of reluctance in the implementation of this flap. Dorsal nasal flaps must be quite out of proportion in size relative to the defect. If such a large flap fails, the resultant disability is enormous compared to the proportions of the original problem. Is it a risk worth taking?

The advantages of this flap are many. Local nasal skin is used to repair a nasal wound. Skin grafts and distant two-stage forehead flaps often do not provide the same match in color, texture, thickness, sebaceous quality, or vascular pattern. The scars of this flap are usually well hidden in advantageous locations—the cosmetic junctions of the alar crease and the nose-cheek border as well as within the glabellar frown lines. Transposition flaps such as rhombic or bilobe flaps will provide matching skin but create unnatural, geometrically shaped scars, which if visible are not hidden within natural junctions or creases.

The disadvantages inherent in the nature of the flap are limited to size and mobility. The issue of risking loss, through necrosis of large amounts of tissue for closure of small defects, must be weighed by each operator. If the flap is properly created, ischemic complications are reported to be rare. The primary problem with the traditional dorsal nasal flap is the limited rotational movement afforded by the pedicle. If this is not anticipated or addressed in the flap design, the free margins of the nose will be displaced. If the defect is on the central nasal tip, the tip will elevate. In an older patient with nasal ptosis, this is not a concern. However, more laterally located wounds may be prone to alar elevation and resultant asymmetry of the nose. Sometimes this corrects with time and sometimes not. This problem may be prevented with use of the Marchac axial flap or by ensuring that the leading edge of the flap extends *beyond* the defect. If the latter is chosen, flap rotation will fill all of the primary wound rather than part of it. This will obviate the need of any secondary movement from the alar rim or tip toward the flap.

The dorsal nasal flap is best used for wounds of the nose 2 to 2.5 cm in diameter or less. Available tissue is not sufficient to make a rotation flap large enough for defects that exceed this size. The wounds may be located on the lower or middle thirds of the nose. On the lower third of the nose, defects are most ideally located centrally on the tip. If tip elevation occurs, it is therefore symmetrical. Defects should be medial or superior to the alar lobule. If the flap crosses the alar crease, the natural concavity is lost and cosmetic junctions are blurred. Furthermore, proximity to the alar rim invites problems with distortion secondary to elevation or compression. The flap should not be used in individuals with thick sebaceous skin because mobility is poor. Obviously, results are better in the older population than in young individuals.

SURGICAL TECHNIQUE

The successful execution of the dorsal nasal flap requires careful planning and design. Since this technique involves extensive tissue movement and undermining, it is important that the patient refrain from consumption of any substances that would interfere with coagulation. Aspirin should be prohibited from 1 week before to 1 week after the procedure. Nonsteroidal antiinflammatory medications are stopped 3 to 7 days before the procedure and are avoided for 3 days after surgery. Alcohol consumption, which causes vasodilitation, should be ceased 1 to 2 days before surgery.

The choice of anesthetic is based on individual preference. Although concern has been expressed about the vasoconstrictive properties of epinephrine, the addition of this substance to the local anesthetic used does not appear to increase the propensity toward ischemic problems.

The design of the flap determines the esthetic success of the procedure. The defect should be no larger than 2.5 cm. The smaller the wound, the less the tendency for anatomic distortion associated with closure of the secondary defect. In drawing the flap, it is helpful to triangulate the defect by addition of the triangle of redundant tissue or standing cutaneous deformity that will be created by flap rotation. The standing cutaneous deformity should be removed above the alar lobule so that the resultant scar is within the alar crease or above. The flap should not be drawn to cross the junction of the lateral nasal sidewall and the ala.

The most important aspect of flap design is the planning of the leading free edge of the flap, that is, the aspect that leads the way in closing the primary defect. Unless movement of the nasal tip or alar rim is anticipated and accepted, the leading edge of the flap should always extend some distance beyond the defect (Figs. 14-1 and 14-2). The rationale behind this is crucial to understand. As previously noted, a rotation

Figures 14-1, 14-2   A 2.5-cm wound on the nasal tip in 42-year-old woman. Dorsal nasal flap designed.

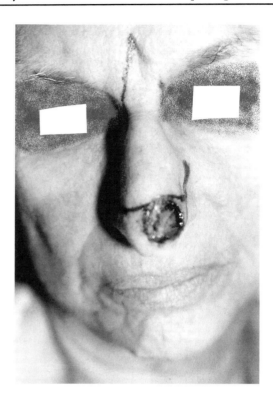

Fig. 14-1

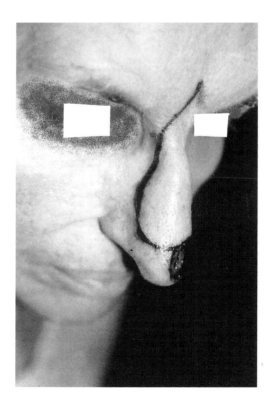

Fig. 14-2

flap moves in a curvilinear path as it pivots around the pedicle. If the height of the flap is equal to the height of the triangulated defect, the flap will not completely fill the primary wound as it rotates in a curved fashion from proximal to distal. This is because the effective height of a rotation flap is progressively diminished as it rotates about its pivotal point. The height of the flap and thus the arc of rotation must be sufficient to compensate for this shortening. If the radius of the arc of rotation is not made large enough, the flap will curve down rather than move straight across, incompletely filling the defect and necessitating advancement of surrounding tissue. This creates wound closure tension. Either the skin will stretch to accommodate this pulling or the surrounding structures must give way and be pulled in toward the flap tip. Since nasal tissue is not elastic, anatomic distortion is the usual outcome. If however, the leading edge of the flap is drawn to extend beyond the defect, it will now fill the primary wound under almost no tension as it follows its curved rotational path. This design is incorporated in every dorsal nasal flap that uses the entirety of nasal skin to repair central defects. The leading edge of the flap is drawn beyond the defect, along the opposite alar crease and then up along the nose-cheek junction. In the heminasal design, the extension of the leading edge must be deliberately added.

From the nose-cheek junction, the flap is drawn through the medial canthus and then up high in the glabella (Figs. 14-1 and 14-2). The higher the flap goes, the greater the length of the rotation flap and the easier it will be to close the secondary defect. The flap design then progresses downward from the highest glabellar point at a 30° angle. If one wishes to incorporate the axial angular vessels within the pedicle, the back-cut must finish superior to the level of the medial canthal tendon. If a random vascular pedicle is acceptable, the back cut may be continued through the inner canthus to the level of the infraorbital crease. As a safe rule, full dorsal nasal flaps should probably incorporate the larger vessels within the pedicle, whereas heminasal flaps may survive well with only the random vascular input.

Once the flap is drawn, anesthesia may be achieved with 1% lidocaine (Xylocaine) with epinephrine (1:100,000) injected along the edges of the flap to be cut and beyond into the tissues to be undermined. The pedicle is injected with 1% lidocaine alone. There is no documentation to support the need for this adjustment for the pedicle. However, since a large flap is being raised on a relatively narrow pedicle, prudence cannot be faulted.

After the anesthetic and hemostatic effects are achieved, the flap is incised. The triangular standing cutaneous deformity associated with the primary

Figure 14-3   **Undermining of flap above perichondrium.**

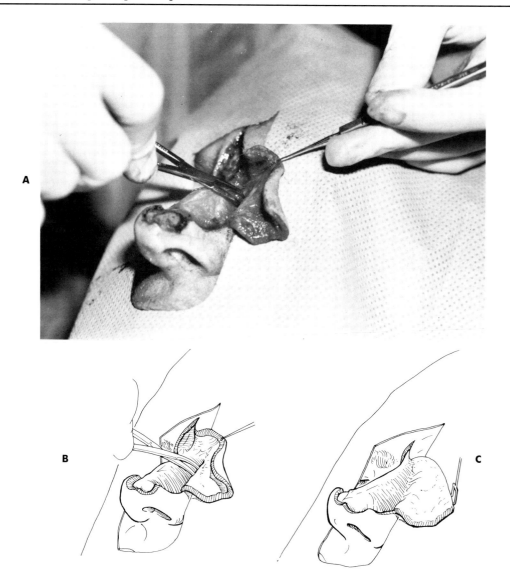

wound is not removed until the amount of redundant tissue anticipated is actually verified after the movement of the flap. If the excisional design is too generous and the standing cone is preexcised before flap movement, closure difficulties may result.

The flap is incised to the relatively avascular plane between the perichondrium and the nasalis muscle. The entirety of the flap is undermined at this level (Fig. 14-3). Extreme care is taken during the undermining of the pedicle. Blunt dissection with a hemostat may be used rather than sharp dissection to avoid injury to the branches of the angular artery. However, the pedicle must be well undermined to permit free rotation.

Bleeding is frequently noted at the nasal tip and the glabellar region. Coagulation is achieved by forceps. The tissue surrounding the flap must be well under-

mined to permit good secondary cheek movement in closure of the secondary defect (Fig. 14-4). At the cheek-nose junction the attachments are often fibrous and vascular. Undermining with a blunt hemostat is again helpful. The fully undermined flap should be freed of most restraining forces in preparation for rotation (Fig. 14-5).

Once the flap and surrounding tissues are fully mobilized, the flap is rotated to close the primary defect (Fig. 14-6). As this occurs, a crescentic secondary wound is visible along the free curvilinear sweep of the flap. A single 5-0 nylon tacking suture is used to visualize placement of the flap and to allow for inspection of alar or tip movement (Fig. 14-7). If distortion is noted, attempts at readjustment of flap position must be attempted. The primary wound is

Figure 14-4   Undermining of peripheral tissues.

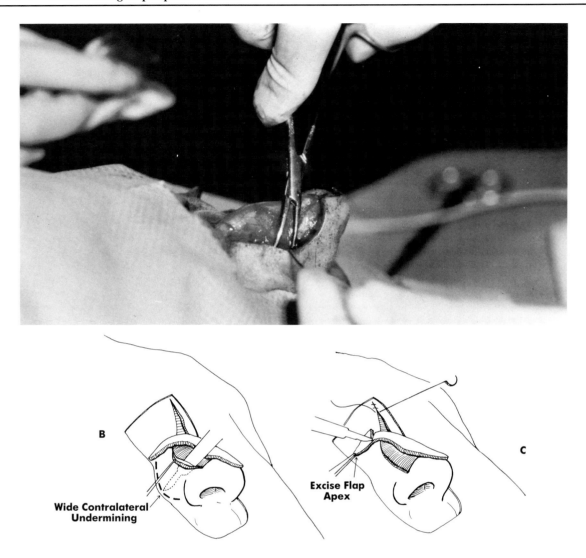

Figure 14-5   Undermined flap mobilized. Forehead donor site closed.

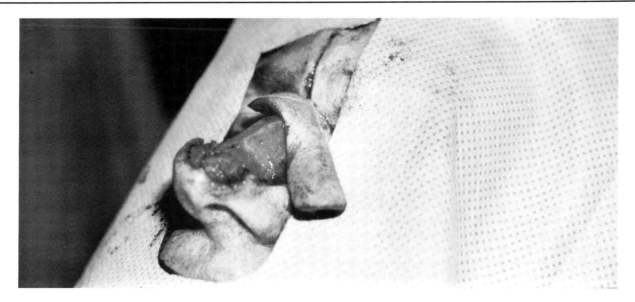

Figure 14-6   Flap draped over defect.

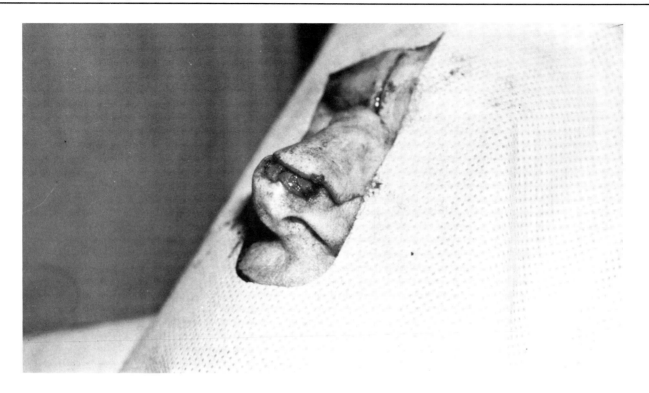

Figure 14-7   Flap positioned with single key suture.

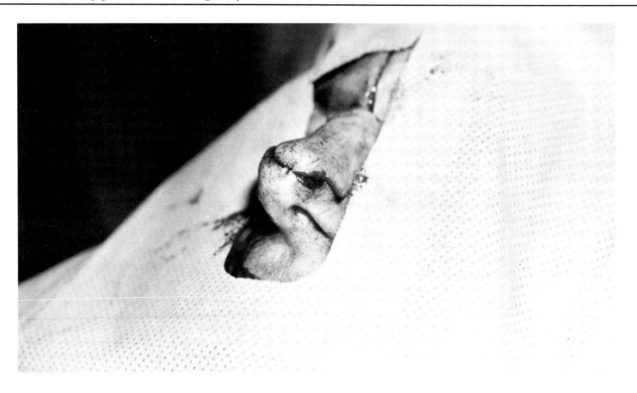

Figure 14-8   Advancement of cheek skin.

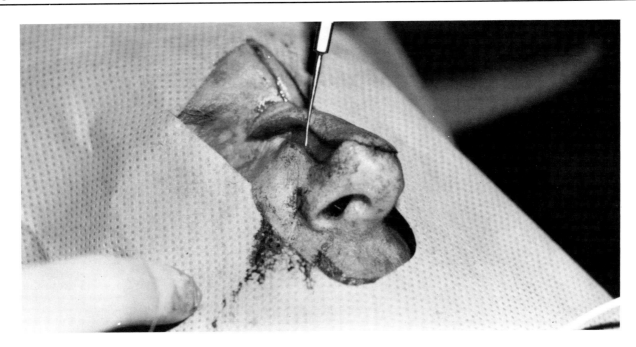

Figure 14-9   Tacking of cheek skin.

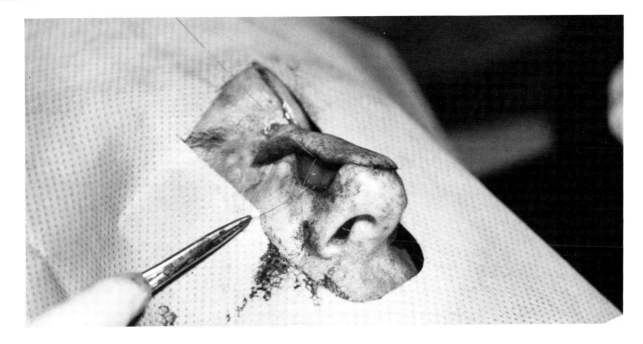

then closed in layers with use of 5-0 polyglactin (Vicryl) sutures for the deep layer and 5-0 nylon sutures for the skin layer.

Attention is next directed to the secondary defect. If the leading edge of the flap has been extended to prevent tension on closure of the primary defect, the secondary defect along the border of the flap will be somewhat wider and irregularly shaped. To prevent distortion of the tip from closure of the secondary defect in this area, it is helpful to try to bring the surrounding cheek tissues in toward the flap with tacking sutures. This is done by pulling the cheek tissue in and tacking to nonmovable fibrous tissue at the pyriform aperture (Fig. 14-8). Tacking is achieved with 4-0 polyglactin interrupted sutures (Fig. 14-9). The secondary defect is then closed with 5-0 polyglactin

Figure 14-10   Sutured flap.

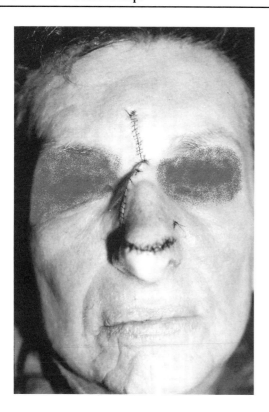

Figures 14-11, 14-12   Six-month postoperative result.

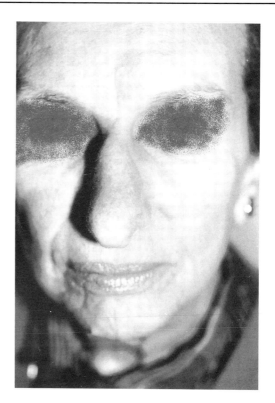

Fig. 14-11

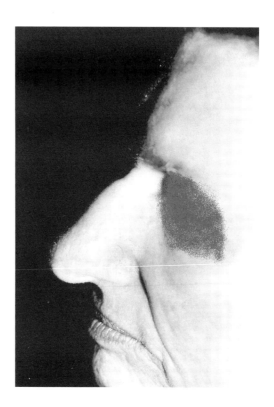

Fig. 14-12

sutures for the deep layer and 5-0 nylon sutures for the skin up to the level of the glabella. It is sometimes helpful to thin the flap edge where it unites with the thinner canthal skin to achieve better opposition. At this point a triangle of glabellar tissue will overlap the proposed closure line. It is simply amputated to achieve a proper fit (Fig. 14-4**C**). The glabellar wound is then closed in a side-to-side fashion (Fig. 14-10). Scars placed at boundaries of cosmetic junctions tend to become less perceptible within 6 months, whereas those within a cosmetic unit or subunit such as the nasal tip may be obvious for a longer period (Figs. 14-11 and 14-12).

CASE EXAMPLES

CASE 1

Fig. 14-13 shows a 1.5-cm defect of the nasal tip in a 45-year-old woman. A laterally based heminasal dorsal nasal flap is drawn. The dotted line represents the area of skin that is undermined to enable flap movement and primary closure of the donor site. The height of the flap was not designed to compensate for the degree of flap pivot. The glabellar back-cut stopped superior to the medial canthal tendon. Fig. 14-14 demonstrates the flap sutured in place after rotation. There was obvious alar elevation due to tethering at the pivotal point, failure to increase the height of the flap, or a

Figure 14-13   A 1.5-cm defect of the nasal tip in 45-year-old woman. Heminasal dorsal flap designed.

Figure 14-14   Heminasal dorsal flap sutured in place.

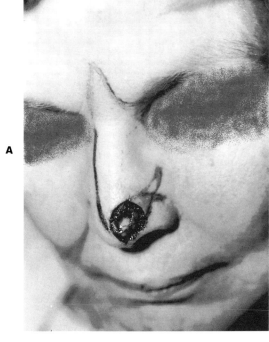

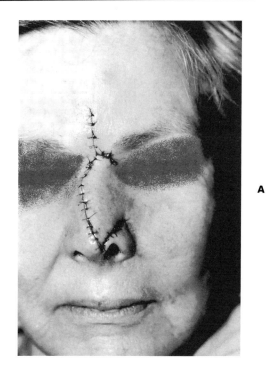

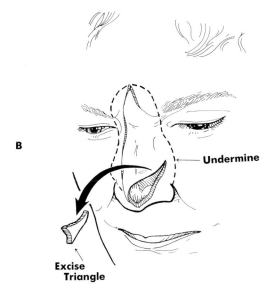

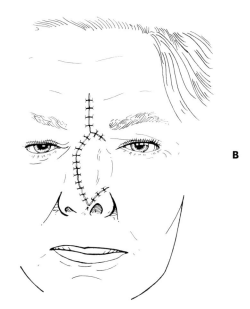

combination of the two. Figs. 14-15 and 14-16 show the 1-year result, with a substantial return of the alar margin to a normal position. The midline nasal scar was visible.

This case demonstrates the mobility problem associated with the dorsal nasal flap. An increase in the height of the flap and thus lengthening of the leading edge would have decreased the closure tension of the primary defect. However, in this patient the defect was so low on the nasal tip that the widest part of the secondary defect was adjacent to the nasal tip. Closure could not take advantage of the distant, more mobile cheek tissue. Therefore extension of the flap's height, which resulted in lengthening of the leading edge, may

still have led to distortion on its own. Fortunately, the elastic pull of the nasal cartilages substantially restored the normal anatomic situation. This is not always the case. Perhaps extension of the back-cut through the medial canthal area would have increased free movement enough to prevent the pull. This removes any axial input to the flap but has been shown to be safe in the heminasal design.

The midline scar is quite visible. Use of all the nasal tissue in the rotational design would have placed the scars in the less obvious cosmetic junction of the nose-cheek boundary. It would have also, by design, increased the length of the leading edge.

Figures 14-15, 14-16   One-year postoperative result. There is excessive elevation of the alar margin.

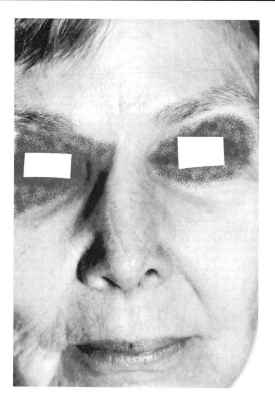

Fig. 14-15

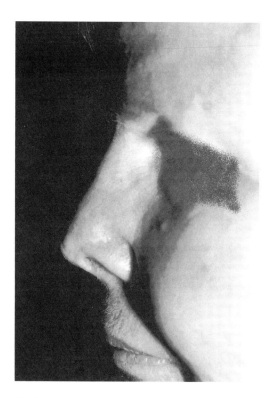

Fig. 14-16

CASE 2

Fig. 14-17**A** and **B** illustrates a 2.5-cm defect on the lateral nasal tip of a 30-year-old man. A laterally based heminasal flap is drawn. The defect is triangulated to demonstrate removal of the standing cutaneous deformity associated with rotation just superior to the alar crease (Fig. 14-17**B**). The leading edge of the flap was not extended. However, the glabellar back cut was shown to extend past the inner canthal region to the level of the infraorbital crease. Fig. 14-18 shows the flap sutured in position. There was no visible alar pull. If there was any lateral deviation of the nasal tip due to closure of the secondary defect, it was not clearly visible. Figs. 14-19 and 14-20 demonstrate the postoperative results. There was no anatomic distortion. The midline scar was not visible.

This case demonstrates successful implementation of the heminasal variant of the dorsal nasal flap. The extension of the back-cut permitted greater flap mobility and prevented alar distortion. The axial input to the flap through branches of the angular artery was cut, but the flap survived well. Extension of the leading edge would not have been successful unless the flap had been converted to a standard dorsal nasal flap design, allowing secondary defect closure to take advantage of the laxity of the cheek. A midline scar deformity was not problematic.

Figure 14-17   **A 2.5-cm defect on nasal tip in 30-year-old man. Heminasal dorsal flaps designed.**

Figure 14-18   **Heminasal dorsal nasal flap sutured in position.**

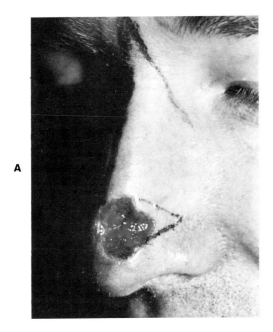

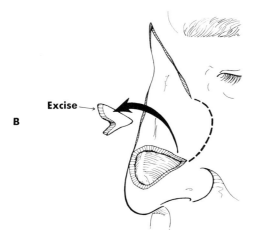

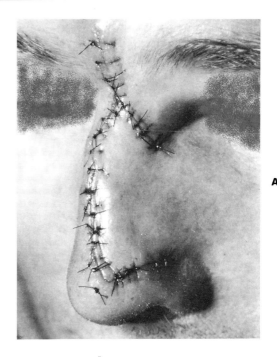

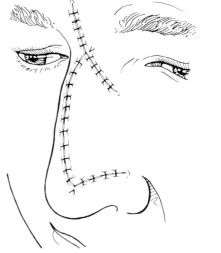

Figures 14-19, 14-20 Postoperative result.

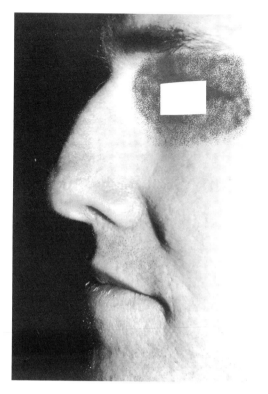

Fig. 14-19

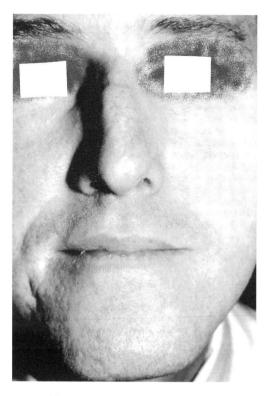

Fig. 14-20

CASE 3

A 70-year-old man had a 1-cm wound located superior to the alar crease. Fig. 14-21 demonstrates a heminasal flap based medially. The back-cut was short and primarily on the nasal bridge, barely reaching the inferior aspect of the glabella. The flap length was therefore relatively short. There was no compensation in the height of the flap. Fig. 14-22 shows the flap sutured into position. Severe alar retraction was seen.

Figure 14-21 Heminasal dorsal flap designed on nose of 70-year-old man with 1-cm wound above alar crease.

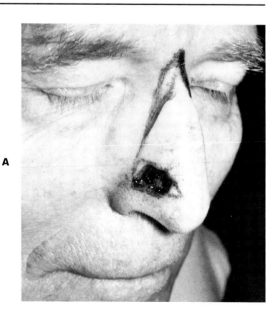

A

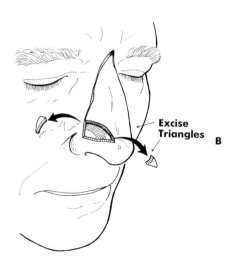

B

Excise
Triangles

Figure 14-22   Flap sutured in place.

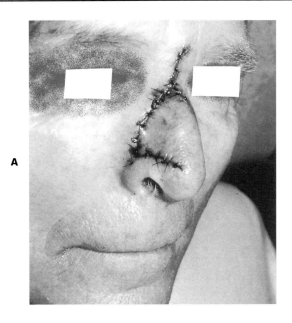

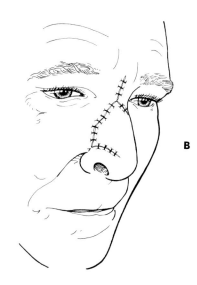

Figures 14-23, 14-24   Three-month postoperative result.

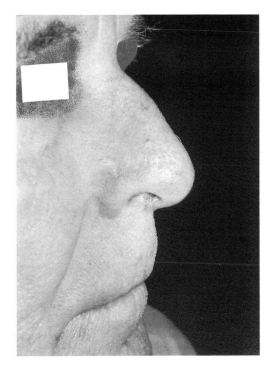

Fig. 14-23

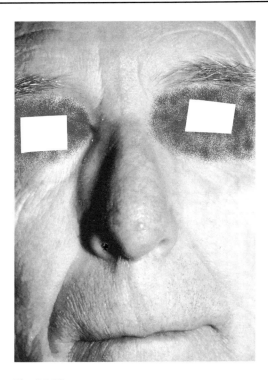

Fig. 14-24

Figs. 14-23 and 14-24 show the 3-month postoperative result. Only partial resolution of the distortion was seen.

This case illustrates several design errors. The primary problem was the length of the flap, which was too short. The flap should extend well into the glabella. The longer the flap, the narrower the secondary defect. The difficulty was compounded by failure to increase the height of the flap. This could have been done quite easily since this flap was medially based. The secondary defect fell just at the nose-cheek junction, providing sufficient laxity for a low-tension closure of the secondary defect. The omission of these design elements led to the problem of alar distortion. Cartilage elasticity did not result in correction of the distortion at 3 months.

CASE 4

Fig. 14-25**A** and **B** illustrates a 1-cm in size wound on the superior nasal tip of a 45-year-old man. A complete dorsal nasal flap was designed. There was obvious compensation of the height of the flap to enable the entire reconstruction of the primary defect without need for secondary movement of the nasal alae or tip. The back-cut was just to the level of the canthal tendon. The wound was triangulated by removal of the standing cutaneous deformity so that closure would result in a scar lying within the alar crease (Fig.

14-25**B**). The flap is seen to be large relative to the size of the defect. The flap and surrounding tissue are widely undermined (Fig. 14-26). Fig. 14-27 demonstrates suturing of the flap. There is no anatomic distortion. Fig. 14-28 shows a 6-month result.

This case demonstrates proper design of a complete dorsal nasal flap. The flap must be large in relation to the size of the wound to create a narrow, easy to close secondary defect. The back-cut extends to but not beyond the inner canthus to maintain an axial input to this large skin flap. Scars are mostly hidden within junctions of esthetic units or subunits.

Figure 14-25   A 1-cm wound on the nasal tip of 45-year-old man. Dorsal nasal flap designed.

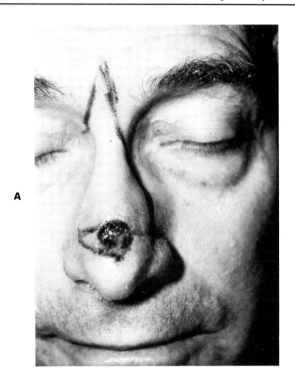

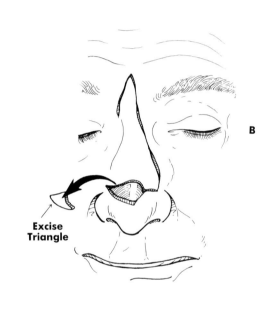

Excise
Triangle

Figure 14-26   Undermining of flap and surrounding tissue.

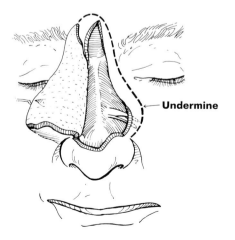

Undermine

Figure 14-27   Dorsal nasal flap sutured in position.

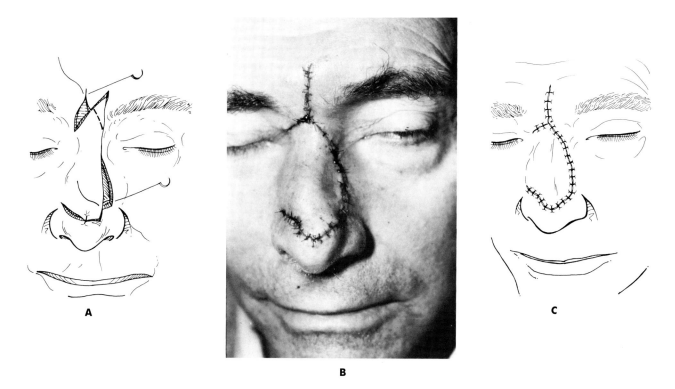

A

B

C

Figure 14-28   Six-month postoperative result.

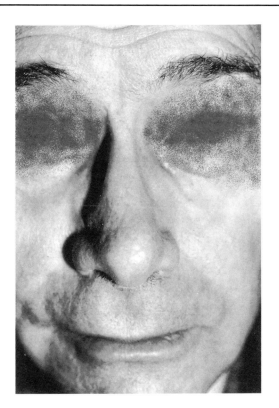

Figure 14-29 A 2.5-cm defect of nasal tip in 62-year-old woman. Dorsal nasal flap designed.

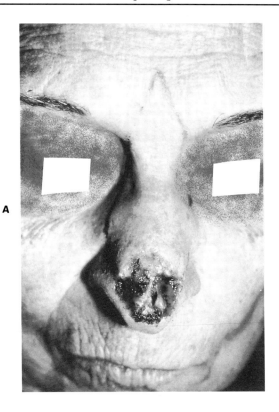

A

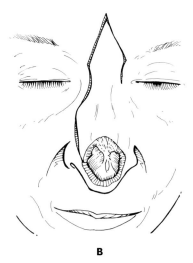

B

CASE 5

Fig. 14-29 illustrates a 2.5-cm wound on the nasal tip of a 62-year-old woman. A dorsal nasal flap with a narrow axial pattern pedicle is drawn. Fig. 14-30 shows repair of the defect without distortion. Figs. 14-31 through 14-33 demonstrate the postoperative result at 6 months. Again, the scar that crossed the nasal tip was apparent.

This case demonstrates more narrowing of the skin pedicle than in the other cases presented. Since the wound on the nasal tip was so large, this was deemed necessary to allow for a low-tension wound closure. Undermining beneath the pedicle was done with blunt dissection to preserve all vascular input.

Figure 14-30 Closure with dorsal nasal flap with narrow axial pedicle.

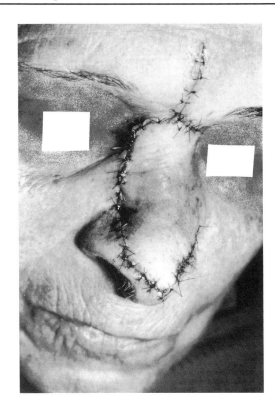

Figures 14-31, 14-32, 14-33   Six-month postoperative result.

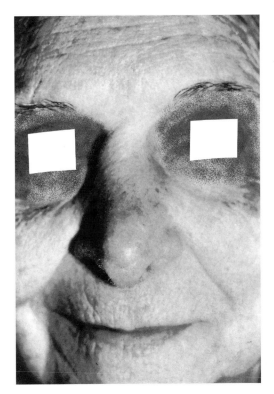

Fig. 14-31

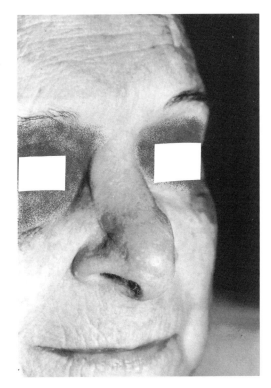

Fig. 14-32

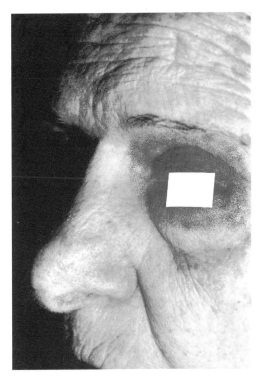

Fig. 14-33

SUMMARY

The dorsal nasal flap is a rotation flap that uses all or part of nasal skin. It allows for the esthetic repair of relatively large lower and midnasal defects with matching adjacent tissue. Many of the scars that result from implementation of this flap can be designed to lie within cosmetic boundaries.

Mobilization of the flap may be achieved by narrowing of the pedicle through which the flap rotates. The pedicle of laterally based heminasal flaps may be shortened by extension of the glabellar back-cut beyond the inner canthal region. Since this reduces the total vascular supply of the flap via branches of the angular artery, it is not advised for the larger complete dorsal nasal flaps. In these instances pedicle narrowing is best achieved by extension of the triangle used to excise the standing cutaneous deformity of rotation up toward the pedicle rather than horizontally along the alar crease. This large flap with a relatively narrow pedicle will survive because of its axial design.

Distortion of the free margins of the alae and tip is prevented by a compensatory increase of flap height in the design of both the complete dorsal nasal flap and the medially based heminasal flap. This cannot be done for the laterally based heminasal flaps because the secondary defect is created along the dorsum of the nose and is too far from the cheek to take advantage of the inherent laxity of that region. In this situation extension of the glabellar back-cut must be relied on to provide additional tissue to assist in closure of the secondary defect.

Finally, all rotation flaps must be designed quite large relative to the size of the associated wound. Although it is emotionally difficult to use such a large flap for a small defect, flap survival is not an issue as long as the patient is not vascularly compromised (for example, by cigarette smoking), closure tension is not excessive and postoperative bleeding and infection are avoided. Although the dynamics of this flap must be well understood to prevent anatomic distortion, the proper use of this reconstructive option can produce esthetic results on the nose that are difficult to match by any other technique.

REFERENCES

1. Elliott RA Jr: Rotation flaps of the nose, *Plast Reconstr Surg* 44:147, 1969.

2. Rieger RA: A local flap for repair of the nasal tip, *Plast Reconstr Surg* 40:147, 1967.

3. Rigg BM: The dorsal nasal flap, *Plast Reconstr Surg* 52:361, 1973.

4. Lipshutz H, Penrod DS: Use of complete transverse nasal flap in repair of small defects of the nose, *Plast Reconstr Surg* 49:629, 1972.

5. Bray DA, Eichel BS: Closure of large nose-cheek groove defects, *Arch Otolaryngol* 103:29, 1977.

6. Bray DA, Eichel BS, Kaplan H: The dorsal nasal flap, *Arch Otolaryngol* 107:765, 1981.

7. Babin RW, Krause C: The nasal dorsum flap, *Arch Otolaryngol* 104:82-83, 1978.

8. Olbourne NA, Kraaijenhagen JH: Rotation flap for distal nasal defects, *Br J Plast Surg* 28:64, 1975.

9. Cronin TD: The V-Y rotational flap for nasal tip defects, *Ann Plast Surg* 11:282, 1983.

10. Marchac D: The naso-frontal rotation flap, *Ann Chir Plast* 15:44, 1970 (translated).

11. Marchac D, Toth B: The axial frontonasal flap revisited, *Plast Reconstr Surg* 76:686, 1985.

EDITORIAL COMMENTS

Shan R. Baker

The dorsal nasal flap, at first glance, may appear too aggressive for the repair of a distal or midnasal defect. On the contrary, it is a very straightforward rotation-advancement flap. Because the flap is primarily a rotation flap, the size must be relatively large compared with the size of the primary defect to maximize tissue movement and decrease wound-closure tension at the flap donor site. It is imperative to assess for adequate skin laxity and to plan for secondary movement at the free margins of the nasal alae and tip before reconstruction with this flap. An oversized flap may be necessary for lateral nasal defects to prevent alar elevation.

Before any surgical repair that involves a dorsal nasal flap, the surgeon should use the pinch test to determine the laxity of the glabellar and dorsal nasal skin. Sufficient laxity is present when the surgeon is able to gather or pinch between the fingers 1 to 2 cm of skin on the nasal dorsum, bridge, and glabella. Once sufficient laxity has been established, the flap is designed as a laterally based rotation-advancement flap. Greater laxity must be present as the defect size increases. The base or pedicle is located superior and lateral to the surgical defect. A curvilinear line is drawn from the defect laterally in the nasofacial sulcus. This line may extend onto the cheek if additional tissue is needed. The line is directed superiorly through the nasal portion of the medial canthus and into the superior aspect of the glabella within a glabellar crease. The distance from the base of the glabella to the superior tip of the glabellar portion of the flap should be approximately 1.5 to two times the vertical height of the nasal defect to ensure adequate tissue movement. At this point the line is directed toward the contralateral medial canthus, creating a 30° to 45° angled back-cut. Incisions can be made before undermining. Alternatively, prior to incisions, undermining bluntly from the defect toward the glabella may be accomplished in the loose areolar plane just below the superficial musculoaponeurotic system of the nose.

Once the flap undermining has been accomplished, incisions are completed in the lines previously drawn. Blunt dissection and undermining beneath the musculature of the nasal sidewall is then completed until the entire flap is elevated from the periosteum and perichondrium. Special emphasis must be placed on complete mobilization of the pedicle of the flap down to the epicanthal ligament as well as to the contralateral nasal-facial sulcus beneath the transverse nasalis muscle. This is necessary to achieve maximum flap mobility and tissue movement. The myocutaneous flap is then advanced and rotated into the primary surgical defect. Before final closure, the flap is secured with a temporary suture to check for any discrepancy of skin thickness or distortion of the alae or nasal tip. If necessary, the underlying adipose tissue and muscle of the flap may be trimmed to maximize skin thickness match. Judicial defatting and debulking of the flap tip does not compromise flap survival due to the excellent vascularity of the flap. In particularly thick sebaceous skin, the flap edges should be beveled in one direction and the adjacent nasal skin beveled in the opposite direction. The defect, if created by Mohs surgery, will already be beveled. In such instances the flap should then be accordingly beveled in the opposite direction for a precise fit. With this technique the wound edges approximate in a sliding fashion. Preparing the skin edges in such a fashion may reduce the risk that the scar incision line will be depressed and will spread.

The secondary glabellar defect may be closed with a V-Y advancement, a Z-plasty, or preferably by primary closure. When primary closure of the donor site is accomplished, the triangular segment of the flap harvested from the glabellar skin is draped over the primary glabellar incision line. The triangular segment of the glabellar skin is then trimmed for a perfect fit, creating a single glabellar incision line that lies in a glabellar crease. Thinning of the flap at the medial canthus is critical because the thicker glabellar skin of the flap is advanced to the medial canthus, where the skin is thinner. This is an important step for maximal cosmesis. The dorsal nasal flap is in part a pivot flap, and, as such, a standing cutaneous deformity occurs at the inferior aspect of the pedicle. The redundant skin is excised laterally, which eliminates the need to back-cut toward the pedicle of the flap which could compromise flap vascularity. The flap is then sutured with a standard layered closure. It may be necessary to undermine and advance cheek skin to assist in the closure of the secondary defect, which occurs in the region of the nasofacial sulcus. In such instances, a periosteal tacking suture may be helpful to maintain the sulcus.

Although the primary motion of the dorsal nasal flap is advancement-rotation, it is critical to be aware that secondary motion also occurs, which can raise the nasal tip or distort alar rim symmetry. This must be anticipated and planned in the flap design; otherwise the nasal free margins will be displaced. In older patients with nasal ptosis and a central nasal tip defect, slight elevation of the nasal tip is of no concern. In younger patients, however, nasal tip elevation may result in an unacceptable cosmetic outcome. Repair of lateral nasal defects with the dorsal nasal flap may result in asymmetric mild to extreme permanent alar elevation in patients without ample lax nasal and glabellar skin. Thus, movement of the flap must be sufficient to completely fill the primary defect without much wound-closure tension to prevent alar retraction. Secondary movement must come from the glabellar and cheek tissue rather than the alar rim or tip.

Two modifications may be performed during the dorsal nasal flap procedure. If any cephalic portions of the lower lateral cartilage are removed during tumor extirpation, the surgeon can similarly trim a corresponding amount from the opposite lower lateral cartilage to maintain symmetry, perhaps with even some refinement of nasal tip definition. In cases in which loss of cartilage may jeopardize support of the nasal airway, auricular or nasal septal cartilage grafts should be used to replace the missing nasal cartilage. Likewise, if the patient has a protruding dorsal nasal hump, this can be directly reduced and optimal cosmesis provided through a reduction rhinoplasty at the time of flap transfer[1] (Fig. 14-34).

Figure 14-34 *A* and *B*, Basal cell carcinoma overlying overprojected convex nasal bridge in 65-year-old patient. *C*, A 2 × 2.4 cm defect of nasal bridge extending to underlying bone following excision of skin cancer. Dorsal nasal flap is designed for repair of defect. *D*, Flap in position after reconstruction and concomitant reduction rhinoplasty. Standing cutaneous deformity was excised in midline of nose. *E* and *F*, Appearance 6 months postoperatively. (From Johnson TM, Swanson NA, Baker SR et al: The Reiger flap for nasal reconstruction, *Arch Otolaryngol Head Neck Surg* [in press].)

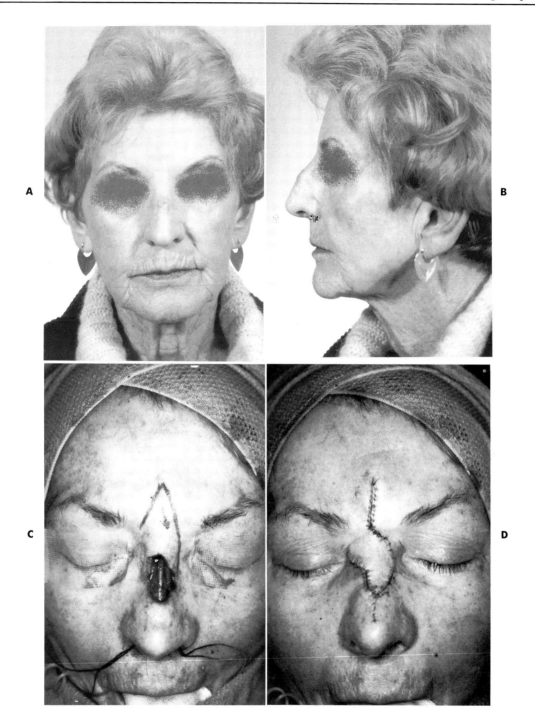

Figure 14-34, cont'd   For legend see opposite page.

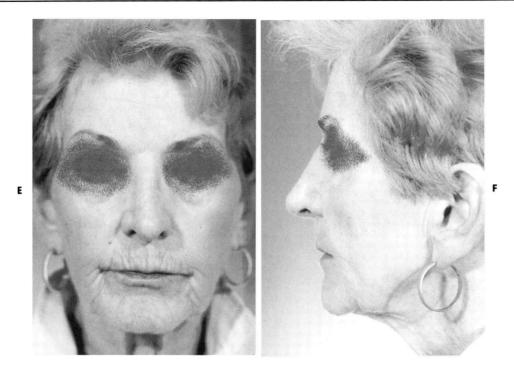

REFERENCE

1. Johnson TM, Swanson NA, Baker SR et al: The Reiger flap for nasal reconstruction, *Arch Otolaryngol Head Neck Surg* (in press).

EDITORIAL COMMENTS

Neil A. Swanson

This is an excellent theoretical discussion of this sliding flap. It is a flap that is a good example of a combination of rotation and advancement. It has been described as a rotational flap with a back-cut, which for the most part may be accurate. Dr. Dzubow presents an excellent discussion of the history and biomechanical design of this flap. He gives a good discussion of how important it is to consider secondary motion with this flap. Generally the secondary motion will elevate the nasal tip or alar rim if the surgeon is not careful. When secondary motion occurs on a ptotic nose, this may actually be of benefit. It can also be of benefit in straightening out a deviated columella.

I agree that the height of this flap into the glabellar area is important to maximize the tissue movement and minimize secondary motion. However, I do not back-cut to the degree that the author does until I have rotated tissue into place to see whether it is necessary. Often extension of the back-cut will augment tissue motion, but it is not always necessary. The level of undermining, as discussed, is important to maintain and maximize the blood flow to this flap.

From a technical standpoint I agree completely with Dr. Dzubow that the resultant standing cutaneous deformity with this flap should be excised after the primary defect has been closed and the flap anchored in place. This should always be done by angling the excision outward and therefore, widening the base of the flap. It is tempting to remove the standing cutaneous deformity in other directions but it really can compromise the vasculature. Wherever possible, I choose to make the incision for this flap laterally at the nose-cheek junction, extending up near the canthus to the glabella. The midline or just-off-midline incision (for example, Fig. 14-13) can leave a less esthetic scar than that hidden in the cosmetic boundary of the cheek and nose. This flap is often placed in a sebaceous nasal tip. It is very difficult to get a good suture line in this skin. One trick is to maintain the tissue bevel from Mohs surgery within the Mohs surgery defect and counterbevel the advancing edge of the flap. This then can be sutured in place, after undermining of the defect itself as a tongue and groove type of fit. This, followed by postoperative dermabrasion, has given me the best chance of a nondepressed, unsightly scar.

15

SKIN GRAFTS

Richard G. Glogau

Ann F. Haas

INTRODUCTION

For centuries skin grafting has been performed to cover certain types of skin defects. The technique involves removal of skin from one location and reattachment at another site. It can be a useful tool for the head and neck surgeon for defects in which flap coverage is not feasible.

Graft viability depends on factors that permit new capillary ingrowth from the recipient bed. These factors include the blood supply to the recipient bed, the microcirculation of the surface of the recipient bed, the vascularity of the donor graft tissue, the contact between graft and recipient bed, and the patient's overall physical health.

Rudolph and Ballantyne[1] state that "most skin graft failures can be ascribed to flaws in the recipient site rather than to technical defects in the skin graft cutting." Certainly a wound without adequate vascular supply will not support a graft. Local factors include nonviable tissue in the wound, such as crushed material or foreign bodies. Irradiated tissue and excessive fibrosis at the base of the defect provide decreased vascular supply. Exposed bone, cartilage, or tendon without periosteum, perichondrium and peritendon are also relatively avascular. Additional procedures may be required to optimize graft "take" in these tissues.

Exposed skull is best treated either by burring off of part of the outer table with a diamond fraise or by making holes through the table to establish communication with the diploë.[2,3] Application of zinc chloride fixative in the traditional Mohs technique will also allow the development of rich granulation tissue after spontaneous separation of the devitalized outer table.[4] A small (2-mm) trephine can also be used to cut holes through cartilage to expose the vascularized perichondrium from the other side. Large areas of exposed cartilage may require coverage with some vascular tissue, such as a muscle flap, before grafting, or, as in

the ear, part of the cartilage can be removed in an area where it is not needed for structural support so that the graft can be placed on the exposed subcutaneous tissue.[5] A graft placed over avascular defects smaller than 1 cm^2 may survive via a bridging effect where nutritional support comes from vessels in the tissue adjacent to the devascularized bed. Grafting can also be delayed until sufficient granulation tissue grows across the avascular tissue to support a graft. The appearance of granulation tissue can be facilitated by covering the defect with either a wet dressing, such as saline-soaked gauze, or antibiotic ointment covered by gauze, or by using a semiocclusive dressings.

The vascularity of the graft is probably of more importance with full-thickness than with split-thickness skin grafts (STSGs). For head and neck defects most donor sites selected for full-thickness skin grafts (FTSGs) are also from the head and neck. Since STSGs have less dermis that need neovascularization, they can be harvested from a variety of locations. We will consider selection of the donor site in more detail in the discussion of the specific grafts.

Contact between graft and recipient bed is of vital importance for establishment of the neovascularization necessary for graft survival. A bleeding or oozing recipient bed can cause graft failure due to formation of hematomas or seromas. Hemostasis can be accomplished by ligation, cautery, or pressure. Hemostatic agents such as hemostatic cellulose (Surgicel™) or hemostatic gelatin sponges (Gelfoam™) provide a nonvascular block between the graft and the recipient bed and therefore should not be used. If bleeding is profuse, grafting should probably be delayed. Hematoma or seroma formation as well as the action of mechanical shear forces that disrupt contact between graft and recipient bed can be minimized with suture techniques and placement of dressings. Hypertrophic granulation tissue accepts a skin graft poorly and needs to be trimmed to the plane of the surrounding tissue. In addition, granulating tissue contains bacteria; consequently, a quantitative biopsy culture of the wound surface and subsequent appropriate use of antibiotics may be necessary to ensure that the graft is not rejected. If the recipient site is truly infected when the graft is placed, graft loss is almost inevitable. However, mere colonization may not be enough to compromise the graft. The number and type of bacterial organisms will determine success or failure.

Although all wounds are contaminated, infection occurs only in wounds in which local defense mechanisms are overwhelmed by the large amount of bacteria or by the bacterial virulence. It has been suggested that the presence of more than 10^5 organisms per gram of tissue usually leads to graft loss.[3] Streptococcal infection can cause total loss of the graft. *Pseudomonas* organisms, because of the resulting exudate, can cause the graft to float off the bed before healing. Topical agents that effectively control wound bacteria include saline dressings, silver nitrate solution, silver sulfadiazine (Silvadene), mafenide acetate (Sulfamylon) cream, acetic acid solutions, vinegar and water, and sodium hypochlorite solutions. Selected enzymatic debriding agents, such as dextranomer beads (Debrisan), fibrinolysin and desoxyribonuclease (Elase), and sutilains (Travase) ointment, are not as effective as is repeated sharp debridement of the wound in preparation for surgery but can be useful in some settings.

The patient's general health may also be a consideration in whether the graft fails. Certain systemic problems can compromise vascularity, such as rheumatoid arthritis, systemic lupus erythematosis and other autoimmune diseases, hematologic disorders, and diabetes. Protein deprivation, metabolic catabolism, severe vitamin deficiency and relative hypoxemia, and corticosteroids and cytotoxic immunosuppressant medications may also have a deleterious effect on the graft, as can the vasoconstriction induced by nicotine.[3]

FULL-THICKNESS SKIN GRAFTS

An FTSG consists of epidermis and the full thickness of dermis (Fig. 15-1). These skin grafts generally resist contraction, and have a texture and pigment appearance more similar to normal skin. They may grow in children. Ideally an FTSG needs a small, well-vascularized, uncontaminated wound bed for survival. Generally an FTSG is preferred over a STSG when wound contraction might result in a functional deformity or when an improved cosmetic result is desired. FTSGs are generally selected over a local flap repair when they offer a better cosmetic result, when there isn't enough surrounding skin to create a local flap, and when a distant flap is inappropriate. Areas for which these

grafts are frequently selected include the nasal tip, nasal ala, lower eyelid, ear, temple, and forehead.

Donor sites for FTSGs are either closed primarily or with a flap or STSG. Because of this, FTSGs are generally used to cover smaller defects. Because FTSGs retain most of the donor site qualities, careful choices regarding these qualities at the time of surgery should minimize any color and texture problems. For facial defects, most FTSGs are taken from the upper eyelid, preauricular and postauricular skin, lateral neck, supraclavicular region, and occasionally the melolabial fold (Fig. 15-2). Postauricular skin is photoprotected and has fewer adnexal structures, so it may not be ideal for repair of nasal defects. Harvesting of preauricular skin unilaterally in men may move the sideburn closer to the ear, leaving a symmetry problem. The supraclavicular area may be thinner or more photodamaged than the face, which could also be a cosmetic problem. It may be a problem to hide supraclavicular donor site scars in women because they tend to wear clothing with lower neck lines. The skin of the melolabial sulcus and fold may be a good donor match for the nose, but excision in one fold may require similar excision in the other fold to yield a symmetrical result. Eyelid defects are best replaced with full-thickness skin commonly harvested from postauricular, upper eyelid, or supraclavicular skin. A unique donor site consideration for FTSGs in children is to avoid later hair growth. The groin is an excellent donor site, but—especially in children—care must be used in selection of an area that will be free of hair when the child matures.

After selection of a donor area, a template is made of the recipient site by pressing sterile surgical gauze, nonadherent bandages (Telfa) or some other flexible sterile material into the wound. The serosanguinous wound fluid adherent to the gauze acts as the template, and the template is trimmed away from the excess gauze. The template is placed, serosanguinous side down, onto the donor area, and a tracing is made around the template with a marking pen. Alternately, painting around the rim of the defect with a sterile marker or gentian violet, then placing the nonadherent pad quickly against the wound, yields an oversized imprint of the defect, which is then cut out and traced onto the donor site.[6] It is necessary to take into account both the natural contractility of a harvested FTSG and the mobility and flexibility of the recipient site. Most FTSGs contract about 10% to 15% after excision from the donor site; therefore a graft approximately 20% to 25% larger than the recipient defect should be harvested.[7] For an area where mobility is not a concern, such as the nose, a graft can be trimmed exactly to the defect size. For an extremely mobile area, such as the

Figure 15-1   Relationship of skin graft type to thickness of skin.

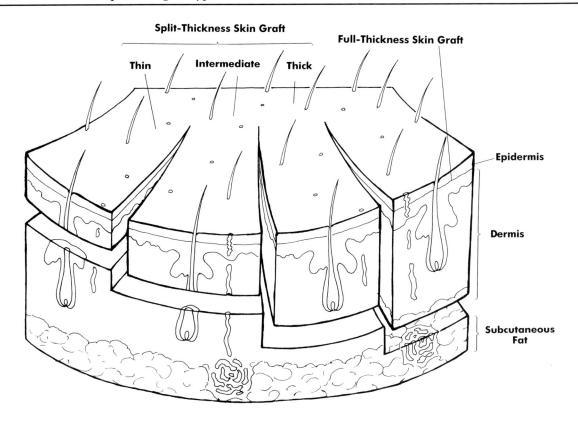

Figure 15-2   Donor sites for full-thickness skin grafts applied to face.

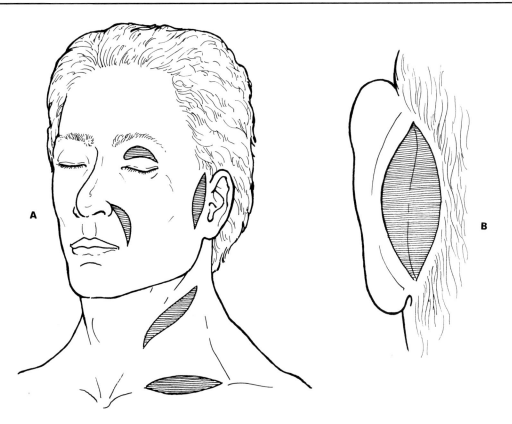

lower eyelid, the graft must be harvested 150% to 200% larger in the vertical direction than is the recipient defect to avoid problems with graft contraction and resulting ectropion.[3] The donor area is then prepared and anesthetized with lidocaine (we prefer the addition of epinephrine). The tracing is then excised to include subcutaneous fat and is placed onto saline-soaked sterile gauze while the donor site is closed.

Customarily, the graft is then defatted by removing the subcutaneous fat from the underside with the use of serrated scissors, such as blepharoplasty scissors. This is most easily accomplished by placement of the graft over the index finger, epidermal side down. Defatting is completed when the shiny dermis is seen uniformly. The graft is then placed dermal side down into the recipient defect. There are circumstances in which it may not be appropriate to trim the fat on the underside of the graft; a thicker graft may be required for better contour in some locations such as nasal defects.

The graft should contact the recipient wound bed in such a fashion to permit maximum surface adherence, allowing no tenting or puckering. This can be accomplished in several ways. Basting sutures, which are placed to bind the graft to the underlying tissue, are very helpful in large or concave sites and serve to eliminate any dead space. A variation of the basting suture calls for placement of the basting suture under direct visualization before the entire perimeter of the graft is sutured into place (Fig. 15-3).[8] This technique permits accurate hemostasis if bleeding is encountered and permits more directed placement of sutures for better approximation of the graft to the wound bed. Either permanent or absorbable sutures can be used. The perimeter of the graft is then sutured in place with either interrupted sutures, or a running suture, or a combination of nonabsorbable interrupted sutures followed by placement of running fast-absorbing gut sutures. The excess graft is carefully trimmed as the perimeter is sutured. Sutures should be placed from graft to skin. If nonabsorbable sutures are used, they may be removed in 1 week.

Dressings can also assist in prevention of hematomas and seromas as well as diminishing of the detrimental effects of mechanical shear forces. Some variation of the tie-over, or bolster-type, dressing is commonly employed (Fig. 15-4). In one variation, one end of each interrupted suture placed (in pairs) at the graft periphery is left long enough to be tied with its other contralateral suture over some sort of bolster. Another variation places interrupted sutures, again in pairs, into the surrounding skin 1 or 2 mm from the actual wound edge. One tie, left long from each suture is tied to its contralateral suture again over some sort of bolster. This method may provide less tension on the actual

Figure 15-3 Placement of visualized basting sutures to secure graft to recipient site.

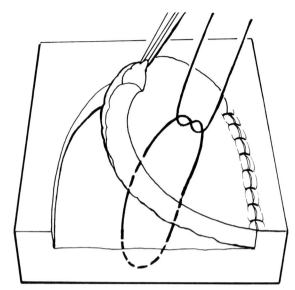

wound edge. Steri-strips have also been placed over a bolster to simulate the tie-down dressing. The bolster itself can be made of various materials, such as sterile foam rubber[9] (which must be gas sterilized).[6] The more traditional bolster is made of sterile cotton or gauze and usually follows placement of bacitracin-coated interpositional surfacing material (N-terface) or a nonadherent (Telfa) interpositional material into the wound bed directly on top of the graft. Some surgeons prefer to dampen the sterile cotton balls or gauze, so they can be more easily molded into any concavity at the graft edge, ensuring graft-bed approximation. Petrolatum 3% bismuth tribromophenate (Xeroform) gauze can also be used directly on the wound as a bolster material. Alternatively, the tie-over sutures could be placed initially at surgery but not secured until 24 hours postoperatively when the risk of bleeding has decreased, and a cotton swab (Q-tip) can be rolled over the graft toward the nearest edge to extract any accumulated fluid. Some surgeons prefer to take the tie-over dressing down at 48 hours to inspect and then replace it with a more traditional dressing; however, most surgeons probably prefer to leave the bolster undisturbed until the time for suture removal.

The advantages to these types of dressings include minimal daily wound care, isolation of the wound from the environment; constant and even compression, which decreases the risk of hematoma formation; and immobilization of the graft. The status of the graft cannot be monitored, however, except in cases when the dressing is removed at 48 hours.

FTSGs routinely go through an evolutionary period, which can be unpredictable for the physician and terrifying for the patient (Fig. 15-5). Initially the graft

Figure 15-4   *A,* Variations of tie-down bolster dressing. Tie-over sutures can be placed at the wound edge as part of the perimeter fixation of the graft. *B-D,* Alternatively, bolster sutures can be placed 1 to 2 mm from wound edge.

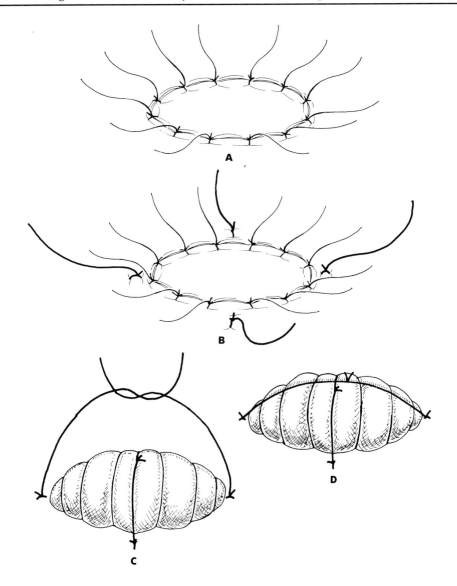

is white and then becomes somewhat cyanotic, and the violaceous color either evolves into a hyperemic stage (which fades over weeks to months to an approximately normal color) or the graft fails and becomes necrotic. Often the entire epidermis will blacken and slough and then reepithelialization occurs. The patient must be informed and prepared for this sequence of events.

All is not lost even with a failing graft. The necrotic graft at the very least acts as a biologic dressing, allowing either healing by second intention, in cases of full graft slough, or it preserves whatever viable dermal portion of the graft exists and consequently permits reepithelialization both from the wound edges and

from adnexal structures. The result is often still cosmetically acceptable.

The advantages of an FTSG compared with the STSG include better color and texture match, better coverage of deeper defects, no need for special equipment, and generally an easier donor site to care for (Fig. 15-6). The major disadvantages of an FTSG compared with the STSG are the reduced survival rate because they are thicker, the need for longer healing time, and the contour changes that can develop.

Significant differences between graft thickness and defect depth although they usually even out with time, can cause a permanent deformity. If this is anticipated with a deep defect, delay of grafting for 7 to 10 days

Figure 15-5 *A,* A 3 × 2.5 cm full-thickness skin defect of nasal tip after tumor resection. *B,* Full-thickness skin graft combined with composite auricular skin cartilage graft harvested from the right ear and preauricular area. *C,* Full-thickness skin graft component is used to repair skin defect of nasal tip. Skin-cartilage composite graft component is used to repair alar margin. *D,* Appearance of full-thickness skin graft 2 weeks postoperatively. Portions of graft appear cyanotic, and others (inferior aspect) appear violaceous. *E and F,* Appearance of nose 6 months postoperatively. Mild notching of alar margin is observed. (Courtesy Shan R. Baker, M.D.)

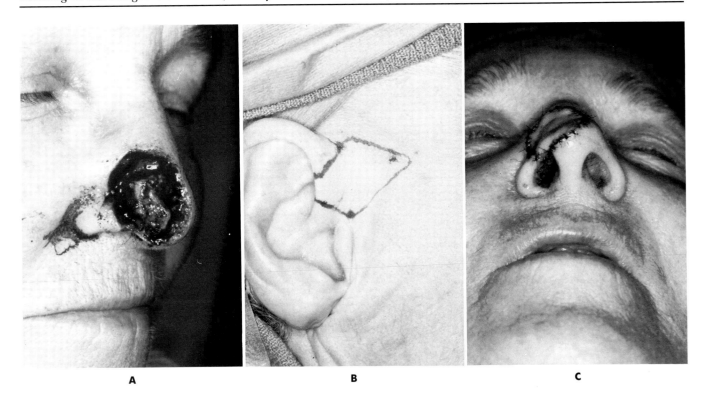

A   B   C

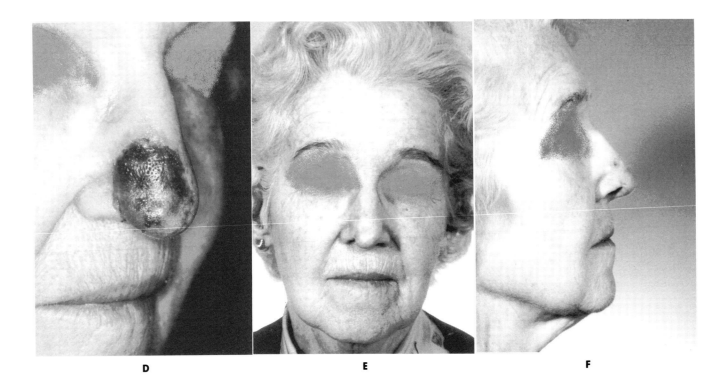

D   E   F

Figure 15-6   *A and B,* A 3 × 3.5 cm full-thickness skin defect of upper nasal dorsum after removal of skin cancer. *C and D,* Five months after repair of nasal defect with full-thickness skin graft harvested from postauricular area. No dermabrasion or other revision surgery was performed. (Courtesy Shan R. Baker, M.D.)

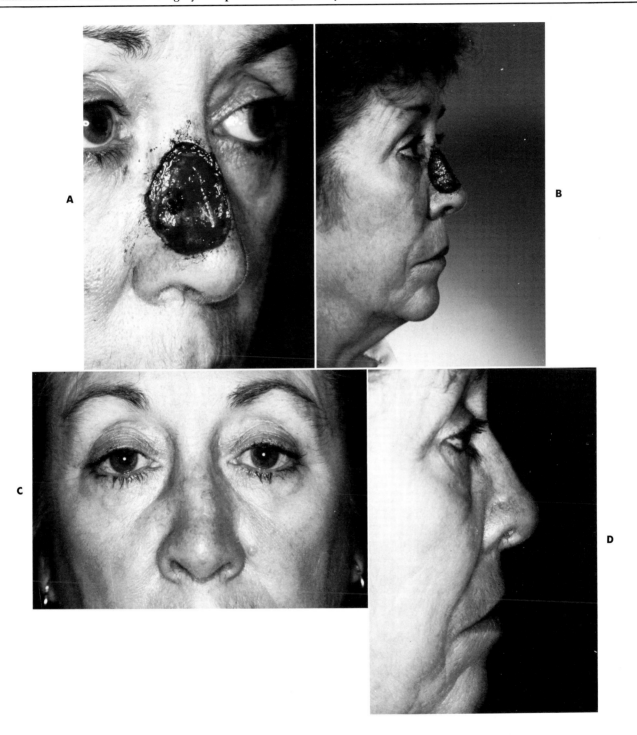

will permit granulation tissue to fill in the defect sufficiently to achieve a better contour (Fig. 15-7). At the time of grafting any reepithelialization of the wound by new epidermis must be removed.

For slight elevation differences between graft and adjacent skin or for slightly depressed suture lines, focal dermabrasion can be rewarding, particularly on the nose[9,10] (Fig. 15-8). The pincushion complication is a function of wound contraction and will resolve to some extent, given adequate time. Intralesional steroids injected beneath the graft may assist in resolution of this problem. Sometimes it is necessary to revise the graft by surgically removing the fibrous layer of scar tissue beneath the graft, thus debulking the graft.

The carbon dioxide laser has been shown to be effective in revision of hypertrophic scars after FTSGs.[11] This laser may be indicated for treatment of small lesions for which scar dermabrasion is difficult because of the large size of the fraise or wire brush or because of a restrictive location of the scar.

SPLIT-THICKNESS SKIN GRAFTS

An STSG consists of a sheet of epidermis and a variable portion of underlying dermis, depending on how "thick" the graft is cut (Fig. 15-1). Most of these skin grafts are of intermediate thickness (.012 to .018 inch) but can vary from "thin" (.008 to .012 inch) to "thick" (.018 to .030 inch). A thin graft has greater potential for survival than a thick graft because of a greater capillary network exposure on the cut undersurface. This permits greater absorption of nutrients from the wound bed. There is also less total tissue that requires revascularization in a thin graft. Both of these factors make a thin graft ideal for a wound that has some degree of vascular compromise. However, thin grafts, because of the smaller amount of protective dermis, do not stand up well in areas of repeated trauma; these areas generally require thicker grafts or flaps.

Generally, STSGs heal with a relatively poor cosmetic result compared with full-thickness grafts. Although the thicker STSGs tend to have a less shiny, atrophic appearance than the thin type, generally STSGs should be viewed as a functional rather than a cosmetic method of reconstruction. Further disadvantages of STSGs include contraction, lack of growth in children, and abnormal pigmentation. A relative contraindication to placement of an STSG is wound contraction that would yield functional compromise.

Relative indications for STSGs include repair of defects too large for FTSGs or flaps after cancer surgery (to more easily evaluate possible recurrence)

Figure 15-7 *A*, A 2 × 1.5 cm full-thickness skin defect of nasal tip after removal of basal cell carcinoma. Wound was allowed to granulate several days before repair with full-thickness skin graft harvested from preauricular area. *B*, Seven months postoperatively. Graft has been dermabraded. (Courtesy Shan R. Baker, M.D.)

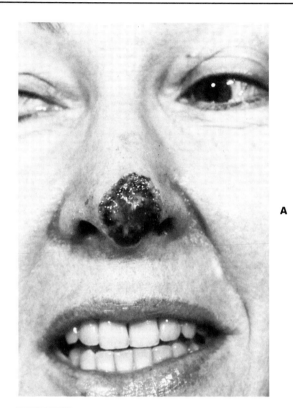

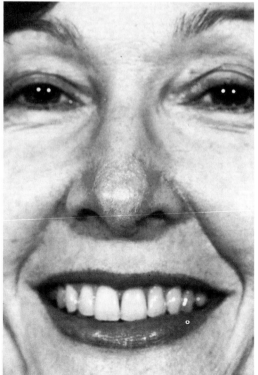

Figure 15-8   *A,* A 2 × 2 cm full-thickness skin defect of upper lateral nose after removal of skin cancer. Wound was repaired with full-thickness perichondrial cutaneous graft harvested from concha cavum. *B,* Nine months postoperatively. Edges of graft were dermabraded 6 weeks and 3 months after surgery. (Courtesy Shan R. Baker, M.D.)

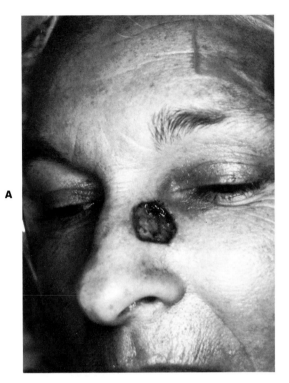

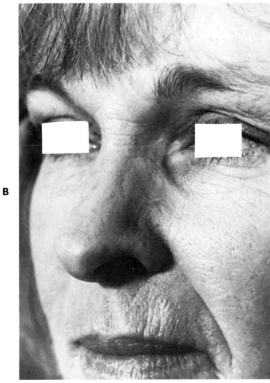

(Fig. 15-9) to provide temporary coverage for a wound when reconstruction is planned at some future time, to provide backing for a flap used to repair through-and-through defects, and to provide coverage to wounds of such a nature that an FTSG would not survive.[3,12]

Selection of the donor site should take into account the cosmetic appearance of the donor site scar, color and texture matching, practicality of wound care, and choice of instrument for harvesting of the graft. For STSGs applied to facial defects, "blush zone" donor sites, such as supraclavicular areas, lateral neck, preauricular skin, and scalp have been effectively used. The scalp can be a source of multiple grafts, and best results are obtained if the STSG is cut superficially, which serves to prevent hair growth at the recipient site and baldness at the donor site. In children, however, excessive blood loss secondary to the extreme vascularity of the scalp may preclude it as an ideal donor site. In pale-skinned individuals, scalp skin may be too hyperpigmented.

In younger women for whom cosmesis may be an issue, a covered area, such as a hip or buttock can be used. Mons pubis has been suggested as a possible donor site in this group, where harvest of a thin graft avoids hair follicles.[13] The anterolateral aspect of the thigh, a common and convenient donor site, lends itself to accessibility for the physician and ease of care for the patient. Other sites with flat surfaces, such as the abdomen, torso, or inner part of the upper arm can also be used in certain circumstances.

Instrumentation

The electric Brown dermatome is probably the most common device used and the most widely available (Fig. 15-10). It permits precise adjustments of graft width. This dermatome must be assembled before use. The screws on the back of the dermatome must be loose before placement of the disposable blade over the projecting rivets. Once the blade is against the casing, the screws are tightened with the sterile wrench that is part of the dermatome set. The thickness dials are marked in thousands of an inch and should be set at a thickness of zero before calibration. Both dials then can be moved clockwise simultaneously or alternately by 0.0005-inch increments (if the thickness dials are moved by an increment larger than this, the dermatome may be put out of alignment). The graft thickness dial is set at 15 thousandths of an inch, which corresponds to the passage of the leveled portion of a Bard-Parker No. 15 blade between the dermatome blade and the casing. Once the "standard set" of 15 thousandths of an inch has been verified, the desired thickness can be set. The width is next set with use of the dial on the side of the casing to correspond to the

Figure 15-9 *A,* Extensive angiosarcoma of scalp, with proposed resection margins marked. *B,* Wound is repaired with split-thickness skin graft harvested from leg. Graft is fixed to adjacent scalp with skin graft staples. *C,* Large bulky tie-over bolster dressing is used to secure graft. *D,* Appearance of graft 4 weeks postoperatively. (Courtesy Shan R. Baker, M.D.)

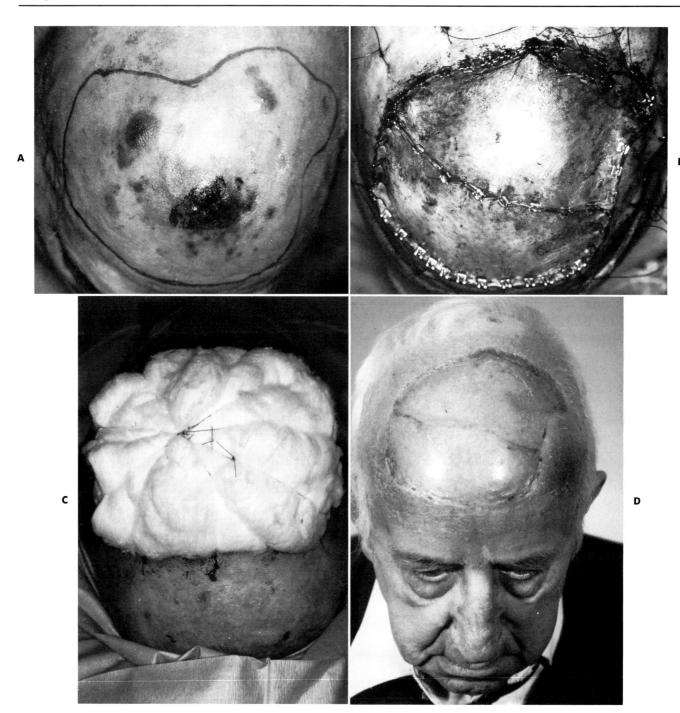

Figure 15-10   Brown dermatome.

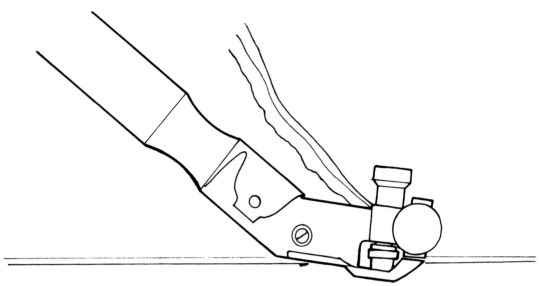

width of the wound as measured perpendicular to the long axis.

The donor skin is marked with a rectangular design selected so that the length of the rectangle is equal to the greatest dimension of the recipient defect plus an extra 25% to compensate for graft shrinkage. Local anesthesia (1% lidocaine with epinephrine at a concentration of 1:200,000) is infiltrated into the selected site. The addition of hyaluronidase (Wydase), 150 units per 30 ml of anesthetic, permits rapid diffusion of anesthetic through the donor area while requiring fewer needle sticks.[14] A spinal needle is useful for uniform infiltration of the entire rectangle. After skin preparation with chlorhexidine (Hibiclens), either sterile mineral oil or lubricating surgical jelly is applied in a thin layer.

An assistant provides traction beyond the proposed donor area either manually or with a tongue depressor or other instrument (Fig. 15-11**A**). The surgeon provides countertraction by placing his or her nondominant hand behind the dermatome and retracting away from the unit as it is placed on the patient's skin so that the flat surface is parallel to the skin surface. Light downward and forward pressure is applied as the surgeon's foot depresses the foot pedal to start dermatome operation. As the dermatome is advanced forward, the assistant gently places hemostats or forceps on each corner of the graft as it appears above the blade (Fig. 15-11**B**). This allows the surgeon to evaluate the thickness of the graft and keeps the graft from getting caught in the blade. When the dermatome has been advanced to the end of the donor area, the dermatome, while still cutting, is lifted up and away from the skin (like an airplane on takeoff), which in most cases tapers the graft and frees it from the donor bed.

A semiocclusive dressing such as Opsite has a use in the harvesting of STSGs. Application of this dressing to the donor site before graft harvesting allows the harvesting of a graft that can be much easier to handle, thus eliminating self-sticking and curling of the graft. It also prevents mistaken application of the graft wrong side down.[15] In addition, the graft with Opsite is much easier to apply to wounds of both irregular contour (such as the conchal bowl) and those of irregular thickness that require extensive thinning. The semiocclusive dressing permits easier trimming and suturing of the graft to the wound bed as well as provides mechanical stability to the graft. The dressing spontaneously separates from the wound over the course of time as it heals. It is not necessary to make adjustments in dermatome settings because the extra thickness of the Opsite is negligible.

The electric Padgett dermatome also yields good skin grafts but is not as common in the office setting because it must be gas sterilized (Fig. 15-12). The Padgett comes with three templates, allowing grafts of widths of 5, 10.1, 15.2 cm (2, 4 or 6 inches) to be harvested. The blade is placed into position against the bottom of the casing; the template of preselected width is then placed on top of the blade and both blade and template are tightened with a screwdriver. The graft thickness is then set by adjustments made on the dial at the side of the dermatome. No calibration is necessary. The technique of graft harvesting is similar to that of the Brown dermatome.

Another instrument, which is particularly useful for small grafts, is the Weck knife. This is a freehand-harvest system and comes with a handle, disposable blades, and several templates used to control graft thickness. The blade is placed onto the handle, after which the template is attached. The skin is prepared, and the assistant provides traction. The blade is placed parallel to the skin surface, and a sawing motion is used as the knife is advanced through the skin (Fig. 15-13). As a graft of sufficient size is obtained, the downward pressure is lightened, and a few more back and forth motions will separate the graft, or the graft edge can be trimmed with a scalpel. Because the edges of grafts obtained by this method are somewhat jagged due to the sawing motion, they are usually trimmed before placement. This must be accounted for in determination of the ultimate size of the graft necessary to cover the recipient wound.

The Davol-Simon dermatome is a battery-operated unit that is also useful for harvesting of small grafts (Fig. 15-14). Because of the fixed nature of the blade, the graft width is limited to 3 cm, and only short grafts can be harvested. The graft thickness is permanently fixed at 15 thousandths of an inch. Because the handle cannot be sterilized, the system comes with a sterile plastic bag and twist tie, as well as a single-use sterile head with blade attached. The Davol-Simon dermatome can be more difficult to use because it requires considerable downward pressure to advance.

The Castroviejo dermatome is a small electric dermatome, which is often used to obtain mucous mem-

Figure 15-11 *A,* Harvesting of split-thickness skin graft with Brown dermatome. Assistant provides traction beyond proposed donor area. *B,* As dermatome is advanced forward, assistant elevates graft away from cutting blade of dermatome. **(Courtesy Shan R. Baker, M.D.)**

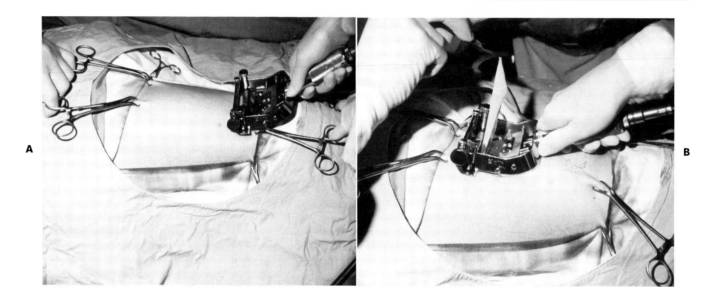

A   B

Figure 15-12 Padgett dermatome.

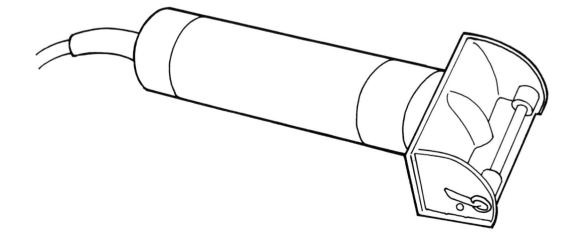

brane grafts for reconstruction of eyelid and eye socket deformities. A motor moves the small cutting head with the blade and controls the thickness of the cut.

The Reese or Padgett-Hood drum dermatomes require the use of special adhesives, are difficult to use, and would probably not rank very high in the armamentarium of most head and neck reconstructive surgeons.

Donor Site Care

Donor site defects from STSGs often cause more pain and problems for the patient than the actual grafted site. Primary problems are pain, drainage, and risk of infection. Hemostatic agents, such as thromboplastin or oxidized regenerated cellulose (Surgicel), can be placed on the donor site before placement of the dressing. Likewise, gauze soaked with 1% lidocaine with epinephrine can also be placed over the donor site temporarily until the permanent dressing is placed. The most popular donor site dressings are the semi-

permeable occlusive dressings. Many surgeons advocate use of a polyurethane-based semiocclusive dressing, such as Opsite or Tegaderm over the wound, followed by application of a strip of tape around the perimeter and a gauze dressing at dependent sites to collect exudate. This gauze dressing can be left in place, and the healing process can then be observed. Any fluid collection beneath the dressing can be drained by insertion of a sterile needle to aspirate fluid, then "patching" the needle hole with a small piece of Opsite. Another approach is to change the dressing after the first 24 to 48 hours, which is the period of greatest production of wound transudate, and leave the second dressing in place for 5 to 7 days. Tincture of benzoin or other skin adhesive has been recommended before application of Opsite to increase adherence.

Semipermeable membrane dressings greatly decrease the amount of pain from the donor site and permit a moist environment, which facilitates wound healing. Infection has not been found to be a problem with these dressings. A few surgeons use the open method of donor site healing, in which no dressing is applied. Although this may be practical for some areas that are difficult to bandage, this method may not effectively control pain. Bulky dressings, which remain in place for 10 days, have also been used for donor site care.

A hydrophilic polyurethane dressing (Allevyn), which is highly absorbable and nonadherent, can also be used for donor site care. The outer layer, which is waterproof, and bacteria-proof, is based on the same material used to make Opsite. This dressing is popular with patients because it is soft and cushioning and the absorbent nature prevents fluid buildup and "leaks" common with Opsite. A recent report by Brodovsky et al[16] suggests that Nobecutane spray is effective as a temporary dressing for skin graft donor sites. It contains a modified acrylic resin in an organic solvent along with the bactericidal-fungicidal agent tetramethylthiuram disulfide (TMTD) and forms a transparent plastic film when sprayed on the wound. The study showed rapid, painless healing, and the dressing was shed spontaneously with epidermal regeneration.

The same principles apply for both FTSGs and STSGs in terms of attachment to the wound bed. Peripheral attachment can be accomplished by absorb-

Figure 15-13 Weck knife freehand system.

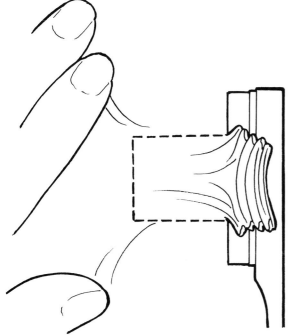

Figure 15-14 Davol-Simon dermatome.

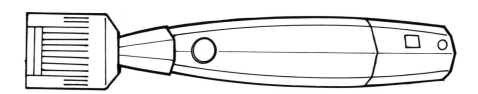

able or nonabsorbable sutures or a combination of these. For grafts of considerable size, the use of staples to attach the graft to the wound may be most practical (Fig. 15-9**B**). Staples must be placed so that the edges as well as the underside of the graft are in good apposition to the wound bed. Care must be used so that the staples don't "gather" the graft at the wound edge and cause potential space for the loculation of fluid.

It should be noted that the tie-down dressing is not mandatory to achieve good apposition between the graft and the wound bed. (The tie-down dressings were discussed extensively in the section about full-thickness skin grafts). A good compression dressing and/or basting sutures can accomplish the same purpose. Basting sutures (simple or interrupted) can be placed in the central portion of the graft to promote adherence to the wound bed and prevent loculated fluid. Small "piecrust" slits can be made in the center of the graft to facilitate drainage. A variation of the basting suture, the spiral basting suture, is particularly useful for STSGs.[15] The suture is started at the edge of the graft with one interrupted suture placed, and the "tail" is left long. The suture is run as a basting suture from the periphery of the graft in a circular fashion to the center of the graft, where the suture is tied to the tail of the initial interrupted suture (Fig. 15-15). The spiral basting suture provides uniform apposition without wrinkling the graft. This suturing technique eliminates the need for a tie-down bolster dressing, permitting observation of the wound 24 to 48 hours after application of a compression dressing. A gel dressing (Vigilon) can provide a moist environment, will allow rapid healing, and will not adhere to the graft when this dressing is changed. Cotton balls can be placed over the dressing to provide even more compression.

MESHED GRAFTS

Meshed grafts are indicated for large defects where there is insufficient skin and the epidermis must be expanded to cover the defect (such as severe burns or scalp defects) as well as for defects where flexibility is required (such as on the elbow). They are also indicated for defects that drain significant amounts of fluid (although if a defect is draining copious amounts of fluid, grafting should probably be delayed). Meshed grafts are probably of limited use in head and neck reconstruction and may in the future be superseded by autologous grafts or allografts. There are several disadvantages to meshed grafts. The spaces between the epithelial bridges must heal by epithelialization, and generally the final result also retains the meshed pattern, which on the face can be cosmetically distressing. The meshing of skin grafts occurs when the STSG is placed on a plastic carrier that has a groove pattern, which defines the size of the holes to be placed in the graft. Carriers are available to allow expansion of the graft to 1.5, three, or six times the original area of the graft. Once the graft is placed onto the carrier, the carrier is advanced through a mechanical mesher by means of a crank. Once the graft is placed, shiny (dermal) side down into the defect, it is secured in place by placement of a few interrupted nylon sutures or staples at various spots along the graft. A gel dressing, such as Vigilon, can be placed over the graft and changed daily, or the traditional tie-down bolster, with use of antibiotic ointment, interpositional surfacing material N-terface, and then sterile cotton balls can be used.

To achieve acceptable cosmetic results, Davison et al[17] suggest the use of nonexpanded machine meshed grafts. The 1:1.5 carrier board is cut in half and, with the graft, is passed sideways through the meshing machine to achieve an even finer skin perforation pattern. The meshed skin is placed on the recipient bed so that the perforations are aligned along the natural skin creases, and then the graft is tensioned longitudinally to close the perforations to slitlike spaces.

PINCH GRAFTS

Pinch grafting is a simple technique, which may eventually be replaced by thin graft harvesting with the Davol-Simon dermatome or the Weck blade. Pinch grafts have traditionally been used on wounds that are draining (the spaces between the grafts after placement permits drainage) and have been suggested for treatment of the hypopigmentation in localized areas of vitiligo. Essentially, the donor skin is held with pickups and then lifted (Fig. 15-16). The elevated bit of skin is then transsected with iris scissors or a scalpel. Multiple grafts (usually less than 1 cm) are harvested and placed almost next to each other, and the spaces in between heal by epithelialization. The major drawback is the unsightly "hillock" surface irregularity when these grafts heal.[12] This results from the irregular depth of the graft, which is due to the tenting effect. (The lateral part of the graft is thin epidermis, whereas the thicker central portion contains more dermis.) One solution to this problem, as proposed by Robinson,[18] is to use a punch biopsy to obtain a specimen of uniform depth by limitation of the downward force, thereby limiting the depth to the deep dermis. The fat is trimmed once the plug is removed, yielding a graft of uniform depth. This technique is probably applicable only to smaller wounds in cosmetically less important areas.

Figure 15-15 Spiral basting suture used to secure split-thickness skin graft to wound bed.

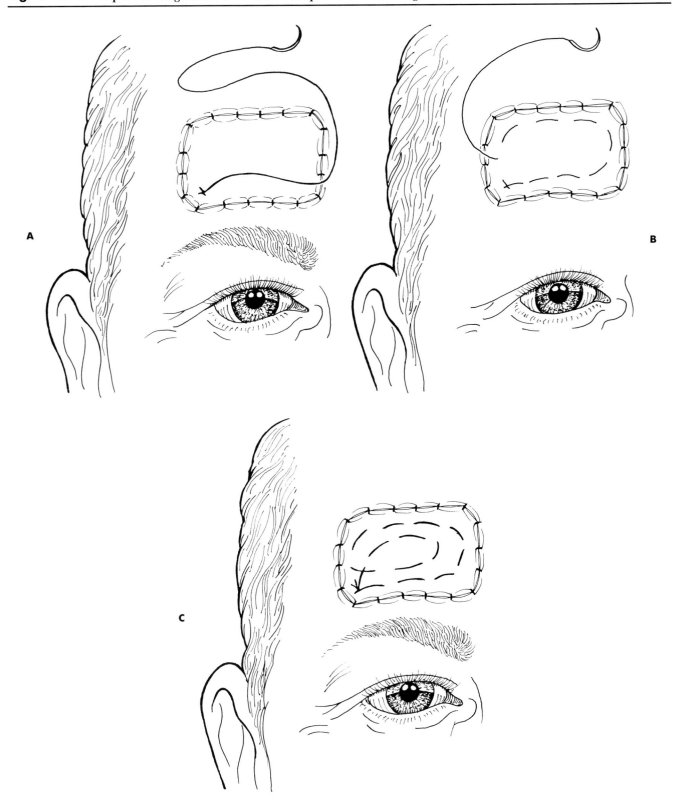

Figure 15-16 **Simple technique for pinch skin grafting.**

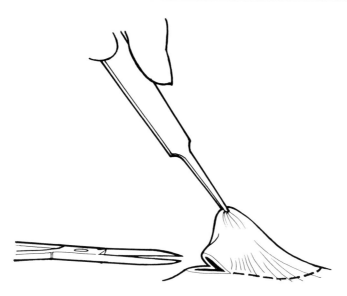

COMPOSITE GRAFTS

Composite grafts contain two or more tissue layers. In head and neck reconstruction, the most common uses for these grafts are for repair of alar rim and auricular defects and for eyebrow reconstruction.

The advantages of a composite graft (usually taken from the ear) for alar rim defects include the ability to maintain the thinness and contour of the alar rim and provision of structure (via auricular cartilage) to the graft to prevent alar contraction. The auricular donor sites most commonly used are the helical crus, the helical rim, the antihelix, tragus, and the earlobe (skin and fat), but any area of the ear can be used depending on the size of the original defect and the necessary contour of the donor area (Fig. 15-17). The helical crus provides a good contour for grafting of small alar rim defects because it is straight and does not have an anterior roll, which can be a problem with the helical rim. (In addition, taking the graft from the helical rim also shortens the ear.) Because the inner part of the helical crus is shallow, other donor sites may be needed for significant alar defects.

The primary disadvantage of composite grafts is that they have a high risk of failure secondary to the high metabolic demands of these grafts. Composite grafts obtain their vasculature from the recipient site at the edges of the graft. The vasculature necessary to support a composite graft that consists of multiple tissue layers is considerable, which is why this type of graft is most successful when transferred from an ear to the nose, which has abundant vascularity. Surgical technique and hemostasis are extremely important

because of the tenuous vascular supply, as is the size limitation for the graft. Because of the need for proximity of the graft to vascular tissue, the composite graft generally should be no larger than approximately 1.5 to 2 cm. However, Avelar et al[19] reported that they successfully used a composite graft containing postauricular skin and almost 70% of the total area of the conchal cartilage and also successfully transferred composite grafts larger than 2 cm for reconstruction of nose and ear deformities. Skouge[3] discusses the "tongue and groove" placement of the graft edge into the recipient site as well as use of a turndown, hinged flap for large defects; both techniques are designed to increase the vascular recipient surface area and to provide an inner lining to the nose.

The defect can be carefully measured and then marked on the donor site, or a template can be made. The graft is harvested and placed into cold saline until it is transferred to the recipient site. The recipient site on the alar rim must be deepithelialized and scar tissue removed to facilitate the amount of surface area that gets exposed to the graft. The graft is sutured in layers, starting with the mucosal layer, using an absorbable suture. The needle should pass through the mucosa and then through the graft edge, so that the knots are tied external to the graft (Fig. 15-18). If the grafts are small (less than 1 cm in diameter), the cartilage does not need to be sutured to the recipient cartilage. For larger composite grafts, placement of small polyglycolic Dexon sutures may add mechanical stability to the graft-wound interface. The skin edges of the wound are sutured to the anterior skin edges of the graft with small, nonabsorbable sutures, which are removed 1

Figure 15-17   Common composite graft with donor sites from auricle.

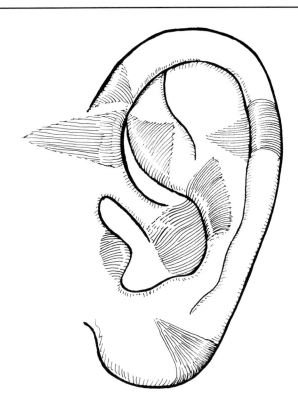

Figure 15-18   Attachment of composite graft to recipient site on nose. Knots should be tied externally to graft.

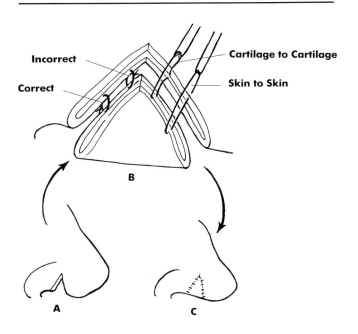

week later. It should be emphasized that there is minimal handling of the graft with small amounts of tissue being incorporated with each suture. The sutures are spaced so as to not strangle the tissue and impede neovascularization.

An ointment-coated nasal packing can be placed gently in the nasal vestibule, and a light coat of antibiotic ointment and nonadherent (Telfa) dressing are placed externally. The perioperative use of antibiotics has been suggested because of the high bacterial colonization encountered in the perinasal area.

The postoperative appearance of these grafts is characteristic. At placement the grafts are blanched, but they develop a pink color at about 6 hours (Fig. 15-19). By 24 hours, they are cyanotic and at postoperative days 3 to 7 they develop a pink color in surviving grafts. In grafts destined to fail, an eschar develops on the epidermis, and either the entire graft or the cartilage necroses and sloughs.

For reconstruction of partial auricular defects, it is possible to use composite grafts from the opposite ear or a cartilage graft combined with a banner flap. In complete reconstruction of the auricle, costal cartilage has been used, as it is available in the quantities needed for structural support, although elastic cartilage provides a better framework for auricular reconstruction. A technique designed to use the chondrogenic capacity

of perichondrium has also been described to reconstruct auricular defects.[20] A skin flap on the posterior part of the auricle is raised in the conchal area. Then a piece of perichondrium that approximates the size of the defect is excised and sutured, chondrogenic surface outward, to the underlying fascia beneath a previously prepared postauricular skin flap. Two months later the postauricular skin flap and cartilage disk (produced by the perichondrial graft) are dissected free. As a composite graft with the overlying skin, the flap and cartilage disk are sutured in a layered fashion to the prepared area of the auricular defect, with the skin flap connected to the anterior skin of the auricle. After 3 weeks, the flap with regenerated cartilage is cut along the base. The skin defect on the posterior auricle is covered by a local flap, and the skin defect behind the ear is covered with a graft, freehand full thickness. This technique permits formation of elastic cartilage without limit in size and without any structural defect at the donor site.

COMPOSITE HAIR-BEARING GRAFTS

Several techniques have been advocated for reconstruction of the eyebrow. Strip grafting, which is actually a type of composite graft that contains skin and fat, generally gives good results.

The most important consideration in the recipient site is the presence of scarring, which, because of the related decreased blood supply, may limit the size of

Figure 15-19   *A and B,* Full-thickness loss of alar margin (2 × 1.5 cm) after removal of basal cell carcinoma.
C, Composite auricular graft consisting of skin, subcutaneous fat, and cartilage is harvested from right antitragus. *D,*
Graft is balanced immediately after transfer to nose. *E and F,* Appearance of composite graft 9 months postoperatively.
No revision surgery was necessary. *G,* Donor site of composite graft 9 months postoperatively.

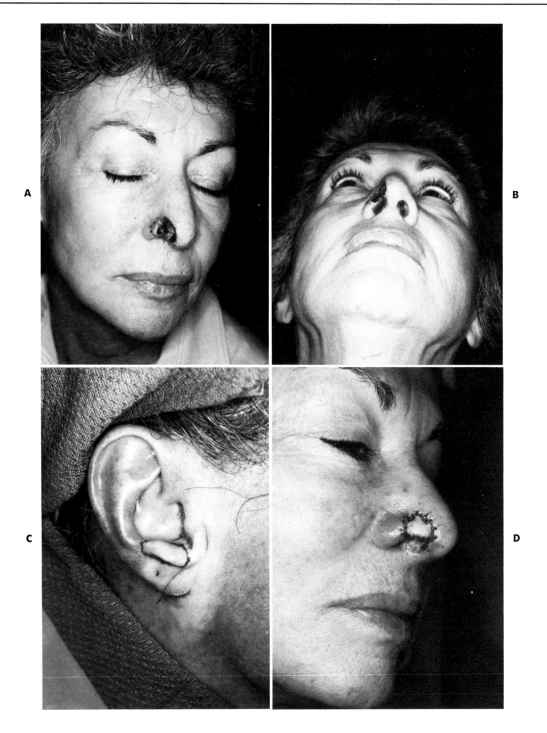

Figure 15-19, cont'd.   For legend see opposite page.

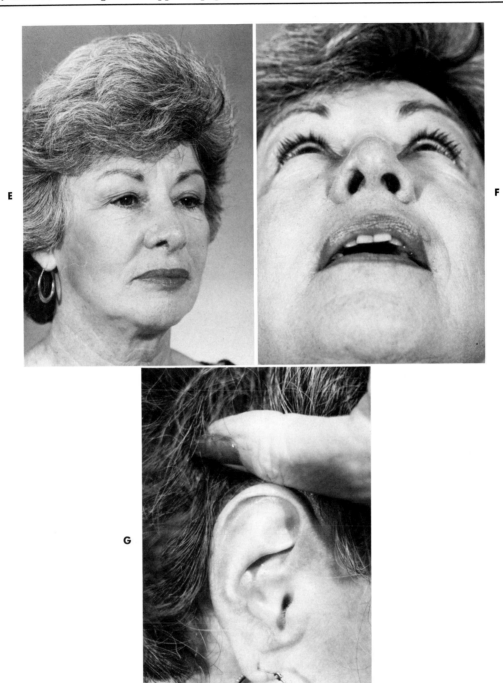

the graft. In a severely scarred area a graft restricted to 5 mm in width has been suggested, as opposed to a graft 1 cm wide, which could survive in an area with no scarring. The contralateral eyebrow assists in texture of the graft and in planning of the shape and height of graft placement.

Strip grafting is performed with the patient under local anesthesia. The donor site is chosen from the scalp, based on hair quality, and is generally planned so that the long axis of the graft runs cephalocaudad, with the medial part of the graft most cephalad (Fig. 15-20). Although this will not yield a pattern of hair growth identical to the multidirectional normal eyebrow (which has predominantly lateral growth) (Fig. 15-21), the graft will be oriented with lateral growth, giving a satisfactory cosmetic result. The proposed brow is measured and marked on the patient with a template. The hair is trimmed (not shaved) to permit visualization of the hair shaft angle. The incision is made parallel to the hair shafts, to prevent injury to the hair follicles, and is carried down through fat and galea to the periosteum. The graft is removed and placed into sterile saline. The donor site is then closed in a layered fashion. The recipient site is prepared and anesthetized. The premeasured strip of skin is excised with careful hemostasis. The graft is trimmed so that there is a small amount of fat below the hair follicles and then placed into the recipient defect. The graft is sutured in place with nonabsorbable sutures, then dressed with antibiotic ointment and a light compression dressing. Sutures are removed in 1 week.

A full-thickness eyebrow graft from the opposite eyebrow can also be used as a type of composite graft to correct a partially resected eyebrow, particularly if the defect is circular or oval, such as those created after Mohs micrographic surgery.[21] If possible, the donor site is taken from the location corresponding to the resected area of the contralateral brow. The donor graft is removed with sufficient depth to avoid damage to hair roots. It is then rotated, so that the orientation of the hair alignment is the same as that of the recipient site (Fig. 15-22). The graft is then sutured in place following undermining of the recipient site. The donor site is closed primarily.

COMPOSITE GRAFTING FROM EARLOBE TO NOSE

The earlobe is another relatively common site for composite donor grafts. Wedge-shaped donor grafts from the lateral earlobe can be "filleted" rather than defatted, to produce a lenticular shaped graft of sufficient bulk to restore the contour of the nasal tip.[22] A full-thickness composite graft can also be taken from the central part of the earlobe and used to repair

Figure 15-20 Orientation of donor strip grafts from scalp.

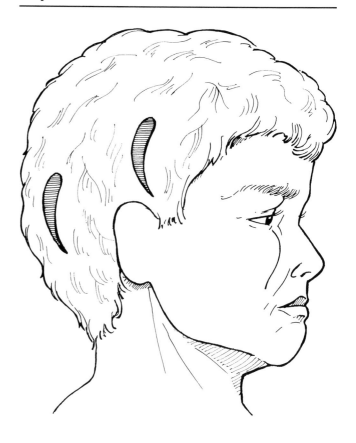

Figure 15-21 Multidirectional orientation of hair of brow.

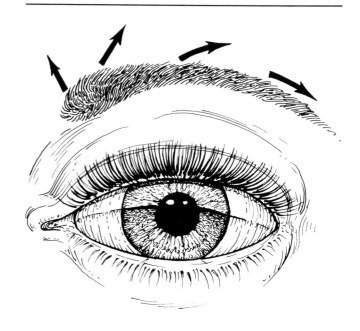

Figure 15-22   Rotation of harvested composite graft from opposite eyebrow. Care is taken to maintain correct hair orientation at recipient site.

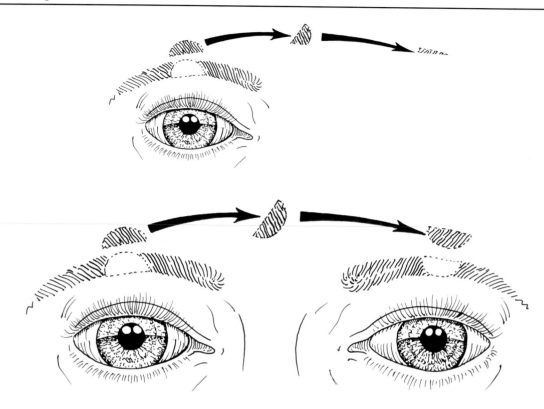

defects of the nose, which include loss of nasal lining (not involving the alar rim). The skin surfaces of the graft are sutured to the respective surfaces of the nasal defect in a layered fashion.[23] Earlobe composite grafts have also been used to reconstruct the columella and unilateral earlobe defects with use of a composite graft from the opposite earlobe.[24]

COMPOSITE GRAFTS IN EYELID RECONSTRUCTION

Composite grafts are also used for reconstruction in eyelid surgery. Free autogenous tarsal grafts have been used for eyelid reconstruction for many years, and a double composite lid graft reconstruction procedure that uses opposing upper and lower lids for reconstruction of extensive lid defects has been described.[25,26]

CULTURED AUTOLOGOUS SKIN GRAFTS

Cultured autologous skin grafts are the most recent advancement in the methods of replacement of lost skin. In this technique a small piece of tissue is harvested from the patient, and the donor tissue is expanded many times in a tissue culture laboratory (with the use of established techniques) to provide large amounts of epithelium, which are eventually returned to the patient. Clinical experience with cultured human autologous keratinocyte sheets was first documented by O'Connor et al[27] in 1981 in burn patients. Subsequently, epithelial autografts have been used to cover burn wounds (including third-degree burns)[28-31] and leg ulcers,[32-34] to cover the defect after excision of a giant congenital nevus,[35] and in the treatment of junctional epidermolysis bullosa.[36] Research has also shown that these types of grafts may be beneficial in reducing recurrences following removal of hypertrophic scars or keloids.[37] They have also been used to correct pigmentation secondary to piebaldism.[38]

Recent advances in keratinocytic cultivation have allowed the generation of sufficient epidermis to cover an entire body surface within 3 weeks.[39] Shave excisions of donor skin of 1 cm^2 or less were expanded in culture in 1 week to cover wounds as large as 90 cm^2, when cultured keratinocytes were applied to a collagen-coated dressing and applied to the wound.[32] Even cultured autologous epithelial cells in suspension have been shown to heal in full-thickness burn wounds when spread onto the prepared wound by use of a sterile spatula.[30] Although only a few studies have reported long-term follow-up of autografts versus STSGs, the preliminary results suggest comparable longevity at 15 months and at 5 years after grafting.[28,31,33] Compton et al,[40] who used cultured keratinocyte autografts on full-thickness burn wounds, observed anchoring fibrils at the dermoepidermal junction 1 month after grafting; the graft required more than 1 year to reach full maturation. This interval of maturation is comparable to meshed STSGs.[40] Rete ridges appeared anywhere from 5 to 18 months after grafting. During the 5-year follow-up period of this study, the underlying connective tissue remodeled and elastin was regenerated, yielding an appearance similar to native dermis.[40] Wound contraction under STSGs and under cultured keratinocyte autografts appeared similar when both methods were used to graft defects that resulted from excision of giant congenital nevi. Some have suggested that the autologous grafts present an esthetically better appearance than comparable sites treated with mesh grafts.[28] This technique could conceivably supersede mesh graft–dermatome treatment of STSGs, especially in patients with limited donor sites.

Problems with keratinocytic sheet attachment and subsequent revascularization after graft placement have been noted and are not unlike the skin fragility and blistering following STSG at donor and recipient sites. Such problems are thought to be due to the delay in epidermal-dermal rete ridge development and the delayed development of anchoring fibrils. To combat the fragility problem, Hansbrough et al[41] prepared a "composite graft" placing cultured autologous keratinocytes onto the surface of a modified collagen-glycosaminoglycan membrane containing autologous fibroblasts. This "composite graft" was placed onto limited areas of excised full-thickness burn wounds, with an acceptable rate of survival. Formation of a basement membrane occurred within 9 days of graft placement. In the future this type of composite graft may help provide a more stable wound closure earlier in the postgrafting period.

There are several factors to consider in the preparation of autologous skin in vitro, including the size and location of the harvested tissue, management of the donor defect, age of the patient, size of the defect to be covered, amount of time needed to culture sufficient tissue, and proximity of facilities that have the expertise for culturing keratinocytes. Because cells obtained from older patients can be more difficult to culture, either a longer time period to permit culture or use of cultured allograft must be considered. A way to circumvent this problem is to freeze cultured epithelium, which remains viable if stored in a skin bank.[30,42,43] Autologous grafting lends itself most easily to the following: (1) relatively small defects, which require less time for keratinocytic expansion; (2) surgical defects for which removal of the lesion can be a preplanned event, such as removal of certain skin cancers, certain epidermal tumors, and (3) congenital nevi; and elective treatment of other conditions, such as aplasia cutis congenita. Indications for a meshed skin graft such as in repair of a large defect of the scalp or burn wound might also be amenable to autologous grafting (if the time to generate the keratinocytic sheet can be managed) or to allografting from a banked source.

ALLOGRAFTS

To bridge the delay in culturing of autologous keratinocytes, cultured keratinocytes or cryopreserved cadaver allografts can be used.[31,43] These allografts are grown from cadaver skin or human neonatal foreskin.[44,45] It was discovered in 1983 that cultured allogenic keratinocytic sheets applied to burn wounds did not result in graft rejection.[44] Further investigation suggests that keratinocytes in culture lose their ability to express HLA-DR and to stimulate lymphocyte production.[46] It now appears that healing occurs because of reepithelialization from the wound margins and stimulation of wound healing.[47,48] Recent studies have shown that the allografts are eventually replaced by host epithelium.[49]

One team successfully treated a full-thickness burn with skin allografts from cadavers, followed by later abrading the allograft to remove the allogenic epidermis, which was resurfaced with autogenous keratinocyte cultures.[42,43] Thus the final grafts were actually composites of allogenic dermis and autologous cultured epidermis. The concept was to use the cadaveric allograft to decrease fluid loss and prevent bacterial invasion during the immediate period of immunosuppression following the burn injury. Before recovery of immunocompetence the allograft epidermis, which is more antigenically active then the dermis, is removed and replaced by host epidermis. The allogenic dermis, like cultured allogenic keratinocytes, eventually gets replaced by host cells, through a slow minimized rejection process.[50]

Cadaveric homografts may be difficult to obtain because of medicolegal, social, or religious reasons. Early coverage of defects, such as burns, with cultured allografts stored frozen could circumvent this dilemma. Both cadaver and culture specimens must be screened for communicable diseases such as acquired immunodeficiency syndrome (AIDS), hepatitis B, cytomegalovirus, and herpes.[51] It should be noted that certain other communicable diseases such as Creutzfeldt-Jakob disease are transmissible in humans after corneal transplantation, after dura mater graft transplantation, and in homografts for repair of the tympanic membrane.[52-54] Unfortunately, there are no routine screening procedures to prevent transmission of Creutzfeldt-Jakob disease.[52-54]

In conclusion, cultured epidermal grafts, either autologous or allografts, can provide permanent or at least long-term coverage in areas either where there is not enough donor tissue for STSGs or when the secondary donor defect might interfere with healing. The final outcome appears at least comparable to or perhaps superior to meshed STSGs. As skin banking and culture facilities become more available, permitting supplies of an antigenically null skin substitute, the head and neck surgeon may become more involved in the use of these types of grafts.

REFERENCES

1. Rudolph R, Ballantyne DL: Skin grafts. In McCarthy JG, editor: *Plastic surgery, vol 1, General principles,* Philadelphia, 1990, WB Saunders.

2. Jensen F, Petersen NC: Repair of denuded cranial bone by bone splitting and free skin grafting, *J Neurosurg* 44:728, 1976.

3. Skouge JW: *Skin grafting,* New York, 1991, Churchill Livingstone.

4. Mohs FE: *Chemosurgery in cancer, gangrene and infections,* Springfield, Ill, 1956, Charles C. Thomas.

5. Mellette JR, Swinehart JM: Cartilage removal prior to skin grafting in the triangular fossa, antihelix and concha of the ear, *J Dermatol Surg Oncol* 16:1102, 1990.

6. Salasche SJ, Feldman BD: Skin grafting: Perioperative technique and management. *J Dermatol Surg Oncol* 13:863, 1987.

7. Hill TG: Reconstruction of nasal defects using full-thickness grafts: a personal reappraisal, *J Dermatol Surg Oncol* 12:995, 1983.

8. Adnot J, Salasche SJ: Visualized basting sutures in the application of full-thickness skin grafts, *J Dermatol Surg Oncol* 13:1236, 1987.

9. Hill TG: Enhancing the survival of full-thickness grafts, *J Dermatol Surg Oncol* 10:639, 1984.

10. Robinson J: Improvement of the appearance of full-thickness skin grafts with dermabrasion, *Arch Dermatol* 123:1340, 1987.

11. Wheeland RG: Revision of full-thickness skin grafts using the carbon dioxide laser, *J Dermatol Surg Oncol* 14:130, 1988.

12. Skouge JW: Techniques for split-thickness skin grafting, *J Dermatol Surg Oncol* 13:841, 1987.

13. Stal S, Spira M: Mons pubis as a donor site for split-thickness skin grafts, *Plast Reconstr Surg* 75:906, 1985.

14. Tromovich TA, Stegman SJ, Glogau RG: *Flaps and grafts in dermatologic surgery,* Chicago, 1989, Year Book Medical.

15. Glogau RG, Stegman SJ, Tromovich TA: Refinements in split-thickness skin grafting technique, *J Dermatol Surg Oncol* 13:853, 1987.

16. Brodovsky S, Dagan R, Ben-Bassatt M: Nobecutane spray as temporary dressing of skin graft donor sites, *J Dermatol Surg Oncol* 12:386, 1986.

17. Davison PM, Batchelor AG, Lewis-Smith PA: The properties and uses of non-expanded machine-meshed skin grafts, *Br J Plastic Surg* 39:462, 1986.

18. Robinson JK: An alternate method of obtaining a punch graft. *J Dermatol Surg Oncol* 8:162, 1982.

19. Avelar JM, Psillakis JM, Viterbo F: Use of large composite grafts in the reconstruction of deformities of the nose and ear, *Br J Plastic Surg* 37:55, 1984.

20. Ohlsen L: Reconstruction of auricular defect with perichondrial graft: a new technique, *Scand J Plast Reconstr Surg* 12:299, 1978.

21. English FP, Forester TDC: The eyebrow graft, *Ophthalmic Surg* 10:39, 1979.

22. Lipman SH, Roth RJ: Composite grafts from earlobes for reconstruction of defects in noses, *J Dermatol Surg Oncol* 8:135, 1982.

23. Breach NM: Repair of a full-thickness nasal defect with an ear lobe "sandwich" graft, *Br J Plast Surg* 32:94, 1979.

24. Kruchinski GV: New method of ear lob plasty using graft taken from lobe of healthy ear, *Acta Chir Plast* 17:242, 1975.

25. Beyer-Machule CK, Shapiro A, Smith B: Double composite lid reconstruction: a new method of upper and lower lid reconstruction, *Ophthalmic Plast Reconstr Surg* 1:97, 1985.

26. Stephenson CM, Brown BZ: The use of tarsus as a free autogenous graft in eyelid surgery, *Ophthalmic Plast Reconstr Surg* 1:43, 1985.

27. O'Connor NE, Milliken JB, Banks-Schlegel S et al: Grafting of burns with cultured epithelium prepared from autologous epidermal cells, *Lancet* 1:75, 1981.

28. Bettex-Galland M, Slongott, Hunziker T et al: Use of cultured keratinocytes in the treatment of severe burns, *Z Kinderchir* 43:224, 1988.

29. Gallico G, O'Connor NE, Compton CC et al: Permanent coverage of large burn wounds with autologous cultured human epithelium, *N Engl J Med* 331:448, 1984.

30. Khalfan HA, Hamza AA, Saeed T et al: Novel method of skin substitution in plastic surgery, *Burns* 15:335, 1987.

31. Munster AM, Weiner SH, Spence RJ: Cultured epidermis for the coverage of massive burn wounds, *Ann Surg* 221:676, 1990.

32. Brysk MM, Raimer SS, Pupro R et al: Grafting of leg ulcers with undifferentiated keratinocytes, *J Am Acad Dermatol* 25:238, 1991.

33. Hefton JM, Caldwell D, Bioles DG et al: Grafting of

skin ulcers with cultured autologous epidermal cells, *J Am Acad Dermatol* 11:650, 1986.

34. Leigh IM, Purkis PE: Culture grafted leg ulcers, *Clin Exp Dermatol* 11:650, 1986.

35. Gallico G, O'Connor NE, Compton CC et al: Cultured epithelial autografts for giant congenital nevi, *J Plast Reconstr Surg* 84:1, 9, 1989.

36. Carter DM, Lin AN, Varghese MC et al: Treatment of junctional epidermolysis bullosa with epidermal autografts, *J Am Acad Dermatol* 17:246, 1987.

37. O'Connor NE, Gallico GG, Compton CC: Modifications of hypertrophic scars and keloids with cultured epithelial autografts, *Proc Am Burn Assoc* 22:7, 1990.

38. Selmanowitz VG, Rabinowitz AD, Orentreich N et al: Pigmentary correction of piebaldism by autografts: I. Procedures and clinical findings, *J Dermatol Surg Oncol* 3:615, 1977.

39. Green H, Kehinde O, Thomas J: Growth of cultured human epidermal cells into multiple epithelia suitable for grafting, *Proc Natl Acad Sci* 76:5665, 1979.

40. Compton CC, Gill JM, Bradford DA et al: Skin regenerated from cultured epithelial autografts on full-thickness burn wounds from 6 days to 5 years after grafting, *Lab Invest* 60:600, 1989.

41. Hansbrough JF, Boyce ST, Cooper ML et al: Burn wound closure with cultured autologous keratinocytes and fibroblasts attached to a collagen-glycosaminoglycan substrate, *JAMA* 262:2125, 1989.

42. Cuono C, Langdon R, McGuire J: Use of cultured epidermal autografts and dermal allografts as skin replacement after burn injury, *Lancet* 1:1123, 1986.

43. Langdon R, Cuono C, Bishall N et al: Reconstitution of structure and cell function in human skin grafts derived from cryopreserved allogenic dermis and autologous cultured keratinocytes, *J Invest Dermatol* 91:478, 1988.

44. Hefton JM, Madden MR, Finkelstein JL et al: Grafting of burn patients with allografts of cultured epidermal cells, *Lancet* 2:428, 1983.

45. Phillips T, Kehinde O, Green H et al: Treatment of skin ulcers with cultured epidermal allografts, *J Am Acad Dermatol* 21:191, 1989.

46. Thivolet J, Faure M, Demidim A et al: Long-term survival and immunological tolerance of human epidermal allografts produced in culture, *Transplantation* 42:274, 1986.

47. Beele H, Naeyaert JM, Goeteyn M et al: Repeated cultured epidermal allografts in the treatment of chronic leg ulcers of various origins, *Dermatologica* 183:31, 1991.

48. Leigh IM, Purkis PE, Navsaria HA et al: Treatment of chronic venous ulcers with sheets of cultured allogenic keratinocytes, *Br J Dermatol* 117:591, 1987.

49. Gielen V, Faure M, Mauduit G et al: Progressive replacement of human cultured epithelial allografts by recipient cells as evidenced by HLA class 1 antigen expression, *Dermatologica* 175:166, 1987.

50. Young D, Langdon R, Kahn R et al: Analysis of the fate of allografted dermis using a DNA printing technique. Paper presented at the 21st Annual Meeting of the American Burn Association, New Orleans, March 1989.

51. Clarke JA: HIV transmission and skin grafts, *Lancet* 1:983, 1987.

52. Duffy P, Wolf J, Collins G et al: Possible person-to-person transmission of Creutzfeldt-Jakob disease, *N Engl J Med* 290:692, 1974.

53. Tange RA, Troost D, Limburg M: Progressive fatal dementia (Creutzfeldt-Jakob disease) in a patient who received homograft tissue for tympanic membrane closure, *Arch Otorhinolaryngol* 247:199, 1990.

54. Willison HJ, Gale AN, McLaughlin JE: Creutzfeldt-Jakob disease following cadaveric dura mater grafts, *J Neurol Neurosurg Psychiatry* 54:199, 1990.

EDITORIAL COMMENTS

Shan R. Baker

The authors have provided an overview of the use of full-thickness, split-thickness, and composite skin grafts for reconstruction of the head and neck. There is no limit on the surface area of a full-thickness skin graft that may survive; thus almost all small and intermediate-sized facial defects that are to be repaired with skin grafts should be covered with a full-thickness graft. This will provide better texture and color match with surrounding facial skin compared with split-thickness skin grafts, and there will be less wound contracture. As the surface area of the defect increases, however, the use of full-thickness skin grafts becomes less practical because of the difficulty in closure of the graft's donor site.

There are many methods of fixation and stabilization of split- and full-thickness skin grafts during the healing phase. Some surgeons prefer the open technique, in which the graft is not covered with a dressing but left exposed so that the graft can be "rolled" to remove accumulated serum beneath the graft. Other techniques use basting sutures as discussed in this chapter. Generally I prefer to use bolster dressings to secure most full- and split-thickness grafts. The dressing is left in place for 5 days, and then the graft is exposed. Any serum is evacuated at that time, and the patient is instructed to frequently compress areas where seromas have developed.

The use of composite grafts from the auricle to repair nasal defects can be helpful at times, but I confine their use to small alar margin or columellar defects (2 cm or less in greatest dimension). Patient selection is important, and I limit the use of these techniques to younger (under 65 years of age) individuals and to persons who do not use tobacco. In my opinion an improved survival rate of composite grafts can be achieved if grafting is delayed until the nasal defect has healed by second intention. Surface contact between the compos-

ite graft and recipient site should be maximized, and this can be accomplished using turnover hinged flaps based on the margin of the nasal defect. The number of sutures that secure the graft should be limited, theoretically to prevent restriction of early neovascularization. Systemic steroids have been shown to enhance survival of composite grafts. I use a 60-mg dosage of prednisone on the day of surgery tapered to 5 mg on postoperative day 7. I also cool the graft, using ice-saline compresses, during the first 3 days after transfer. Theoretically this reduces the biological requirements of the graft in the early postoperative period before neovascularization has occurred.

EDITORIAL COMMENTS

Neil Swanson

This is a very complete and comprehensive chapter on all types of skin grafting. The chapter begins with an excellent description of some basic concepts of skin grafting. The authors stress the importance of adherence to a clean, relatively sterile and well-vascularized bed to maximize survival of the graft. Also mentioned is the concept of delaying a graft to promote granulation tissue and enhance vascularity. If this is allowed, it provides the additional benefit of filling in the depth of a defect so that the contour by skin grafting can be enhanced. One technical point is in preparation of the granulating bed. With delayed grafting, the bed must be scored or crosshatched to interrupt the myofibrils and other contractile elements, which have begun to form as part of the wound healing process. This will enable not only a better graft survival but also less contraction of the graft and graft bed.

Some other technical points are interesting and worth stressing. I usually place basting sutures regardless of the type of dressing to be used. As mentioned in the chapter, these are almost always placed under direct visualization so as to prevent inadvertent bleeding. There is nothing more frustrating than meticulously suturing a graft in place, then placing a basting suture

that nicks a small vessel. One then has to undo the entire graft, reestablish hemostasis, and resuture. Placement of the basting suture under direct visualization eliminates this risk. I usually place the basting suture with rapidly absorbing cat gut and use the same suture material to suture the graft edges to the site. N-terface is an excellent first layer of the layer dressing regardless of whether it is tied or taped in place. It does not stick to anything and allows for easy, nontraumatic removal of the dressing. If I place a tie-over dressing, which has become rarer each year of my practice, I place the ties for the tie-over away from the edge of the graft. I think this allows for much better contour and less trauma on the edges of the graft.

Dermabrasion is very useful to blend the edges of the graft into the surrounding skin as well as to help blend the color and texture of the graft. In this regard, I will often enlarge the defect if it does not fit a fully esthetic unit so that I'm grafting the entire esthetic unit. That entire esthetic unit is dermabraded usually at approximately 8 weeks.

The chapter also ends with an excellent discussion of cultured autologous skin grafting. This technique is becoming more routine and is applicable not only in burn patients but also in reconstructive surgery.

Section II

Reconstruction of Facial Structures

16

RECONSTRUCTION OF THE EYELIDS

Bhupendra C. K. Patel

Patrick M. Flaharty

Richard L. Anderson

INTRODUCTION

There are accounts of extraordinary plastic surgery in India in the fourth century BC. The techniques described antedate all other such surgery and were unparalleled in Europe for almost 2000 years. Early methods of reconstruction of the nose are of particular interest because similar methods were subsequently used for eyelid reconstruction. Mutilation of the eyelids was a form of punishment in Roman times; when the Roman chief Regulus was captured by the Carthaginians, they tore off his eyelids.[1] Caron du Villards refers to the destruction of the eyelids of the Christian Crusaders by their captors.[2] The adage of Celsus Cornelius (25 BC to 50 AD), *"Se nimium palpebrae deest nulla id curatio restituere potest"* (if the least portion of the lid is gone, no cure can restore it), was accepted as incontrovertible until the Renaissance.

In the 14th century the elder Branca of Catania, Sicily, and Antonio, his son, are said to have repaired nasal defects using a pedicle graft from the arm. This method came to be known as the Italian method. The first recorded use of the Italian method for lid reconstruction was in 1934 by Sichel.[3] Paul Berger[4] in 1896 devised a leather harness to improve patient comfort, as the patient had to maintain the position shown in Fig. 16-1 for 12 to 20 days.

In 1646 Marcus Aurelius Severinus reconstructed a lid with use of healing by second intention when he excised scar tissue and packed the wound with lint. This is often called the Celsus method. A similar method of reconstruction by second intention was described by Guillon-Dolois in 1678, and similar procedures have also been attributed to Demosthenes and Ali ibn 'Isa.[5] In 1739 le Dran[6] reported the use of the skin on the side of the nose for the repair of a medial lower lid defect.

Carl von Graefe[7] opened a new era of plastic surgery in 1818 when he described the repair of a lower lid that had been destroyed by gangrene. He used a pedicle cheek flap much the same as the flaps used centuries earlier in India and later in the 15th century by the elder Branca. Dieffenbach, the father of plastic surgery, after much animal experimentation, reported extensively on ophthalmic reconstruction, including the use of a pedicle graft in 1835. The term *Blepharoplasty* (Greek, *blepharon*, eyelid, and *plasos*, formed) was originally used by von Graefe in 1818 to describe a case of eyelid reconstruction he had performed in 1809,[7] and this term prevailed for the next 150 years. Partial tarsorrhaphy, which is frequently used in the reconstruction of eyelids, was first reported by von Walther in 1826.

In 1829 J. C. G. Fricke[8] of Hamburg described the use of a flap from the temple for repair of the upper lid and a flap from the zygomatic region for the repair of the lower lid. Similar pedicle flaps from nearby areas for the replacement of eyelid skin were described by Eduard von Graefe[9] in 1830.

Baronio reported the first successful free grafting of skin in animals in 1804. In 1869 Jacques Reverdin[10] made his revolutionary contribution to reconstructive surgery by demonstrating conclusively that a completely detached piece of human epidermis would continue to live and grow if placed on a proper bed. In 1870 several surgeons used free skin grafts for lid repairs, including Lawson,[11] Holmes, Lee, and Pollock.[12] Five years later Wolfe[13] of Glasgow published a report of a free full-thickness skin graft from the forearm used for correction of ectropion in a miner. Wolfe's report gained more circulation in the English literature, and full-thickness grafts are commonly referred to as Wolfe grafts. The first report of a free graft in the American literature was from Wadsworth[14] of Boston in 1876.

Gradenigo[15] made the astute observation in 1870

Figure 16-1   **Berger's harness for improvement of patient comfort during lid reconstruction (1895).**

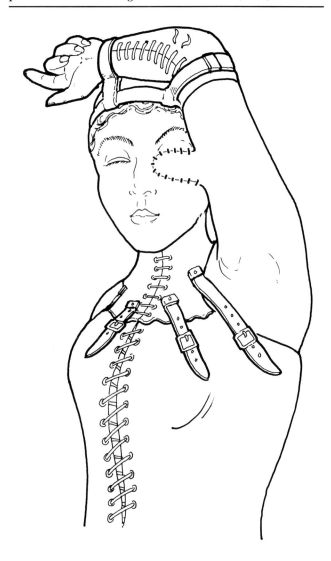

that nothing will satisfactorily reconstruct eyelids as well as normal lid tissues themselves, and he used the structures of one eyelid to rebuild the opposite lid. A single pedicle flap from the upper lid to supply additional skin for the lower lid was used by Valude in 1889. Landolt[16] in 1885 used a double pedicle or bridge flap to provide skin to the entire lower lid. It was only after the work of Dantrelle and Tartois[17] in 1918 and Wheeler[18] in 1925 that free grafting of large areas of upper lid skin was given proper emphasis. Wheeler made the important observation that only rarely is there insufficient skin in one of the upper eyelids when needed.

Full-thickness skin from various distant parts of the body has been used to supply skin for the eyelids. Skin of the arm has been used both with a pedicle, as in the Italian method, and as a free graft. Scrotal skin was first used by Tartois, whose results were variable. Skin from the back of the ear was first used by Blair[19] in 1932.

The first original American article on eyelid reconstruction was by Monks[20] of Boston in 1893. He used a pedicle flap from the scalp to reconstruct the lower lid. John M. Wheeler is widely regarded as the father of oculoplastic surgery in the United States and published widely on eyelid reconstructive procedures in the 1920s and 1930s. His student Wendell L. Hughes was the next major force in oculoplastic and reconstructive surgery, followed by Hughes's students Alston Callahan, Byron Smith, and Crowell Beard.

ANATOMY

Before the surgical concepts of eyelid reconstruction can be grasped, a clear understanding of eyelid anatomy is essential. The palpebral fissure measures 10 to 12 mm in the vertical dimension and 25 to 30 mm in the horizontal dimension. In the primary position of gaze the upper eyelid is 1 to 2 mm below the superior limbus and tends to get lower with age. The peak of the upper lid is nasal to the center of the pupil. The lower eyelid margin is usually at the inferior edge of the corneal limbus. The lowest portion of the lower eyelid margin is just temporal to the pupil. The upper eyelid crease is 8 to 12 mm above the eyelashes and is formed by the subcutaneous insertion of the terminal fibers of the levator aponeurosis muscle. The skin overlying the orbital septum has no levator aponeurotic subcutaneous extensions and folds over the eyelid crease. The lower eyelid has a poorly defined crease 2 to 3 mm below the lid margin nasally and 5 to 6 mm temporally.

The upper eyelid has six layers: skin, obicularis oculi muscle, levator aponeurosis muscle, Müller's muscle, tarsus, and conjunctiva.[21] However, the number of layers depends on the level of the eyelid examined (Fig. 16-2). The eyelid has a thin epithelial layer, which attaches to the orbicularis muscle by a loose connective tissue devoid of dermal-like tissue.

The concentrically arranged orbicularis muscle is the protractor of the eyelids and is divided into pretarsal, preseptal, and orbital sections. The orbital portion overlaps the orbital rims and interdigitates with the eyebrow muscles superiorly.

The pretarsal and preseptal orbicularis muscles contribute to the superficial and deep portions of the medial and lateral canthal tendon. The medial canthal tendon supports the nasal aspect of the eyelids and has superficial and deep components that anchor the lids nasally and posteriorly against the globe. A superior branch of the medial canthal tendon extends from the anterior portion of the tendon to insert onto the frontal

Figure 16-2   Schematic cross section of upper eyelid.

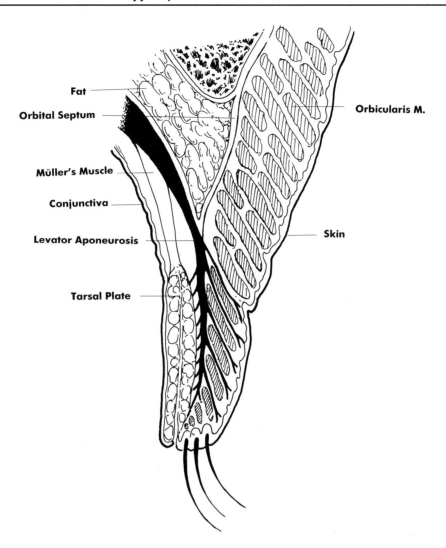

Fat

Orbital Septum

Orbicularis M.

Müller's Muscle

Conjunctiva

Levator Aponeurosis

Skin

Tarsal Plate

bone.[22] The lateral canthal tendon has a tendinous portion from the pretarsal orbicularis and a ligamentous component, which is a direct extension of the tarsus. They attach to the lateral orbital rim at Whitnall's tubercle. The lateral canthal tendon draws the eyelid laterally and posteriorly, approximating the eyelids to the globe, and this must be considered during surgical reconstruction of this tendon.[23,24] The orbital septum forms the anatomic boundary between the eyelid and the orbit. It originates at the arcus marginalis of the orbital rim, extends toward the tarsus, and fuses with the levator aponeurosis and the lower lid retractors before their insertion into the tarsus.[25] Recognition of the septum and preaponeurotic fat is important in eyelid reconstruction.

The upper lid tarsal plate is 10 to 12 mm at its maximum height, tapers toward the medial and lateral borders, and attaches to the orbital rims by the medial and lateral canthal tendons. The levator palpebrae superioris muscle is redirected by Whitnall's ligament and begins to transform into an aponeurotic extension. The aponeurotic fibers attach into the subcutaneous tissues as well as into the anterior surface of the tarsal plate.

The lower lid tarsal plate ranges from 3 to 5 mm in height. The lower lid structure is much the same as the upper lid, except that the lower lid retractor is a fibrinous extension from the inferior rectus, and the fibers do not extend into the subcutaneous tissues of the eyelid or anterior tarsal plate. The lower lid crease is therefore poorly formed, and the lower lid has a range of motion of only 3 to 5 mm.

ANESTHESIA

Eyelid reconstructive procedures may be carried out with use of local or general anesthesia. Most operations are performed with the patient under local anesthesia combined with intravenous sedation to reduce anxiety associated with the procedure. Local anesthetic agents with epinephrine are preferred, to enhance vasoconstriction of the highly vascular eyelids if there is no medical contraindication. Lidocaine hydrochloride (2%) with epinephrine at a concentration of 1:100,000 is used for most reconstructive procedures. For procedures of longer duration, an equal mixture of 2% lidocaine hydrochloride with epinephrine and 0.5% bupivacaine hydrochloride with epinephrine is used. A 30-gauge needle is used to inject subcutaneously between eyelid skin and orbicularis muscle. For minimal formation of hematomas, visible vessels are avoided, as is the penetration of the orbicularis muscle. Diffusion of the anesthetic agent anesthetizes deeper tissues. For the periorbital region excluding the eyelids, a 25- or 27-gauge needle facilitates entry into the thicker tissues. Regional nerve blocks are seldom used in eyelid surgery because eyelids have an overlapping sensory distribution.

Intravenous diazepam or midazolam is useful to reduce patient anxiety and is also a potent amnestic agent. Intravenous thiopental or methohexital will temporarily sedate the patient. These agents are titrated until the patient achieves an adequate level of anesthesia without respiratory suppression. Topical 1% tetracaine hydrochloride drops provide anesthesia of the ocular surface.

RECONSTRUCTION

Causes of loss of eyelid tissue include trauma, surgical excision of neoplasms, congenital colobomas, periocular infections that cause necrosis, irradiation, and burns. The aim of eyelid reconstruction is to reestablish functional eyelids with adequate protection of the eyeball and reasonable cosmesis. The requirements of an adequately reconstructed eyelid are as follows:

• A smooth mucous membrane internal lining to maintain lubrication of the ocular surface and avoid corneal irritation

• A skeletal support equivalent to the normal tarsus to provide adequate lid rigidity and shape but also allow molding to the globe

• A stable eyelid margin to keep lashes and skin away from the cornea

• Proper fixation of the medial and lateral canthal attachments of the lids for eyelid stability and orientation

• Adequate muscle to provide tone and power for closure

• Supple, thin skin to allow eyelid excursion

• Adequate levator action to lift the upper lid above the visual axis

The eyelids may be considered anatomically to consist of an anterior and posterior lamella, both of which must be adequately repaired. The anterior lamella, which consists of skin and orbicularis muscle, provides dynamic closure of upper and lower lids and contributes to the lacrimal pump mechanism. It may be reconstructed with advancement, transposition, or rotation musculocutaneous flaps or with full-thickness skin grafts. The posterior lamella is made up of the tarsus and its conjunctival lining. Reconstruction of this layer may include tarsal-conjunctival transposition, advancement or rotation flaps, free autogenous composite tarsal grafts, or tarsal substitute grafts including sclera, auricular cartilage, nasal septal chondromucosa, and hard palate mucosa. In the reconstruction of both anterior and posterior lamellae, at least one must have its own blood supply. The technique used to reconstruct eyelids depends on the size, location, configuration, and depth of the defect (Tables 16-1 and 16-2). When the defect is superficial, only the anterior lamella needs to be repaired. Full-thickness defects require reconstruction of both layers.

PRIMARY CLOSURE AND LOCAL SKIN FLAPS

The concept of relaxed skin tension lines (RSTLs) is a useful one.[26] In general, these lines will be the same as the lines of facial expression[26] (Fig. 16-3). Scars that follow RSTLs are less conspicuous, and, whenever possible, incisions should be placed in these lines during reconstruction of the eyelids.

Although elliptical facial excisions should be oriented with the long axis of the ellipse parallel to RSTLs of the face, there is a risk of cicatricial ectropion if this approach is used in the upper or lower eyelid. Generally, wound-closure tension must be directed parallel to the lid margin. In standard blepharoplasty incisions, deformation of the lids is spared by the redundant lid skin and muscle.

Fig. 16-4 shows some of the common orientations of ellipses used to excise tumors in the eyelids and periorbital region. The simple ellipse excision sacrifices normal skin in up to 160% of the surface area of the

Table 16-1   Lower Eyelid Reconstruction

Size of Eyelid Margin Defect (% of eyelid width)	Repair
<25%	Direct closure
25%-50%	Lateral cantholysis
Temporal 50%	Periosteal strip
≤66%	Full-thickness unipedicle flap
≤75%	Tenzel flap
<95%	Hughes tarsoconjunctival flap
100%	Hughes tarsoconjunctival flap with periosteal strips; free tarsoconjunctival grafts with periosteal strips; or full-thickness bipedicle flap

Table 16-2   Upper Eyelid Reconstruction

Size of Eyelid Margin Defect (% of eyelid width)	Repair
<25%	Direct closure
25%-50%	Lateral cantholysis
Temporal 50%	Periosteal strip
Up to 50% lateral defects	Tarsal rotation flap
Up to 66% medial defects	Tarsal rotation flap
50%-75%	Free tarsoconjunctival grafts
75%-100%	Cutler-Beard flap or free tarsoconjunctival grafts with periosteal strips

Figure 16-4   Periorbital ellipse orientations to facilitate minimal wound-closure tension and camouflage scars.

Figure 16-3   Periorbital wrinkle lines.

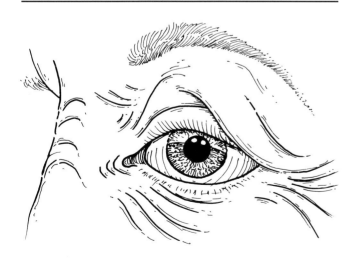

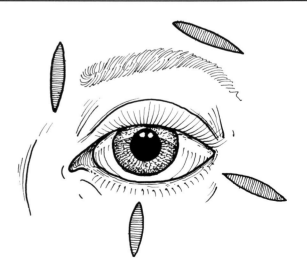

Figure 16-5 *A*, Double "S" ellipse, in which alternate halves of the ellipse are excised (shaded area), thus sacrificing less normal tissue. *B*, Remainder of ellipse is mobilized to obtain O-to-S repair. *C*, O-Z plasty. Curved incisions are made from opposite tangents of circular defect. *D*, Wound repair assumes Z configuration.

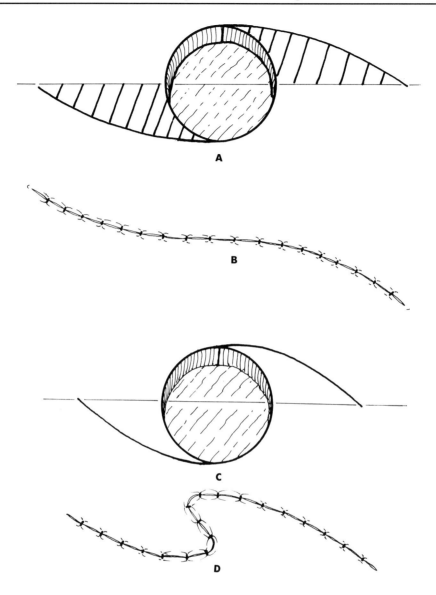

lesion being excised. For this reason modified ellipses (Fig. 16-5) can be designed to minimize the amount of normal skin sacrificed and prevent a straight-line configuration of the final scar. The double-S ellipse sacrifices half the normal tissue of a simple ellipse. O-Z double rotation flaps allow closure of circular defects with minimal wound-closure tension. They allow redirection of the tension of wound closure along the long axis of the ellipse and are particularly useful in lower eyelid defects in which tension should be directed parallel to the lid margin.

The use of skin flaps for the repair of anterior lamellar defects of the eyelids and periorbital region is preferred to free skin grafts.[27] These can be designed as transposition (Fig. 16-6) or advancement flaps. Skin flaps maintain their color and texture after transfer, and local flaps best match the eyelid and periorbital skin. Skin flaps also undergo less contraction than skin grafts. The richly vascular periorbital region allows the use of flaps whose design would be inappropriate in other areas of the body. However, extensive previous surgery or irradiation may diminish collateral circulation. The availability and local extensibility of eyelid skin and anatomic landmarks are important considerations in flap design.

Figure 16-6   Transposition flap used to repair anterior lamellar defect of lower eyelid. This can be designed as either cutaneous or musculocutaneous flap.

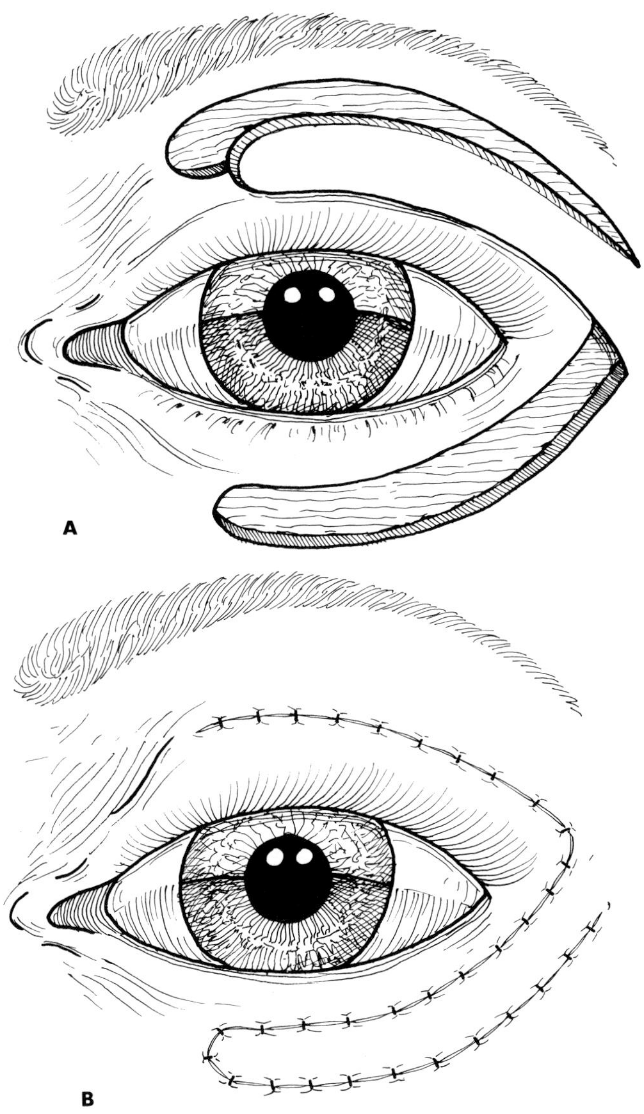

Figure 16-7   Unipedicle advancement flap used to repair pretarsal skin defect.

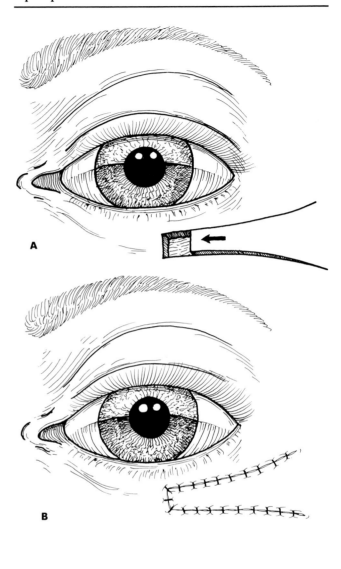

Advancement Flaps

Advancement flaps are used mostly in the periorbital region and include the standard unipedicle rectangular flaps as well as V-Y and Y-V flaps. The unipedicle rectangular advancement flap used in the periorbital region is a skin-muscle flap that takes advantage of the elasticity of the skin in this region and can repair defects up to 25 cm^2. This technique is particularly useful for the repair of defects of the eyebrows and medial upper and lower eyelids.[28] Defects that affect the pretarsal and preseptal skin can be closed with similar incisions used for blepharoplasty (Fig. 16-7). The resulting parallel scars avoid deformities of the lid margins and use the available skin in the lateral periorbital region (Fig. 16-8). V-Y advancement flaps may be used to lengthen structures or close donor sites.[21] Y-V advancement flaps may be used to repair epicanthic folds[29] or release skin contracture.

Rhombic Flap

The rhombic flap is the most useful transposition flap for periorbital repairs. The principles of design are well known and will not be discussed here.[30] In the periorbital region, these flaps are particularly useful for the repair of medial canthal[31] and lateral periorbital defects. The rhombic flap leaves less scarring than does the glabellar transposition flap when used to repair medial canthal defects.[32]

In the periorbital region the design of the rhombic flap is important to avoid distortion of the eyelid margin or eyebrow. The maximum wound-closure tension vector should be determined to properly design the flap. In the lower lids this vector should be parallel to the lower lid margin to minimize vertical tension. In the medial and lateral canthal regions vertically oriented wound-closure tension is acceptable, provided that it is not transmitted to the lid margin. The elasticity and distensibility of the periocular tissue allow the reconstruction of rhombic defects with use of a rhombic flap and wide undermining of adjacent

tissue. Common flap orientations in the periorbital region are shown in Fig. 16-9.

DIRECT CLOSURE WITH OR WITHOUT LATERAL CANTHOLYSIS

Direct closure of the anterior and posterior lamellae with or without cantholysis can be used to repair lower lid defects that measure up to 50% of the width of the lid margin.[33] The advantage of this technique is that it is a single-stage repair that maintains normal eyelid anatomy, including preservation of the eyelashes.

Technique

The borders of the defect should be perpendicular to the eyelid margin. The defect is made into a pentagon by excision of the tissues below the tarsus in a wedge. Each end of the defect is held with skin hoods, and approximation is attempted. If this can be achieved without undue wound-closure tension, a primary repair may be performed (Fig. 16-10). If the edges cannot be easily brought together, a lateral cantholysis is necessary (Fig. 16-11). A horizontal cut through skin, muscle, and tendon is made at the lateral canthus with use of straight utility scissors. The lateral part of the lid is pulled medially to place the lateral canthal tendon on tension, and this crus is then divided by making a vertical cut (Fig. 16-12). Exact vertical alignment of the tarsus is imperative to a satisfactory lid margin repair. Three interrupted 5-0 polyglactin sutures on a spatulated needle are passed through the anterior two thirds of the tarsal plate to avoid corneal irritation.

The lid margin is then closed by placement of a vertical mattress suture for proper anteroposterior

Figure 16-8   Musculocutaneous advancement flap is directly advanced into defect. When combined with lower lid and cheek advancement flaps, large medial canthal defects can be successfully repaired.

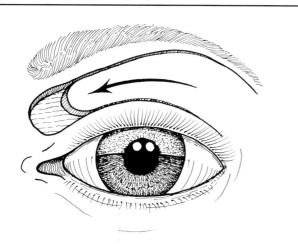

Figure 16-9   Proper orientation of rhombic flaps in periorbital region.

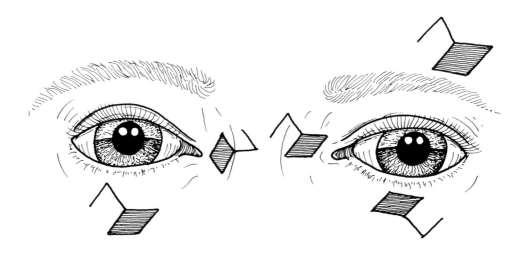

Figure 16-10   *A,* Left upper lid basal cell carcinoma in a 59-year-old man. *B,* Anterior and posterior lamellar defects after Mohs surgical excision. *C,* Polyglactin sutures (5-0) are passed through anterior two thirds of tarsal plate. *D,* Musculocutaneous flaps are dissected, and eyelid margin is closed. *E,* Appearance 6 months after reconstruction.

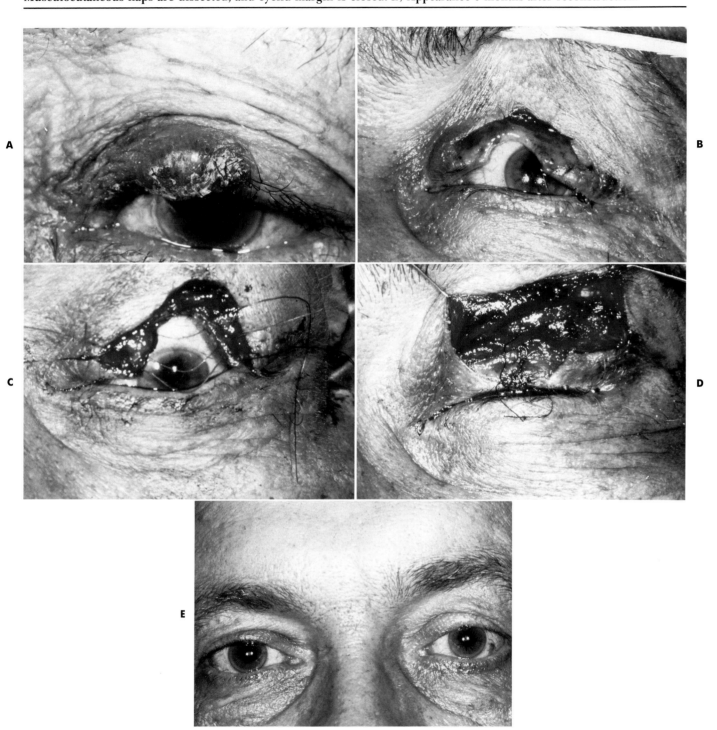

Figure 16-11 *A,* Lateral cantholysis is performed to facilitate primary wound closure of lower lid defect. *B,* Sutures are passed through the anterior two thirds of tarsal plate to avoid corneal irritation. *C and D,* Precise approximation of lid margin is achieved with vertical mattress sutures.

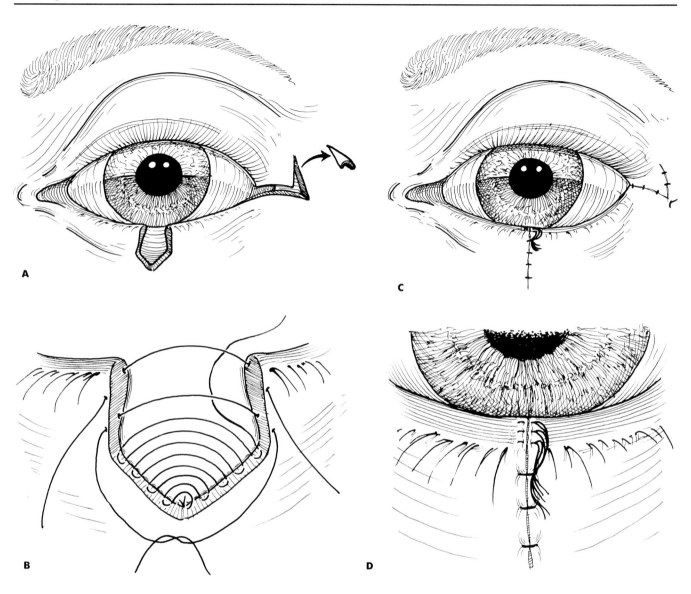

alignment (Fig. 16-11). A 7-0 silk suture is entered through a meibomian gland orifice 3 mm from the wound edge and exited from the tarsal plate 3 mm from the lid margin; it then enters the opposing tarsal fragment 3 mm from the lid margin and exits in a gland orifice 3 mm from the cut edge. The suture is then passed through the lid margin 1 mm on either side of the wound edge. This suture is tied firmly enough to achieve moderate eversion of the lid margin. The ends of this suture are cut long. An additional interrupted suture is passed through the gray line and another through the lash line. These sutures are also cut long. The orbicularis muscle is closed with inter-

rupted 7-0 buried polyglactin sutures, and the skin with interrupted 7-0 nylon or silk sutures. The long sutures from the lid margin are incorporated into the third knot of the lower skin sutures to prevent them from irritating the eye.

The Tenzel flap is a musculocutaneous flap in conjunction with a lateral cantholysis and allows closure of lower lid defects that involve up to 75% of the width of the lid margin.[34] A semicircle is drawn, approximately 20 mm in diameter, beginning at the lateral canthal angle, arching superiorly and temporally no further than the lateral extent of the brow (Fig. 16-13). A No. 15 Bard-Parker blade is used to make an

Figure 16-12   *A,* Squamous cell carcinoma of right upper lid. *B,* Loss of medial half of upper eyelid after micrographic surgical excision. Lateral eyelid remnant is lifted, and superior crus of lateral canthal tendon is cut. *C,* Residual upper lid is mobilized. *D,* Medial part of residual tarsus is sutured to medial canthal tendon with 4-0 polyglactin suture. Skin defect is closed with advancement musculocutaneous flap.

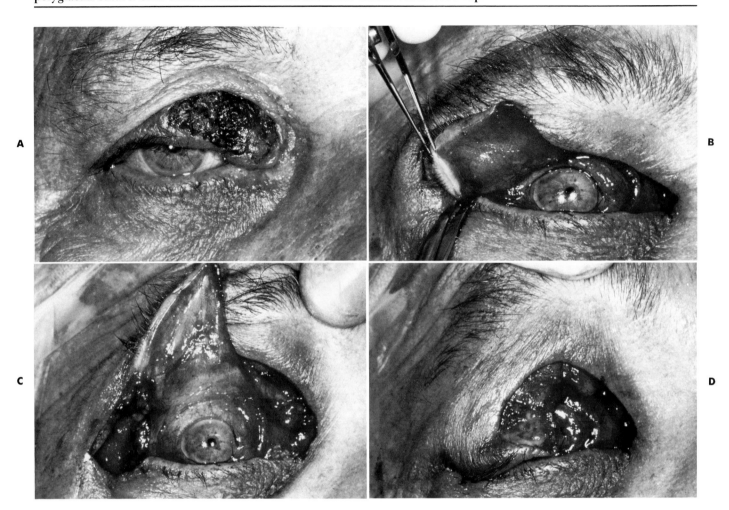

incision along this mark. A flap that consists of skin and orbicularis muscle is elevated and widely undermined inferiorly to mobilize the flap medially. A lateral canthotomy is performed with use of sharp straight scissors, and the inferior crus of the lateral canthal tendon is divided. If the lateral portion of the lid still cannot be easily approximated to the medial portion, the inferior retractors and orbital septum are divided. This is done by passing one blade of sharp straight scissors under the conjunctiva and the other under the orbicularis muscle. The retractors are divided from the inferior border of the tarsus until the flap is adequately mobilized to suture the medial remnant as previously described.

The deep edge of the musculocutaneous flap is sutured to the inner aspect of the lateral orbital rim with a 4-0 polyglactin suture on a small strong half-circle needle. This suture provides adequate lateral and posterior forces to the lateral part of the lower lid. After the free conjunctival edge of the medial remnant and lateral flap are sutured together, the orbicularis layer is approximated with interrupted 6-0 polyglactin sutures, and the skin is approximated with 6-0 nylon sutures.

This technique uses the residual fragment of lateral tarsus to reconstruct part of the lower lid; the remainder of the lid is composed of the musculocutaneous flap with no tarsus or tarsal substitute. Mustarde's[35] cheek flap suffers from the same deficiency even when a mucous membrane graft is used to line the inside of the flap. Postoperative complications of a Tenzel flap for lid reconstruction include lateral canthal webbing, ectropion, lid notching, and symblepharon formation.[36]

Figure 16-13 *A*, Tenzel flap is incised. *B*, Flap consisting of skin and orbicularis muscle is elevated and widely undermined. *C*, Lateral canthotomy and cantholysis are performed *(dotted line)*. Lid defect is then repaired as in primary wound closure.

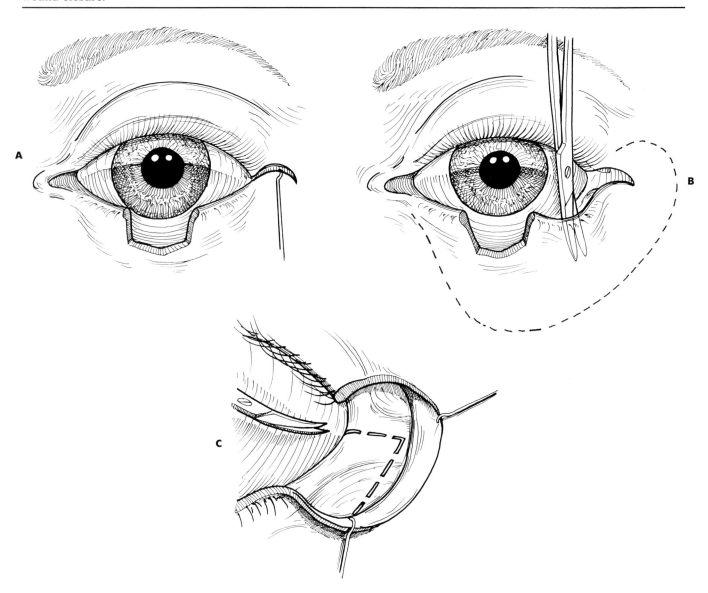

COMPOSITE TRANSPOSITION FLAP FOR LOWER EYELID RECONSTRUCTION

The composite transposition flap harvested from the upper eyelid is a useful flap for repair of full-thickness lower lid defects that involve up to two thirds of the width of the lower lid (Fig. 16-14). This unipedicle transposition flap repairs both the anterior and posterior lamellae. The primary indication for this flap is repair of full-thickness temporal lower eyelid defects. The major advantage of this method of eyelid repair is the one-stage surgical procedure, which avoids the need for more distantly located flaps or grafts. Other advantages are that the flap uses tarsus for structural support, and the pedicle suspends and supports the eyelid, reducing the incidence of lower eyelid retraction, laxity, and ectropion. This method avoids surgery on other structures to obtain free grafts, such as from the nose or ear. It also eliminates the need to close the visual axis. A thorough working knowledge of eyelid anatomy and particularly the vascular supply of the eyelid is necessary for the success of this technique. If a

Figure 16-14   *A*, Full-thickness transposition flap is outlined on upper eyelid. *B*, Flap is elevated and made ready for transposition. *C*, Base of flap is shown before its transfer into position. *D*, Flap is sutured into position. *E*, Appearance of reconstructed eyelid 6 months after surgery.

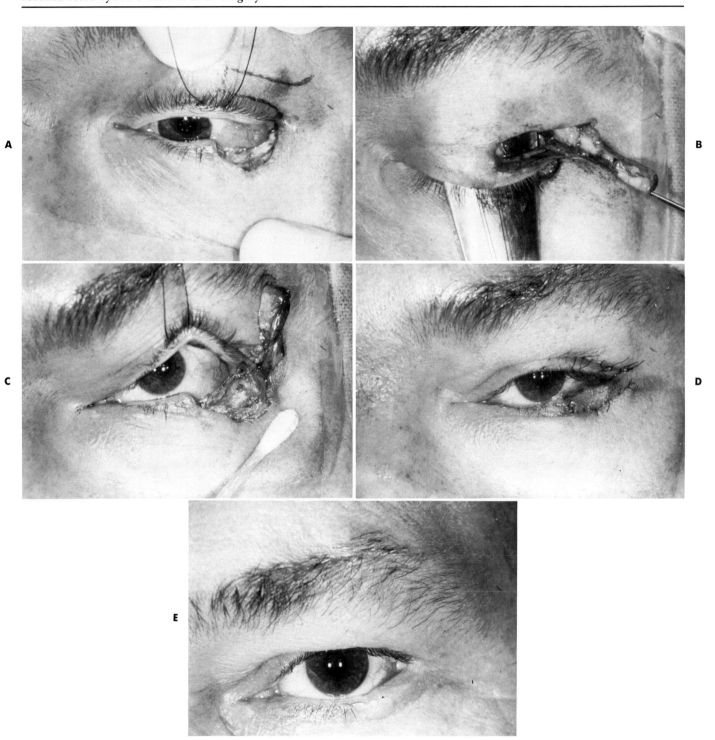

temporal stump of the lower eyelid remains, other reconstruction methods should be used.

Technique

The eyelid defect is examined and measured. The transposition flap is outlined in the upper eyelid[23] (Fig. 16-14). The lower incision is placed 4 to 5 mm above the eyelash line to avoid the marginal arcade, which is the major arterial supply to the lower portion of the upper eyelid. The higher incision line is placed approximately 6 mm superior to the lower incision at the upper tarsal border. The upper border of the flap is extended lateral to the lateral canthus and angles upward, creating a relaxing incision for transposition.

A protective eyelid plate is placed between the upper lid and the globe, and a No. 15 scalpel blade is used to make a full-thickness incision along the upper border of the flap. It is important to stabilize the anterior lamella tautly over the posterior lamella to avoid rolling of the tissues. Stevens scissors are used to complete the incision. A similar maneuver is then performed for the lower incision, again with care taken to stabilize the anterior and posterior lamellae.

The lateral portion of the lower incision is carried further inferiorly as a skin-only incision, usually continuing to the canthal defect. The lateral portion of the upper incision is extended superiorly in a plane just deep to the orbicularis muscle. Careful dissection to isolate the lateral palpebral vessels is necessary before completion of these incisions.

In some cases the full-thickness upper eyelid flap can now be transposed to the lower eyelid. In other cases further dissection and elevation of the orbicularis muscle lateral to the pedicle are necessary to transpose the flap. Care must be taken to avoid transection of the lateral extent of the deep orbicularis fibers that form the base of the pedicle and that provide support and vascular supply to the transposed flap.

The flap is carefully handled to avoid damaging its blood supply while it is sutured into the lower eyelid. The tarsal edges are approximated with 5-0 polyglactin sutures as in the standard repair of an eyelid margin defect. The conjunctiva of the lower border of the flap is sutured to residual fornix conjunctiva with a running 7-0 chromic suture. It is important to recess the lower eyelid retractors from the lower fornix conjunctiva and to elevate the conjunctiva superiorly to reduce the wound-closure tension on the conjunctiva. The skin edges are approximated with 7-0 silk suture.

The levator aponeurosis and Müller's muscle are recessed at the lateral upper eyelid to prevent postoperative lagophthalmos and lateral lid retraction. The conjunctiva is ballooned away from the levator aponeurosis and Müller's muscle with a subconjunctival injection of local anesthetic. A subconjunctival dissection is carried upward to the superior fornix, which separates Müller's muscle and levator aponeurosis en bloc from the conjunctiva. The superior free conjunctival edge is sutured to the superior border of the tarsus with a running 7-0 chromic suture. It is sometimes necessary to cut the lateral horn of the levator aponeurosis to avoid temporal eyelid retraction. The position and contour of the eyelid are assessed, and additional recession or advancement performed as necessary. The skin edges of the upper eyelid wound are approximated with 7-0 silk.

COMPOSITE ADVANCEMENT FLAP FOR LOWER EYELID RECONSTRUCTION

The composite advancement flap for lower eyelid reconstruction, or Hughes tarsoconjunctival flap, is a lid-sharing procedure in which a tarsoconjunctival composite flap from the upper lid is advanced into a defect in the lower lid (Fig. 16-15). This is an excellent method for repair of lower lid defects that are greater than 60% of the width of the lid margin. The main advantage of this flap is that it replaces lost posterior lamella with the same type of tissue. Disadvantages are that it is a two-stage procedure that requires a second operation to separate the eyelids, and it involves temporary closure of the eyelid for 4 to 6 weeks. The technique is contraindicated in children, because of the risk of deprivation amblyopia, and in monocular patients.

Technique

The medial and lateral edges of the defect are made perpendicular to the upper eyelid margin, and the inferior border of the defect is squared off to make it rectangular.[37,38] The edges of the defect are advanced centrally using two hooks, and the width of the defect is measured by calipers. A 4-0 silk traction suture is passed through the upper eyelid margin, and the upper lid is everted over a Desmarres retractor (Fig. 16-16). A three-sided flap is marked on the central portion of the tarsal conjunctiva using light diathermy. This location for the flap is irrespective of whether the defect is located medially or laterally. The horizontal border of the flap should be at least 4 mm superior to the lid margin to avoid upper lid entropion, trichiasis, loss of lashes, and contour defects. The vertical borders of the flap should extend perpendicular to the lid margin into the fornix.

An incision is made with a No. 15 surgical blade through conjunctiva and tarsus, and the flap is separated from the overlying levator aponeurosis and

Figure 16-15   *A,* Hughes technique for reconstruction of lower eyelid. Hooks are used to approximate wound edges, and width of persistent defect is measured. *B,* Three-sided flap consisting of conjunctiva and tarsus is incised. Horizontal border of flap is at least 4 mm superior to lid margin. *C,* Composite flap is mobilized into lower lid defect so that upper border of tarsus contained within flap is in alignment with remaining lid margin. *D,* Anterior lamella is reconstructed with advancement cutaneous or musculocutaneous (if orbicularis muscle is present) flap. *E,* Superior edge of advancement flap is sutured to conjunctiva 1 to 2 mm above upper border of tarsus contained within tarsoconjunctival flap. *F,* Pedicle of tarsoconjunctival flap is divided 4 to 6 weeks after initial reconstructive stage.

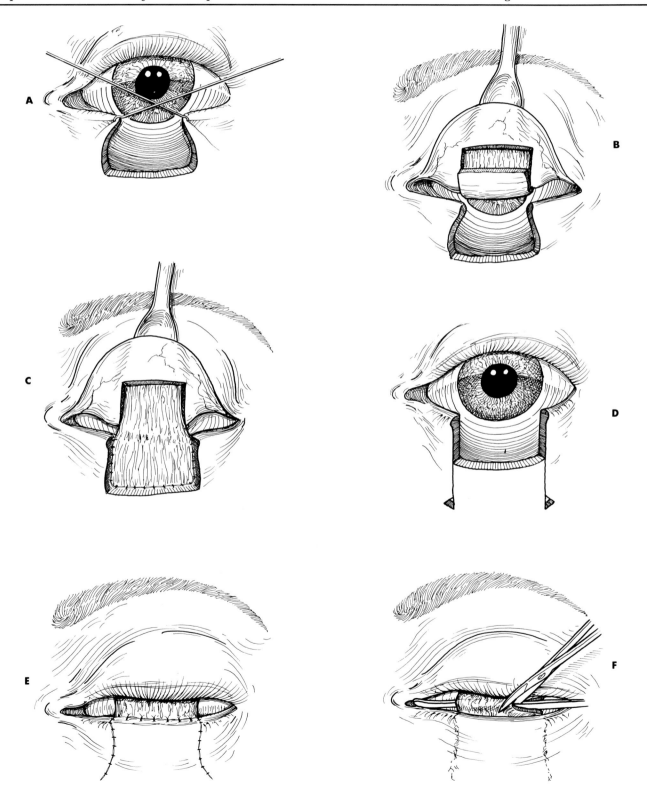

orbicularis muscle by sharp and blunt dissection. The dissection is carried beyond the superior border of the tarsus between conjunctiva and Müller's muscle toward the upper fornix. A small volume of 2% lidocaine with a 1:100,000 concentration of epinephrine injected through a 30-gauge needle subconjunctivally helps to separate these planes and improves hemostasis. Incorporation of Müller's muscle in the flap provides a better blood supply, especially when the anterior lamella is repaired with a skin graft, but it results in a higher risk of delayed upper eyelid retraction. When the anterior lamella is to be repaired with a flap, the conjunctiva alone provides an adequate blood supply for repair of the defect.

The tarsoconjunctival flap is mobilized into the lower lid defect so that the upper border of the tarsus contained in the flap is in alignment with the remaining lower lid margin. The lateral and medial edges of the tarsus are secured to the adjacent stumps of lower lid tarsus with interrupted 5-0 polyglactin sutures on a spatula needle. These are passed through the anterior two thirds of the tarsus to avoid rubbing of the sutures on the globe. The tarsus can be sutured, in the absence of a lateral tarsal stump, to the periosteum of the lateral orbital rim and, in the absence of a medial stump, to the medial canthal tendon with 4-0 polyglactin sutures. The inferior edge of the tarsus is sutured to the inferior conjunctiva and retractors with a 6-0 continuous poly-

glactin suture. The anterior lamella can be reconstructed using a full-thickness skin graft or a musculocutaneous flap as previously discussed. The skin overlying the tarsoconjunctival flap is sutured to the conjunctiva 1 to 2 mm above the upper border of the tarsus with a continuous 6-0 chromic suture. If a local flap cannot be used, we prefer to take full-thickness skin grafts from the upper eyelid of either eye. Although postauricular skin may be used, eyelid skin gives the best color and texture match. The graft is sutured to the skin edges of the defect with interrupted 7-0 nylon or silk sutures.

Second-Stage Hughes Procedure

The pedicle of the tarsoconjunctival flap is divided 4 to 6 weeks after the initial surgery to ensure time for the flap to develop a blood supply from the lower eyelid and to allow local tissue contraction. After local anesthesia is administered, sharp straight scissors are used to divide the flap 1 mm above the proposed new lid margin (Fig. 16-16 **F** through **H**). Care is taken to tilt the scissor blades so that more of the posterior lining of the flap is left. A small wedge of tissue is excised, and the conjunctiva is sutured to the skin with a running 7-0 polyglactin suture. This ensures that stratified squamous epithelium does not come into contact with the ocular surface. The upper segment of the flap is

Figure 16-16   *A,* Defect of left lower lateral eyelid and lateral canthal area after micrographic excision of basal cell carcinoma in 62-year-old woman. *B,* Horizontal incision of upper eyelid tarsus 4 mm from eyelid margin. *C,* Tarsoconjunctival flap advanced after dissection into superior fornix. *D,* Tarsoconjunctival flap is mobilized into lower lid defect. Upper border of tarsus contained within flap is in alignment with remaining lower lid margin. Lateral and medial edges of tarsus have been sutured to lateral orbital rim and residual medial tarsus, respectively. Inferior edge of tarsus has been sutured to inferior conjunctiva. Musculocutaneous flap has been raised to repair anterior lamella. *E,* Appearance 1 week after reconstruction. *F,* Appearance of reconstruction 6 weeks postoperatively. *G,* Tarsoconjunctival flap is cut with scissors angled so as to leave more conjunctival surface than skin. *H,* Appearance of reconstructed eyelid 6 months postoperatively.

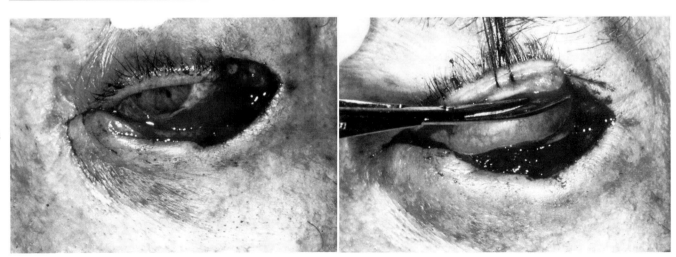

A   B

Figure 16-16, cont'd.   For legend see opposite page.

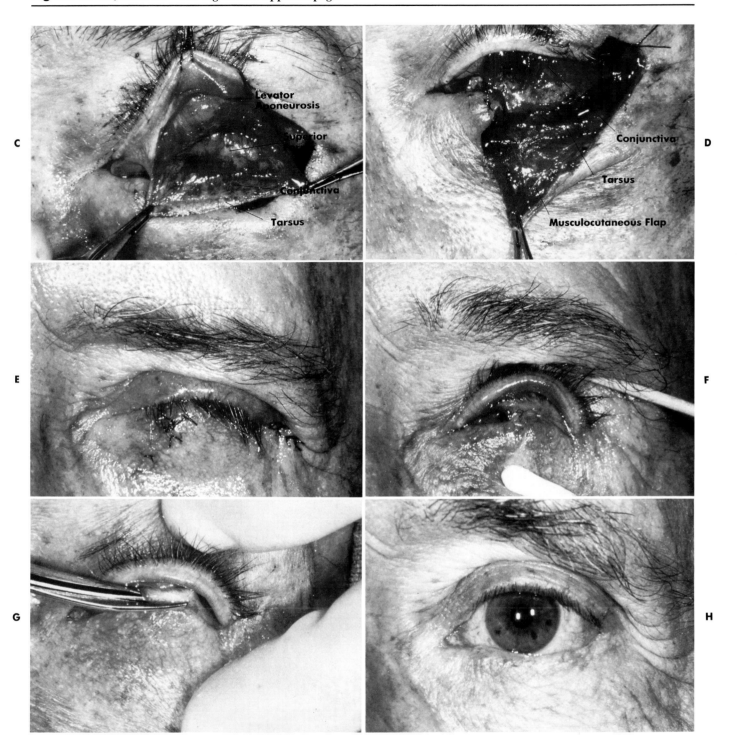

allowed to retract. If Müller's muscle has been incorporated in the flap, blunt straight scissors are used to undermine between Müller's muscle and the levator aponeurosis until the desired lid height and contour are obtained.

Modified Hughes Flap

In patients with vision in only one eye, the Hughes flap is impractical because of the necessity to keep the eye occluded for up to 6 weeks. We have modified the Hughes flap for use in these patients. We buttonhole the center of the conjunctival component of the tarsoconjunctival flap in these patients approximately 1 week after the initial surgery (Fig. 16-17). This has not resulted in any failed flaps or loss of full-thickness skin

grafts placed on the external surface of the flap. In addition to allowing the patient to see, this buttonhole allows examination of the cornea in patients with corneal disease. More recently we have started to buttonhole these flaps at the time of the primary surgery.

COMPOSITE BIPEDICLE ADVANCEMENT FLAP FOR TOTAL LOWER EYELID RECONSTRUCTION

A full-thickness composite bipedicle advancement flap can be used to reconstruct a total lower eyelid, restoring both the anterior and posterior lamellae (Fig. 16-18). Its use is indicated in cases of full-thickness

Figure 16-17   *A,* Appearance of Hughes flap 10 days after stage 1 and just before central buttonhole is made. *B,* Appearance of central opening 4 weeks later.

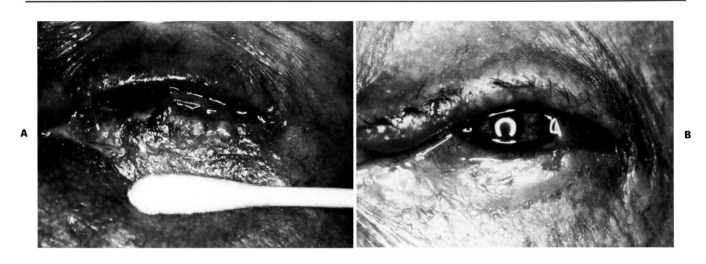

Figure 16-18   *A,* Loss of total right lower eyelid after excision of lower eyelid basal cell carcinoma. *B,* Tarsal incision is made with Bard-Parker blade.

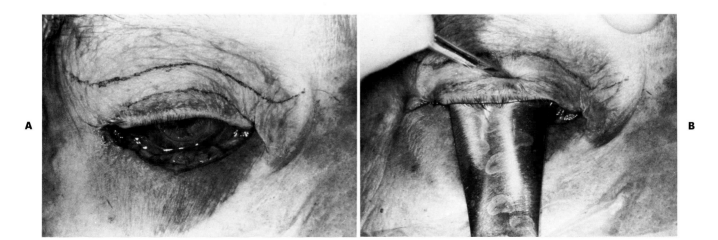

Figure 16-18, cont'd   *C*, Lower full-thickness eyelid incision is completed in tarsal portion of upper eyelid. Medial and lateral regions are left intact at this point to avoid major vessels. *D*, Upper incision completed with Stevens scissors. Incisions are made superficially in medial and lateral canthal regions to avoid deep vessels. *E*, Lower lid retractors are recessed to reduce inferior tension on conjunctival fornix. *F*, Bipedicle flap has been advanced into lower eyelid and sutured into position. Patient is raised to sitting position to adjust height and contour of upper eyelid. Upper eyelid is adjusted to slightly ptotic position to compensate for some elevation after surgery and to provide better eyelid closure. *G*, Appearance 1 year postoperatively. Medial ptosis is present, but patient did not desire correction. *H*, Everted lower eyelid. Note good support to lower lid, with normal tarsal tissues forming posterior lamella of reconstructed eyelid.

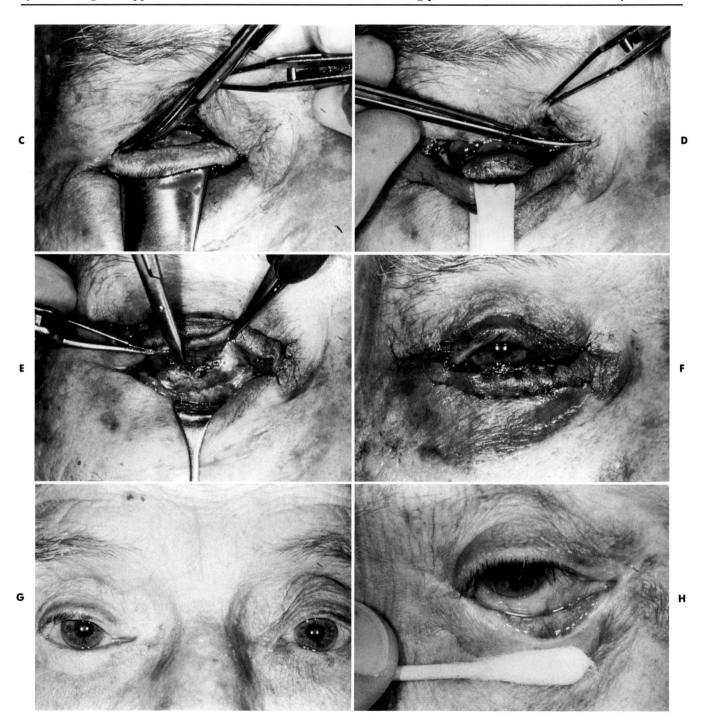

defects of the temporal lower eyelid that involve up to two thirds of the width of the lid. The technique provides excellent tissue match and cosmesis in a single-stage reconstruction, which avoids the need for more distal flaps and grafts. Like the Hughes flap, it uses tarsus for structural support rather than substitutes. Similar to composite transposition flaps, the bipedicle advancement flap suspends and supports the eyelid, reducing the incidence of lower eyelid retraction, laxity, and ectropion. Other advantages of this technique are that it is a one-stage reconstruction, so it avoids surgery on the other eyelids or the nose or ear, and it eliminates the need to close the visual axis. As with the Hughes flap, a thorough working knowledge of eyelid anatomy is necessary. This method of eyelid reconstruction should not be used if the temporal stump of the lower eyelid remains.

Technique

The bipedicle flap is first outlined on the upper eyelid.[39] The skin and anterior lamella are placed on superior tension, and the lower incision line is marked 5 mm above the lash line. This avoids the marginal arcade, which is the major arterial supply to the lower part of the upper eyelid. The upper incision is marked 5 to 6 mm above and parallel to the lower mark (the approximate level of the central upper lid). The higher line is angled up medially and laterally beyond the medial and lateral canthi to allow advancement.

After placement of a lid plate between the eye and the upper eyelid, a No. 15 Bard-Parker scalpel blade is used to make an incision along the lower mark. The anterior lamella is stabilized on the tarsus to avoid "rolling" while all incisions are being made. The lid is everted to ensure that the cut is at the desired level on the tarsus. The incision is then completed with use of Westcott scissors. The upper mark is incised in a similar fashion.

The medial and lateral portions of the lower incision are skin-only incisions. The upper incision is extended superiorly through skin and orbicularis oculi muscle. Careful dissection to isolate the medial and lateral palpebral vessels is necessary before completion of these incisions. The medial and lateral extent of the deep orbicularis fibers forms the base of the bipedicle flap and provides support and vascular supply to the flap. Blood is also supplied by subcutaneous and conjunctival vessels. In some cases it may be necessary to cut the conjunctiva at the medial and/or the lateral base of the flap to allow advancement.

The bipedicle flap is handled carefully with a small Penrose drain. After advancement into the lower lid defect, the lower conjunctival border of the flap is sutured to the residual inferior fornix conjunctiva with a running 7-0 chromic suture. It is important to recess the lower lid retractors from the lower fornix conjunctiva before suturing of the conjunctiva.

If the flap cannot be transposed into the lower lid defect without compromise of the blood supply, the flap is mobilized as close as possible to the desired position, and a minor canthal revision is performed several months later. When there is a residual stump of medial or lateral lid remaining, a strip of skin and muscle may be removed to avoid the transposed flap lying over canthal or lid skin.

The flap's donor site is repaired as follows. The levator aponeurosis and Müller's muscle are recessed to prevent postoperative lagophthalmos and eyelid retraction. The conjunctiva is ballooned away from the levator aponeurosis and Müller's muscle with a subconjunctival injection of local anesthetic. A subconjunctival dissection is carried superiorly into the fornix. The free conjunctival edge is sutured to the upper border of the remaining tarsus with a running 7-0 chromic suture. The levator aponeurosis and Müller's muscle are recessed by an amount slightly greater than that of the transposed flap and are sutured to the conjunctiva with an interrupted 6-0 chromic suture. The lid height and contour are evaluated with the patient sitting up, and intraoperative adjustments are made. The skin is closed using a continuous 7-0 nylon suture. An antibiotic-steroid ointment is placed in the eye. A firm patch may compromise blood supply and is avoided. No dressing is applied.

PERIOSTEAL STRIP FOR EYELID RECONSTRUCTION

Strips of periosteum pedicled from the zygoma can be used for repair of posterior lamellar defects of the temporal upper or lower eyelid. This technique is indicated in cases of temporal eyelid defects that spare half of the medial tarsus. The procedure provides excellent fixation of the posterior lamella to the lateral orbital rim, resulting in a satisfactory lateral canthal angle contour. It is a one-stage reconstruction, which avoids surgery on the other eyelids or the nose or ear. It also provides a method of simultaneous reconstruction of combined upper and lower temporal eyelid defects and eliminates the need to close the visual axis. A disadvantage of this technique is that the periosteal strip is less rigid than tarsus. This method of repair cannot be used with a tarsal rotation flap.

Technique

The lateral orbital rim is exposed, and a rectangular periosteal strip with an intact base is incised with a

Figure 16-19   Periosteal and temporalis fascial strip can be used to reconstruct posterior lamella of temporal eyelid defects. Strip is angled 45° so that lower eyelid contour is followed after strip is reflected inferomedially.

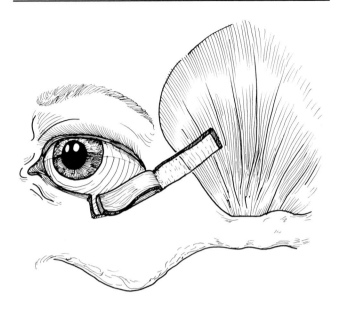

scalpel blade and separated with a Freer elevator.[40] The strip is directed 45° upward for lower eyelid reconstructions and 45° downward for upper lid reconstructions, so as to follow the contour of the lids. The strip should be at least 1 cm wide and long enough to reach the residual tarsal stump (Fig. 16-19).

For lower eyelid reconstructions the small strip of periosteum overlying the narrow frontal process of the zygoma is supplemented with contiguous temporalis fascia by extension of the periosteal incisions laterally. The temporalis fascia is firmly attached to the periosteum, allowing the creation of a single strip of tissue with good strength. The strip is reflected nasally with the outer periosteum against the globe and sutured to the anterior surface of the residual tarsus with 5-0 polyglactin sutures.

Upper and lower temporal eyelids may concurrently be reconstructed by use of two strips of periosteum that overlap at the base (Fig. 16-20). The anterior lamella is reconstructed with musculocutaneous flaps. When sufficient conjunctiva is available, it is sutured to the new eyelid margin. Otherwise the conjunctiva is sutured to the border of the strip, and the surface of the periosteal strip is left to reepithelialize.

TARSAL ROTATION FLAP FOR UPPER EYELID RECONSTRUCTION

The tarsal rotation flap involves the horizontal rotation of a vertical segment of tarsus to repair medial or lateral upper eyelid defects (Fig. 16-21). It may be used to reconstruct defects up to two thirds of the width of the medial upper lid and one half of the lateral upper lid. Advantages of this method include an intact pedicle at the eyelid margin, which allows good mechanical support and a natural lid contour. It is a one-stage reconstruction that avoids surgery on the other eyelids or the nose or ear. It retains tarsus and conjunctiva as posterior lamella, which is more physiologic than sclera or cartilage grafts. Like the periosteal strip technique, it eliminates the need to close the visual axis and avoids complications associated with harvesting of a flap from the lower eyelid. Disadvantages of this flap are a possible noticeable step-off at the pivotal point along the eyelid margin, which improves with time; temporary ptosis due to tightness of the reconstructed lid; and possible dehiscence of the lid repair. The tarsal rotation flap should not be used with a periosteal flap.

Technique

The tarsus at the edge of the defect is freed from the conjunctiva and Müller's muscle at its superior border for 3 to 4 mm. A vertical tarsal strip 3 to 4 mm wide is created using Wescott scissors. This gives a vertical strip 7 to 10 mm long and 3 to 4 mm wide. This vertical strip is turned downward into a horizontal orientation after the anterior tarsal surface has been freed of attachments to the levator aponeurosis. The strip is then attached to the canthal tendon remnants or periosteum with 4-0 polyglactin sutures.

In reconstruction of extensive medial upper eyelid defects, a lateral canthotomy, superior cantholysis, and skin and muscle advancement are used to mobilize the temporal eyelid stump medially. Residual conjunctiva in the superior fornix can be undermined and freed from Müller's muscle, and advanced and sutured to the superior border of the rotated tarsus. Alternatively a free conjunctival graft or mucous membrane graft may be used for conjunctival replacement. However, adequate healing has occurred in cases in which this area was left bare.

The anterior lamella is repaired by undermining and advancement of musculocutaneous flaps from adjacent areas. If there is insufficient skin available, a muscle flap can be used to cover the tarsal flap and a free-skin graft can be applied to this.

TARSAL COMPOSITE GRAFTS

A free tarsoconjunctival composite graft can be harvested from the contralateral upper lid and used to provide posterior lamellar support and mucous membrane lining for reconstruction of the upper lid (Fig.

Figure 16-20 *A*, Extensive lateral canthal basal cell carcinoma of right eye. *B*, Defect after micrographic excision of tumor. *C*, Single strip of temporalis fascia and periosteum has been elevated at 45° angle and has been sutured to residual lower eyelid tarsus. Upper eyelid was also reconstructed with periosteal strip. *D*, Appearance 1 year postoperatively.

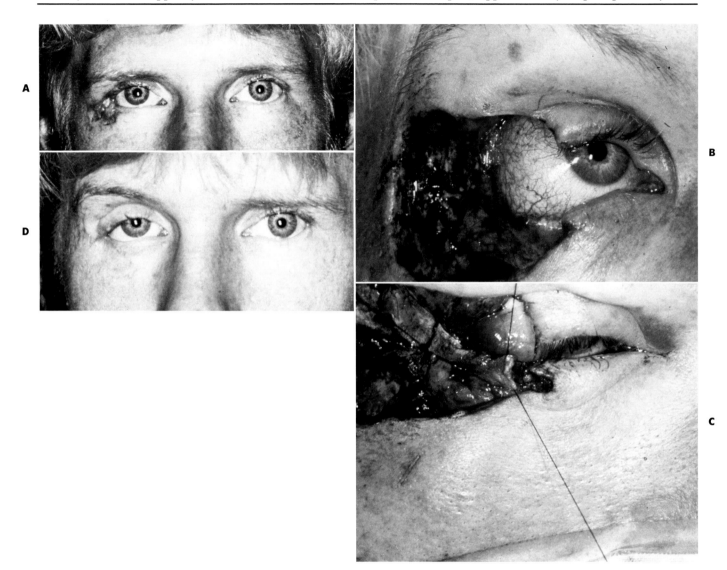

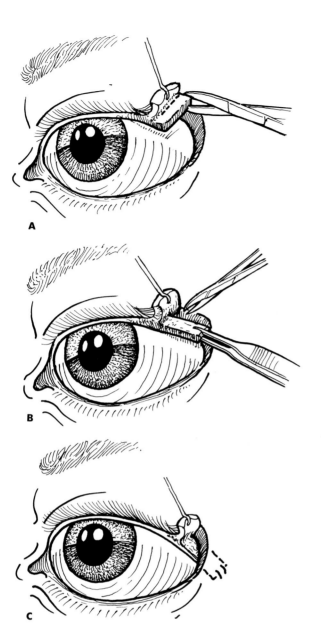

Figure 16-21   *A,* **Tarsus and conjunctiva are freed from anterior lamella at border of defect. Vertical incision** *(dotted line)* **creates strip of tarsus and conjunctiva 3 to 4 mm wide, sparing 2- to 3-mm pedicle at eyelid margin.** *B,* **Tarsal conjunctival flap is turned downward 90° to horizontal orientation.** *C,* **Flap is sutured to periosteum of orbital rim at lateral canthal tendon.** *D,* **Medial upper eyelid defect. Tarsal rotation flap has been fashioned and is being rotated to suture to remnant of medial canthal tendon. Anterior lamellar defect was repaired with use of musculocutaneous flap.**

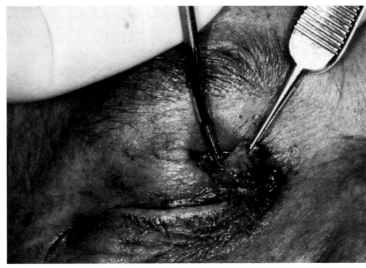

Figure 16-22 *A*, Contralateral eyelid is everted, and incision is made 4 mm from eyelid margin. *B*, Vertical cuts have been made to mobilize tarsoconjunctival graft. Levator aponeurosis has been separated from anterior surface of tarsus. *C*, Conjunctiva is cut 2 mm above superior border of tarsal plate. *D*, Defect of total upper eyelid after tumor excision. *E*, Tarsoconjunctival graft is sutured to remnants of medial and lateral canthal tendons with conjunctival frill along new eyelid margin. Anterior lamellar defect is closed with use of a musculocutaneous flap.

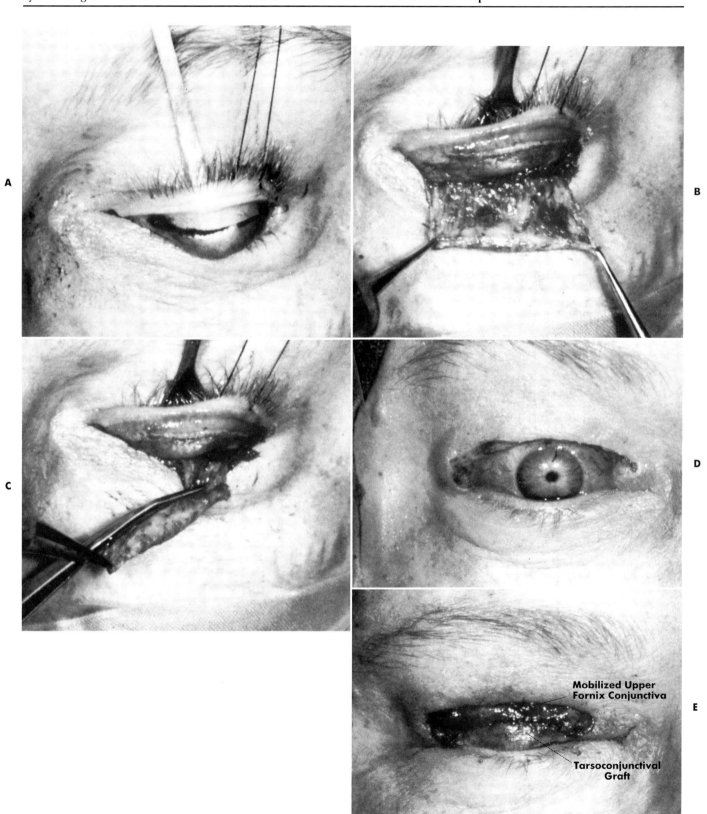

16-22). Grafts can be used to repair up to two thirds of the width of the eyelid and to replace lost posterior lamella with the same type of tissue. The major disadvantage of this technique is that it violates the normal contralateral eyelid.

Technique

The size of the defect to be repaired is assessed by holding the lateral part of the upper lid with a skin hood and pulling it toward the lateral canthus.[41] A 4-0 silk suture is passed through the lid margin of the contralateral upper lid, which is then everted over a Desmarres retractor. A light cautery is used to mark the tissue to be excised. The lower incision is marked at no less than 4 mm from the lid margin. The vertical marks are extended to the top of the tarsus and onto the adjoining conjunctiva. The graft is harvested by cutting of the tarsus with a No. 15 Bard-Parker blade and completion of the dissection with Westcott scissors. The anterior tarsal surface is separated from the levator aponeurosis by blunt and sharp dissection. A 2-mm frill of conjunctiva is left at the superior border of the tarsal graft. The graft is placed on a moist gauze pad, and the donor site is left to heal spontaneously after careful cautery of all bleeding points.

The tarsoconjunctival composite graft is then transferred into the defect. The conjunctival frill is placed inferiorly at the site of the proposed reconstructed upper eyelid margin. The lateral end of the tarsus is sutured either to the lateral canthal tendon or to the periosteum if no tendon is available, with a 4-0 polyglactin suture on a small half-circle needle. The medial end of the graft is sutured to the lateral border of the remnant upper eyelid. Partial-thickness interrupted 6-0 polyglactin sutures are used to avoid corneal irritation. The upper border of the tarsus is sutured to the superior conjunctival fornix, Müller's muscle, and levator aponeurosis. A musculocutaneous flap is fashioned to re-form the anterior lamella.

CUTLER-BEARD PROCEDURE

The Cutler-Beard procedure is a lid-sharing technique in which a skin-muscle-conjunctiva flap from the lower lid is advanced into a defect in the upper lid (Fig. 16-23). It is indicated for large defects and for total absence of the upper lid. The technique provides a useful means of total eyelid reconstruction when no other alternatives are available. The major disadvantage of the Cutler-Beard procedure is that the tarsus is not replaced with a rigid structure, leading to possible instability of the reconstructed lid margin.[42] It also involves temporary closure of the eyelids for 4 to 6 weeks.

Technique

The borders of the full-thickness defect are trimmed to make them perpendicular to the lid margin.[43] The edges of the defect are advanced toward each other with use of skin hooks, and the size of the remaining defect is measured. A horizontal line is marked 5 mm below the lower eyelid margin and 2 mm wider than the measured horizontal defect. The 5-mm margin ensures an intact blood supply to the lower lid remnant. Vertical lines are then drawn from either end of the horizontal mark and extended inferiorly for approximately 15 mm. A 4-0 silk traction suture is passed through the gray line of the lower lid, and the eyelid is placed on traction over a lid guard. With the lid guard protecting the eyeball, a horizontal full-thickness incision is made with a No. 15 Bard-Parker blade. Sharp straight scissors are then used to make the vertical cuts, and the incision is carried to the inferior fornix on the conjunctival side. Beyond that, skin and orbicularis are undermined.

The flap is passed under the bridge of the lower lid and sutured to the remnants of the upper lid. The conjunctiva and lower lid retractors along the medial and lateral borders of the flap are sutured to the residual tarsus. The 6-0 polyglactin sutures are passed through the anterior two thirds of the tarsus to avoid corneal irritation. If no residual medial or lateral tarsus remains, the sutures are passed through the medial and lateral canthal tendons respectively. If the upper lid has a superior remnant of tarsus, the conjunctiva and the lower lid retractors are sutured to this remnant. The orbicularis muscle layer is then closed with interrupted 7-0 polyglactin sutures, and the skin is closed with interrupted 7-0 nylon sutures.

Second-stage Cutler-Beard Procedure

The pedicle of the flap is divided after 6 to 8 weeks to allow the tissues to stretch and develop a new vascular supply. The time period needs to be longer in patients who have undergone radiation therapy or whose flaps are under marked tension. A horizontal mark is made with a pen 2 mm below the desired lid margin. The flap is cut with scissors, which are held angled so that more of the conjunctival surface than skin is left in the new upper lid margin. The conjunctiva is advanced over the edge of the flap and sutured to the skin with a continuous 7-0 polyglactin suture. It may be necessary to excise a wedge of tissue between the skin and the conjunctiva and some additional skin to ensure that the lid margin has a smooth conjunctival lining and not a keratinized epithelium. The inferior border of the lower lid bridge is freshened, and the conjunctiva and the retractors are sutured to the inferior edge of the tarsus with interrupted 7-0 polyglactin sutures. The

Figure 16-23 *A*, Total loss of left upper eyelid after excision of basal cell carcinoma. *B*, Horizontal incision has been made 5 mm below lower eyelid margin, and vertical marks have been made to outline borders of flap. *C*, Cutler-Beard flap is elevated. *D*, Residual conjunctiva of upper eyelid is dissected free to superior fornix (at lower forceps). Levator aponeurosis edge is identified (at upper forceps). Flap is sutured to these structures. *E*, Appearance 1 week after surgery. *F*, Flap is divided 6 weeks after initial surgery. Scissors are angled to leave more conjunctiva than skin at new eyelid margin. *G*, Appearance of reconstructed left eyelid at 6 months postoperatively.

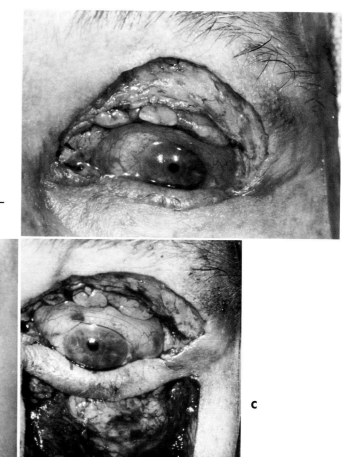

A

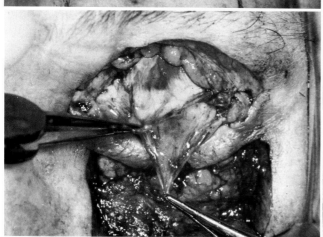

B

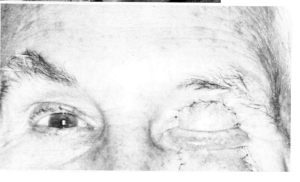

C

D

E

Figure 16-23, cont'd.   **For legend see opposite page.**

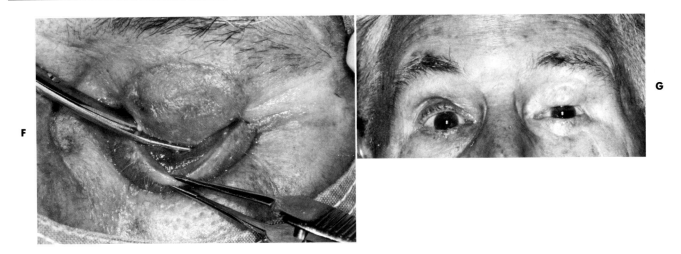

skin is closed with continuous 7-0 nylon sutures. Undermining of the skin and orbicularis may be necessary to prevent a lower lid ectropion. If there is horizontal lid laxity, a lateral tarsal strip procedure should be carried out.

REFERENCES

1. Serre M: *Traite sur l'art de restaurer les difformités de la face, selon la méthode par déplacement, or méthode française,* Montpellier, 1842, L Castel.

2. Velpeau AALM: Paupières: II. Maladies des paupières. *Dict Med* 23:279, 1841.

3. Sichel A: Une discussion sur la blepharoplastique, *Gaz Hop* 8:276, 1834.

4. Berger P: Rhinoplastie par la methode italienne, *Bull Acad Med* 35:204, 1986.

5. Ali ibn 'Isa (Jesus Hal): *Memorandum book of a tenth century oculist,* Chicago, 1936, Northwestern University (translated by CA Wood).

6. le Dran: Sur un oeil eraille, *Mem Acad Ro Chir* 1:440, 1743.

7. von Graefe CF: *De rhinoplastice,* Berlin, 1818, Reime.

8. Fricke JCG: *Die Bildung neuer Augenlider (Blepharoplastik) nach Zerstörungen und dadurch hervorgebrachten Auswartswendungen derselben,* Hamburg, Germany, 1829, Perthes & Besser (French review and part translation by FJ Riester: In *J Prog Sci Inst Med* 3:56, 1830).

9. von Graefe E: Blepharoplastik, *Encucl Worterb Med Wiss* 5:578, 1830.

10. Reverdin JL: Greffe epidermique: expérience faite dans le service de M. le docteur Guyon, a l'hôpital Necker, *Gaz Hop* 43:15, 1870.

11. Lawson G: On the transplantation of portions of skin for the closure of large granulating surfaces, *Trans Clin Soc Lond* 4:49, 1870-1871.

12. Pollock GD: Cases of skin-grafting and skin transplantation, *Trans Clin Soc Lond* 4:37, 1870-1871.

13. Wolfe, JR: A new method of performing plastic operations, *Br Med J* 2:360, 1875.

14. Wadsworth OF: A case of ectropion treated by transplantation of a large flap without pedicle, *Boston Med Sci J* 95:747, 1876.

15. Gradenigo P: *Scritti oftalmologici del Conte Pietro Gradenigo,* Padua, Italy, 1904, Stabilimento della Societa Cooperativa Tipografica.

16. Landolt: De quelques operations pratiquées sur les paupieres, *Arch Opthalmol* 5:481, 1885.

17. Tartois E: *Nouveau procédé de blepharoplastie sans pedicule,* Paris thesis, 1918.

18. Wheeler JM: Correction of cicatricial ectropion by use of true skin of upper lid, *JAMA* 77:1628, 1921.

19. Blair VP: Repairs and adjustments of the eyelids, *JAMA* 99:2171, 1932.

20. Monks GH: The restoration of a lower eyelid by a new method, *Boston Med Surg J* 189:385, 1893.

21. Doxanas MT, Anderson RL: *Clinical orbital anatomy,* Baltimore, 1984, Williams & Wilkins.

22. Anderson RL. Medial canthal tendon branches out, *Arch Ophthalmol* 95:2051, 1977.

23. Anderson, RL, Gordy DD. The tarsal strip procedure, *Arch Ophthalmol* 97:2192, 1979.

24. Jordan DR, Anderson RL: The lateral tarsal strip revisited, *Arch Ophthalmol* 107:604, 1989.

25. Anderson RL, Beard C. The levator aponeurosis: attachments and their clinical significance, *Arch Ophthalmol* 95:1437, 1977.

26. Grabb WC, Smith JW: *Plastic surgery*, ed 3, Boston, 1979, Little Brown.

27. Patrinely JR, Marines HM, Anderson RL: Skin flaps in periorbital reconstruction, *Surv Ophthalmol* 31:249, 1987.

28. Anderson RL, Edwards JJ: Reconstruction by myocutaneous eyelid flaps, *Arch Ophthalmol* 97:2358, 1979.

29. Callahan MA, Callahan A: *Ophthalmic plastic and orbital surgery*, Birmingham, 1979, Aesculapius.

30. Limberg AA: Design of local flaps. In Gibson T, editor: *Modern trends in plastic surgery*, London, 1966, Butterworth.

31. Shotton F: Rhombic flap for medial canthal reconstruction, *Ophthalmic Surg* 14:46, 1983.

32. Bullock JD, Koss N, Flagg SV: Rhomboid flap in ophthalmic plastic surgery, *Arch Ophthalmol* 90:203, 1973.

33. Anderson RL, Ceilley RI: A multispecialty approach to the excision and reconstruction of eyelid tumors, *Ophthalmology* 85:1150, 1978.

34. Tenzel RR, Stewart WB: Eyelid reconstruction by the semicircle flap technique, *Ophthalmology* 85:1164, 1978.

35. Mustarde JC: *Repair and reconstruction in the orbital region*, New York, 1971, Churchill Livingstone.

36. Miller EA, Boynton JR: Complications of eyelid reconstruction using a semicircle flap, *Ophthalmic Surg* 18:807, 1987.

37. Cies WA, Bartlett RE: Modification of the Mustarde and Hughes methods of reconstruction of the lower lid, *Ann Ophthalmol* 7:1497, 1975.

38. Hughes WL: A new method for rebuilding a lower lid, *Arch Ophthalmol* 17:1008, 1937.

39. Anderson RL, Jordan DR, Beard C: Full-thickness unipedicle flap for lower eyelid reconstruction, *Arch Ophthalmol* 106:122, 1988.

40. Weinstein GS, Anderson RL, Tse DT et al: The use of a periosteal strip for eyelid reconstruction, *Arch Ophthalmol* 103:357, 1985.

41. Stephenson CM, Brown BZ. The use of tarsus as a free autogenous graft in eyelid surgery, *Ophthalmic Plast Reconstr Surg* 1:43-50, 1985.

42. Carrol RP: Entropion following the Cutler-Beard procedure, *Ophthalmology* 90:1052, 1983.

43. Cutler NL, Beard C: A method for partial and total upper lid reconstruction, *Am J Ophthalmol* 39:1, 1955.

44. Anderson RL, Weinstein GS: Full-thickness bipedicle flap for total lower eyelid reconstruction, *Arch Ophthalmol* 105:570, 1987.

45. Kersten RC, Anderson RL, Tse DT et al: Tarsal rotational flap for upper eyelid reconstruction, *Arch Ophthalmol* 104:918, 1986.

EDITORIAL COMMENTS

Shan R. Baker

Reconstruction of the eyelid requires meticulous surgical technique and a knowledge of the anatomy and physiology of the eyelids, cornea, and conjunctiva. Loss of a large portion of the lower eyelid may be associated with relatively uncompromised eye function; however, even small defects of the upper eyelid can result in corneal exposure and subsequent permanent impairment of the vision. Thus the repair of upper eyelid defects presents a greater challenge. Reconstruction of the upper eyelid requires sufficient tissue to cover the cornea when the eye is closed and must possess sufficient mobility to elevate above the pupil when the eye is opened. Reconstruction must provide muscle power to elevate the lid and be sufficiently thin to allow elevation and conformation to the topography of the globe.

Similar to nasal reconstruction, both upper and lower eyelid reconstruction requires restoration of internal lining (posterior lamella), structural support and external lining (anterior lamella). Repair of eyelid defects call for special considerations that are not applicable to reconstruction of other areas of the face, such as certain suture techniques, the relative lack of importance of RSTLs, and the common use of composite flaps. The authors have discussed these special considerations and have provided a systematic approach to eyelid reconstruction. They succinctly describe a number of useful techniques for the repair of eyelid defects of varying severity.

EDITORIAL COMMENTS

Neil A. Swanson

When I first read this superb chapter, I wasn't sure whether I was reading a chapter or a textbook! The chapter is incredibly complete, with a particularly excellent section on the anatomy of the lids. The concept of anterior and posterior lamellae and the importance of separate closure of each within reconstructive entities is clearly stated. This fits, with the lids as anesthetic unit, within the broad concepts of a closure within a cosmetic unit wherever possible.

The flaps warrant a mention. The rhombic transposition flap used in eyelid reconstruction is an excellent choice. As the authors state, the lines of tension to close the secondary defect with the rhombic flap must approach parallel to the lid margins. If not, secondary motion of closure of the secondary defect will pull down and cause ectropion. I usually measure and cut the rhombic flap for an eyelid approximately 20% larger than the defect. If properly designed, the oversized flap will set into a defect with no tension and actually push up on the lid margin.

I've been privileged to work with two sets of excellent oculoplastic surgeons in Michigan (Bart Frueh, M.D., and Christine Nelson, M.D.) and in Oregon (Jack Wobig, M.D., and Roger Dailey, M.D.). The flap used by all four surgeons, which continues to give reproducible superb results and which is well described in this chapter, is the Hughes tarsoconjunctival flap. It is well worth becoming familiar with the usefulness of this flap.

17

RECONSTRUCTION OF THE NOSE

Frederick J. Menick

A CONCEPTUAL HISTORY

Although cartilage, bone, soft tissue, and mucous membrane lining are lost in major nasal defects, the most obvious tissue deficiency is skin. Well vascularized and lying adjacent to the nose, the forehead has been acknowledged as the best donor site because of its superb color and texture match. The earliest nasal reconstructions used an unlined forehead flap to rebuild the nose. The classic Indian flap carried midline tissue on paired supraorbital and supratrochlear vessels. Its base lay at or above the eyebrows. However, when so designed, its length was quickly limited by the hairline, its reach by the pedicle's high arc of rotation. A 180-degree twist also produced a kink at the nasal root that could impair blood flow.

Between 1840 and World War I, it became apparent that the results of reconstructions using unlined flaps were poor. The external shape of the nose and its airways became distorted by the contracting scar on the underlying raw surface of the covering flap. Surgeons realized that they must provide lining. Ideally, missing tissues should be replaced in kind and quantity, but residual intranasal mucous membranes seemed inadequate for the task. One solution was to line the cover flap by folding its distal end onto itself, thus creating its own inside and outside. In a major nasal reconstruction this formed, in a manner of speaking, the tip, ala, and columella while eliminating raw areas in the lower part of the reconstructed nose. However, a normal hairline position limited available flap length unless hair was to be transferred to the nose. When one third of the flap was used for lining as well as cover, midline forehead tissue could not provide sufficient skin to create a long columella that maintained projection, allowed infolding of the covering flap for lining, and avoided unnecessary tension that might diminish flap vascularity. Auvert, in 1850, designed a longer flap by slanting it across the forehead at an angle of 45 degrees. Such "oblique" flaps came into general use in the latter part of the nineteenth century and were designed to follow

the hairline into the temple recess. German surgeons of the same period positioned forehead flaps horizontally. Gillies, in 1935, described a radical departure from oblique forehead flaps. His up and down flap ascended over one supraorbital pedicle into the hair-bearing scalp and then descended back into the forehead. This provided greater flap length and was sufficiently wide to ensure blood supply. In 1942, Converse modified the up and down flap by creating a long pedicle that was camouflaged within hair-bearing skin and that included the major vascular supply of the scalp. However, it was called the "scalping" flap for good reason. After a formidable operation, a large hairy pedicle hung across the eye for weeks prior to division.

These forehead flap variations were designed solely to provide additional length. Each created a forehead defect that was harder to close. Surgeons were caught in a predicament. On the one hand, they worried about forehead scarring. On the other hand, they bemoaned insufficient tissue not only for nasal reconstruction but also for adjacent defects. Neighboring cheek, lip, and nose defects in the midface were filled with even larger forehead flaps. Frequently a single plump lump replaced the three-dimensional contour of these multiple contiguous facial units. Too often the forehead was scarred beyond repair.

Rather than folding the forehead flap, others eliminated the raw area on the deep surface of the covering flap by other methods. Volkmann, in 1874, turned down portions of residual nasal skin adjacent to the defect, hinged on scar, to provide lining. Thiersch transferred flaps from other facial areas in 1879, and more recently, Millard advocated rolling over bilateral melolabial flaps to line both the ala and columella. In 1898, Lossen first applied skin grafts for lining. Most often grafts of split- or full-thickness skin were placed under the covering flap during a preliminary operation. Weeks later, once the viability of the grafts was assured, these prelaminated flaps were transferred with the forehead flap to the nose. In this way, cover

305

and lining were supplied simultaneously after a preliminary operation. In 1943, Gillies popularized the placement of composite chondrocutaneous grafts to simultaneously provide lining and support. In 1956, Converse suggested a septal mucoperichondrial cartilage graft as an alternative. The advantages Converse ascribed to the use of his septal composite graft for lining are equally applicable to all methods that do not fold the covering flap for intranasal lining. Less flap length is required because skin is used only for cover. The blood supply is heartier because the covering flap is not folded on itself. Thick and shapeless alar margins formed by flap infolding are also avoided.

Traditionally, lining has been supplied by folding the distal covering flap upon itself, by hinging over adjacent skin based on scar along the wound edge, by the use of a secondary flap (a second forehead flap or a melolabial flap), or by preliminary placement of chondrocutaneous or chondromucosal grafts. Unfortunately, each method provides lining that is thick, stiff, and avascular. Lining distorts external shape and crowds the airway. Necrosis, infection, and the extrusion of a supportive framework are common. The best combination of lining and cartilage support comes from either the ear or the septum as a composite graft. However, these techniques require one or two preliminary stages performed weeks before the nose can be constructed. At best they make a satisfactory alar margin. Unfortunately, their shape is fixed by their natural configuration and by the scar that surrounds them as they sit on the forehead awaiting transfer to the nose. When the nose is finally assembled, little can be done to shape the cartilage fragments so that they resemble the normal subcutaneous architecture of a nose. They are glued to the undersurface of the flap and fixed in whatever position they assumed on the forehead.

It also became obvious that without a skeletal framework, the soft tissue of cover and lining collapse, impairing the airway and limiting nasal projection. A rigid skeleton is needed to provide support, projection, and contour. However, most lining methods preclude its successful placement. A single covering flap cannot be folded into the three-dimensional shape of a normal nose. The alar rims and tip become thick and, without support, shapeless. Accurate placement of primary columella, alar, and tip support is precluded. Hinge flaps of skin that border the defect are stiff and poorly perfused. Only after soft tissues have healed can bone and cartilage pieces be placed as cantilevered grafts to lift the dorsum and tip. Because of their bulk and the risk of extrusion, they are not used primarily but must be added months later in final touch-up operations. Unfortunately, once gravity and the contractural effects of the healing process have distorted nasal contour, it can never be regained. Covering skin becomes constricted and stiff. Multiple late revisions are required to sculpt subcutaneous tissue into a semblance of a nasal shape. Very few surgeons have the skill required to accomplish this.

Primary cartilage grafts are not routinely placed when most useful, that is, when the nose is first assembled. The common lining choices are not vascular enough to support primary cartilage grafts, and because they are thicker than normal, the lining itself distorts shape and crowds the airway, creating a "blob stuffed with lining." Traditionally, support has been provided to the nose secondarily after soft tissues are healed (and contracted). Most often such support is incomplete and unaesthetic. At best, a bulky dorsal cantilever strut is fixed to the nasal root and a cartilage graft positioned along the alar rim.

A MODERN APPROACH

The questions remain: Can we restore contour and create symmetry to the contralateral normal? Can we blend scars? Can we control the contractual forces of wound healing and avoid multiple late revisions?

A different technical and conceptual approach to nasal reconstruction helps to overcome previous cover, lining, and support limitations. The forehead is perfused by an arcade of vessels supplied by the supraorbital, supratrochlear, infratrochlear, dorsal nasal, and angular branches of the facial artery. A rich anastomotic plexus centered on the medial canthus can supply a unilaterally based paramedian forehead flap (Fig. 17-1). This paramedian forehead flap is abundantly perfused by a vertically oriented axial blood supply. Its arc of rotation is near the medial canthus. It reaches the columella and can be aggressively thinned prior to inset. It is sufficient in size to resurface part or all of the nasal surface.

At first glance, residual intranasal mucous membrane seems to be inadequate to line a major nasal reconstruction. But a broad expanse of residual and well-vascularized intranasal mucosa is available to provide lining for lateral, heminasal, and total nasal defects. Burget and Menick have studied the blood supply of the septum (Fig. 17-2). The septal branch of the superior labial artery will allow elevation of the entire ipsilateral septal mucoperichondrium on a narrow pedicle. If both right and left septal branches are included, the entire septum can be shifted as a composite flap containing a sandwich of cartilage between the two leaves of the mucous membrane. Such flaps of septomucoperichondrium, cartilage, and bone extend from the nasal floor below to the level of the medial canthus above, and posteriorly beyond the

Figure 17-1   Vasculature of the forehead. A rich anastomotic plexus centered on the medial canthus can supply a unilaterally based paramedian forehead flap. It is abundantly perfused by a vertically oriented axial blood supply.

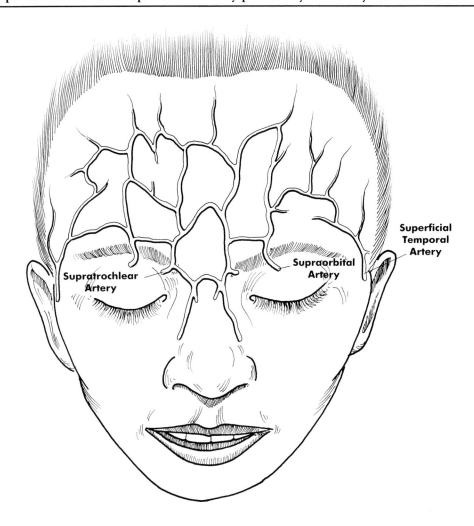

Superficial
Temporal
Artery

Supraorbital
Artery

Supratrochlear
Artery

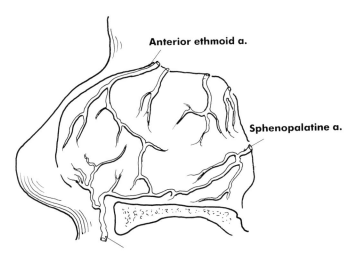

Anterior ethmoid a.

Sphenopalatine a.

Septal br. of superior label a.

Figure 17-2   Vasculature of nasal septum. The septal branch of the superior labial artery will allow elevation of the entire ipsilateral septal mucoperichondrium on a narrow pedicle. The entire septum can be shifted upward as a composite flap based on both septal branches.

ethmoid perpendicular plate. Burget and Menick have also described a bipedicle flap of residual vestibular skin based medially on the septum and laterally on the nasal floor that can be advanced inferiorly to line the ala and the nostril margin. More importantly, these lining flaps are thin and reliably viable. Neither external shape nor airway patency is distorted by the excessive bulk associated with other methods of lining. Loss of lining, the chief enemy of nasal reconstruction, seldom occurs. Just as important, this well-vascularized lining allows the primary placement of cartilage grafts in the missing tip, ala, sidewall, or dorsum.

In the normal nose, dorsal support is supplied by the nasal bones and leading edge of the septum. The sidewall is supported by the nasal bones and upper lateral cartilages, and the tip by the medial and lateral crura of the alar cartilages. The lateral crus provides projection of the domes and the sculpted facets of the aesthetic tip. If missing, the normal cartilaginous framework of each must be replaced. Primary cartilage grafts must replace missing support to the dorsum, tip, and lateral sidewall. Additionally, a strip of cartilage must be placed along a reconstructed nostril margin, even though the normal alar lobule contains no cartilage. This serves to brace the alar rim and prevent constriction inward, contraction upward, and collapse during the healing stages. These support grafts must be placed at the time of initial reconstruction. Primary support grafts serve many functions. They provide support, maintain airway patency, create a nasal shape, and brace soft tissues against the forces of myofibroblastic contraction associated with normal wound healing. They fix the soft tissues of the new nose in "concrete" by virtue of the cartilage that backs both lining and cover, and simulate the normal shape and aesthetic lines of the nose. When covered by a thin and conforming skin flap, the shape of this subcutaneous skeletal architecture shows through. The nose has a nasal shape from the outset. The need for multiple late revisions is markedly decreased.

AESTHETIC AND FUNCTIONAL CONSIDERATIONS

The primary function of the face is to look normal. Many patients wish more than a healed wound. They want their nose restored as it was before being injured. They want to look normal, not peculiar or different. The nose also functions physiologically as an air conduit. Its airways must be patent, without constricting scar and not stuffed by thick, unsupported soft tissues. Unfortunately, the physiologic function of the nose is often worse after traditional reconstructions. Past methods of nasal reconstruction, due to their bulk

and scar, neither recreate a normal-appearing nose nor allow easy nasal breathing.

At the outset, the patient and the surgeon must define their goal. A healed wound can be obtained by secondary intention healing or by the simple placement of a skin graft or flap. Some patients will be satisfied, but many will request that their nose be restored to its prior appearance. Unfortunately, it is impossible to reconstruct a nose lost to injury or cancer. Bits and pieces of other expendable tissue can only be put together to create a facsimile of a nose, which will give the illusion of normality. Such an aesthetic reconstruction requires that the missing facial units be restored to the expected color, texture, thickness, hair-bearing quality, and contour. Although not every patient or every wound lends itself to the restoration of normality, this chapter assumes that this is the objective.

REGIONAL FACIAL UNITS

The face can be divided into adjacent regions, each with its own characteristic skin color and texture, skin thickness, hair quality, and surface contour. The nose is made up of concave and convex surfaces, which are separated from one another by ridges and valleys. The nose is a major facial unit, and its smaller parts may be considered topographic subunits (Fig. 17-3). Each subunit may be exaggerated or understated, but its general shape is relatively constant from nose to nose. The surface of the nose, made up of these slightly convex or concave surfaces, can be divided into the subunits of the tip, dorsum, paired sidewalls, alar lobules, and soft triangles.

The shape of the tip subunit is determined by the contour of the underlying alar cartilages. Each side of the tip has a bulge or dome that reflects a point of light. Superior and lateral to the dome is a slight drop-off in the level of the skin surface, which is marked by a shadow. This gentle valley separates the tip subunit from the nasal sidewall and ala. The supratip depression marks the border between tip and dorsum. The dorsum of the nose extends from the supratip depression to the glabella superiorly, where a transverse wrinkle perpendicular to the procerus muscle may mark its upper limit. The lateral borders of the bony and cartilaginous dorsum are defined by ridges, which are visible, palpable, and grow heavier with age. Each lateral ridge reflects a line of light and casts a shadow, which separates the dorsal subunit from the nasal sidewall. The nasal sidewall unit sweeps laterally from the edge of the dorsum to form an almost unbroken concave slope with the cheek. The C-shaped alar groove, shallow medially and deep laterally, sets off the alar lobule from the sidewall, tip, cheek, and lip. The

Figure 17-3   Nasal topographic aesthetic subunits.

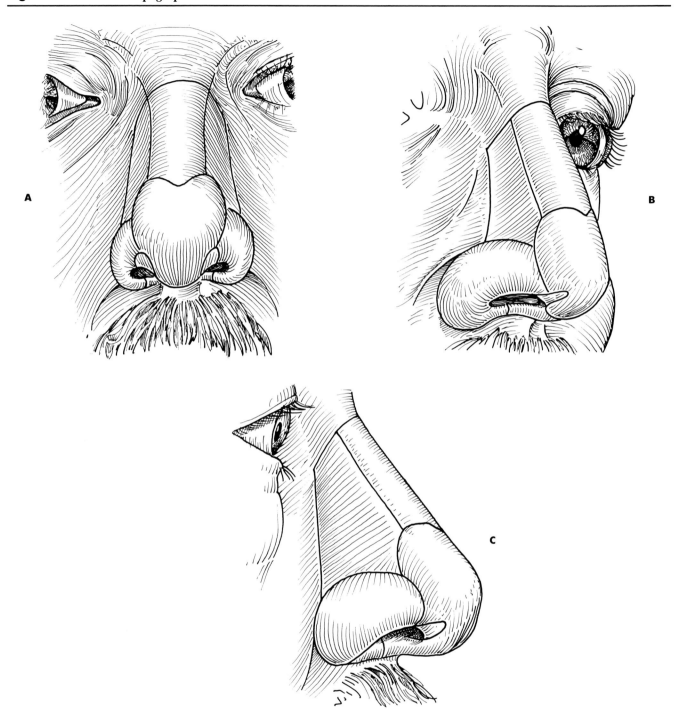

alar subunit is a smooth bulge that reflects a spot of light. The soft triangle is itself a small subunit visible as a shadow depression between the arched caudal border of the alar cartilages and the nostril margins.

Regional unit concepts have important implications to the surgeon. Nasal units are covered by skin with a specific color, texture, and thickness. Each unit has specific contours determined by underlying soft and hard tissue. If the nose is to look as it did before injury, it must be restored as a major facial unit composed of each subunit.

"Normality" is recreated by the establishment of expected nasal subunits, each with its characteristic covering skin and contour. With normality in mind, we must analyze a defect and determine what is missing, both anatomically and aesthetically. Although we cannot control wound healing or prevent scars, we can select the color, texture, and thickness of donor tissues so that they match the recipient site. We can also control the size, shape, and direction of our incisions and excisions and so manipulate the scars that are produced. Scars should be camouflaged by strategically positioning them in the borders between subunits. If scars are positioned in the joins that separate the hills and valleys of the normal nasal surface, such scars will be perceived as normal fold or contour lines and not as distracting deformities.

Our goal is to restore the nose (nasal subunits), not simply fill defects. Wounds should be altered in size, shape, depth, and position to better recreate subunits. If a large part (more than 50%) of a subunit is lost, replacing the entire subunit rather than patching a defect frequently gives a superior result. Adjacent normal tissue that remains within a subunit should often be discarded. This positions border scars in the joins between units where they will mimic the shadowed valleys and lighted ridges. It also takes advantage of inevitable trapdoor contraction, which will cause the entire subunit to bulge, simulating the normal contour of the tip, dorsum, dorsal hump, and alar lobule.

Remember that the tissues must be replaced exactly, in both kind and quantity. The contralateral normal or ideal should be used as a guide for these designs. A fresh wound is distorted by wound tension, edema, and anesthetic injection. A healed wound is distorted by old scar or a previous reconstruction. Thus, neither accurately describes the true tissue loss. An exact pattern should be made of the contralateral normal tip, ala, or sidewall and used to create a pattern for the necessary covering skin. If a contralateral normal is missing, a pattern from an ideal nose can be utilized.

The surgeon must also choose donor materials so that materials nearly identical to the missing tissues are resupplied. Like tissue is always the first choice. A forehead flap or melolabial flap is used for cover, septal or ear cartilage grafts for support, and intranasal lining flaps to resupply the internal nasal surface.

Also, if the three-dimensional quality of a regional unit is to be restored, contour must be integrated into each and every step. The nose must be built on a stable platform. If the cheek and lip are missing, they should be restored separately. Primary framework grafts must be positioned prior to wound healing to support and shape the new nose. Soft tissue and scar should be sculptured and contoured.

Application of the subunit principle of nasal reconstruction helps to define an intellectual scheme effective in improving the aesthetic result. It points to specific techniques and suggests appropriate materials and donor sites that will best resupply the recipient defect with ideal missing tissue.

DEFECT CLASSIFICATION

Nasal defects can be divided according to site, size, and depth. The upper two thirds of the nose (dorsum and sidewalls) and the columella are covered by thin, shiny, and slightly mobile tissue, which is present in slight excess. In contrast, the tip and ala are covered by thick, pitted, and sebaceous skin, which is adherent to the underlying tissues. A local flap or skin graft is satisfactory for smaller defects in the upper two thirds. A single lobe flap (Banner flap) rotates easily in the area of slight excess, and its closure is supplemented by the moderate mobility of the wound margins. Skin grafts, although at risk for hypo- or hyperpigmentation, normally heal with a smooth and shiny surface, which blends satisfactorily into the smooth and shiny surfaces of the dorsum and sidewalls. Skin grafts are a poor choice, however, in the tip and ala, where they appear as an island or patch of shiny skin sitting within the thick, pitted skin of the tip and ala. Such thick, stiff skin also rotates poorly when utilized as a single lobe flap. In the tip and ala, single lobe transposition flaps are also associated with distortion of adjacent free margins and excessive wound-closure tension, as well as standing cutaneous deformities, which develop about the point of pivot. The bilobed flap of McGregor and Zitelli can overcome these problems. It moves adjacent matching skin to the area of deficiency while filling the secondary defect with a second flap taken from the upper two thirds of the nose in the area of slight excess. A skin graft or single lobe transposition is useful for defects in the dorsum, sidewall, or columella. Bilobed flaps are best for small defects in the tip or ala.

The depth of the defect governs the choice of material for reconstruction. In superficial defects, when only skin and a small amount of subcutaneous tissue are missing, a full-thickness preauricular skin graft can be selected for repair. When bone or cartilage is exposed, a local or distant flap will be chosen according to the size of the defect. However, if the underlying nasal support is missing and a cartilage framework must be restored with primary cartilage grafts, a local flap is no longer applicable. A delicate cartilage reconstruction will collapse under the tension of wound closure and be distorted. In such circumstances a distant flap (a melolabial or forehead flap) will be required.

The size of the defect frequently determines the choice of local or distant flaps for nasal resurfacing. If the defect is greater than 1.5 cm in its largest dimension, there is rarely enough residual tissue to redistribute over the entire reconstructed nose. Local transposition flaps are precluded, and distant tissue (a melolabial or forehead flap) will usually be required.

A small amount of extra skin is available in the melolabial fold. Its skin matches the nose, but its underlying fat has a strong tendency to contract. The melolabial fold can supply enough skin to resurface the ala, and the contractility of the melolabial flap can be utilized to simulate the round, expected bulge of the normal ala. The dimensions of the flap, its arc of rotation, and its contractility, however, make it a poor choice for resurfacing other nasal areas. A midline forehead flap is always employed to replace dorsal, tip, hemi, or total nasal units, while a superior based melolabial interpolation flap is often used to replace the alar subunit. A superiorly or inferiorly based cheek rotation flap designed along the melolabial sulcus, or a skin graft can be used to repair defects of the nasal sidewall.

THE MELOLABIAL INTERPOLATION FLAP

A small amount of excess tissue that matches the ala in color and texture lies near the melolabial fold. This soft, gelatinous tissue contracts too much for reconstructing the nasal tip or dorsum. However, it is ideal for the ala where its soft fat contracts into a "blob" that resembles the normal alar contour. Unfortunately, melolabial tissue is present in limited amount, and its excision can excessively flatten the melolabial fold. The arc of rotation and length of the flap are relatively short. It cannot comfortably be transferred to the nasal dorsum or tip.

First, an exact pattern of the contralateral normal ala is positioned just superior to the melolabial sulcus. The flap is based on vessel perforators from the facial artery centered above and below the zygomatic major muscle. Because the musculocutaneous perforators supply its base, it is an axial flap with an excellent blood supply. The base is tapered superiorly to keep the standing cutaneous deformity off the nose and to facilitate transposition. Standing cutaneous deformity excision is marked distally. The flap is designed as an interpolation flap in which the final scar of donor site closure will lie exactly in the melolabial sulcus. The flap is traced 1 mm larger in all dimensions to allow for postoperative contraction. The inset is thinned distally, leaving only 1 to 2 mm of subcutaneous tissue in the area of inset. The donor site is closed by undermining adjacent cheek skin and advancing it inferiorly and medially. Three weeks later the pedicle is divided. The flap inset is partially elevated, and excess subcutaneous tissue and scar are sculpted from the alar base, lip, and cheek join. It is then wrapped around the alar lobule and inset into the alar sill. The residual pedicle, which served as a vascular carrier, is discarded, and the cheek is closed by advancement so that the final scar lies exactly in the alar facial sulcus and melolabial sulcus. A melolabial interpolation flap is easily performed under local anesthesia with sedation on an outpatient basis.

THE PARAMEDIAN FOREHEAD FLAP

The central forehead is perfused by a rich plexus of vessels supplied by the supraorbital, supratrochlear, infratrochlear, dorsal nasal, and angular arteries. Axial, vertically oriented vessels extend superiorly toward the hairline. A unilateral paramedian forehead flap can be based on either the right or left supraorbital-supratrochlear complex. Its base lies close to the defect between the medial brow and medial canthus. Its axial and vertically oriented blood supply allows a narrow pedicle base design as well as aggressive thinning of the distal flap prior to inset. Forehead skin is used only for nasal cover and not for adjacent lip or cheek defects. The central vertical component is employed to resurface the dorsum, tip, and columella, and its lateral wings are employed to wrap around the ala and to curve into the nostril floor and alar sill if a total nasal resurfacing is required. Redundant tissue is removed from the forehead in both horizontal and vertical directions when closing the donor site. This facilitates primary closure of the vertical component as an inconspicuous vertically oriented paramedian scar and the lateral wings as scars that lie in the natural transverse wrinkle lines of the forehead. The forehead flap is transferred using general anesthesia with an overnight hospital stay. The pedicle is later divided using local anesthesia on an outpatient basis.

First, an exact three-dimensional pattern is made of the defect. Most often this is designed on the contralateral normal or on an ideal model. Forehead skin does not contract, so the pattern is designed exactly. If too much skin is supplied, it will contract postoperatively and obscure the detailed contour created by the underlying support framework. If inadequate skin is supplied, it will cause the underlying cartilage grafts to collapse. The three-dimensional foil pattern, which has been cut, bent, and crimped to fit the defect exactly, is then flattened and traced at the hairline directly above either the right or left supratrochlear and supraorbital blood supply. This is located just lateral to the glabella frown crease and may be specifically identified with the use of a Doppler. The pedicle is designed with a base 1.2 to 1.5 cm wide. A narrow pedicle allows easy pivoting without strangulation. A narrow pedicle does not distort the eyebrow on donor site closure and does not need to be replaced at the time of pedicle division. The arc or rotation is checked with a gauze sponge. If additional length is needed to reach the defect, the pedicle can be positioned closer to the defect by extending the pedicle base incisions across the supraorbital rim and bluntly separating the underlying corrugator muscle fibers while preserving vessels to the flap. Alternately, to increase length, the extension for the columella can be extended into the hair-bearing scalp. Because of its excellent axial blood supply in nonsmokers, the distal 1.5 cm of the flap can be thinned almost to dermis so that the forehad flap skin corresponds to the thickness of nasal skin. This maneuver is risky in smokers, however. Axial vessels, which can be seen coursing through the subdermal subcutaneous fat, are preserved. When elevated, the hair-bearing columella extension of a vertical flap may be thinned of fat and frontalis and each hair follicle clipped from behind, diminishing the transfer of hair to the nose. The distal 1.5 to 2 cm of the flap are elevated off the frontalis muscle (in nonsmokers), and then dissection passes deeply between the frontalis muscle and periosteum. The frontalis muscle is included with the proximal pedicle. The flap is transferred to the nose and sutured to the defect with fine cutaneous silk sutures. The forehead donor defect is closed by undermining in the subfrontalis plane into both temple areas. No galeal scoring is performed. The wound edges are advanced and the wound closed. A few #3-0 nylon tension sutures are placed percutaneously, just through the wound edge, so that the suture marks will be minimal. These simple sutures approximate the wound under moderate wound-closure tension. Attempts to approximate the tissue under extreme wound-closure tension are unnecessary and can create tissue ischemia. A layered wound closure is then performed. Skin sutures are removed in 3 to 4 days and the heavier nylon retention sutures at 9 to 10 days. Because of the narrow pedicle width, the inferior forehead wound always closes easily. Depending upon the flap dimensions, a

gap may remain high on the forehead below the hairline. It should be covered with a petroleum bandage and allowed to heal secondarily. If skin grafted, it will appear forever as a shiny, discolored forehead patch. Incisions along the hairline or into the scalp to rotate tissues for forehead closure are unnecessary.Similarly, the use of prior skin expansion only delays reconstruction and increases the patient's discomfort and social isolation. It also adds uncontrollable shrinkage of expanded forehead skin to the complexities of nasal reconstruction. Any gap that remains in the forehead after transfer of the paramedian forehead flap should be allowed to heal by secondary intention. Over the ensuing 3 to 4 weeks, it will fill with granulation tissue, contract, and epithelialize. The residual defect after flap transfer is rarely wider than 1½ to 2 cm. When healed, it will shrink to one third the original size. Further revision is rarely necessary.

Once the flap inset is well vascularized and adherent, the pedicle can be divided at 3 weeks. Excess tissue in the proximal pedicle is not returned to the forehead. The proximal base is unrolled, sculpted of excess subcutaneous tissue and scar, and inserted as a small inverted *V* in the medial brow where it will simulate a glabella frown crease. The distal flap inset can be reelevated to within 1 to 1½ cm of the alar margin and tip. Subcutaneous tissue and scar are then excised from both the flap and the recipient bed until the nasal contour is correct. The thinned flap is then trimmed to fit a subunit shape and inset in a normal join between adjacent units or in a normal wrinkle line present across the nasal bridge. If the original defect extends high into the nasal root, it may be possible to preserve the supratrochlear vessels under the reconstructed skin at the root of the new nose, maintaining a permanent blood supply to the transferred forehead skin.

In major reconstructions, wound contracture may cause unpredictable changes. Primary cartilage grafts may shift in position, or additional grafts may be needed to increase projection. In such cases, it may be wise to delay pedicle division. At 3 weeks, once the reconstructed lining and cartilage grafts are stable, the flap can be lifted proximally from the recipient bed, maintaining a columella and rim inset. The underlying subcutaneous tissue and scar are then sculpted and additional cartilage grafts placed as necessary. The flap is then resutured to the defect. Three weeks later (a total of 6 weeks after flap transfer) the pedicle is finally divided. Such an intermediate operation allows aggressive revisional modifications, which can be safely performed while the pedicle is intact and the flap maximally vascularized. Such a sequence improves vascular safety and minimizes late postoperative revision.

SUPPORT

In the normal nose, dorsal support is supplied by the nasal bones and the leading edge of the septum. The sidewall is supported by the nasal bones and upper lateral cartilage, and the tip by the medial and lateral crura of the alar cartilages. The lateral crus provides projection of the domes and sculpted facets of the aesthetic nasal tip. If missing, the normal cartilaginous framework of each unit must be replaced. Primary cartilage grafts can replace the dorsum, tip, and lateral sidewalls. Additionally, a strip of cartilage must be placed along the new nostril margin, even though the alar lobule contains no cartilage. It is required to brace the alar rim and prevent constriction inward, contraction upward, or collapse during healing stages.

The soft tissues of cover and lining collapse without a skeletal framework, impairing the airway and limiting projection. A rigid skeleton must be provided to provide support, projection, and contour and to brace the reconstruction against the force of myofibroblast contraction. Primary cartilage grafts fix the form of the new nose by virtue of the cartilage that backs lining. They simulate a normal shape and reestablish the aesthetic lines of the nose. The major function of the framework is to achieve and maintain airway patency and profile.

A microform of the external nose must be created by fabricating primary cartilage grafts into the contour of the missing units. Each graft is reduced in all dimensions by 2.5 mm to accommodate the thickness of forehead skin. Each graft fixes the underlying mucous membrane lining into position and imparts an external shape to a specific subunit. The reconstructed nose should stand erect and feel rigid to touch at the end of the initial procedure.

Four different hard tissue grafts are available to fix the underlying mucosa in position and impart a specific subunit surface shape.

1. **Dorsal buttress**—A bridge buttress of layered septal cartilage, costal cartilage, or rib, iliac, or cranial bone can be installed along the dorsum to prevent upward contraction and postoperative shortening. It provides shape and projection to the bridge and creates a dorsal subunit shape.

2. **Sidewall brace**—A sidewall brace of septal cartilage and bone can be harvested and trimmed to a trapezoidal shape. Positioned on the sidewall, it replaces the missing upper lateral cartilage and nasal bone. It supports the midvault against collapse and braces it against upward contraction. It serves as a platform for glasses.

3. **Columellar strut**—A columellar strut of septal or conchal cartilage, 4 mm wide, is scored and bent to replace one or both alar cartilages. These alar cartilage replicas are fixed to the stumps of residual medial crura, scored and bent laterally, and then sutured to the lining of the residual or reconstructed vestibule. They support the dome and recreate the nasal tip. Additional projection can be provided by adding one or two Peck-type, 4- × 9-mm cartilage grafts, which are anchored to the tops of these newly reconstructed columellar struts (Fig. 17-4).

4. **Alar batten**—An alar rim batten consisting of a 4-mm-wide strip of septal or conchal cartilage is placed along the leading edge of the lining sleeve from the alar base to the nostril apex (Fig. 17-5). Buried in a pocket laterally and attached medially to the tip framework, it fixes a new alar rim in position and creates a normal bulging contour to the alar lobule.

The surgeon must determine what part of the internal chassis is missing and replace it. Each graft is shaped, carved, bent, and fixed to mirror exactly the ideal or contralateral normal as regards rim position and arch, projection, contour, and symmetry. The surgeon's goal is to create a "fabricated composite flap" of lining tissue and primary cartilage grafts, which will create a microform of the external nose.

LINING FLAPS

A broad expanse of residual and well-vascularized intranasal lining is available to line lateral, heminasal, or subtotal nasal defects. Only flaps from intranasal donor sites (the vestibule, middle vault, and septum) are thin and supple. Such highly vascularized lining will support primary cartilage grafts.

An understanding of the arterial supply to the septum is of vital importance. The septum is vascularized posteriorly through the sphenopalatine artery and anterosuperiorly through the ethmoid artery. Minimal vascular supply is provided by the continuation of the greater palatine artery through the incisive foramen. The major anterior inferior blood supply of the septum enters through the upper lip (see Fig. 17-2). A branch of the facial artery, the superior labial artery, winds medially through the orbicularis oris muscle at the level of the vermilion roll. Lateral to the philtrum column, it gives off a septal branch that passes vertically upward and enters the septum lateral to the nasal spine before breaking up into the septal plexus. In fact, the entire ipsilateral septal mucous membrane can be elevated on a 1.3-cm-wide pedicle based on the superior labial

Figure 17-4   *A,* Columellar strut and alar cartilage replacement grafts can be harvested from nasal septal cartilage. *B,* The grafts are scored and bent to simulate the contour of the lower lateral nasal cartilages. *C, D,* The grafts are fixed to the stumps of residual medial crura and to the lining of the residual or reconstructed vestibule. *E, F,* Additional projection of the nasal tip can be provided by adding one or two Peck-type cartilage grafts, which are anchored to the tops of the newly reconstructed columellar struts.

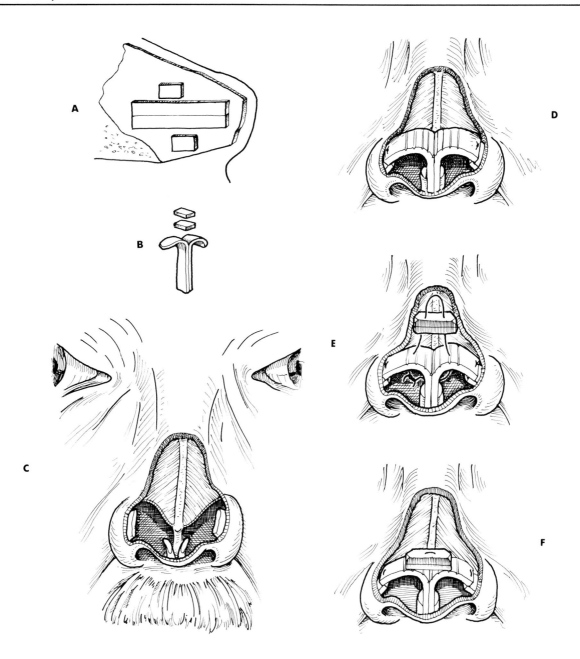

Figure 17-5   An alar rim batten *(A)*, consisting of a 4-mm-wide strip of conchal cartilage, is placed along the leading edge of the lining sleeve from alar base to nostril apex. Conchal cartilage grafts can also be used to replace the lateral crus of the lower lateral nasal cartilage *(B)*.

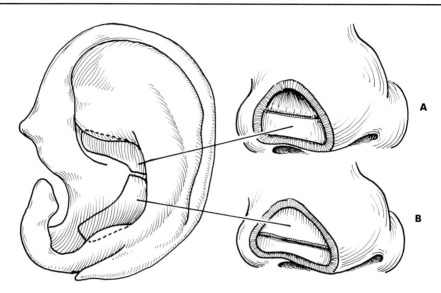

artery in the zone between the anterior plane of the upper lip and the anterior-inferior edge of the pyriform aperture. This knowledge of the vascular supply of the septum allows the successful transfer of well-vascularized intranasal mucosal lining flaps to reconstruct the nose. Several options are available.

In small lateral defects, residual vestibular skin frequently remains at the superior margin of the defect. If residual vestibular skin is intact, it can be incised as a bipedicle flap approximately 8 mm wide. Based medially on the septum and laterally on the nasal floor, it can be advanced inferiorly to line the nasal margin. However, a defect remains in the area of the lateral midvault. The residual sidewall defect, which exists above the vestibular flap, is resurfaced with a transposed septal flap in one of two ways. A modified contralateral septal mucoperichondrial flap, as originally described by de Quervain and popularized by Kazanjian, can be employed. This hinge flap is based on the dorsal nasal septum and receives its blood supply from the anterior ethmoidal artery. It is approximately 2 cm wide and 2.5 cm long. First, the ipsilateral mucoperichondrium is incised and reflected and the septal cartilage harvested as in an SMR. Such exposure is obtained by incising the mucoperichondrium horizontally below the dorsum and vertically posterior to the caudal septum. These incisions lie in the area of the inner aspect of the remaining L-shaped septal strut. The ethmoid bone and septal cartilage, exposed in the septal donor site during flap elevation, are removed as graft material. An L-shaped septal strut support is preserved. The contralateral mucosa is incised along

three sides but kept intact dorsally. It is transposed laterally across the contralateral nasal airway to line the upper vault. It is also sutured inferiorly to the bipedicle vestibular flap. As originally described, this was a composite flap composed of septal cartilage and mucous membrane. However, the cartilage of the septum is more efficiently removed as a single large piece. This abundant harvest of septal cartilage can then be fabricated into the necessary components of struts, buttresses, battens, and braces that are required to reconstruct nasal support and shape. Once these linings are positioned and sutured together, cartilage grafts are sutured in place external to the flaps. Using a taper needle, 5-0 or 6-0 nylon sutures are passed through the cartilage grafts to the underlying raw surface of the lining flaps to anchor the flaps to the cartilage, thus creating a "composite" flap of lining and cartilage. The lining flaps vascularize the primary cartilage grafts, while the cartilage grafts give shape and support to the underlying lining flaps. The ipsilateral septal mucosa is repositioned to restore the septal partition. Frequently a fistula persists superiorly.

The other way of resurfacing the sidewall lining defect is by use of an ipsilateral septal mucous membrane flap. After infiltrating both sides of the septum with local anesthesia with epinephrine, the mucoperichondrium of the ipsilateral septum is elevated. On transfer, the ipsilateral septal flap must be both wide and long enough to reach and line the sidewall defect (Fig. 17-6). Normally it is approximately 2 cm high and 2.5 cm deep. It is incised on three borders but left attached by a 1.3-cm-wide pedicle based in the zone

Figure 17-6 In small lateral nasal defects, residual vestibular skin is mobilized downward as a bipedicle flap *(A)*. An ipsilateral septal mucosal flap *(B)* is incised on three borders but left attached by a 1.3-cm-wide pedicle based in the zone between the anterior inferior edge of the pyriform aperture and the anterior plane of the upper lip. This flap is turned laterally to repair the donor site of the bipedicle vestibular skin flap. Septal cartilage left exposed by the septal flap is harvested and used to fabricate the necessary components of struts, buttresses, battens, and braces required to reconstruct nasal support and shape.

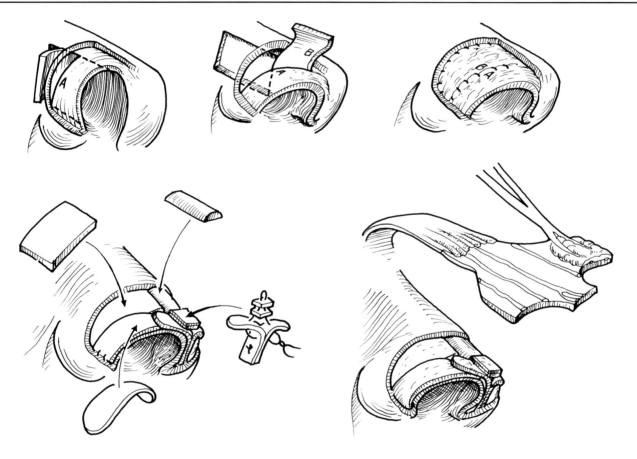

between the anterior inferior edge of the pyriform aperture and the anterior plane of the upper lip—the region of the nasal spine. Mucosal attachments of septal mucoperichondrium to septum, not employed for transfer, remain untouched. The septum receives its major anteroinferior blood supply through the septal branch of the superior labial artery. When left attached in this strategic zone, the septal mucoperichondrium may be twisted and transposed laterally. The ipsilateral septal flap is turned laterally and sutured to the residual lateral lining defect. The flap pedicle will temporarily obstruct the nasal airway, but 3 weeks postoperatively, at the time of forehead flap division, it can be sectioned and the airway opened.

In heminasal defects, the tissue loss extends superiorly toward the nasal bone. Residual vestibular skin is not present, and a bipedicle flap is unavailable to line the alar rim. In such cases, an ipsilateral septal mucous membrane flap based on the ipsilateral superior labial artery can be transposed laterally and pivoted anteriorly to provide lining to the proposed ala and alar rim. The sidewall lining defect that exists above this first flap is supplied by a contralateral septal mucous membrane hinged flap vascularized dorsally on the anterior ethmoidal vessels. Thus, the lining for a heminasal defect is supplied inferiorly by an ipsilateral septal flap based on the superior labial artery and superiorly by a contralateral septal mucous membrane flap based on the anterior ethmoidal arteries. A permanent septal fistula remains. Although crusting may occur for several months, the large septal fistula that remains is rarely symptomatic. In central nasal defects, when the tip and dorsum are missing, residual septal lining and support remain within the residual septum. A long full-thickness composite septal flap can be incised along three borders and pivoted from the septal donor site to supply support and lining for the columella and the tip of the nose. Its base is centered in the region of the nasal spine and upper lip and contains the septal branches of the superior labial arteries, which ensure good vascularity. Depending on the requirements for missing support and lining, a flap of appropriate dimensions is outlined and incised with a stout straight scissors, a right-angle scissors, and a scalpel or right-angle knife. Such flaps of septal mucoperichondrium, cartilage, and bone may extend from the nasal floor below to the level of the medial canthi above and posteriorly behind the ethmoid perpendicular plate, depending upon the requirements of the defect—tip or tip and entire dorsum (Fig. 17-7). The 1.3-cm-wide pedicles of mucous membrane located at the lower edge of the pyriform aperture, which contain the septal branches of the superior labial arteries, must be maintained. However, the flap remains fixed at the nasal spine due to its cartilaginous

attachments. To allow easy rotation, the septal leaves must be gently separated above the nasal spine and the mucoperichondrium elevated with a Freer elevator. A strip of septal cartilage, a few millimeters wide, is then resected from the cartilaginous base of the flap between the bilateral soft tissue perichondrial flaps. This permits the flap to rotate up and out to reach the tip and dorsum. Vascularity through the soft tissues of the mucoperichondrium remains unaltered.

The flap is designed overly wide to create an intentional excess. As the flap pivots into position, its distal end pops over the exposed stump of the nasal bones and locks into position, maintaining dorsal nasal skeleton. The extra lining is folded laterally to line the dorsal nasal vault and tip. The excess cartilage and bone harvested with the composite flap is removed and used where needed as grafts for structural support (Fig. 17-7**C**). In one stage, a stable platform and ample lining can be supplied to the lower middle and upper nasal vaults.

SUMMARY

The residual nose is a storehouse of materials, which can be emptied as necessary, both for lining and hard tissue support needs. Such cover and lining supply a soft tissue canopy. A primary cartilage framework provides rigidity and resilience for support, protection in space, airway patency, and nasal shape and braces the reconstruction against contraction. Support grafts depend on cover and lining for vascularization. Lining depends on a framework for rigidity, support, and shape. Support must be provided before the completion of wound healing to prevent soft tissue collapse and myofibroblast contraction. Because tissue is replaced in kind and quantity, multiple secondary subcutaneous thinning or secondary replacements of added skeletal support are not required. Thin vascular lining flaps and primary cartilage grafts, carved as replicas of the normal cartilaginous support, allow the surgeon to shape a nose in a single stage. An ideal contour is established at the outset, and the relentless force of myofibroblast contraction is resisted. This method of nasal reconstruction emphasizes the use of thin, supple, and vascularized local vestibular skin and septal flaps for lining. Support, contour, projection, and bracing are provided by primary ear and septal cartilage grafts fabricated to recreate dorsal, tip, sidewall, and alar support framework. Thin and well-vascularized forehead or melolabial flaps are positioned for the replacement of surface subunits. Well-matching skin forms an envelope that allows the underlying shape of the support framework to show through and recreate the expected nasal surface subunit contour.

Figure 17-7 *A,* A full-thickness composite septal flap for reconstruction of the internal lining and structural support of the nasal tip and lower nasal dorsum can be incised along the marked borders and can include septal cartilage and bone. To allow rotation, septal mucosal leaves are separated from the nasal spine, and a strip of septal cartilage a few millimeters wide is resected from the base of the flap. *B,* As the flap pivots into position, its distal end pops over the exposed stump of the nasal bones and locks into place, maintaining dorsal nasal support. The extra mucosal lining is folded laterally to line the dorsal nasal vault and tip areas. *C,* The excess cartilage and bone are harvested from the composite flap and used where necessary as grafts for structural support.

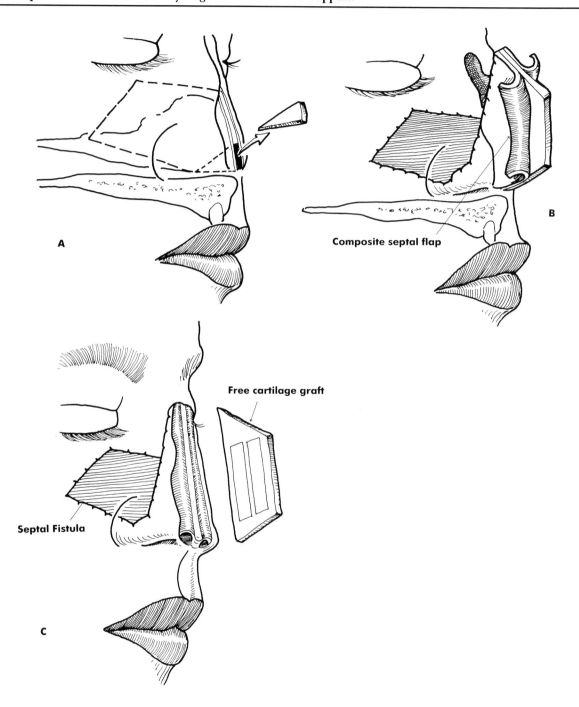

Figure 17-8   *A, B,* A 5- × 6-cm skin defect of nasal dorsum and a 3- × 2-cm skin and soft tissue defect of left ala. *C,* A left melolabial interpolation flap is designed using a foil template of the contralateral normal right ala to create an exact pattern of the skin necessary to replace the entire left alar subunit. *D,* Melolabial interpolation flap transposed. A paramedian forehead flap is designed to replace the entire dorsal subunit following excision of residual normal skin. *E,* Paramedian forehead flap and melolabial flaps in place.
(From Menick FJ: Artistry in aesthetic surgery: aesthetic perception and the subunit principle, *Clin Plast Surg* 14:729, 1987.)

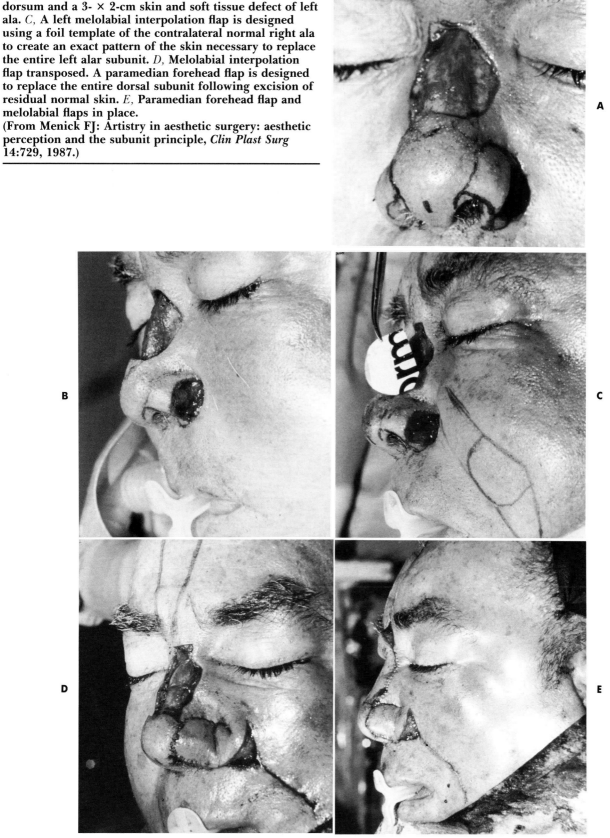

Following are examples of implementation of the reconstructive surgical concepts outlined in the preceding portion of this chapter.

Fig. 17-8 shows defects of the nasal bridge and left ala after excision of basal cell carcinoma. The dorsal defect encompasses part of the dorsal subunit and extends into both nasal sidewalls. Approximately 60% of the left alar skin is missing. Outlines of the nasal subunits are marked with ink. Residual normal adjacent skin within the dorsal and alar subunits will be excised and discarded. The skin of each lateral nasal sidewall will be advanced so that the border of the resulting dorsal defect will conform to the expected join of the dorsal and sidewall units.

A left melolabial interpolation flap is designed and positioned lateral to the left melolabial fold (Fig. 17-8**C**). A foil template of the contralateral normal right ala is used to create an exact pattern of the skin necessary to replace the entire left alar subunit after excision of residual normal skin. The melolabial inter-

polation flap is transposed to resurface the left ala (Fig. 17-8**D**). The original dorsal defect has been modified by advancing the residual sidewall skin to the expected join of the dorsal and sidewall units. A paramedian forehead flap based on the right supratrochlear vessels is designed to replace the surface of the entire dorsal subunit. Paramedian and melolabial interpolation flaps are seen in place in Fig. 17-8**E.**

Although postoperatively there are extensive and inevitable scars at both donor and recipient areas of the forehead, nose, and cheek, they are not apparent (Fig. 17-9). Scars are strategically placed so that the flap joins resemble the ridges and valleys of the expected facial and nasal units. The cheek scar is exactly positioned in the left melolabial sulcus. The forehead flap pedicle base, after division, is replaced by a small inverted *V* that simulates the glabellar frown crease. Scars outlining the dorsal and left alar units are hidden in the joins between the expected hills and valleys of each subunit.

The patient in Fig. 17-10 presents with a defect that

Figure 17-9 Six months postoperative. Scars are strategically placed so that the flap joins resemble the ridges and valleys of the expected facial and nasal units. (From Menick FJ: Artistry in aesthetic surgery: aesthetic perception and the subunit principle, *Clin Plast Surg* 14:729, 1987.)

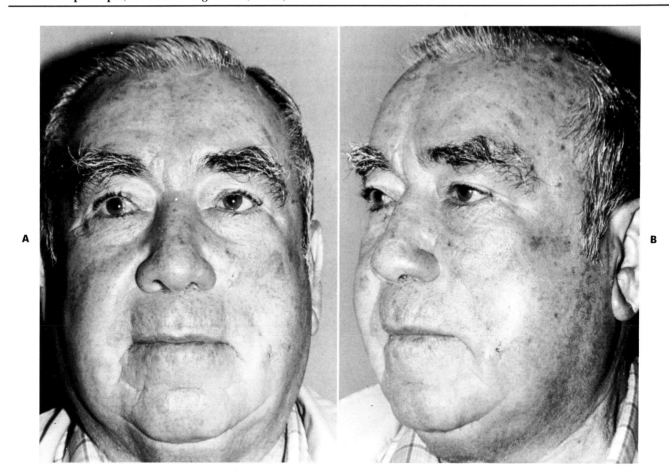

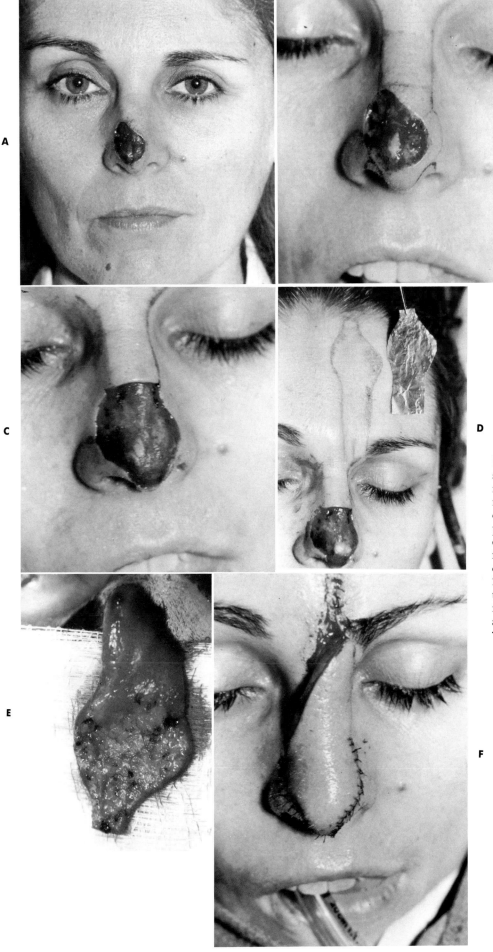

Figure 17-10 *A,* A 4- × 3-cm skin defect following skin cancer removal. *B,* Nasal subunits are marked. *C,* Residual normal skin covering the remaining tip and portions of the dorsal subunit are discarded. *D,* Paramedian forehead flap is designed using a foil pattern of the surface defect. *E,* The distal 2 cm of the flap is thinned nearly to dermis. *F,* The paramedian forehead flap resurfaces the dorsal and tip subunits.

Figure 17-11   Three months postoperative. The scars on the nose are camouflaged by positioning them along the joins of the nasal subunits.

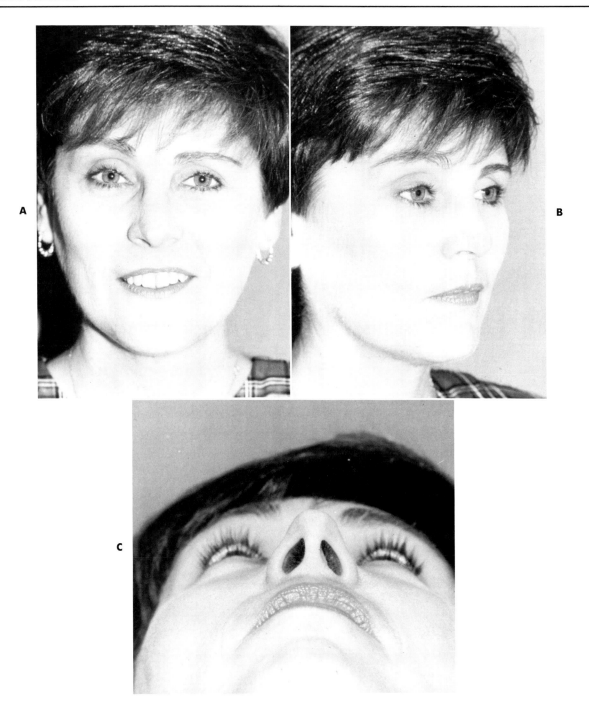

encompasses the skin of part of the nasal tip, dorsum, and right sidewall after skin cancer excision. The nasal subunits are marked with ink. Nasal tip cartilages are exposed. Residual normal skin within the tip and part of the dorsal subunits is discarded (Fig. 17-10**C**). The right sidewall is advanced a few millimeters to better position the final scar at the junction of the dorsal and sidewall subunits. An exact foil pattern of this surgically designed defect is positioned at the hairline directly above the left supratrochlear vessels to assist in the design of a paramedian forehead flap (Fig. 17-10**D**). In this nonsmoker, the distal 1½ to 2 cm of the flap is thinned nearly to dermis by excision of frontalis muscle and subcutaneous tissue (Fig. 17-10**E**). The bulbs of any hair follicles are clipped from the deep surface of the flap and coagulated. The thin forehead flap resurfaces the dorsal and tip subunits. Fig. 17-11 shows the results 3 months following surgery. Scars are nicely camouflaged in the joins of the nasal subunits.

The patient in Fig. 17-12 shows an 8- × 4-cm defect after excision of recurrent basal cell carcinoma involving the left cheek, upper lip, and ala. Rather than restore this three-dimensional defect involving multiple aesthetic units with a single flap, the donor defect is shared and each individual unit reconstructed separately. The nasal subunits are drawn, and the left melolabial fold marked with ink (Fig. 17-12**B**). The upper lip and alar base are resurfaced by medial advancement of residual lip skin after making an incision along the left melolabial fold (Fig. 17-12**C, D**). The standing cutaneous deformity formed by the advancement of lip tissue is trimmed parallel to the normal lip wrinkle lines, and the wound is sutured. Residual skin on the left ala is excised and the defect resurfaced with a superiorly based melolabial interpolation flap designed by using an exact template of the contralateral normal ala (Fig. 17-12**E**). After secondary division of the pedicle, the residual cheek defect will be closed by cheek advancement. The melolabial interpolation flap is designed exactly above the left melolabial sulcus (Fig. 17-12**F**). It has a subcutaneous base fed by axial perforators, which pass above and below the zygomatic major muscle. After excision of residual skin within the left alar subunit, the lining is supported and shaped by a conchal cartilage alar batten (Fig. 17-12**G, H**).

Distally the inset is thinned, leaving only 1 to 2 mm of subcutaneous tissue, which corresponds to the normal thickness of alar skin (Fig. 17-13). The superior subcutaneous base of the flap transposes easily (Fig. 17-13**B**). The donor site is closed by undermining adjacent cheek skin and advancing it inferiorly and medially. Three weeks later, the pedicle is divided. The flap inset is partially elevated, and excess subcutaneous tissue and scar are sculpted from the alar base, lip, and cheek join (Fig. 17-14). The flap is wrapped around the alar lobule and inset into the nasal sill. The medial cheek defect is closed so that the final scar lies exactly in the alar facial and melolabial sulcuses (Fig. 17-14**C, D**).

Following reconstruction of the lip, nose, and upper lip, the three-dimensional character of these structures has been restored (Fig. 17-15). Scars lie hidden in subunit joins. The alar margin is well supported by the auricular cartilage graft.

A young woman presented with a full-thickness defect of the distal columella, dome, and parts of the right sidewall and ala secondary to a human bite (Fig. 17-16**A**). Replacement of the lost tissue as a composite graft had been unsuccessful. In this patient, it was decided to resurface the missing skin only and not to discard residual normal adjacent covering skin within subunits. Thin and highly vascular vestibular skin remains at the superior aspect of the wound. A bipedicle flap of vestibular lining based medially on the membranous septum and laterally on the nostril floor is advanced inferiorly to restore lining to the proposed alar rim (Fig. 17-16**B, C**). A dorsally based hinge flap of contralateral septal mucous membrane and cartilage is swung laterally to fill the defect above the reconstructed alar margin. The flimsy bipedicle vestibular flap is held with forceps (Fig. 17-16**D, E**). The exposed septal cartilage of the Kazajian flap has been scored to create a more vaulted contour to support the lateral sidewall. A conchal cartilage graft is positioned along the alar rim to provide support to the airway and shape to the alar margin (Fig. 17-16**F, G**). The dorsal and tip subunits are outlined. A second conchal graft was placed atop the alar margin batten and overlaps the nasal sidewall cartilage graft to create the contour of the missing lateral alar crus and is attached to the nasal tip (Fig. 17-16**H**). A paramedian forehead flap thinned nearly to dermis is transposed to resurface the external cover defect exactly (Fig. 17-16**I**).

In Fig. 17-17 the patient is shown 3 weeks following the initial reconstruction and just before pedicle division. The flap pedicle is divided, and the distal inset partially reelevated to allow further sculpting of excess subcutaneous tissue and scar prior to completion of the inset (Fig. 17-17**B**). Healthy conchal cartilage grafts are visible in the depths of the wound. Results are seen three months postoperatively (Fig. 17-17**C, D**).

The case shown in Fig. 17-18 represents a right full-thickness heminasal defect of the tip, ala, and nasal sidewall. Residual normal vestibular skin remains at the superior aspect of the defect. The lining of the alar margin is replaced with a bipedicle flap of residual

Text continued on page 331.

Figure 17-12 *A,* An 8- × 4-cm skin defect following removal of skin cancer. Defect involves portions of the ala, lip, and cheek. *B,* Nasal subunits marked. *C, D,* Upper lip and alar base are repaired with an advancement of the residual lip skin. *E,* Foil template used to design interpolation cheek flap to resurface entire ala. *F,* Interpolation flap outlined. Medial cheek defect will be reconstructed by cheek advancement following detachment of melolabial flap. *G, H,* Residual skin of ala excised, and conchal cartilage alar batten in place. (From Menick FJ: Nasal reconstruction—creating a visual illusion, *Adv Plast Surg* 6:193, 1989.)

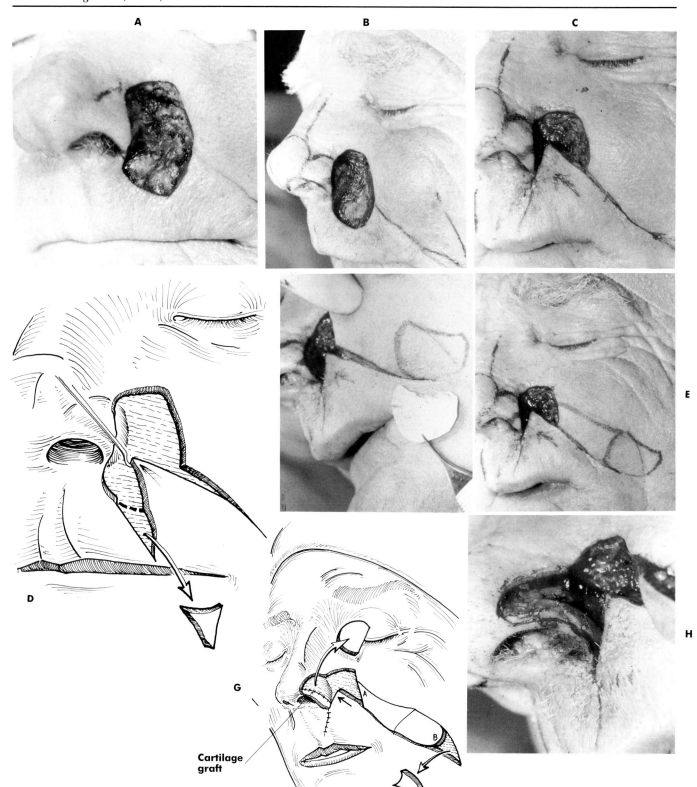

A   B   C

D   E

G   H

Cartilage
graft

Figure 17-13   *A, B,* Interpolation flap is dissected, maintaining a substantial subcutaneous pedicle medially. *C, D,* Distal portion of melolabial interpolation flap is thinned to normal thickness of alar skin and sutured in place.

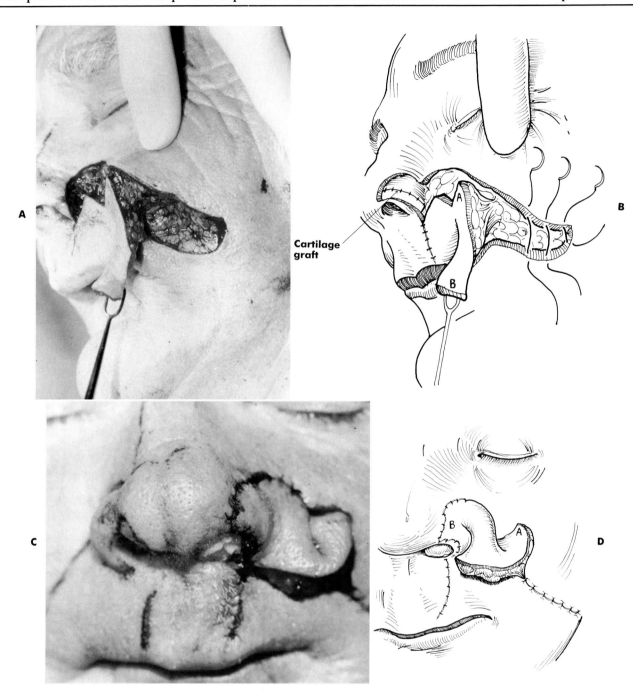

Cartilage graft

Figure 17-14 *A, B,* Three weeks later the pedicle is divided. The flap inset is partially elevated and thinned. *C, D,* The flap is inset by wrapping it around the alar lobule and attaching it to the nasal sill. The original medial cheek defect is repaired by advancing cheek skin medially so that the final scar of wound closure will lie exactly in the alar facial and melolabial sulcuses. (From Menick FJ: Nasal reconstruction—creating a visual illusion, *Adv Plast Surg* 6:193, 1989.)

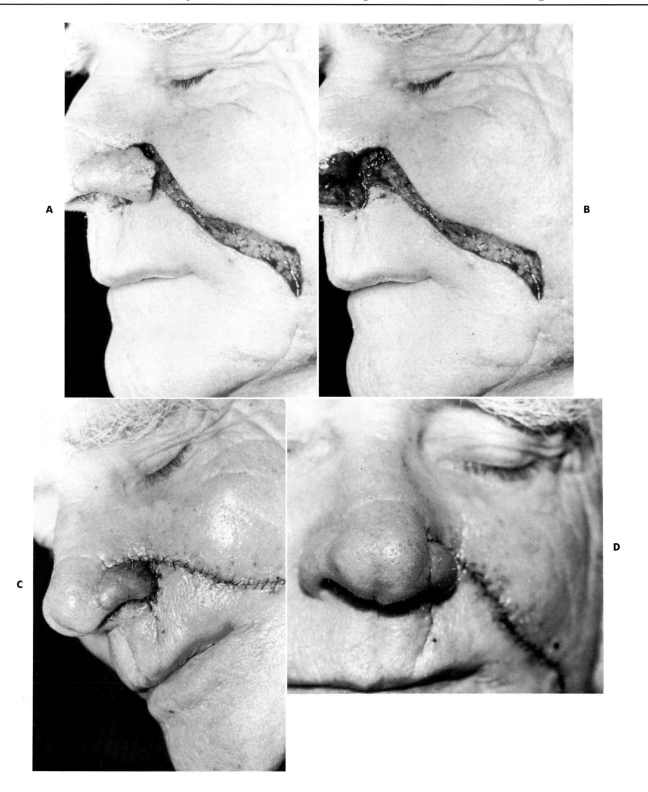

Figure 17-15   Six months postoperative. The three-dimensional character of the cheek, lip, and nose has been restored. (From Menick FJ: Nasal reconstruction—creating a visual illusion, *Adv Plast Surg* 6:193, 1989.)

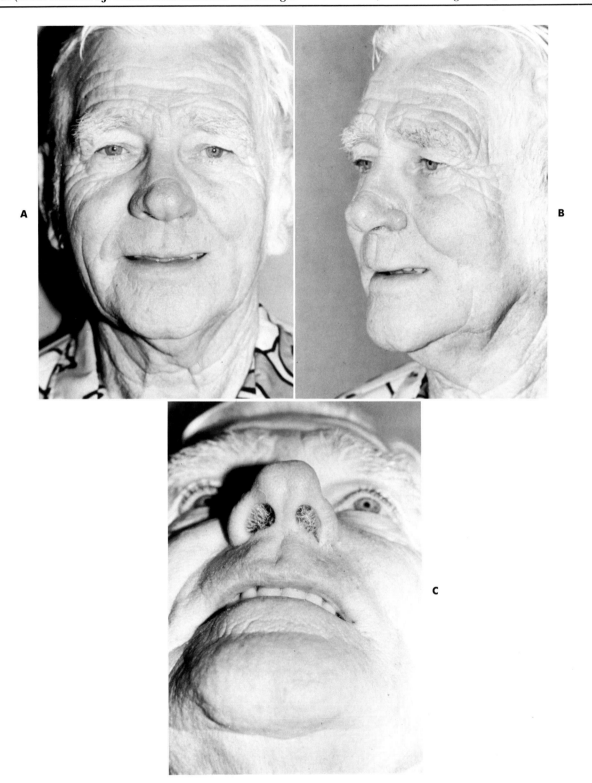

Figure 17-16 *A,* A full-thickness defect of the ala and a portion of the tip, columella, and nasal sidewall secondary to a human bite. *B, C,* Bipedicle flap of vestibular lining is advanced inferiorly to resurface the interior of the alar rim. A dorsally based hinge flap of contralateral septal mucosa and septal cartilage is turned laterally to provide lining and structural support above the reconstructed alar margin. *D, E,* The exposed septal cartilage of the hinge flap is scored to create a more vaulted contour to support the lateral sidewall. *F, G,* Conchal cartilage graft is positioned along alar rim to provide support. *H,* A second conchal graft placed on top of the alar margin batten and hinge septal flap creates the contour of the missing lateral alar crus. *I,* A paramedian forehead flap provides cover for the external surface defect. (*Probl Gen Surg* 6:455, 1989.)

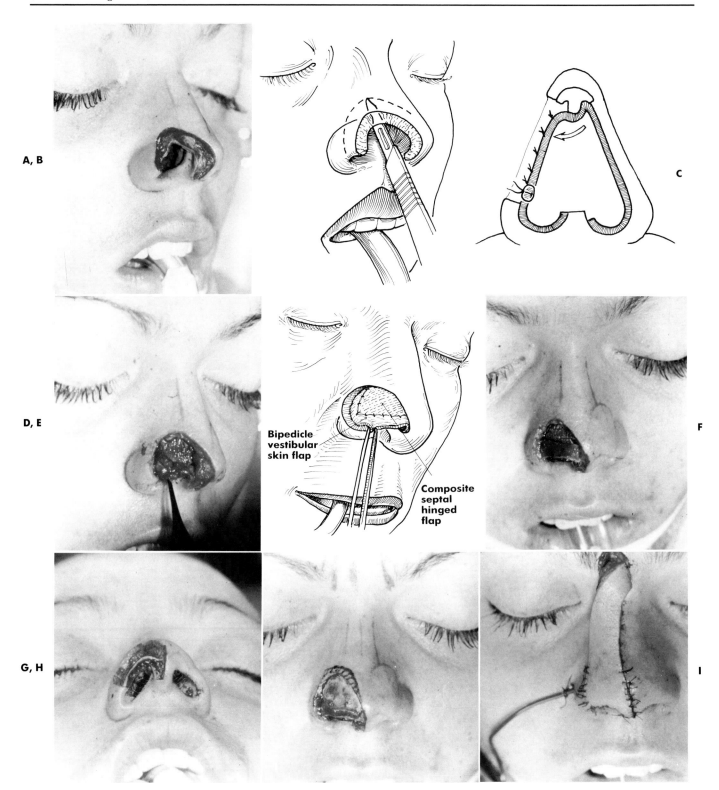

Figure 17-17   *A,* Three weeks following initial reconstruction and just prior to pedicle division. *B,* Distal flap is partially elevated from recipient site, and excessive subcutaneous tissue and early scar tissue are removed. *C, D,* Three months following completion of reconstruction. (*Prob Gen Surg* 6:455, 1989.)

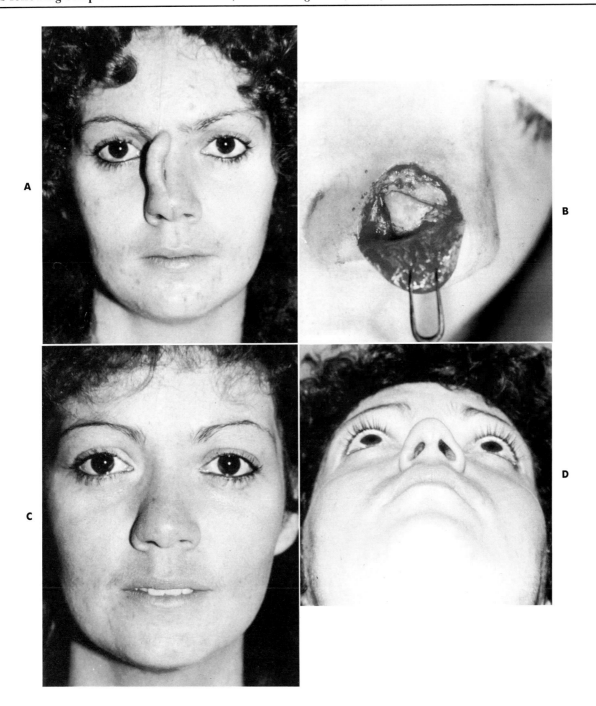

Figure 17-18 *A*, Full-thickness heminasal defect of the tip, ala, and portion of nasal sidewall. *B*, A bipedicle flap of remaining vestibular lining is incised. *C, D*, An ipsilateral septal mucoperichondrial flap held by forceps (A) is used to resurface the donor site for the bipedicle vestibular lining flap held by forceps (B). *E, F*, Vestibular flap and septal flap sutured in place. The flimsy nasal lining being held by the forceps requires cartilage grafts for structural support. *G*, Septal cartilage grafts consisting of an alar margin batten, sidewall brace, and hemitip graft are sutured in position. *H*, Foil template aids in designing paramedian forehead flap by representing the exact pattern of the missing surface defect. *I*, The paramedian forehead flap is thinned and transposed. *J*, Forehead flap transposed. (From Menick FJ: Aesthetic refinements in use of forehead for nasal reconstruction, *Clin Plast Surg* 17:607, 1990.)

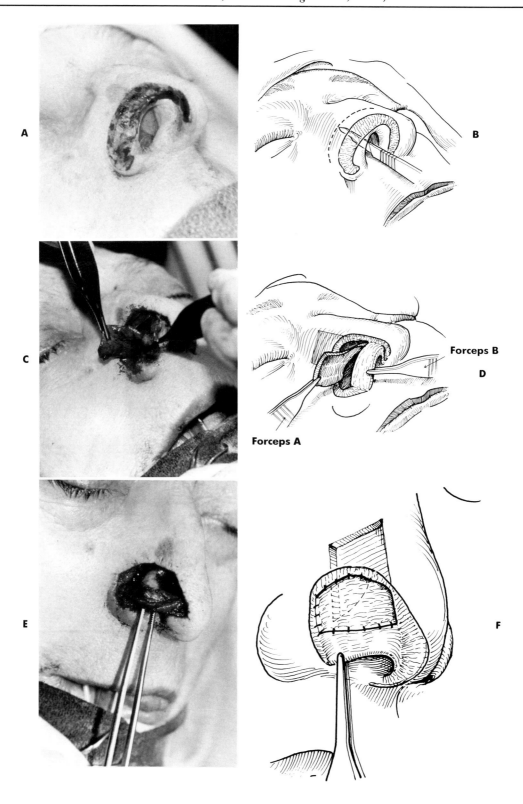

Figure 17-18, cont'd   For legend see opposite page.

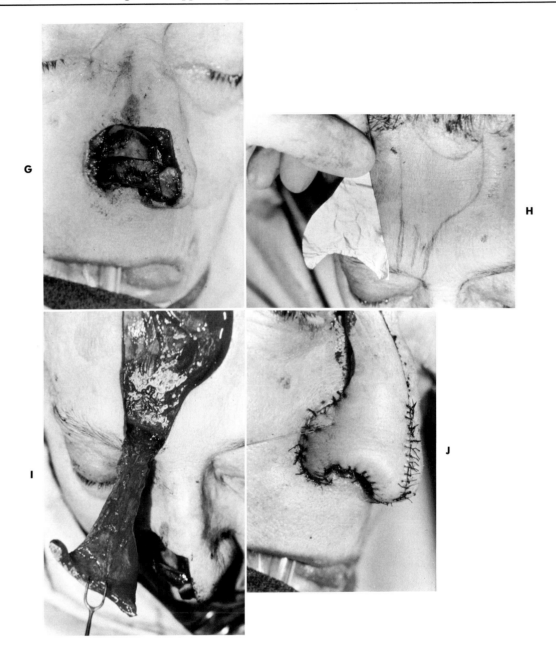

vestibular lining, similar to the method used in the previous example. The flap is based medially on the septum and laterally on the nasal floor. The more superior aspect of the lining defect, which is the donor site for the bipedicle vestibular lining flap, is replaced with an ipsilateral septal mucoperichondrial flap based on the septal branch of the superior labial artery. This flap is being held by forceps marked *A* in Fig. 17-18**D**. The vestibular flap is pulled inferiorly to supply lining to the alar rim. The ipsilateral septal flap is swung laterally to replace the lining in the superior

aspect of the defect. After suturing of the septal and vestibular flaps, the restored nasal lining is flimsy and is supported by forceps (Fig. 17-18**E, F**). Support, contour, and a bracing effect against myofibroblast contraction is supplied by an alar margin batten placed along the proposed alar rim, a sidewall brace of septal cartilage to restore the sidewall unit, and a hemitip graft (Fig. 17-18**G**). Using the contralateral left normal heminose as a guide, an exact foil pattern of the missing right heminose is created and positioned vertically above the right supratrochlear vessels for the

Figure 17-19 *A*, Three weeks following transposition of forehead flap. *B*, Pedicle of flap divided. A portion of the distal flap is partially elevated from the recipient site to allow subcutaneous sculpturing. *C*, The nasal inset is recontoured to create the sidewall and nasal alar groove. The proximal flap has been discarded and the pedicle base replaced at the medial brow as a small inverted *V*. (From Menick FJ: Aesthetic refinements in use of forehead for nasal reconstruction, *Clin Plast Surg* 17:607, 1990.)

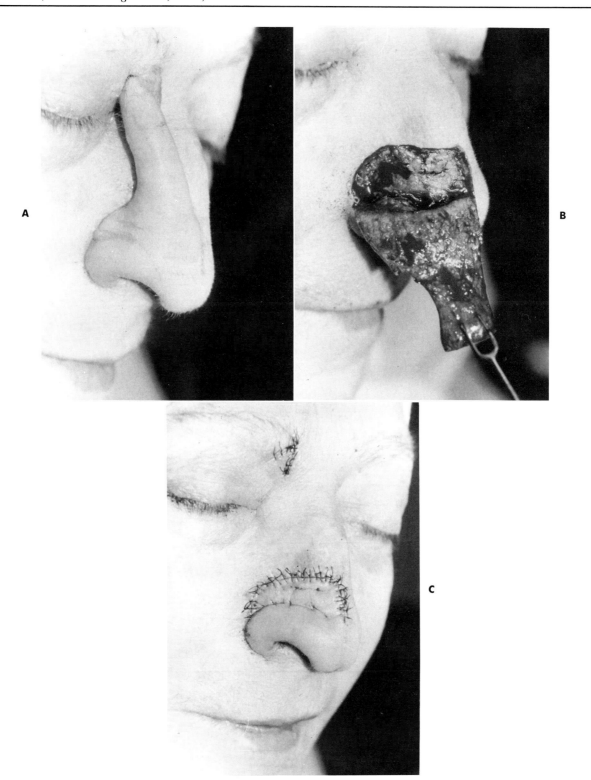

purpose of designing a paramedian forehead flap (Fig. 17-18**H**). The pedicle base is 1.3 cm in width. The flap is thinned in its distal 1½ cm almost to dermis and elevated inferiorly across the brow. The forehead flap is transposed and sutured (Fig. 17-18**I, J**). Three weeks later, prior to pedicle division, the right alar subunit is outlined in ink, and excessive subcutaneous tissue and scar will be sculpted to improve the nasal shape after pedicle division (Fig. 17-19**A**). The pedicle is divided and the flap inset partially reelevated to allow subcutaneous sculpturing (Fig. 17-19**B, C**). The pedicle base has been discarded and replaced at the medial brow as a small inverted *V*. The nasal inset is recontoured by subcutaneous sculpturing to recreate the sidewall and nasal alar groove contour. The results six months postoperatively are seen in Fig. 17-20. The contour of the nasal alar groove has been nicely restored. There is some distortion of the left nostril on base view.

Fig. 17-21**A** shows a heminasal defect after the excision of a previously irradiated recurrent basal cell carcinoma. All layers of the left nasal dome, ala, and sidewall are ablated. The defect extends onto the cheek. At the initial operation, raw areas of the nasal surface were skin grafted. The left cheek skin was

Figure 17-20   Six months postoperative. (From Menick FJ: Aesthetic refinements in use of forehead for nasal reconstruction, *Clin Plast Surg* 17:607, 1990.)

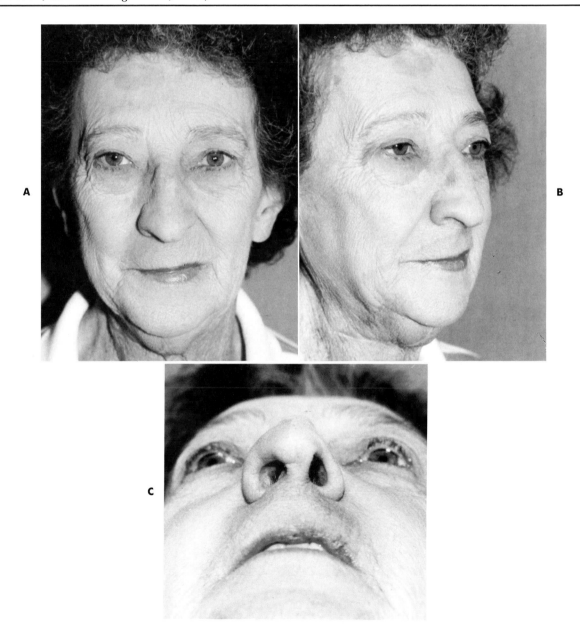

Figure 17-21 *A,* Defect of the left nose and cheek following removal of recurrent basal cell carcinoma. The left nasal dome, ala, and sidewall are resected. *B,* A flap of ipsilateral septal mucosa is outlined for the purpose of providing lining to the alar rim. A previously delayed melolabial flap is outlined. *C,* Ipsilateral mucosal flap is turned downward to provide lining to the nasal vestibule. An auricular cartilage graft is placed along the alar margin for structural support. *D,* Mucosal flap transposed. A strip of cartilage is held over the lining with forceps to simulate repair that will be used to support the alar rim. A previously delayed melolabial flap is incised and will be discarded. *E, F,* A contralateral mucoperichondrial hinge flap is swung across the nasal passage and secured to the pyriform aperture to provide internal lining to the superior portion of the defect. Septal cartilage grafts are placed over the hinge flap and along the alar rim to create an alar margin batten and sidewall brace. *G, H,* An additional cartilage graft harvested from the auricle is positioned on top of the medial aspect of the batten and sidewall cartilage grafts to replace the missing left lateral crus.

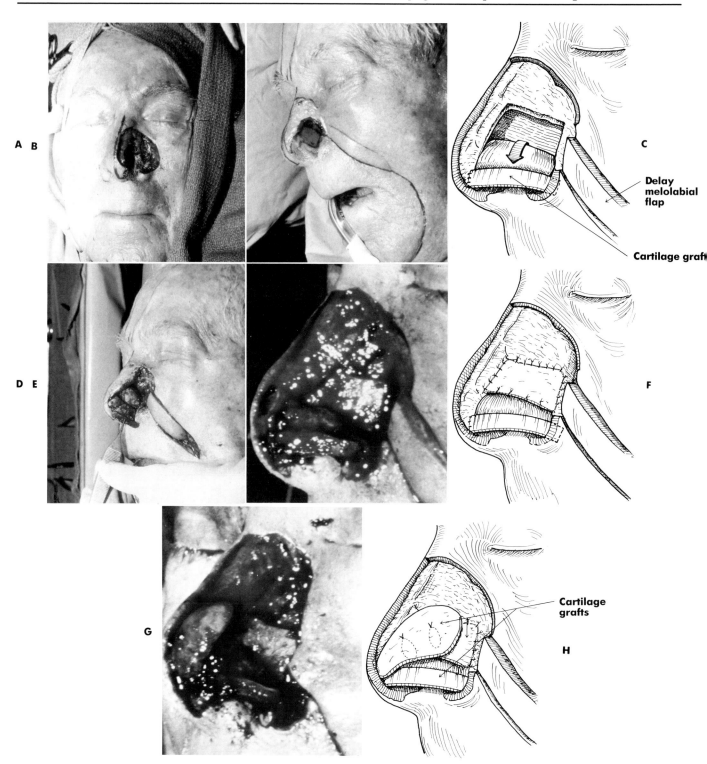

advanced, and a left melolabial flap (which would later be discarded) was delayed. Because tissue loss extends to the nasal bones, a bipedicle flap from above the defect is unavailable (Fig. 17-21**B**). A flap of ipsilateral septal mucosa is outlined based on the septal branches of the superior labial artery in the region of the nasal spine. Unilateral septal mucosa, left attached by a 1.5-cm pedicle, is twisted and transposed to fill the lining defect along the vestibular rim (Fig. 17-21**C**). A strip of cartilage is held over the lining with forceps to simulate the planned repair, and exposed septal cartilage is visible at the septal donor site (Fig. 17-21**D**). Based on the dorsal septal blood supply, a contralateral Kazanjian septal mucoperichondrial hinge flap is swung across the airway and fixed to the pyriform aperture (Fig. 17-21**F**). Septal cartilage grafts are placed along the alar rim and sidewall to create an alar margin batten and a sidewall brace (Fig. 17-21**E, F**). Using the contour of the normal contralateral right dome as a guide, a large conchal cartilage graft is fabricated to resemble the missing left lateral crus and positioned at the tip over the alar margin graft (Fig.

17-21**G, H**). Based on a foil template designed on the contralateral normal right heminose, a paramedian forehead flap is transposed to resurface the entire left heminasal unit. A 1½- × 2-cm forehead defect located near the hairline is left to heal by secondary intention after coverage with a Vaseline gauze dressing (Fig. 17-22). To resurface the defect in units, the cheek was advanced and the nose restored as a heminasal reconstruction. All scars lie between topographic units and should be less visible. The melolabial flap was unnecessary and was discarded.

Fig. 17-23 shows the patient three months postoperatively. Cover, lining, and support have been replaced in an aesthetic manner. The restoration of normal landmarks, highlights, and contour reestablishes the "expected normal." Thin vascular lining and cover flaps are supported, contoured, and braced by primary cartilage grafts. Scars are camouflaged because they lie hidden within the expected contours of the face. The three-dimensional facial contour of the lip, cheek, and nose has been recreated.

Figure 17-22   Paramedian forehead flap transposed to cover heminasal surface defect.

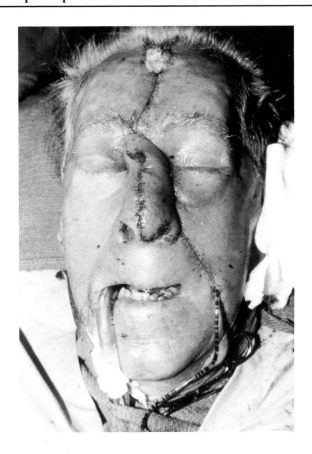

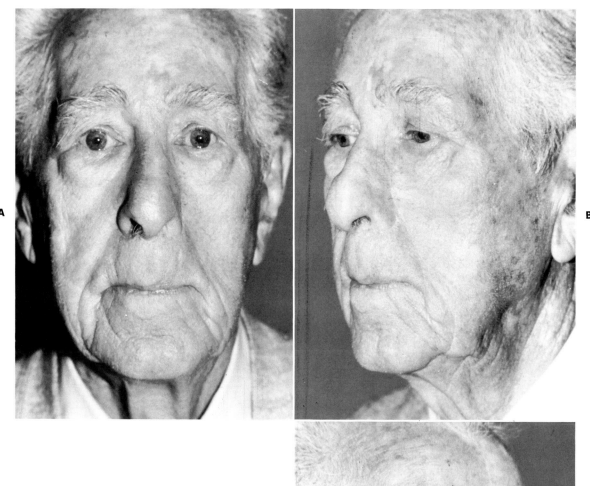

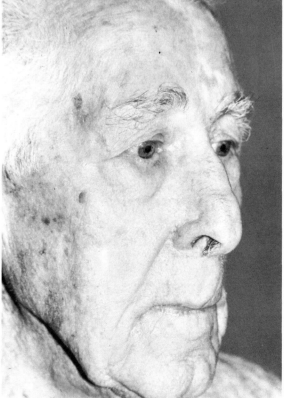

Figure 17-23 Three months postoperative. The three-dimensional topographic contour of the lip, cheek, and nose has been recreated.

SUGGESTED READINGS

1. Adamson JE: Nasal reconstruction with the expanded forehead flap, *Plast Reconstr Surg* 81:12, 1988.

2. Antia NH, Daver BM: Restructive surgery for nasal defects, *Clin Plast Surg* 8:535, 1981.

3. Burget GC, Menick FJ: The subunit principle in nasal reconstruction, *Plast Reconstr Surg* 76:239, 1985.

4. Burget GC, Menick FJ: Aesthetic restoration of one-half the upper lip, *Plast Reconstr Surg* 78:583, 1986.

5. Burget GC, Menick FJ: Nasal reconstruction: seeking a fourth dimension, *Plast Reconstr Surg* 78:145, 1986.

6. Burget GC, Menick FJ: Nasal support and lining: the marriage of beauty and blood supply, *Plast Reconstr Surg* 84:189, 1989.

7. Burget GC, Menick FJ: *Aesthetic reconstruction of the nose*, St. Louis, 1993, Mosby.

8. Converse JM: Composite graft from the septum for nasal reconstruction, *Trans Am Cong Plast Surg* 8:281, 1956.

9. Converse JM: Introduction to plastic surgery. In Converse JM, editor: *Reconstructive plastic surgery*, ed 2, vol I, Philadelphia, 1977, WB Saunders.

10. Converse JM: Full thickness loss of nasal tissue. In Converse JM, editor: *Reconstructive plastic surgery*, ed 2, vol 2, Philadelphia, 1977, WB Saunders.

11. Converse JM, McCarthy JB: The scalping flap revisited, *Clin Plast Surg* 8:413, 1981.

12. Delpech JM: *Chirurgie Clinique de Montepellier: Observations et Reflexions Tires des Travauc de Chirurgie de Cette Ecole*, Paris, 1823–1828, Gabon.

13. de Quervain F: Ueber Partielle Sietliche Rhinoplastik, *Zentralbl Chir* 29:297, 1902.

14. Gillies HD: *Plastic surgery of the face*, London, 1920, Frowde, Hodder, and Stoughton.

15. Gillies HD: A new free graft applied to reconstruction of the nostril, *Br J Surg* 30:305, 1943.

16. Gillies HD, Millard DR: *The principles and art of plastic surgery*, Boston, 1957, Little, Brown.

17. Gonzalez-Ulloa M, Castillo A, Stevens E, et al: Preliminary study of the total restoration of the facial skin, *Plast Reconstr Surg* 13:151, 1954.

18. Jackson IT: Local flaps in head and neck reconstruction, St Louis, 1985, The CV Mosby Co.

19. Kazanjian VH: The repair of nasal defects with a median forehead flap: primary closure of forehead wound, *Surg Gynecol Obstet* 83:37, 1946.

20. Kazanjian VH, Converse JM: *Surgical treatment of facial injuries*, Baltimore, 1949, Williams & Wilkins.

21. Labat M: De la Rhinoplastic, Art de Restaurer ou de Refaire Completement la Nez, doctoral dissertation, Paris, 1834.

22. Mallard GE, Montandon D: The Washeo tempororetroauricular flap: its use in twenty patients, *Plast Reconstr Surg* 70:550, 1982.

23. McCarthy JG, Lorenc ZD, et al: The median forehead flap revisited: the blood supply, *Plast Reconstr Surg* 76:866, 1985.

24. McDowell F: *The source book of plastic surgery*, Baltimore, 1977, Williams & Wilkins.

25. Mendelson BC, Masson JK, Arnold PG, et al: Flaps used for nasal reconstruction: a perspective based in 180 cases, *Mayo Clin Proc* 54:91, 1979.

26. Menick FJ: Artistry in aesthetic surgery: aesthetic perception and the subunit principle, *Clin Plast Surg* 14:723, 1987.

27. Meyer R, Kessebring V: Reconstructive surgery of the nose, *Clin Plast Surg* 8:435, 1981.

28. Millard DR: Various uses of the septum in rhinoplasty, *Plast Reconstr Surg* 81:112, 1988.

29. Millard DR Jr: Hemirhinoplasty, *Plast Reconstr Surg* 40:440, 1967.

30. Millard DR Jr: Reconstructive rhinoplasty for the lower half of a nose, *Plast Reconstr Surg* 53:133, 1974.

31. Millard R: Total reconstructive rhinoplasty and a missing link, *Plast Reconstr Surg* 37:167, 1966.

32. Millard RJ: Reconstructive rhinoplasty for the lower two-thirds of the nose, *Plast Reconstr Surg* 57:722, 1978.

33. Miller TA: The Tagliacozzi flap as a method of nasal and palatal reconstruction, *Plast Reconstr Surg* 76:870, 1985.

34. Orticochea MA: A new method for total reconstruction of the nose: the ears as donor areas, *Clin Plast Surg* 8:481, 1982.

35. Ortiz MF, Musolas A: Nasal reconstruction using forehead flaps, *Perspect Plast Surg* 3:71, 1989.

36. Richardson GS, Hanna DC, Gaisford JC: Midline forehead flap nasal construction in patients with low browlines, *Plast Reconstr Surg* 49:130, 1972.

37. Sawhney CP: A longer angular midline forehead flap for the reconstruction of nasal defects, *Plast Reconstr Surg* 58:721, 1976.

38. Shaw WW: Microvascular reconstruction of the nose, *Clin Plast Surg* 8:471, 1981.

EDITORIAL COMMENTS

Shan R. Baker

Dr. Fred Menick and his colleague Dr. Gary Burget have brought reconstructive rhinoplasty to a higher level, by emphasizing the importance of replacing missing nasal tissue with like tissue. Deficiencies of internal nasal lining are replaced with mucosal flaps harvested from the remaining nasal interior. Absent cartilage is replaced with septal or chonchal cartilage, positioned, trimmed, and shaped to match as closely as possible the missing cartilage. Great emphasis is placed on thinning and sculpturing the cartilage grafts so that they replicate the exact configuration of contralateral cartilage, if present, or the form one might expect in an ideally shaped nose. This detailed attention to refabricating the structural support of the nose combined with the concept of using mucosal flaps rather than skin grafts or skin flaps for internal nasal lining is the primary source of the superb results Dr. Menick has achieved in reconstructing the nose. Additional factors contributing to his success are the emphasis on isolating the nasal defect as a separate entity from any extension of the defect onto the cheek or lip, and utilizing individual flaps for repair of the different components of the defect. This maintains scars in major aesthetic unit junction zones and prevents blunting or obliteration of these zones while maximizing scar camouflage. Other factors contributing to Dr. Menick's success are the importance he places on providing a surface cover of the entire aesthetic subunit affected by the nasal defect, use of paramedian forehead and melolabial interpolation flaps, and aggressive thinning of these flaps when they are inset. The paramedian forehead flap provides a more effective length compared to the midline forehead flap (see discussion in Chapter 13). Use of melolabial interpolation flaps maintains the alar nasal groove and nasal facial sulcus when present.

Too often in the past, the alar facial sulcus has been violated by transposition flaps harvested from the cheek to reconstruct lower lateral nasal defects. When it has been violated by surgery, a completely natural appearing sulcus is extremely difficult to restore. For this reason, an alternative method of reconstructing the alar lobule is suggested by Dr. Menick. The method utilizes an interpolation flap from the cheek, the pedicle of which crosses over, but not through, the alar facial sulcus. The pedicle may consist of skin and subcutaneous fat or subcutaneous fat only, and is detached from the cheek 3 weeks following the initial transfer to the nose. Although 3 weeks is a lengthy time for the patient to endure the deformity caused by the flap, this interval allows the surgeon to aggressively defat and sculpt the distal flap both at the time of the flap transfer and at the time of pedicle detachment and flap inset. Upon detachment of the flap, the patient has a completely natural appearing alar facial sulcus because no incision or dissections have been made in this region. The interpolation cheek flap is indicated when a pivotal cheek flap is planned to reconstruct a defect of the alar lobule.

The technique of reconstructing the alar lobule using an interpolation cheek flap is as follows. Usually, reconstruction of the entire lobule is planned by removing any remaining skin of the lobule and freshening all margins if the defect results from Mohs surgery. Full-thickness defects are reconstructed by restoring the internal nasal lining deficit with a vascularized mucosal flap. For defects consisting of the alar lobule only, a bipedicle mucosal flap, discussed by Dr. Menick, is developed along the lateral nasal wall. The flap is based on its attachments to the skin of the lateral floor and medial dome of the nasal vestibule. The flap is created by making an extended intercartilaginous incision from the nasal dome to the lateral floor of the vestibule (Fig. 17-24). Depending on the width of the flap required to cover the mucosal defect, this incision may need to be placed cephalad to the standard intercartilaginous incision, sometimes under the upper lateral cartilage. The mucosal flap is mobilized inferiorly, and the inferior edge is sutured to the inferior border of the nasal vestibular skin defect. If the vestibular skin defect extends to the alar rim, then the inferior aspect of the intranasal flap is sutured to the edge of the cutaneous flap used to provide external coverage of the defect. The superior edge of the bipedicle mucosal flap is sutured to the soft tissue of the superior edge of the internal nasal defect. I suggest the use of a full-thickness skin graft to cover the donor site of the bipedicle flap. This is in contrast to the recommendation of Dr. Menick, who advocates the use of a second intranasal flap harvested from the septum to cover the residual sidewall lining defect. The skin graft is obtained from the standing cutaneous deformity that occurs with primary closure of the cheek donor site of the interpolation cheek flap. In my experience, this skin graft survives very well and eliminates the need for septal mucoperichondrial flaps and the associated sequelae of prolonged crusting and/or septal perforation.

Following reconstruction of the internal nasal lining defect with a bipedicle mucosal flap, the next step is to completely replace all missing nasal cartilage with free cartilage grafts harvested from the nasal septum or preferably from the auricle. If the inferior edge of the lateral crura has been removed, not only must the missing cartilage be replaced with a free cartilage graft, but additional grafts should be placed along the alar margin inferior to the position of the original lateral crus (Fig. 17-25). This prevents notching and/or upward contraction of the alar rim. Likewise, when the fibrofatty tissue of the lateral portion of the alar lobule is missing, it should also be replaced with free cartilage grafts because this tissue, although not rigid, provides structural support and contour to the lobule. If the surgeon depends strictly on a skin flap to replace the fibrofatty tissue in the alar lobule, less structural support is provided, and scar contracture causes an

Figure 17-24   *A,* A 3- × 2-cm full-thickness defect of left alar lobule following removal of a basal cell carcinoma. *B,* A bipedicle mucosal flap is developed by making an extended intercartilaginous incision from nasal dome to the lateral floor of the vestibule (photograph is of another patient). *C,* An interpolation cheek flap is designed to resurface the entire alar lobule. *D,* Interpolation flap transposed following placement of an auricular cartilage graft along margin of reconstructed ala. The inferior edge of the cheek flap is sutured to the inferior edge of the bipedicle mucosal flap. The donor site of the mucosal flap is resurfaced with a full-thickness skin graft harvested from the standing cutaneous deformity of the cheek. *E, F,* Front and base view of nose 1 year postoperative. Note symmetry of the upper melolabial fold as a result of returning the proximal pedicle of the interpolation flap back to the cheek at the time of flap inset. *G, H,* Oblique view of right and reconstructed left alar lobule 1 year postoperative.

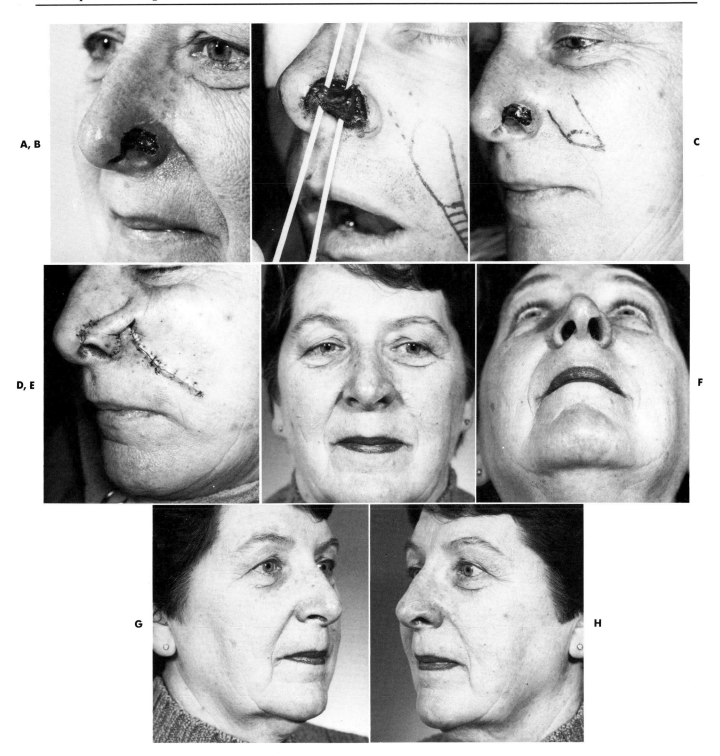

A, B

C

D, E

F

G

H

Figure 17-25 *A,* A 3- × 2.5-cm defect of left alar lobule with loss of fibrofatty tissue in lobular base and alar rim below lateral crus. *B,* Free auricular cartilage graft is placed along inferior edge of lateral crus *(arrows)* to provide structural support of the reconstructed alar rim. An interpolation melolabial flap is designed to resurface the entire lobule. *C,* Three weeks after initial flap transfer and just before flap inset, the pedicle is divided, and the proximal portion is returned to its origin to restore the upper melolabial fold. *D,* Three months after pedicle detachment. No additional revision surgery was performed. Note maintenance of the left nasal facial sulcus and melolabial fold. *E, F,* Profile of right and reconstructed left alar lobule. Note that the left nasal facial sulcus and alar nasal groove are symmetrical with their contralateral counterpart.

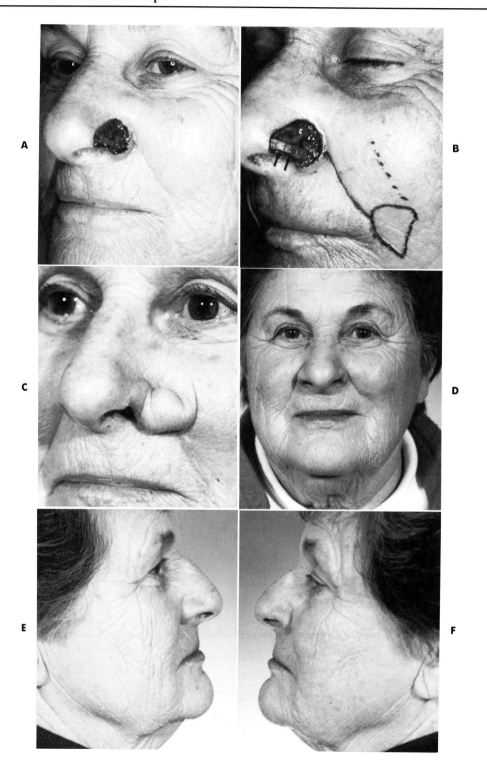

unnatural appearance to the restoration, usually with some notching of the alar rim and partial collapse of the external nasal valve.

Once the structural support to the alar lobule has been secured, a cheek flap is planned to resurface the lobule and cover the restored skeletal support (see Fig. 17-25). A template is fashioned to exactly represent the size and shape of the surface defect. This template is then used to design a superiorly based melolabial interpolation flap. Dr. Menick stresses that he designs the flap so that the medial border falls in the melolabial sulcus. The flap is elevated in the subcutaneous plane and may be lifted on a skin and subcutaneous fat pedicle or based on subcutaneous fat only. I believe a skin pedicle enhances the vascularity of the flap. The flap donor site is closed primarily by undermining the skin of the cheek. The standing cutaneous deformity that occurs with advancement of the cheek skin medially is excised, and a portion of it is used as a full-thickness skin graft to cover the donor site of the intranasal bipedicle mucosal flap, when utilized. The graft is defatted and sutured to the superior aspect of the bipedicle flap below and the remaining mucosa of the lateral nasal wall above. The raw side of the graft lies against the undersurface of the upper lateral cartilage and any remaining lateral crus. The graft is secured to the cartilage by a unilateral nasal pack left in place for 24 hours. The interpolation flap is transposed over the alar facial sulcus, and the distal two thirds of the flap thinned appropriately so that the flap will drape over the cartilage grafts in such a manner that the contour of the alar lobule and alar nasal groove are replicated. This may require thinning of the flap to the level of the dermis in the area along the alar rim in order to restore the delicate topography of the rim. In instances where the defect involves the alar rim and internal nasal vestibular skin, the inferior border of the flap is sutured to the inferior border of the bipedicle mucosal flap developed to replace the missing internal nasal lining. The proximal one third of the interpolation cheek flap is left with an ample amount of subcutaneous tissue to ensure flap vascularity. At the time of pedicle detachment, the proximal portion of the flap to be inset is defatted and contoured.

Maintaining the pedicle attachment for 3 weeks is important to allow the distal flap sufficient time to develop enough collateral vascularity to enable aggressive defatting and contouring of the proximal one third of the flap when the pedicle is divided and the flap is inset. The remaining proximal subcutaneous or cutaneous pedicle is inset into the cheek by opening the upper portion of the wound resulting from closure of the cheek donor site. This is in contrast to Dr. Menick's

approach, which is to discard the remaining tissue and close the donor site so that the resulting scar lies in the upper melolabial sulcus. Reinserting the tissue of the proximal pedicle into the upper cheek restores additional substance to the melolabial fold, minimizing the flattening of the fold that occurs to some degree with all melolabial pivotal flaps. This improves facial symmetry at the expense of having a Y-shaped scar at the superior aspect of the melolabial fold. In my experiences, this scar, which does not lie completely within the melolabial sulcus, is minimally visible and is acceptable because of the improved symmetry of the superior melolabial fold gained by returning all of the proximal pedicle back to the cheek.

The main advantage of the melolabial interpolation flap is that it does not violate the aesthetically important alar facial sulcus. It also minimizes distortion of the melolabial fold, since the only skin removed from the cheek is skin located at the inferior aspect of the fold (see Fig. 17-24). All the skin of the proximal pedicle is preserved and returned to the cheek. Another significant advantage of the interpolation flap is that, in instances where the distal portion of the flap necroses, the flap may on occasion be completely detached from the recipient site, the necrotic tissue removed, and the flap reattached by advancing additional flap tissue toward the recipient site.

The major disadvantage of this technique is that it is a two-staged procedure. However, when standard transposition cheek flaps are used to reconstruct the alar lobule, revisional surgery is frequently necessary to restore the superior portion of the alar facial sulcus. This is because using the more common technique of a one-stage cheek transposition flap to reconstruct the alar lobule almost always deforms the superior portion of the alar facial sulcus, even when the pedicle of the flap is designed well above this structure in an attempt not to deform it.

When tissue defects extend into the alar facial sulcus, the task of restoring this area of complex topography to its natural appearance, identically symmetrical to its counterpart, is a difficult challenge. When confronted with this problem, it is often preferable to reconstruct the medial cheek and alar facial sulcus component of the defect with an advancement cheek flap and reconstruct the alar lobule either with a separate cheek or forehead interpolation flap. This allows each flap to reconstruct the independent aesthetic units of the nose and cheek and places the junction of the borders of the two flaps along the restored alar facial sulcus (Fig. 17-26). When such defects are reconstructed with a single transposition cheek flap, partial or complete

Figure 17-26   *A,* A 6- × 6-cm skin and soft tissue defect of the nose involving the nasal facial sulcus and medial cheek. *B,* A free auricular cartilage graft has been placed along the alar rim for structural support *(arrows).* A cheek advancement flap has been incised to advance into the nasal facial sulcus. A paramedian forehead flap is designed to resurface the nasal component of the defect. *C,* At the time of flap inset, it is aggressively debulked of subcutaneous fat. In spite of this, restoration of the alar nasal groove may require secondary revisional surgery (in this case, 2 months after detachment of forehead flap) consisting of appropriate sculpturing of the flap and the use of tie-over bolster sutures placed full-thickness through the reconstructed alar lobule and lateral nasal wall. *D, E,* Oblique view of right and reconstructed left nasal facial sulcus and alar nasal groove 6 months after detachment of forehead flap. Note excellent symmetry achieved by using two separate flaps to reconstruct separate aesthetic regions of the central face.

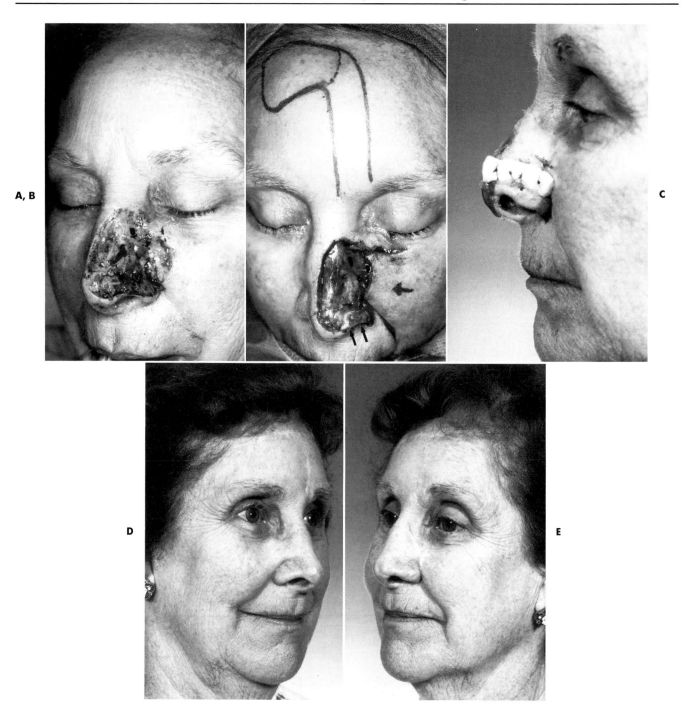

A, B

C

D

E

Figure 17-27   *A,* A 6- × 8-cm defect of the lateral lower nose involving the alar nasal groove and nasal facial sulcus following resection of a basal cell carcinoma. A transposition flap from the cheek is designed to reconstruct the defect. An auricular composite graft is sutured in place to repair a small defect of the internal nasal lining and upper lateral cartilage. *B,* The flap transposed, a portion of the standing cutaneous deformity is excised at the superior aspect of the flap. *C, D,* Five months postoperative. Note persistent standing cutaneous deformity and marked distortion of the nasal facial sulcus. *E,* Proposed incision line to recreate the alar nasal groove and nasal facial sulcus. *F,* Following removal of fibrofatty tissue, the cephalic edge of the wound is advanced under the caudal edge and sutured to deep tissue. The caudal edge of the wound is allowed to heal by second intention. The incision near the lower eyelid is the result of excising the remaining standing cutaneous deformity.

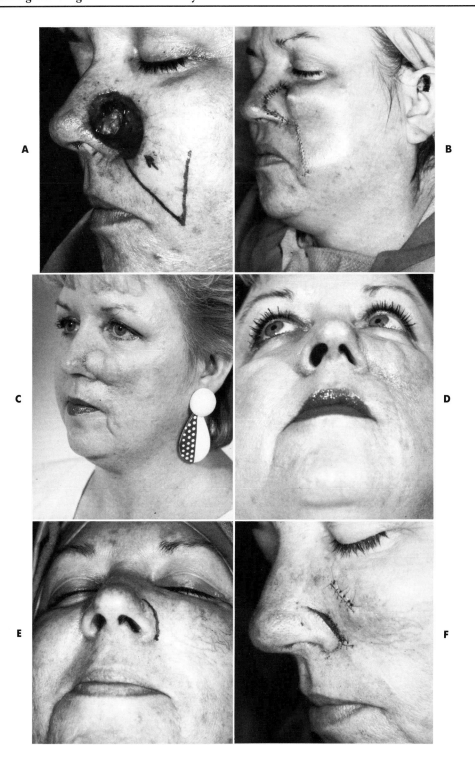

Continued.

Figure 17-27, cont'd   *G, H,* **About 2½ years after revision surgery.** *I, J,* **Oblique view of right and reconstructed left nasal facial sulcus 2½ years after revision surgery. Resemblance of the nasal facial sulcus is noted, but the appearance is not completely natural.**

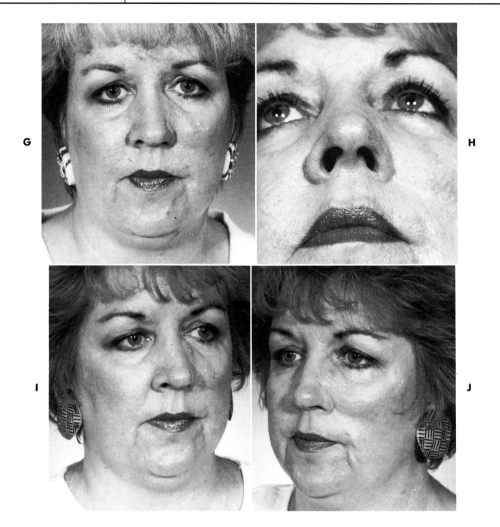

obliteration of the alar facial sulcus will occur, and it must be restored through additional operations. This usually involves multiple surgical procedures and only limited success.

The need to restore the nasal facial sulcus occurs when a cheek flap is placed across the sulcus in situations where the flap has been used to reconstruct the sulcus and portions of the lateral nose. Attempts to restore the contour of the nasal facial sulcus can begin approximately 3 to 6 months after transfer of the flap. An incision is made in the skin of the flap corresponding to the identical position and configuration of the contralateral nasal facial sulcus and alar nasal groove. The cephalic skin edge is undermined for 2 to 3 cm, and scar and fibrofatty tissue is removed in the region corresponding to the proposed nasal facial sulcus and alar-nasal groove. The cephalic edge of the wound is

then advanced under the caudal edge and sutured to deep tissue. The caudal edge of the wound is allowed to heal by secondary intention (Fig. 17-27). It may also be helpful to use deep sutures tied over bolsters in an attempt to eliminate dead-space after debulking of scar and fibrofatty tissue. This helps to create a concavity simulating the alar facial sulcus and nasal alar groove.

In other instances, the inferior border of standard transposition cheek flaps used to repair lateral nasal defects often causes a webbing or bridle scar across the nasal facial sulcus. This is best managed by Z-plasty combined with debulking of underlying scar and soft tissue. The long diagonal arm of the Z should be designed to lie along the linear axis of the bridle scar or web; 60-degree triangular flaps are then designed, incised, and transposed.

18

RECONSTRUCTION OF THE LIP

Gregory Renner

The upper and lower lips comprise a distinct anatomic unit that is the principal feature of the lower face and has great functional and aesthetic importance. Restoration of the lip can sometimes present a considerable challenge to the reconstructive surgeon who seeks excellence in both cosmesis and function. Descriptions of lip reconstruction date back to at least 1000 B.C., where surgical procedures have been found in the eastern Sanskrit writings of Susruta.[1,2] Early reports of lip reconstruction in the Western literature date back to at least the first century (Fig. 18-1).[1] Initial description of the classic V-shaped lip repair is credited to a writing by Louis in 1768, though it is almost certain that such repair was performed much earlier.[1] Reconstructive procedures for the lip received a great deal of attention during the nineteenth century, when most of the basic designs for lip repair were reported. Nearly all of the designs for lip reconstruction that are in current use have origins that date back to that time.

ANATOMY

Lip tissue is a composite of skin, muscle, and mucosa (Fig. 18-2). The hallmark feature of lip tissue is the vermilion, which covers the rounded free margin of the mouth opening. Vermilion is a modified mucosa that is adapted to the external environment. The submucosal plane of the vermilion is devoid of minor salivary glands, in contrast to the buccal submucosal plane, which has numerous glands. The anterior limit of the vermilion is defined by the mucocutaneous or "vermilion" line. The posterior limit of the vermilion is defined by the innermost point of contact between the opposing upper and lower lips when the mouth is closed. Labial vermilion is characteristically red among those of light skin color and is pigmented among blacks. Fullness of the rounded vermilion is considered a mark of beauty in many cultures.

Figure 18-1   A method of reconstruction for a large defect of the lower lip as described by Celsus in the first century A.D. (From Fritze HE, Reich OFG: Die Plastische Chirurgie, Berlin, 1845, Hirschwald.)

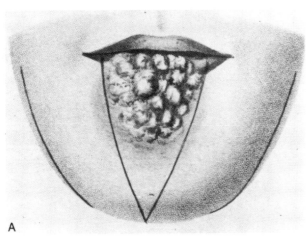

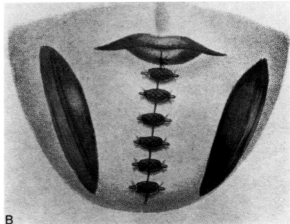

A

B

The body of the lip is made up principally of the orbicularis oris muscle. Orbicularis muscle fibers of the upper and lower lip decussate as they meet on each side at the oral commissures, which allows the muscle to form a functional sphincter around the mouth opening. The many different muscles of facial expression are distributed as bilaterally paired sets, which are mirror imaged on each side of the face and oriented in a radiant fashion around the orbicularis oris muscle sphincter. Each muscle set is attached at specific points along the outer margin of the orbicularis oris muscle, and their selective contractions cause modification in the shape of the lips, producing the many different lip configurations. Since it has no direct skeleton, lip tissue tends to be very elastic and can normally be stretched to a remarkable degree, a trait that is very favorable for reconstructive surgery.

The outline of the upper lip is well defined by the base of the nose centrally and on each side by the melolabial sulcus (Fig. 18-3). The inferior margin of the lower lip is defined by the mental crease. These peripheral crease lines may be barely discernable in infants and very young children but become much more pronounced with advancing age and, in general, are very well-established natural lines on the face. The melolabial sulcus and mental crease lines closely approximate the sites where the different muscles of facial expression attach to the orbicularis oris muscle. They also approximate the points where the lip tissue has indirect connection to the facial skeleton. These

lines are strongly favored sites for placement of the incisions that are necessary for wide excision of lip tumors and for various reconstructive flaps of the lip.

Also important to aesthetic planning of lines for surgical incisions are the relaxed skin tension lines about the lip (see Fig. 18-3). The lines of relaxed skin tension of the lip are oriented in a radiant fashion about the mouth opening, extending from the vermilion to the melolabial sulcus and mental crease lines in a pattern similar to the spokes of a wheel. They are vertical in central portions of the lip and progressively more oblique in more lateral portions of the lip. The lines of relaxed skin tension are reflected in the rhytids, which are commonly seen about the lips with more advanced age. The raised filtrum of the upper lip is oriented vertically and is compatible also with the relaxed skin tension lines of that region. Elective incisions made across the body of either lip are much more likely to be natural appearing and camouflaged if they are made in parallel with the relaxed skin tension lines.

The lips have several motor functions, which include the many different facial expressions, continence of food and liquids in the mouth, articulation of speech, and the actions of whistling and kissing. They are also important in facial aesthetics. The lips have the important functions of sensing touch, pain, and temperature and serve to monitor materials that are about to enter the mouth. The most ideal reconstructions of the lip

Figure 18-2 Composite lip structure showing *(from right to left)* skin, muscle, and mucosa.

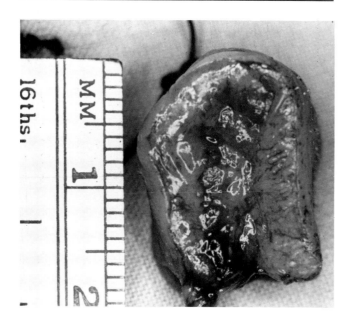

Figure 18-3 Closeup view of the lip unit. Anatomic borders of the lip are strongly represented by the melolabial sulcus on each side and by the mental crease inferiorly. Rhytid lines about the lips parallel lines of relaxed skin tension, which have a radiant pattern about the mouth opening.

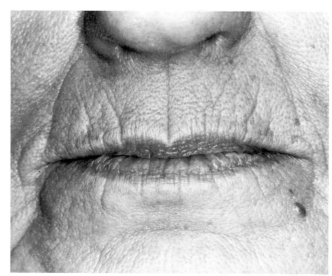

are those that best preserve or restore these many different functions. Restoration of the orbicularis muscle sphincter is highly desirable, particularly in the lower lip. As a general rule it is best if reconstructions of the lip can be designed from within the lip unit itself unless doing so would create excessive microstomia. Patients who require dentures may have a greater need for mouth opening. Reconstructions of slightly more than one half of either lip can in most cases be accomplished satisfactorily using tissues from within

the lip unit alone. When the need for additional tissue exceeds this, the most common reconstructions involve the use of local flaps harvested from the adjacent cheeks or chin. With current designs, any flap tissue taken from outside the lip unit is not able to restore a full, functional orbicularis oris muscle. For the sake of oral continence, muscle restoration in the upper lip is a little less important than it is in the lower lip because the upper lip functions more like a curtain, while the lower lip functions more like a dam.

Figure 18-4   *A,* Lower lip with vermilion defect following micrographic resection of superficial squamous cell carcinoma and surrounding zone of in situ changes. There is also some loss of lower lip skin. *B,* Labial mucosal flap is being elevated and readied for anterior advancement. Dissection is deep to the minor salivary glands and immediately above the orbicularis muscle. *C,* Mucosal flap is now advanced forward to anterior skin margin. In this case it was felt that the skin margin would migrate cephalad as scar tissue matured beneath the flap, which would result in a reasonably natural placement of the anterior vermilion line. *D,* Surgical result at 4 months. There has been considerable retraction of the wound and mucosal flap. Vermilion line is acceptably placed for this elderly male. Continued maturation should further flatten vermilion line scar.

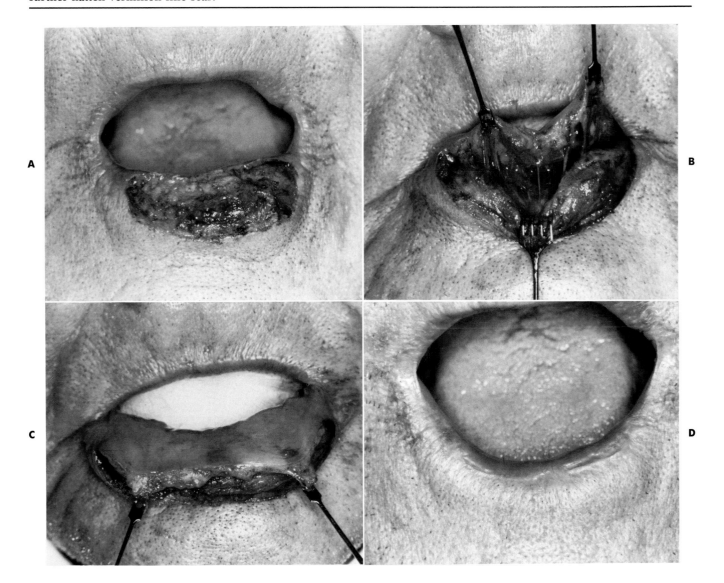

LOCAL FLAPS FOR RECONSTRUCTION OF THE VERMILION

Labial Buccal Advancement Flap

The most favored method of restoration for the vermilion surface is with forward advancement of the labial buccal mucosa (Fig. 18-4).[3] This is most commonly accomplished following a resection of the anterior vermilion for what is determined to be premalignant or very superficial malignant disease. This flap is created by undermining beneath the labial buccal mucosa in a plane deep to the minor salivary glands and immediately above the posterior surface of the orbicularis oris muscle. With careful dissection, the labial artery can be preserved and kept attached to the muscle tissue. If necessary, dissection can be continued down the entire vertical length of the lip into the apex of the buccal sulcus. The mucosal flap is then advanced forward over the free margin of the lip and brought to the anterior vermilion line, where it is sutured. Care should be taken while approximating the wound margins so that the anterior vermilion line will have a natural appearance after full wound maturation.

Replacement of the vermilion with a labial buccal advancement flap can produce an immediately pleasing aesthetic restoration to either lip. However, there are numerous difficulties encountered with this technique, which must be understood when selecting and designing this method of repair. Many times the vermilion line cannot be easily restored to its exact original position because the needs for resection may have required encroachment into the area of the lip skin.[3] Elderly patients who have had a great deal of ultraviolet light exposure tend to have fading of the vermilion line over time, which makes it less defined. The reconstructed vermilion will have a reddish color, similar to vermilion, but will often have an even deeper erythema. A deeper red color is rarely of concern in females but can be a problem in males, especially if the restoration results in a wider vermilion surface.

The larger the vermilion defect, the greater the demand upon the advancement flap. With a greater amount of dissection there will be more fibrosis beneath the flap, which will tend to cause retraction of the restored vermilion as scar maturation occurs. In some cases this will produce a more rounded appearance to the lip. As the vermilion line is pulled inward, whisker hairs may also be turned in and become a source of irritation to the opposing lip when the mouth is closed.

One of the most common complaints made by patients who have had vermilion reconstruction is that the sensory return is never quite perfect. Though they regain usable sensations of touch, pain, and temperature, it is common that many years later patients are still bothered by a relative sense of numbness in the reconstructed vermilion. This holds true for virtually any repair of vermilion using a flap.

Mucosal V-Y Advancement Flap

Small volume deficiencies of the vermilion can be augmented to some degree with vertical V-Y advance-

Figure 18-5 *A,* **A triangular advancement is planned for correction of a small deficiency of the vermilion.** *B,* **With direct closure behind the advancement flap, a Y-shaped pattern is developed.**

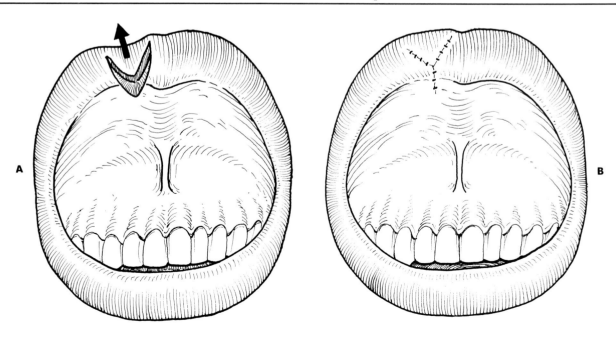

ment of buccal mucosa (Fig. 18-5).[2] The tissue to be mobilized is outlined with a V-shaped incision, of which the apex is placed along the posterior limit of the site that is deficient. Release of the tissue within the V is done by raising up a flap of mucosa above the plane of the orbicularis muscle and labial artery. This triangular unit of tissue is then advanced forward to augment the deficient region with additional soft tissue. Closure of the donor site is in a primary fashion with side-to-side approximation that serves to push the V-shaped flap forward and create the shape of a Y configuration as the wound closure is completed.

Cross-Lip Mucosal Flap

Defects of the labial vermilion can also be restored utilizing a cross-lip transfer of labial buccal mucosa.[2] These transfers may be accomplished using a single pedicle for smaller defects and a double or bilateral "bucket handle" type of pedicle for larger defects involving most of the length of the lip (Figs. 18-6, 18-7). A cross-lip mucosal flap is typically elevated as a linear band of mucosa harvested from an area behind the posterior vermilion line of the donor lip. The width

of this band is determined by the width of the vermilion defect. The mucosal flap is elevated at the level of the orbicularis muscle. For larger repairs the labial artery can be incorporated into the flap for an axial circulation. The flap is transferred across the open mouth and into the opposing vermilion defect. It is fixed into place with interrupted surface sutures, and the donor site is closed primarily. The pedicle can be taken down in approximately 2 weeks as a simple second procedure.

Tongue Flap

The mucosal surface of the anterior tongue can also be used to restore vermilion (Fig. 18-8).[4,5] When taken from the dorsal and lateral surfaces of the tongue, the glossal mucosa will contain the many fine papilla that are characteristic of the tongue surface. Still it will replace vermilion with a red-colored mucosal surface and can be surprisingly satisfactory for vermilion restoration. In restoration of the lower lip it is more common to design the flap from the under surface of the tongue and utilize a superior pedicle. The leading edge of the flap is then sewn to the anterior portion of

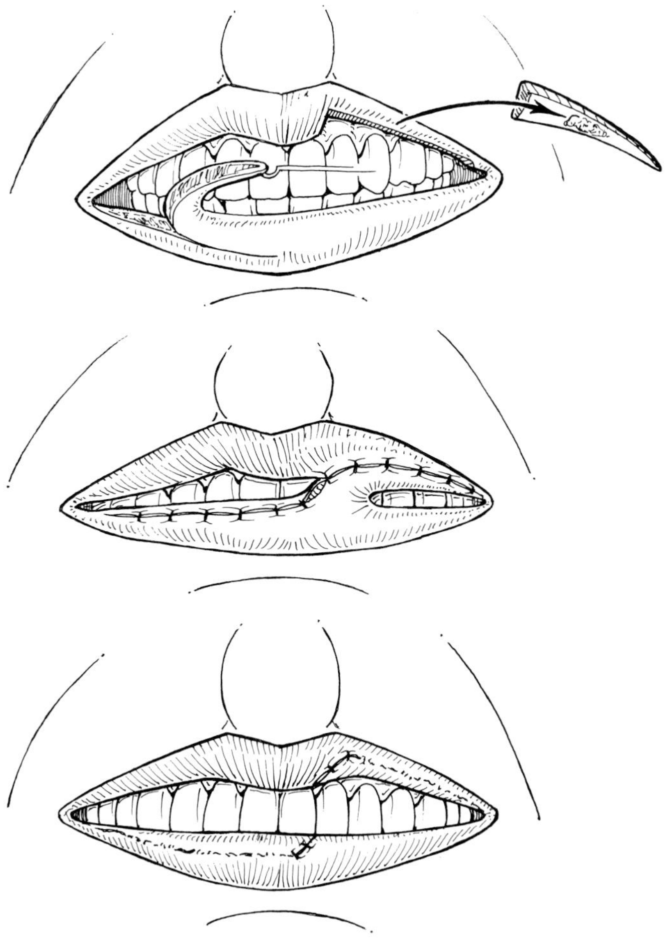

Figure 18-6   *A,* **Vermilion flap with a single pedicle being raised and about to be transferred to the opposing lip.** *B,* **Cross-lip vermilion flap sutured in place with vascular pedicle left intact.** *C,* **Surgical result following later transection of the pedicle.**

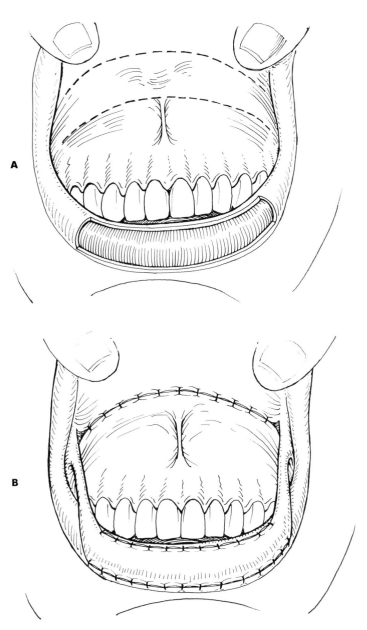

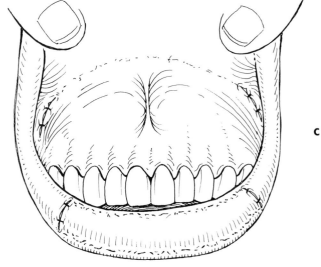

Figure 18-7 *A,* Wide defect of lower lip vermilion. A flap is designed with dotted outline for harvest of labial mucosa from the upper lip with bilateral pedicles. *B,* Bipedicled flap transferred to lower lip defect and sutured into place. Pedicles will be released at a second stage. *C,* Lower lip and donor site upon completion of mucosal transfer.

the vermilion defect. Complete attachment to the posterior portion of the defect is only possible after division of the tongue pedicle at a second stage. The donor site on the tongue is typically allowed to granulate. In replacement of vermilion defects of the upper lip, an inferiorly based tongue flap would typically be used, which would be pedicled on the ventral surface of the tongue.

Tongue flaps in general are awkward and are difficult for the patient. They are not usually considered as a first-line choice for vermilion reconstruction. Still they hold a useful place in the armamentarium of local flaps for vermilion repair.

Vermilion Advancement Flap

Full-thickness defects of only the vermilion portion of the lip are not common. When they involve less than one third the width of the lip, it is possible to perform reconstruction with a sliding advancement of the remaining vermilion (Fig. 18-9).[2,6] A full-thickness incision is made at the vermilion line anteriorly and immediately beneath the labial artery posteriorly. This flap will then include the vermilion portion of the orbicularis muscle. The release for this flap may have to be relatively long in order to allow for the appropriate stretch of the vermilion. A meticulous closure is important to achieve a relatively natural look.

Figure 18-8   *A,* Defect of lower lip vermilion and outline for superiorly based tongue flap. *B,* Lower margin of tongue donor site can be anchored to inner margin of lip defect. *C,* Tongue flap is placed into vermilion defect and secured with sutures. The superiorly based pedicle is maintained. *D,* In a few weeks the pedicle is transected, and the tongue flap is completely transferred to the lip.

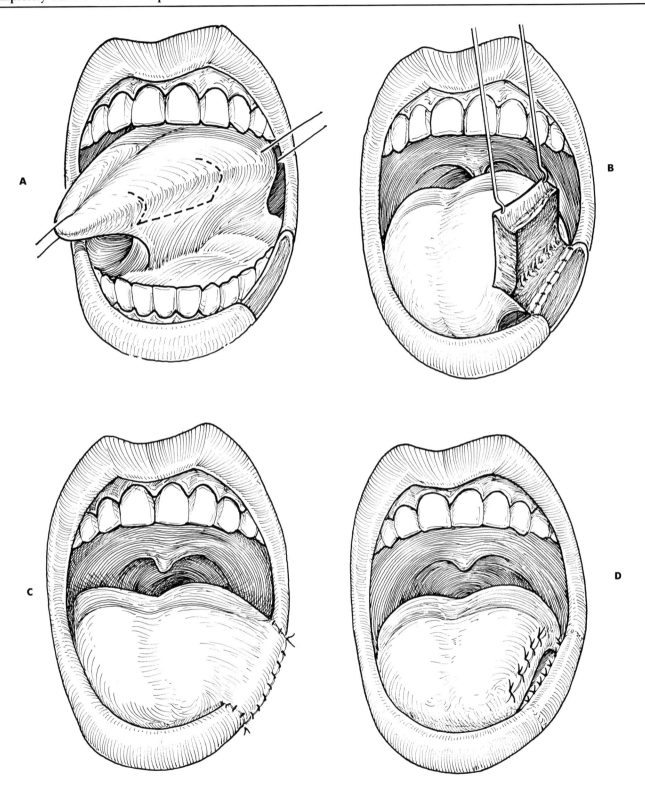

Figure 18-9   *A,* Full-thickness defect of vermilion. Reconstruction is accomplished with direct advancement of the remaining full-thickness vermilion from the side of the lip with greater length. A long releasing incision is made. *B,* Full-thickness vermilion flap is advanced to opposite wound margin and sutured into place. *C,* Full-thickness defect of vermilion, which includes superior portion of orbicularis muscle and some lip skin. Full-thickness lip flap incised to repair skin and muscle defect. A second vermilion flap is incised to repair vermilion defect. *D,* Lip flap transposed. Vermilion flap is advanced. *E,* Lip repair completed.

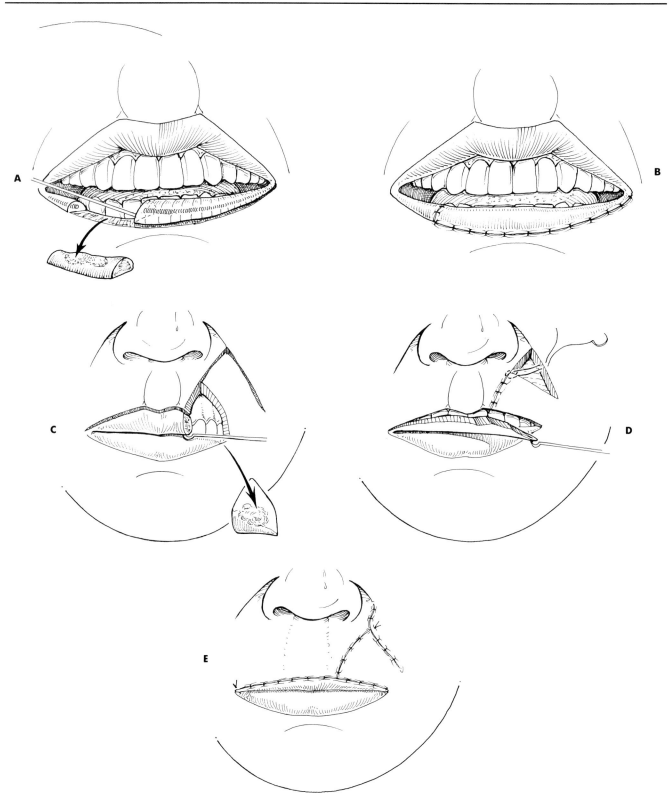

LOCAL FLAPS FOR CUTANEOUS AND FULL-THICKNESS LIP RECONSTRUCTION

When planning excisions of malignancies of the lip it is important to determine whether adequate resection can be accomplished with full-thickness excision or with excision that is more limited in depth. Most cancers that arise in the skin of the lip require resection of only skin and some amount of subcutaneous tissue. Reconstructions of the skin of the lip are performed following principles similar to those applied in cutaneous surgery at other sites. Similar principles apply also to full-thickness lip repair. Respect for anatomic units and for the relaxed skin tension lines is very important as the principles of facial aesthetics are applied to reconstructive surgery of the lip.

Fusiform Repair

Fusiform excision and direct repair remains the preferred method for dealing with simple cutaneous lesions of the lip. Ideally, fusiform design on the lip should be oriented so that the long axis is in parallel with the relaxed skin tension lines (Fig. 18-10).[3] For the sake of aesthetics it is best when the fusiform design can be confined to within lip borders, avoiding extension beyond the melolabial sulcus or mental crease. When there is demand for larger excisions, the need to extend the fusiform-shaped excision beyond the crease lines can often be avoided with the use of M-plasty design (see Fig. 18-10).[3] In this fashion the closure of two smaller adjacent triangles can be accomplished within the lip unit, avoiding the need for extension beyond the borders of the lip. M-plasty may also be used to avoid extending a fusiform excision beyond the mucocutaneous line and onto the vermilion. In some cases, however, the relative redundancy that is left in the vermilion may present more of an aesthetic problem than if the fusiform excision had included a portion of the vermilion.

Labial Transposition Flap

Repair of small cutaneous defects located in the lower part of the upper lip can be accomplished with the use of a transposition flap involving the more lateral portion of the lip.[4] The lateral margin of this flap is made along the melolabial sulcus, while the medial margin is made along the lateral side of the defect and extends upward to meet the lateral margin of the flap at a point higher along the melolabial sulcus (Fig. 18-11). The pedicle remains in the lower lateral portion of the upper lip in the area above the oral commissure. Skin from the upper portion of the lip is then

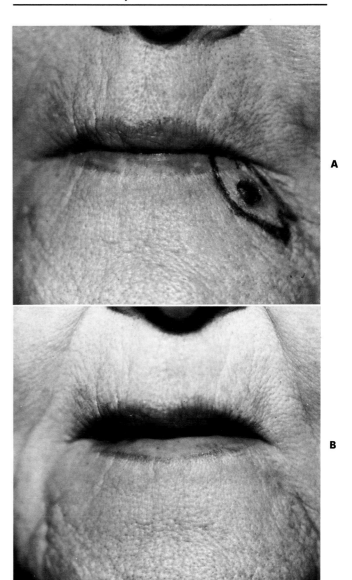

Figure 18-10   *A,* **Elderly female with cutaneous malignancy in the lateral portion of her lip. A fusiform-shaped excision with a small M-plasty on the lower end is planned. The superior margin of this excision is extended into the vermilion to allow for a more natural angle of closure.** *B,* **Surgical result at 1 year. Since the fusiform design was oriented parallel to the relaxed skin tension lines of the lip, the scar blends in well with her natural cutaneous rhytids.**

transposed into the defect on the lower part of the lip. The donor site is closed primarily, drawing the more medial portion of the upper lip skin and tissue along the melolabial sulcus together. The melolabial sulcus will commonly deviate medially to some degree as a result of the reconstruction but usually maintains a reasonably good contour unless the amount of tissue

Figure 18-11 *A,* Cutaneous defect in lower portion of the upper lip and outline for a labial transposition flap. *B,* Immediate result after transfer of the flap. The donor site scar is placed within the melolabial sulcus. *C,* Surgical result at 3 years. Melolabial sulcus is only slightly deformed, but the flap has transferred nonhair-bearing skin into the hair-bearing region of the upper lip in this male.

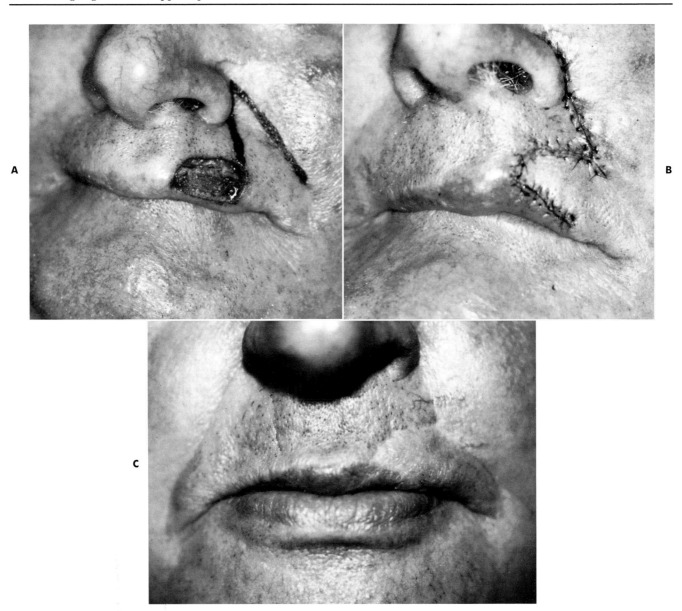

transposed is excessive. The biggest drawback to use of this flap in males is that the skin from the superior portion of the upper lip may be less bearded than skin in the lower portion of the upper lip and may present contrast.

Perilabial Transposition Flaps

Reconstruction of the lip can be done with transposition of tissues from sites immediately adjacent to the lip. Most transposition flaps involve transfer of only

skin and varying amounts of subcutaneous tissue. The facial musculature should not be violated, because it offers no significant advantage to the reconstruction and its disruption can cause considerable impairment to the motor functions of the lip.

Reconstruction of cutaneous defects in the lower lip can be accomplished using a simple transposition flap from the chin or submandibular region. These flaps can be designed with various pedicle positions (Fig. 18-12). The chin unit is a very visible structure. Careful assessment should be made as the flap is planned so

Figure 18-12   *A,* Patient with cutaneous defect of the lower lip and upper chin. A plan is drawn using a laterally based transposition flap from the chin. A second (bilobe) flap is considered if distortion of the chin should become a problem. *B,* The flap is transposed. A single flap is used.

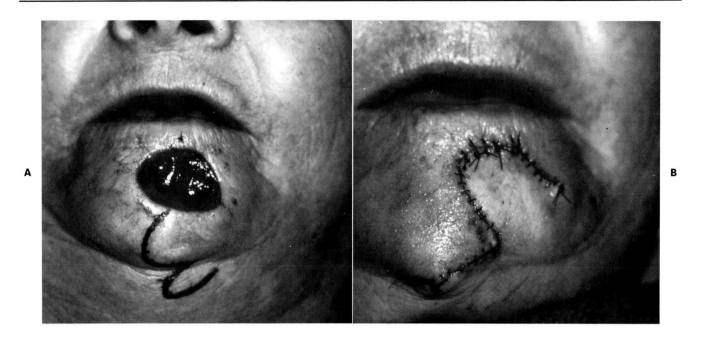

that scar lines are well placed and there is minimal distortion of the chin. Transposition flaps from the chin or submandibular region are not often a first choice for reconstruction.

The medial portion of the cheeks is immediately adjacent and readily available for lip reconstruction. The cheek has the largest size and greatest redundancy of all facial soft tissues. Transposition flaps from the cheeks are preferably designed along the melolabial sulcus. This sulcus, or crease, which separates the cheek from the lip, has been more commonly referred to as the nasolabial sulcus, but the term *melolabial* is more anatomically correct and is used in this text. The medial border of the flap is placed directly along the melolabial sulcus, and the lateral margin is placed at a desired position within the cheek (Fig. 18-13). The lateral wound margin is then advanced medially to the outer margin of the lip as the donor site is closed, and the melolabial crease line is restored.

Melolabial flaps are random in pattern with respect to their subdermal circulatory supply. Though there are sizable blood vessels that course along the side of the nose, they lie in a very deep plane and are not typically included in most melolabial flaps. A majority of melolabial flaps have a fairly long, narrow triangular design. A generous amount of subcutaneous tissue should be included with the flap in order to optimize its viability. Since most melolabial flaps involve the skin of the actual melolabial fold, there is an abundance

of subcutaneous tissue. It is best to avoid removing all of this, however, because there must continue to be sufficient subcutaneous tissue in this region to restore the balance to the face as the new melolabial fold is created. A change in one melolabial fold is easily compared to the unaltered fold on the opposite side.

Melolabial flaps may be pedicled superiorly for reconstruction of defects in the region of the base of the nose and central upper lip. The pedicle may be designed inferiorly for flaps to be used in reconstruction of defects involving the more lateral portions of the upper lip. Unfortunately, with either design there is disruption at some point along the melolabial sulcus due to the flap pedicle. This is much more pronounced in cases where the superior pedicle is used, because the sulcus is normally much more sharply defined in its superior portion (Fig. 18-14). There is also a considerable tendency for the triangular transposition flap to become slightly raised in a "trap-door" fashion as scar tissue matures beneath the flap and along its margins. The "trap-door" deformity can be minimized by wide undermining around the margins of the wound prior to flap transfer. A meticulous inset of the flap with wound edge eversion also helps to minimize this effect. Obliteration of the melolabial sulcus by the flap pedicle can be corrected for by later placing an incision across the pedicle and surgically recreating a sulcus, or at least a line of scar that simulates the melolabial sulcus.

When there is need for more tissue, melolabial

Figure 18-13 *A*, Plan for wide excision of nodular basal cell carcinoma of the upper lip and for reconstruction with an inferiorly based melolabial cheek flap. *B*, Immediate result after transposition of the flap. The donor site is oriented within the melolabial sulcus.

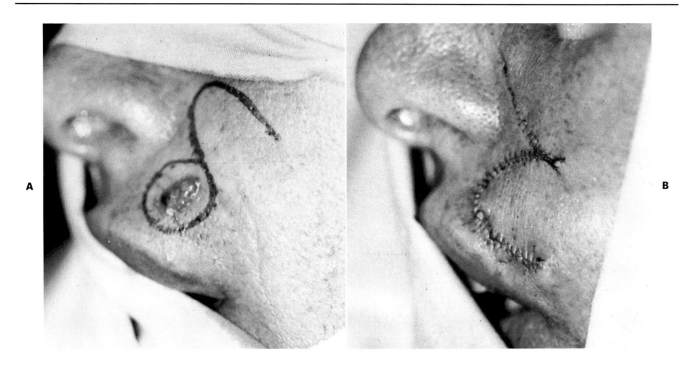

Figure 18-14 Significant deformity of the melolabial sulcus has resulted with transposition of this superiorly based melolabial flap.

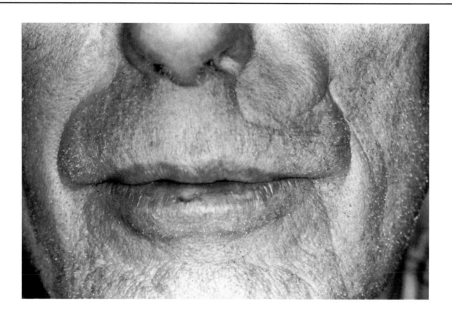

transposition flaps can be designed in a larger size. When an inferiorly based pedicle is used, the distal portion of the flap can be extended upward, lateral to the nose, to gain additional length. Flaps that have a superiorly based pedicle can be designed with even greater length by continuing the design below the level of the oral commissure. The line of the melolabial sulcus can be followed down below the commissure all the way to the submandibular region if necessary. In situations where there is concern about the vascular integrity of an extended melolabial flap, it is possible to go through one or more stages of delay prior to complete flap mobilization and transfer. When full-thickness lip reconstruction is required, a flap should be made as thick as possible, yet with avoidance of disruption to the facial musculature. Surfacing of the underside of the flap can be accomplished with various forms of mucosal flaps or grafts or with placement of a skin graft. When a delay is made prior to actual flap transposition, a graft can be buried on the undersurface for a period of 1 to 2 weeks and then transferred as a composite with the flap (Fig. 18-15).

Transposition flaps from the cheek can also be used for reconstruction of the lower lip (Fig. 18-16). Flaps can be designed with either inferiorly or superiorly based pedicles, similar to those for reconstruction of the upper lip. Those made with superiorly based pedicles have a greater pivotal arc. They can give a greater degree of upward support to the oral commissure, which offers some advantage when there is deficiency of the orbicularis muscle. Sedillot (1848) describes superiorly based flaps that were vertical in their orientation. It is preferable if the flaps can be contoured with a gentle curve to reflect the downward extension of the melolabial sulcus into the submandibular region, separating the cheek from the chin. In general, reconstruction with transposition flaps from the cheeks is less satisfactory for the lower lip than for the upper lip in situations where there is deficiency of orbicularis muscle.

Labial Rotation/Advancement Flaps

A method for reconstruction of cutaneous defects of the upper lip that provides a more natural appearance than can be achieved with most melolabial flaps involves a combination of rotation and advancement of tissue from the region of the lip lateral and inferior to the defect.[3] This flap is designed by extending an incision from the melolabial sulcus downward below

Figure 18-15   *A,* A superiorly based melolabial flap designed with a delay stage. This patient has had high doses of radiotherapy to his face for earlier treatment of upper lip malignancy. The distal portion of the flap is left attached as a second pedicle during the initial delay. A skin graft has been buried beneath the flap to provide internal lining for the full-thickness lip defect. *B,* Transposition of the composite melolabial flap. There is considerable tissue redundancy at the pedicle as the flap is transposed. This can be corrected with revision surgery in a later stage. This patient has other deficiencies still present in the nasal tip and upper lip vermilion. The donor site scar of the flap is well camouflaged along the melolabial sulcus.

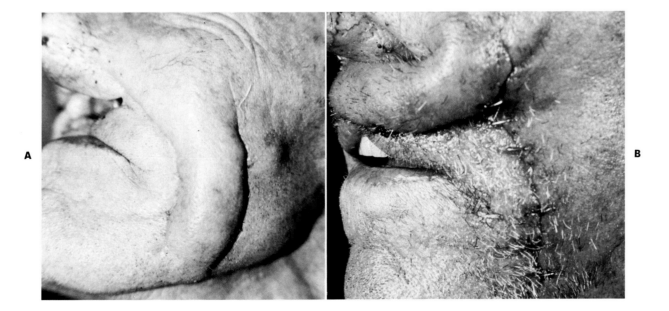

A   B

Figure 18-16 *A*, Illustration of a patient with full-thickness loss of the lower lip and plan for reconstruction with bilateral inferiorly based melolabial flaps. These flaps should be designed with as much thickness as possible while avoiding violation of the underlying facial musculature. *B, C*, Transposition of the flaps is secured, and vermilion restoration is achieved by mucosal advancement from the buccal mucosa.

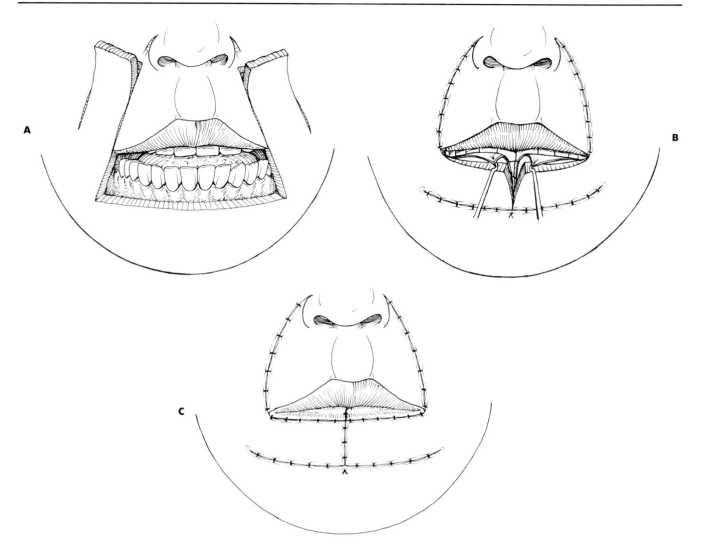

the level of the oral commissure on the involved side (Fig. 18-17). In those situations where the melolabial sulcus comes very close to the commissure, it may be necessary to extend the flap outline a short distance out into the cheek, while still attempting to create the effect of a melolabial sulcus. Careful measurement should be made of the vertical length of the lip in the area of the defect because the transferred lip tissue must at least roughly approximate this height. The lip has a natural gradual taper to its vertical length in the more lateral portions. The outline of the flap may extend a considerable distance below the commissure so that there is an easier release of tissue for the necessary

rotation and advancement of the flap into the upper lip defect.

Dissection of the flap is in a deep plane, harvesting a considerable amount of subcutaneous tissue with the flap. For repair of cutaneous defects, the flap is dissected above the plane of the facial musculature and motor nerves to the lip. Orbicularis oris muscle and buccal mucosa may be included with this flap when there is need for restoration of deep tissues.

Excessive redundancy may be noted along the cheek side of the melolabial sulcus as the flap is transferred. This can be accommodated for with resection of a small Burow's triangle of skin from the cheek at the lowest point of the incision. This flap design is best suited for repair of cutaneous defects of lateral portions of the upper lip, though it can also be used for defects that extend all the way to the philtrum. The oral commissure may be pulled upward, or a slight hooding of skin may occur over the commissure when the flap is initially transferred. Later revision of the commissure may be required; however, if the distortion is not excessive, these problems are often self-correcting as scar maturation occurs and the lips are repeatedly used in facial expression and motor activity.

The surface area requirements for the lateral labial rotation/advancement flap can be lessened by designing a simultaneous rotation/advancement flap involv-ing the skin located in the medial portion of the upper lip. The outline for this second flap is made by placing an incision medially along the melolabial sulcus and base of the nose. Tissue movement of the medial flap should be less aggressive than that of the lateral flap to reduce possible distortion of the labial philtrum and base of the nose. The simultaneous use of these two opposing flaps should be in such a fashion as to maximize the natural appearance of the lip once reconstruction is complete. When there is tissue loss that extends above or lateral to the melolabial region, that portion of the defect can be easily corrected with direct advancement of cheek skin to the position of the melolabial sulcus.

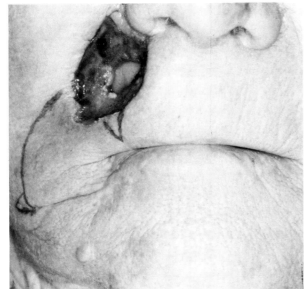

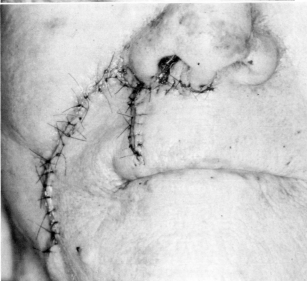

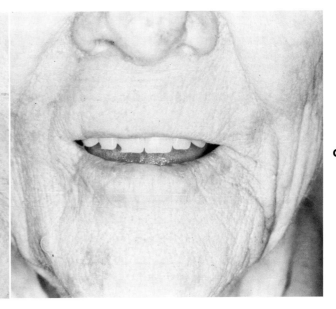

Figure 18-17 *A,* **Patient with a defect of right upper lip from micrographic resection of a cutaneous malignancy. A portion of the defect is full thickness. Mucosal tissue can be closed primarily. Most of her orbicularis muscle remains intact. Cutaneous reconstruction is achieved with a laterally based labial rotation/advancement flap. The primary movement of this flap is by rotation, although some degree of advancement also occurs.** *B,* **The flap is transferred. A minimal degree of advancement of tissue from the central portion of the upper lip has also been utilized. Only a minimal amount of tissue movement is permissible from the central region of the upper lip; otherwise distortion of the labial philtrum and base of the nose can result. Note that the oral commissure has been turned up considerably with this flap because the pivot point was a short distance medial to the actual commissure.** *C,* **Surgical result at 1 month. Outlines of the flap have fallen well within natural lines of the lip unit. Oral commissure has returned to its natural position, and nasal base is not distorted.**

Full-Thickness Reconstruction of the Lip with Direct Closure

Full-thickness reconstruction of the lip requires replacement of skin, muscle, and mucosa. It is highly desirable that there be restoration of the orbicularis oris muscle sphincter, particularly in the lower lip. Preservation and restoration of sensory function should also be considered when confronted with the need to achieve full-thickness reconstructions.

The wedge, or V-shaped, lip excision has long been the standard method for surgical removal of lip malignancies followed by reconstruction with direct approximation of the remaining wound margins (Fig. 18-18). This method of closure can be used with satisfactory results in most situations for defects that may be as large as one third of the width of either lip. For the sake of aesthetics, closure of the V-shaped defect should be designed in congruence with the relaxed skin tension lines of the lip. The base of the V is placed along the vermilion, and a line drawn from the center of this base to the apex should then be made parallel with the relaxed skin tension lines. In the central lip, this line would be oriented vertically with equal length given to the two lateral lines of the V. In

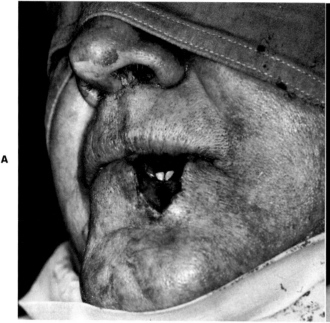

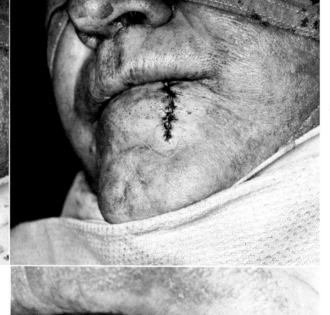

Figure 18-18   *A,* Wedge excision of a lip malignancy. V-shaped defect is closed by direct approximation of wound margins. Accurate approximation should be made of the mucosa, orbicularis muscle, subcutaneous tissue, and skin. *B,* Closure is accomplished. It would have been better if the apex of the V had been oriented in a more oblique manner compatible with the relaxed skin tension lines in this portion of the lip. *C,* In the central lip, a vertical orientation of the wedge excision is proper, but a more oblique orientation is preferred laterally.

sites more lateral in the lip, these lines become more skewed, which produces a more angulated final closure line (see Fig. 18-18**C**).

In repair of a full-thickness lip defect, specific attention should be given to approximation of the mucosa, muscle, subcutaneous tissue, and finally the skin surface, resulting in a four-layer closure. Repair of the mucosa may be done either directly or with sutures placed in a submucosal fashion. It is very important that the muscle layer be approximated well, preferably with slowly absorbed sutures. A specific approximation of the subcutaneous tissue is then performed, preferably with sutures that include a portion of the deep reticular dermis. Skin surface closure is then accomplished and should be performed in such a way as to secure a slight eversion of the edges for ideal appearance.

Early in the course of wound closure, it is best to clearly identify the anterior vermilion line so that repair can be symmetrical with respect to this point. A 6-0 nylon or silk suture is placed through the anterior vermilion line on either side of the defect, though not necessarily tied immediately. The suture can be tagged, allowing the wound margins to be either held open or closed as necessary in order to maintain a reference point as the deeper tissue layers are approximated.

Of almost equal importance is satisfactory approximation of the posterior limit of the vermilion so that there is not a visible disparity in size and shape from one side of the closure line to the other (Fig. 18-19). The lip naturally becomes thinner in its more lateral portions. This disparity can be accommodated for by a slight forward advancement of the buccal mucosa in the lateral segment and, to a lesser degree, posterior advancement of vermilion from the medial segment as the vermilion portions are approximated. It is very important that the distance between these anterior and posterior reference sutures be the same for both segments.

Careful approximation of all tissue levels is important to minimize the tendency for later contraction in the scar line. It is particularly important to obtain accurate approximation of the muscle. It should be recognized that a portion of the orbicularis oris muscle lies beneath the vermilion and gives the rounded appearance to this portion of the lip. The portion of the orbicularis muscle that lies immediately above the plane of the anterior vermilion line should be carefully approximated as well. Failure to do so will significantly increase the chance for later notching or retraction of the free margin of the lip as maturation of the scar tissue occurs.

The V-shaped excision is best designed in such a way that it extends from the vermilion all the way to the mental or melolabial sulcus in order to make for a

relatively easy angle of closure. In some cases maintaining the V-shaped design within these borders could compromise adequate tissue margins laterally, making modifications of the V design necessary. A slightly larger unit of tissue can be resected by modifying the design into a shield shape or U shape. Closure is performed in a similar manner to that of the V-shaped excision. The outline for resection of a greater amount of tissue can be accomplished while maintaining the integrity of the mental and melolabial sulcus with use of an M-plasty design, which produces the effect of a W-shaped excision in the lip and is more often referred to as W-lip excision (Fig. 18-20).[3] The two apex points of the W may be placed along the outer lip crease lines. If there is need to extend the resection beyond this point, then the reversed central apex of the W should be placed along the crease line so that this point makes a natural break between the single proximal line crossing the lip and the two divergent distal lines of the closed W. In some situations it may be preferable that the two angles of the W be of dissimilar size. With W-shaped excision in lateral portions of the lip, the most favored angulation of the closure line may be more easily accomplished using a smaller angle medially and a slightly larger one laterally (Fig. 18-21).

Figure 18-19   Patient 1 year following *V*-shaped excision of a malignancy from the right lower lip. Vermilion of the lateral lip is not as thick as that of the central portion. This disparity has been well accommodated for in this *V*-shaped repair. Note also that orientation of the scar line is oblique and compatible with the rhytid lines in this lateral portion of the lip.

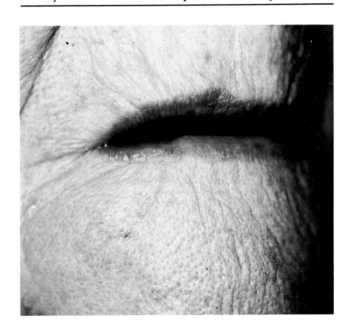

Figure 18-20   *A,* Patient with squamous cell carcinoma of right lower lip. A *W*-shaped design is planned for his resection. Primary wound repair is planned, but a dotted line shows a potential alternate reconstruction with advancement flaps. The central apex of the *W* has been placed at the point of the mental crease, which is a natural point from which the two lateral apex lines can diverge. *B,* Primary wound closure of the *W*-shaped defect is performed. A 6-0 nylon suture has been placed in the anterior vermilion line of both segments. It is not tied initially but serves as a useful reference point in assessing approximation of adjacent tissues.

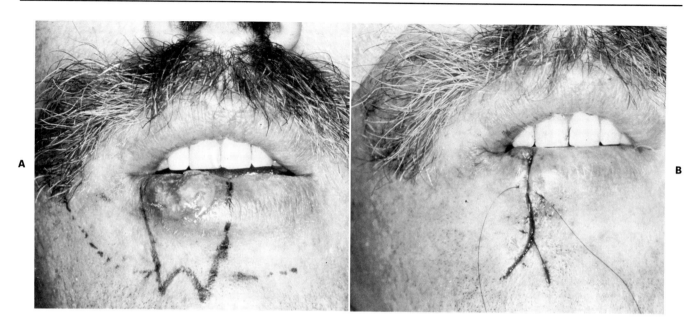

Figure 18-21   *A,* Elderly female who had radiotherapy to the lip as a child for a hemangioma. She is shown here in later life with atrophy of the left side of her lower lip and a large vascular lesion. A plan is made for removal with a *W*-shaped excision. Note that apexes of the *W* are of different sizes and are skewed laterally to be kept congruent with the relaxed skin tension lines in this region. *B,* Surgical result at 6 months. There is still some asymmetry in her lower lip, but much less than had been present preoperatively. The *W*-shaped scar is reasonably well camouflaged.

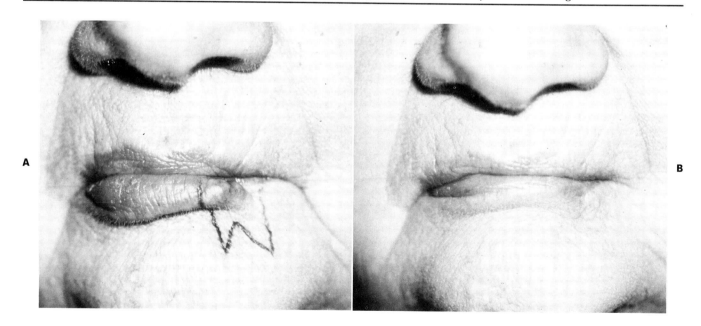

Opposing Lip Advancement Flaps

Reconstruction of rectangular full-thickness defects of either the lower or upper lip may be achieved with simultaneous opposing advancement of the remaining lip segments.[3,7] Bilateral opposing advancement flaps of the lower lip are created by releasing the remaining lip tissue with an incision made along the mental crease (Figs. 18-22, 18-23).[8] The incision should curve gently downward on each side following the upper margin of the chin unit. A full-thickness incision is traditionally made at this site, though it is generally not necessary to complete the incision through mucosa for more than half the distance, because the mucosa stretches remarkably well. Approximation of the two flaps is in a manner similar to that described for V-shaped lip repair. If excessive redundancy appears to be present along the upper margin of the chin as the lip flaps are advanced, it can be accommodated for with removal of a small Burow's triangle from the chin side of the incision at one or both sides.

A similar procedure with bilateral opposing advancement flaps can be used for reconstruction of the upper lip. To facilitate advancement of upper lip tissue, small crescent-shaped excisions of skin lateral to the nasal ala are necessary on each side (Fig. 18-24).[1,9] This maneuver in essence is the removal of Burow's triangles, which facilitates advancement of the flaps beneath the base of the nose to produce a natural appearance in the lip. Traditional advancement flap reconstruction of the upper lip does not provide restoration of the philtrum.

Bilateral opposing advancement flaps are best suited for restoration of central defects of the lower or upper lip and less ideal for repair of defects in more lateral locations. The reconstructed lip will tend to be tighter than the opposing lip, which may become more obvious when the lips are closed. The tightness will tend to lessen over time as the reconstructed lip stretches. If the disparity is excessive, it can produce an unpleasant aesthetic effect. Patients who are edentulous will tend to display a stronger tendency for the reconstructed lip to turn inward. Defects of up to 40% of the width of the lip can usually be restored very well with this method of repair. When defects are greater than 40% of the width of the lips it is usually best to consider methods of reconstruction that add more tissue to the lip. With experience one can assess whether closure with simple advancement flaps will be acceptable. Some clinicians use a prosthetic lip stretching appliance or employ a regular program of manual lip stretching to help improve upon lips made excessively tight with this method of repair.

Figure 18-22   *A,* **Rectangular-shaped excision from central lower lip. Plan is for reconstruction with bilateral opposing advancement flaps of the remaining lip segments.** *B,* **Opposing advancement flaps are brought together in the midline, and a sutured closure is begun. It is often surprising how much stretch is possible with these bilateral flaps, with only a limited releasing incision along the mental crease. The natural chin unit is preserved with this design.**

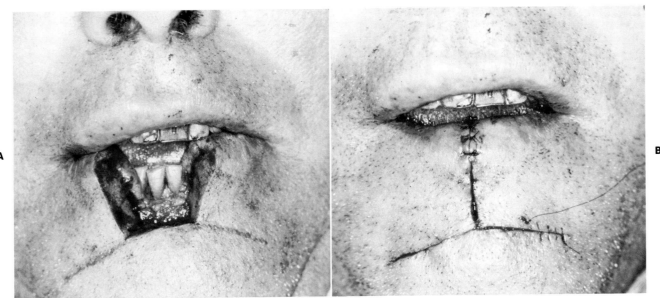

Figure 18-23   *A*, Elderly male with exophytic squamous cell carcinoma of the central lower lip. *B*, Same patient 1 week after a rectangular shaped excision of this lesion and reconstruction with bilateral opposing advancement flaps. The lower lip is slightly tighter than the upper lip, but not seriously so.

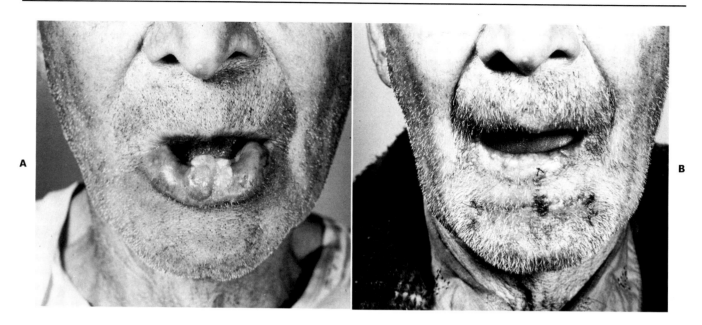

A variation on classic advancement flap repair of the lower lip employs a bilateral stair-step design (Fig. 18-25).[10,11,12] This method of repair was first reported by Isaksson and Johanson.[1] The lip tumor is removed in a rectangular-shaped excision. A series of squares or rectangular excisions is made, connected in a downward diagonal fashion. At the termination of the outline on each side is a small triangular excision. As the lip segments are advanced medially for wound closure, the series of rectangles and terminal triangles are closed in a "stair-step" design. Straight line scar contracture is prevented. This is a novel and functional method of repair but creates a scar that is not as natural to the lower face as one placed along the mental crease.

Circumoral Advancement-Rotation Flaps

Full-thickness or composite lip tissue can be transferred around the oral commissures either unilaterally or with bilateral opposing flaps. Such a method of reconstruction was first described in 1857 by von Bruns (Fig. 18-26).[1] It is more commonly employed in lower lip reconstruction but may also be used for reconstruction of the upper lip. The incision for this repair is placed along the mental crease and then carried around the oral commissures and into the melolabial sulcus on each side. This can also be accomplished in a reverse direction for upper lip repair. The lip flaps are designed so that the width of the flaps from the vermilion line to the outer incision is similar in each

Figure 18-24   *A*, Patient with large squamous cell carcinoma of the nasal columella and upper lip with plan for surgical resection. Resection will include a portion of the nasal columella and the premaxilla, though sparing the alveolar process and gingiva. An immediate reconstruction was not performed because it was determined best to wait for permanent section studies to be more certain of the surgical margins. *B*, Reconstruction with bilateral opposing advancement flaps is planned. Small crescents have been drawn lateral to the nasal ala on each side. Tissue within these crescents is normally resected to allow easy advancement of flaps beneath the nose. *C*, Advancement flaps are approximated. In this case, tissue within the crescents was preserved and transferred with the flaps to help reconstruct the anterior nasal floor. *D*, Completed reconstruction. Some areas within the nose are left to heal by second intention. *E*, *F*, Two months postoperative. Scars are well camouflaged along lateral borders of nose and melolabial sulcuses. This patient wears a beard, which provides even better scar camouflage.

Figure 18-24   For legend see opposite page

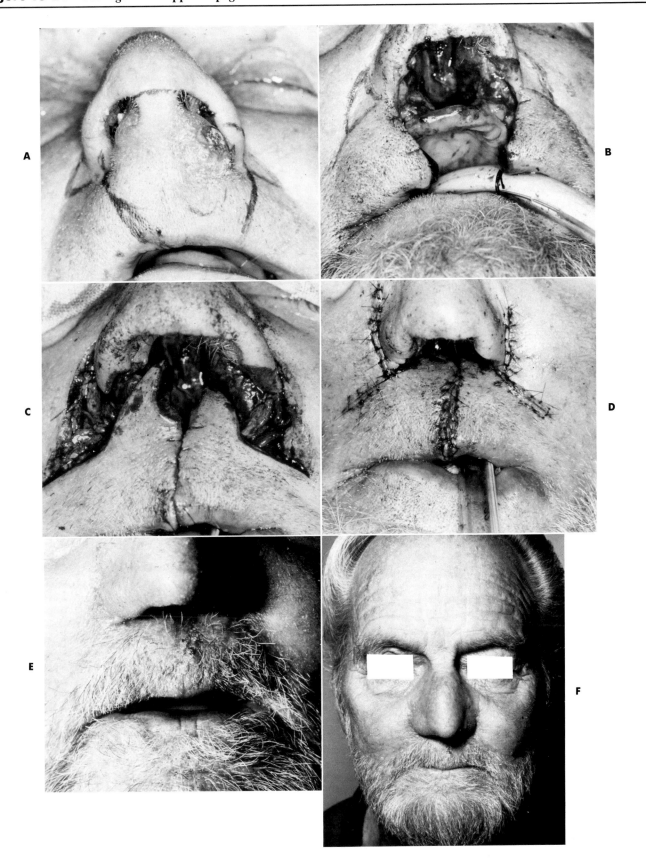

Figure 18-25   *A*, Rectangular-shaped excision of a malignancy is performed from central portion of lower lip. A bilateral stair-step repair is designed. *B*, Closure of stair-step repair.

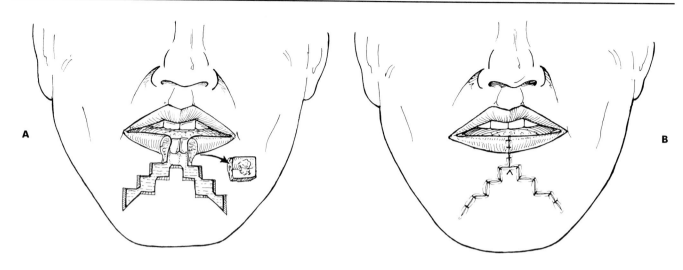

Figure 18-26   Reconstructive surgery of the lip using circumoral advancement-rotation flaps as originally described by von Bruns in his *Chirugischer Atlas* in 1857. (From von Bruns V: *Chirugischer atlas: Bildliche Darstellung der cirurgischen Krankheiten und der zu ihrer Heilung erforderlichen Instrumente, Bandagen und Operationen*, II Abt.: Kau-und Geschmaks-Organ, Tubingen, 1857/1860, Laupp.)

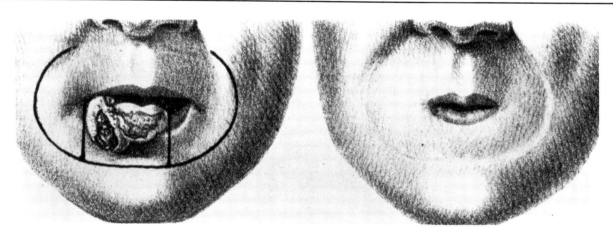

along the length of the flaps, with changes being only gradually increased or decreased. This results in an oval outline around the lip unit. The oval pattern can be adjusted slightly to accommodate for the slight progressive downward turn in the mental crease laterally and for the progressive increase in distance across the upper lip medially. Special attention must be given to maintaining appropriate width of the flap adjacent to the oral commissure. The melolabial sulcus normally comes very close to the commissure, and it is inappropriate to place incisions for the flap at this point. Near the commissure, the outline for the flap is made a short

distance out into the cheek, maintaining a similar width as in the horizontal portion of the flap.

This method of reconstruction is most ideal for restoration of central defects of the lower lip and, to a lesser degree, also of the central upper lip. Whether defects are located centrally or more laterally on the lower lip, it is my preference to create scar lines that are symmetrical with respect to the face. The opposing flap on the contralateral side of the defect can be made longer or shorter than its counterpart. In reconstruction of eccentrically located lower lip defects, it is preferable to make a longer flap of the remaining

Figure 18-27   Note rounded scar about peripheral border of lip unit with this reconstruction. Scars must be flat so that they can be well hidden, particularly where they pass around the oral commissures. The commissures also become more rounded as the musculocutaneous flaps are transferred, but this does not usually produce a significant long-term deformity.

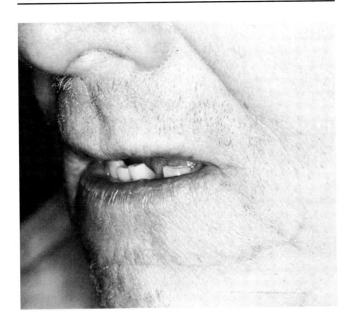

contralateral lower lip than to rotate an equal amount of tissue around the oral commissure from the ipsilateral upper lip. Once the flaps have been released, it is best to first secure the anastomosis of the two opposing flaps and then adjust the repaired lip as ideally as possible with respect to the surrounding facial parts. Care is taken to reattach the muscles of facial expression to the orbicularis oris muscle as much as possible in anatomically appropriate locations along the mobilized orbicularis oris muscle. Failure to perform meticulous wound repair will result in circumoral scars that can appear clownlike on the face (Fig. 18-27). There is a rounding or blunting of the oral commissures as the composite lip tissue is rotated around the corners of the mouth. In many, this problem will become less deforming with time. Because changes of the commissure are bilateral, they are less noticeable than if only one commissure is changed.

A significant modification of the circumoral advancement-rotation flap was described by Karapandzic in 1974.* The feature that is unique to this form of reconstruction is that a more careful dissection is made

*References 1, 2, 3, 7, 13, 14, 15.

during the separation of the deep subcutaneous tissue and the orbicularis oris muscle from the surrounding tissues. During this maneuver a dissection is made that identifies and preserves neural and vascular structures (Figs. 18-28, 18-29). With meticulous dissection, these neurovascular structures can be freed up enough to be stretched and carried with the flap. This allows patients to maintain optimal motor and sensory functions. Circumorally opposing advancement flaps can be used to reconstruct defects in some patients of as much as 60% of the width of either lip (Figs. 18-30, 18-31). However, there is some variability among patients in how easily the lip tissue can be stretched without causing excessive distortions of the oral commissures or creating microstomia. Lip tissue in older patients tends to be more redundant and more tolerant to stretching. A smaller mouth opening may not be acceptable for the patient who wears dentures and must be able to pass them in and out of the mouth easily. A small mouth opening can be stretched wider with persistent effort. This can be accomplished by having the patient place a finger in the mouth at the oral commissure on each side and make repeated attempts at stretching the mouth opening over time. Lip stretching can also be achieved with placement of a prosthetic lip expander, which can be progressively enlarged over time.[8]

Transoral Cross-Lip Flaps

Sabatinni (1836) appears to have been the first to describe a cross-lip transfer of lip tissue for full-thickness reconstruction.[1] By the turn of the century several modifications of design in cross-lip flap reconstruction had been reported. The flap design described by Sabatinni and later by Abbe (1899) involves the transfer of a triangular flap of full-thickness lip tissue from the lower lip to a defect of slightly larger size in the upper lip.[1,16,17] It is more common that there is need to use a flap from the upper lip to reconstruct a defect of the lower lip (Figs. 18-32, 18-33). The labial artery is preserved on one side of the flap to ensure viability of the tissue until it is healed in place. The flap tissue is turned 180 degrees on its pedicle, inserted into the defect of the opposing lip, and sutured into place. The donor site is then closed primarily. After 2 to 3 weeks the pedicle can be released as a minor second procedure.

Cross-lip flap design may be modified to include *W* and rectangular shapes (Figs. 18-33, 18-34, 18-35).[3,7,18,19] Determination of which side to leave pedicled seems to make little difference in most cases. The labial artery courses between the labial mucosa and orbicularis muscle just posterior to the vermilion. The pedicle necessarily includes the labial artery and a small cuff of surrounding tissue near the free margin

Text continued on p. 377.

Figure 18-28 *A,* Patient with two adjacent squamous cell carcinomas of the lower lip with plan for rectangular-shaped excision and circumoral flap repair. *B,* Reconstruction is begun with dissection of bilateral flaps. Complete incision is made through skin and immediate subcutaneous tissue. The circular fibers of the orbicularis muscle are carefully separated from the various attached facial muscles with a slow, careful dissection that preserves as many of the neural and vascular structures in this region as possible. The mucosal incisions are performed separately and not usually made more than 2 to 3 cm in length along the course of the lower lip. Note that width of the flap is kept similar throughout its length. *C,* Neurovascular structures are preserved in this dissection. The largest of these are found in the region near the commissure. Dissection of the muscles is much more difficult around the commissure because of the decussation of orbicularis muscle fibers from the upper and lower lip. *D,* Surgical result at 3 months. Size of mouth opening is adequate. The long scars are reasonably flat and inconspicuous at this point and should improve further with wound maturation.

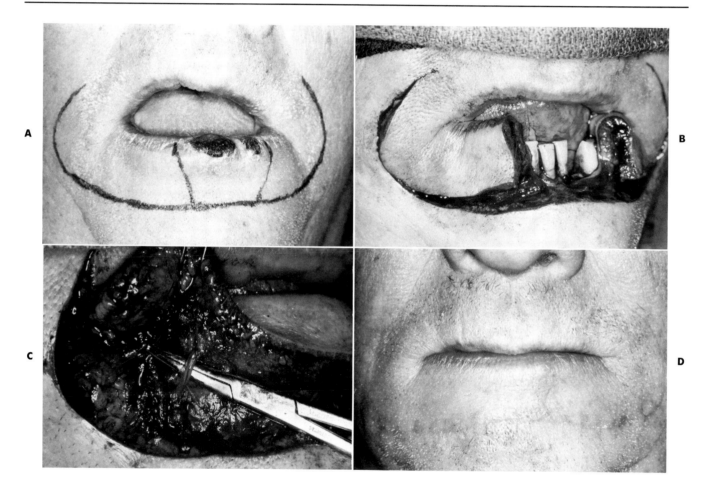

Figure 18-29   *A,* Large defect of the lower lip and commissure with plan for reconstruction with flaps as described by Karapandzic. Note that the outline for these flaps is not bilaterally symmetrical. There is also a fusiform excision planned for removal of a basal cell carcinoma near the nose in this patient. *B,* Same patient with lip defect viewed obliquely. *C,* Surgical result at 1 month. This patient has maintained good motor and sensory function during this time, and the aesthetic result is good in this early phase. *D,* Surgical result at 1 month.

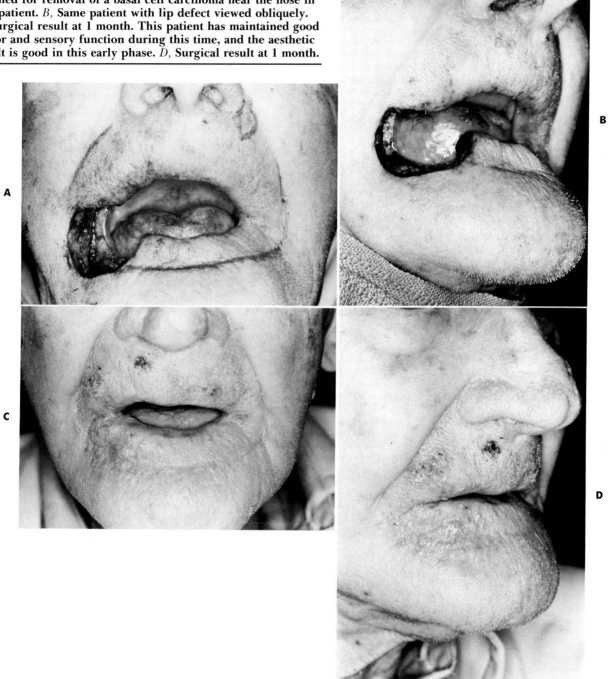

Figure 18-30 *A,* Large surgical defect of lower lip and commissure with plan for Karapandzic type of flap repair. This defect involves more than half of the lower lip. This man does not wear dentures. *B,* The flaps are dissected, and anastomosis of the lip segments is accomplished first. *C,* Much more advancement is obtained with the remaining lower lip segment than the ipsilateral upper lip segment in this case so that there will be minimal distortion of the reconstructed commissure. *D,* After anastomosis of the lip flaps, the repaired lip unit is adjusted so that there is minimal overall asymmetry or distortion prior to its attachment to the surrounding facial tissues.

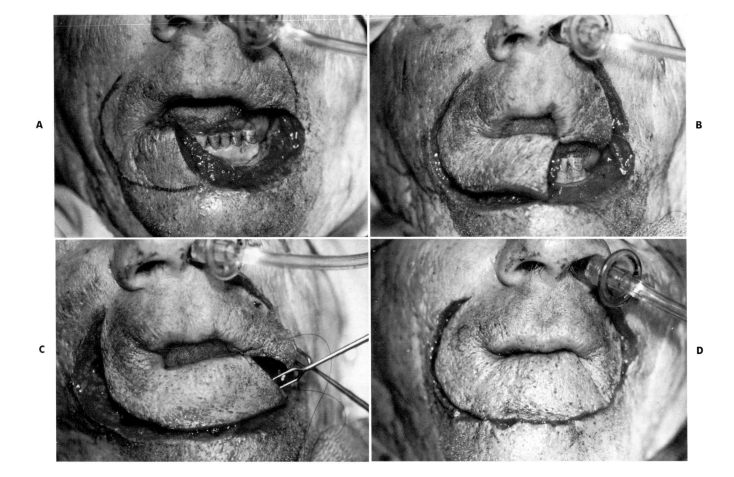

Figure 18-31   *A,* Patient who has undergone numerous previous surgeries and radiation to the midface. Karapandzic flaps are being used to help fill in a large defect of the upper lip. *B,* Immediate closure. This method of reconstruction can provide excellent tissue with motor and sensory functions. It does not offer restoration of the philtrum unless additional procedures are done.

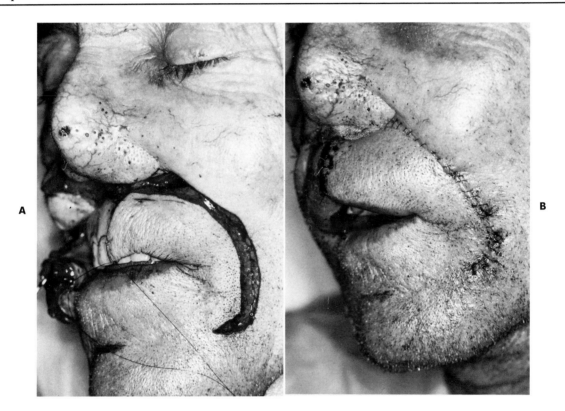

Figure 18-32   *A*, Patient with invasive squamous cell carcinoma of the lower lip with plan for wedge-shaped excision and for cross-lip flap, which is usually made of smaller size. *B*, Initial transfer of the cross-lip flap using a medially placed vascular pedicle. *C*, Illustration of the cross-lip flap in place with the vascular pedicle still preserved. *D*, Illustrated result after later stage release of the vascular pedicle.

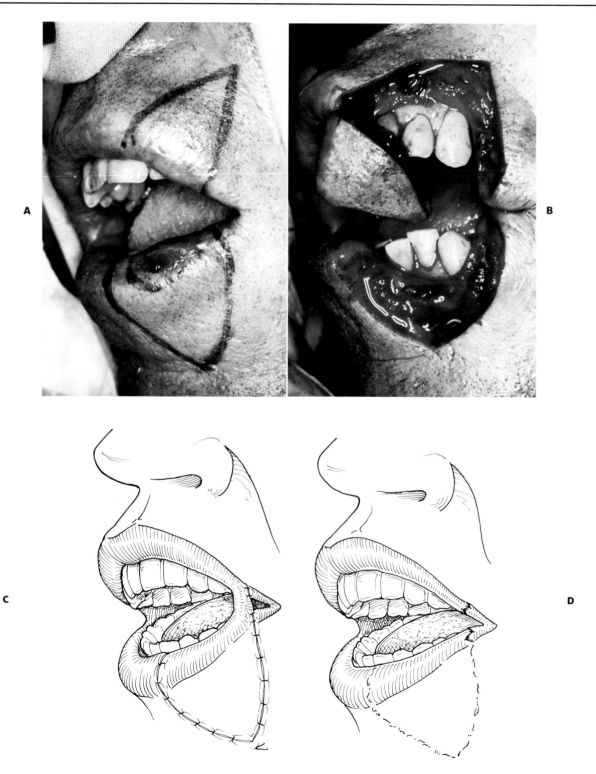

Figure 18-32, cont'd   *E-G,* Cross-lip flap used to repair right lower lip defect. Vermilion is advanced on flap to match width of vermilion at recipient site.

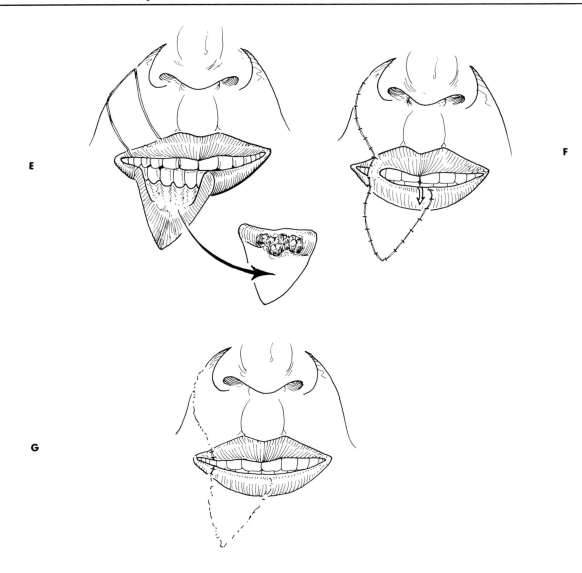

Figure 18-33 *A*, Elderly male with large squamous cell carcinoma of the lower lip. He had a vermilion resection with mucosal advancement done several years earlier. *B*, A large *W*-shaped excision is accomplished. A small area of vermilion resection was also necessary in the right part of the lip. The two points of the *W* are to be closed directly, and a triangular flap from the upper lip will be used. *C*, Surgical result at 6 months. Donor site can hardly be detected in the left upper lip. Vermilion of the cross-lip flap is more white than that of the right lower lip, which had the mucosal advancement flap placed earlier. *D*, Result at 6 months with lips in repose. Whiskers of the cross-lip flap are now directed upward because this upper lip tissue has been turned 180 degrees. Donor site scar is faintly seen in midportion of left upper lip.

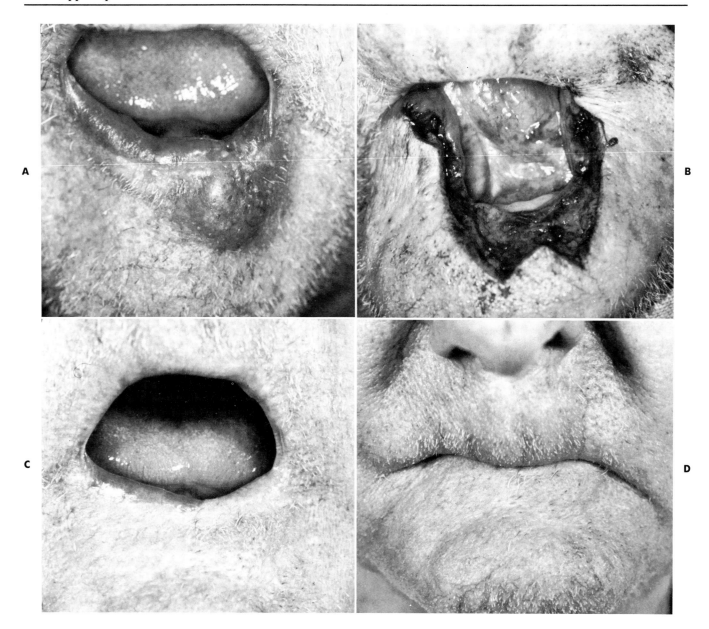

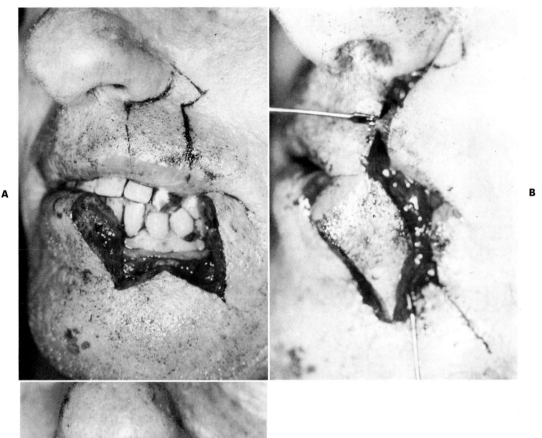

Figure 18-34   *A, W*-shaped excision has been accomplished. A rectangular-shaped flap is designed in the upper lip, lateral to the philtrum. A small crescent is also drawn lateral to the nasal ala because removal of this tissue allows more natural advancement of lateral portion of the lip for donor site closure. *B,* Cross-lip flap is turned. Lateral apex of *W*-shaped excision has been closed directly. Lateral portion of the upper lip is advanced medially for closure of donor site. Note that the perinasal crescent has not yet been removed. *C,* Cross-lip flap in place, and donor site closed. Judgement is required when suturing in the side of the flap that bears the vascular pedicle. Since it cannot be sutured in completely, an estimation is required as to where the vermilion landmarks will be connected when the pedicle is later divided in a second stage.

Continued.

Figure 18-34, cont'd *D*, Surgical result several months after division of pedicle. Flap tissue appears slightly thickened, which is common with this type of flap repair. With its surrounding full-thickness scar and interval denervation, the flap tissue does not distend and relax as well as the adjacent unviolated lip tissue. *E*, Same patient showing the squamous cell carcinoma of his left lower lip. *F*, Surgical result at 6 months with lips in near repose. *G*, Surgical result at 5 years. This patient's face has thinned considerably with aging over this time. There has been further contraction of the scar tissue. The flap does not appear so natural in repose at this point.

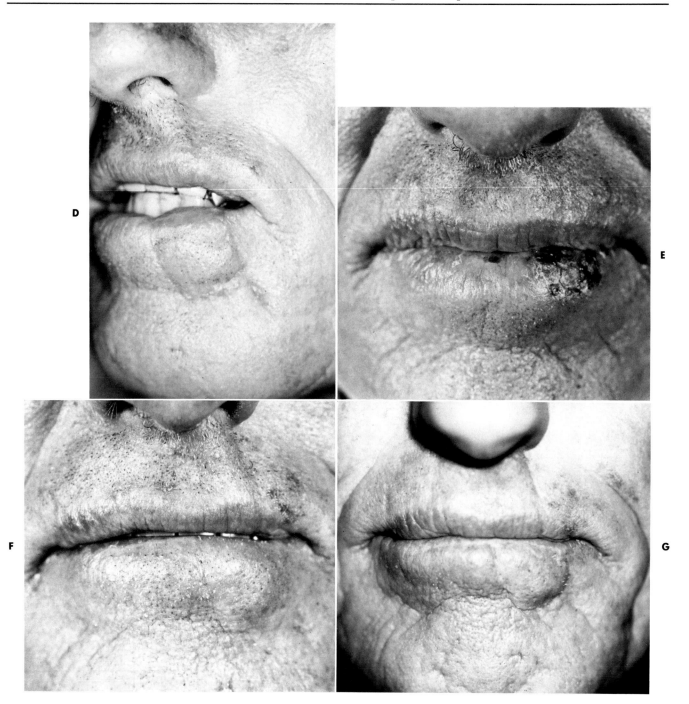

Figure 18-35   *A,* Patient with *W*-shaped excision from the lower lip. Various methods of advancement flap repair were considered, but a cross-lip flap was thought to be the best for this patient. Central apex of the *W* was later excised. *B,* Result of 6 months with use of a rectangular-shaped cross-lip flap. A slight notching is present in the vermilion of the donor site and could stand correction.

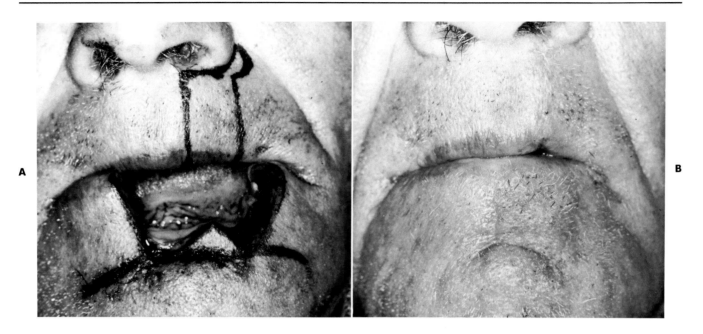

A   B

of the lip. There is no single large associated venous structure in this area, and enough tissue must be left to allow for venous return. Attempts to transfer full-thickness lip tissue to the opposite lip as a free composite graft without a vascular pedicle can sometimes be successful but in general have proven to be undependable.[20] Composite lip grafts should not be much larger than 1 to 1.5 cm in width. Lip tissue hair loss is more likely to occur with composite grafts than with pedicled flaps.[21]

Since cross-lip flap reconstruction involves transfer of composite lip tissue, there is restoration of defects of the orbicularis oris muscle. The first signs of motor reinnervation begin to appear at approximately 6 to 8 weeks and are maximized during the first postoperative year (Figs. 18-36, 18-37).[12,22,23] The quality of motor return to the lip that has received the cross-lip transfer is variable. Some patients do very well, while others demonstrate various degrees of persistent oral incontinence, principally to liquids. It is my observation that problems with continence are more likely to be found in those who are edentulous and of advanced age and also in cross-lip flap reconstructions involving the central portion of the lower lip.

Cross-lip flaps also sustain loss of their sensory functions as they are transferred. Return of sensory function begins after several months and returns in the order of pain, touch, and temperature (cold, then hot). Some patients may complain of hypersensitivity in the

first year or two following reconstruction, especially in cold weather. This problem normally dissipates over a longer period of time.

There is a strong tendency for cross-lip flaps to appear thickened, even after many years. This is for several reasons. The scar tissue that surrounds these flaps is full-thickness and completely encircles the flap except along the free margin of the lip. This presents a classic "trap-door" type of deformity. The establishment of lymphatic drainage from the cross-lip flap to the surrounding tissues is difficult because of the full-thickness scar. If the orbicularis muscle layer is not carefully approximated, there is a greater tendency for retraction in the scar lines. It can be noted in many patients that the cross-lip flap is appropriately thin when the lip is stretched with activities such as smiling but then appears thickened when the lips are relaxed. Overall, the greatest drawbacks to cross-lip flaps relate to the prolonged phase of denervation and to the problems of dealing with a transoral pedicle.

Cross-lip flaps can sometimes be combined with labial advancement flaps to collectively achieve reconstruction in situations of major lip loss. At the present time, cross-lip flaps have lost much of their popularity in favor of the Karapandzic circumoral advancement flap reconstruction, which is generally a one-stage procedure and optimizes preservation of sensory and motor functions.

Figure 18-36 Comparison of electromyograph recordings from an unviolated region of the lip to that from a cross-lip flap at 5 years.

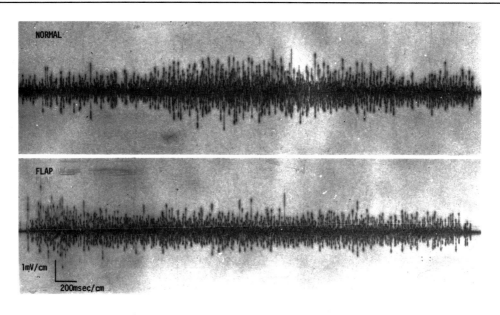

Figure 18-37 *A*, Result at 4 years with cross-lip flap to central lower lip. *B*, With pursing of lips, there is active contraction of muscle within the flap shown by wrinkling of the vermilion.

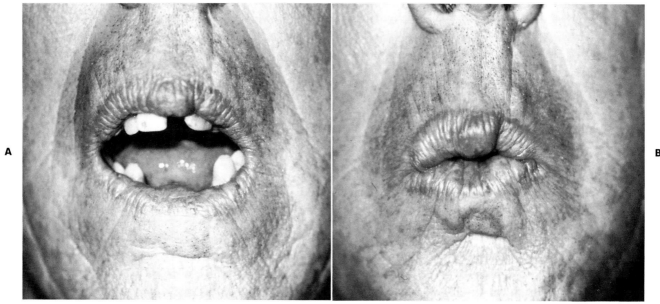

Circumoral Cross-Lip Flaps

Estlander (1872) is credited with first describing a method for lip repair that involved transfer of a full-thickness unit of lip as a pedicled transposition flap brought around the oral commissure (Fig. 18-38).[24] Similar to other cross-lip flaps, this unit of lip tissue is normally designed to be approximately half the width of the defect present in the opposite lip. Some surgeons make the flap slightly larger than half the size of the defect. The flap is brought around the oral commissure on a small vascular pedicle, which contains the labial artery. Originally this was described as a single-stage repair. This technique can produce a significant blunting of the oral commissure resulting in distortion, particularly when the mouth is open (Fig. 18-39). This distortion is enhanced by the fact that it is unilateral and thus stands in contrast to the natural or unviolated commissure on the opposite side of the lip. Some form of commissuroplasty is commonly performed later to minimize this disparity. The circumoral cross-lip flap is a method of repair that is only suited for correction of defects in the lateral portion of the lip.

Defects involving the more central portions of the lip can be repaired with a two-flap method that was originally described by Buck (1876) (Fig. 18-40).[1] The first flap involves the use of a releasing incision extending downward from the oral commissure in such fashion that the remaining lip segment on one side can be brought to the central part of the lip for anastomosis with the opposing lip segment. The defect created after transfer of the lateral lip segment is repaired with cross-lip transfer of a pedicled flap similar in nature to that described by Eslander.

In a further stage of evolution of the circumoral type of cross-lip flap, Gilles[1] described a design that is quadrilateral in shape and serves to simultaneously transfer the remaining lip segment on one side of a defect in combination with a portion of the opposing ipsilateral lip (Fig. 18-41).[1] This has often been referred to as a "fan flap," with analogy to an old-fashioned, collapsible, hand-held fan that is opened.[1] Several variations of this flap design have been described.[2,4,5,12,14] In general, most of the orbicularis oris muscle is not incised but is pulled around the commissure as part of the pedicle. The pedicle is made significantly larger in this flap than in other forms of cross-lip pivotal flaps. Some have used the principles of Z-plasty to help in making the turn about the commissure and resetting of the lateral outline of the flap (Figs. 18-42, 18-43).[4,8] The feature that most distinguishes this method of repair from the circumoral advancement flaps of von Bruns and Karapandzic is the vertical releasing incision made in the donor lip.

Figure 18-38   Estlander type of cross-lip flap, shown here with a more rounded apex of the donor flap; most are triangular in design.

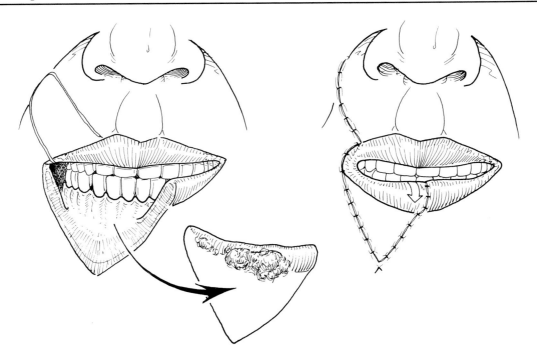

Figure 18-39   *A,* Patient with Estlander type of repair to the left lower lip with lips in repose. *B,* Blunting of the commissure is noted when mouth is open.

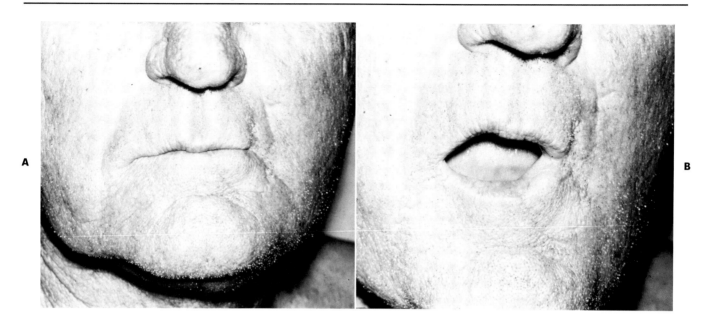

Figure 18-40   Illustration of two-flap technique described by Buck.

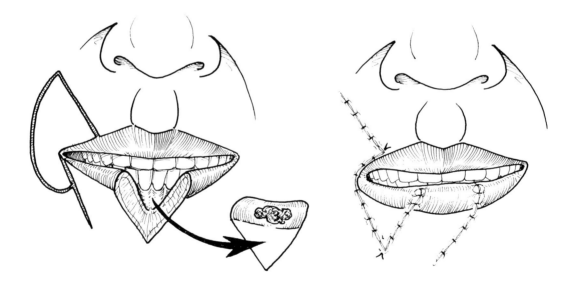

Figure 18-41   *A, B,* **Gillie's "fan flap" for repair of lower lip defect.** *C, D,* **Similar flap with Z-plasty to facilitate transfer to repair upper lip defect.**

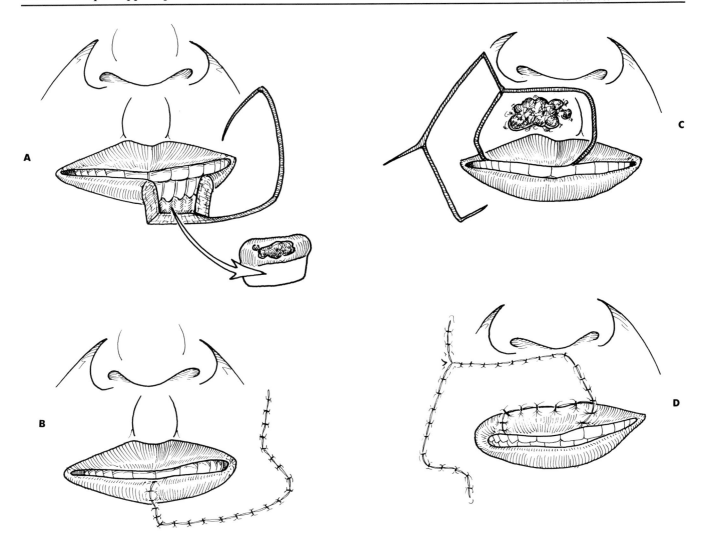

Figure 18-42   **Bilateral Gillie's type of repair with use of Z-plasties to help turn the flaps in reconstruction of the lower lip.**

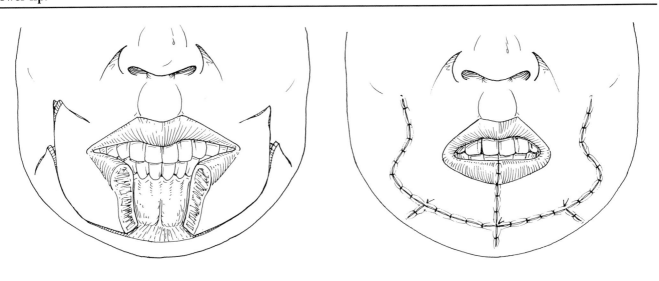

Figure 18-43   Gillie's flaps with use of Z-plasties in bilateral reconstruction of the upper lip.

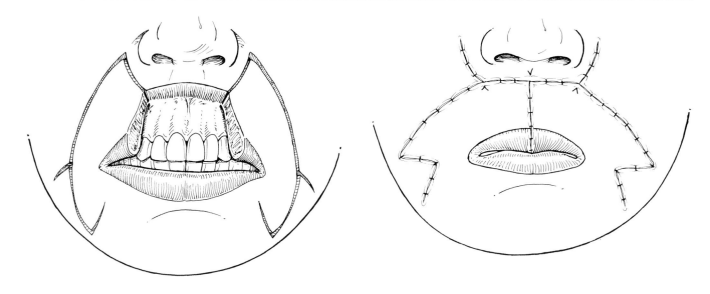

Commissure Revisions

With all of the unilateral cross-lip flaps that involve transfer of tissue around the oral commissure, a common problem is found with distortion of the involved commissure. Some form of commissuroplasty is commonly performed as a secondary procedure.[2] Several types of commissuroplasty are possible. The simplest method of revision involves the horizontal transection of the blunted portion of the commissure to a point similar to that of the natural commissure of the opposite side. Buccal mucosa is advanced forward on each side of the transection to restore a vermilion surface. It may be found necessary to remove a triangular unit of skin and subcutaneous tissue from the blunted region for a more natural result (Fig. 18-44). This should be done cautiously, however because deficiency of the orbicularis muscle tissue in this region can result in oral incontinence.

An alternative method of reconstruction makes use of small flaps of vermilion and orbicularis muscle to enhance the reconstruction. After a triangular unit of skin and subcutaneous tissue has been excised from the blunted region, a small vermilion flap is created from one side of the lip, pedicled from the opposite lip (Fig. 18-45). Horizontal transection is made through the muscle tissue in the middle of the commissure. A small flap of buccal mucosa is made from the region deep to the excised tissue and taken from above or below the horizontal line of the muscle transection. The severed ends of the orbicularis muscle are then pulled laterally into the new commissure. The pedicled vermilion is then placed over the muscle and into the commissure

on one side, and the buccal flap is used to restore vermilion on the other side.

Horizontal Cheek Advancement Flaps

Two nineteenth-century surgeons, Bernard (1852) and von Burow (1853–1855), are credited with originally describing lip reconstructions with a gracefully fitted horizontal advancement transfer of cheek tissue.[1] In a radical departure from simple advancement with no accommodation made for the disparities in redundancy of tissues, both of these authors describe the resection of strategically placed triangles of redundant soft tissue in regions immediately adjacent to the transferred flap. This method of lip repair is generally referred to as the "Bernard cheiloplasty," while the triangular excisions of adjacent redundant tissue are commonly referred to as "Burow's triangles."[1]

Reconstruction of the upper lip with bilateral horizontal advancement flaps is accomplished with excision of four triangles of cheek skin, which were originally described as full-thickness incisions (Fig. 18-46).[9] On each side, a triangle of skin is removed from the portion of the cheek that is above the flap and lateral to the nasal ala. A triangle is also removed from the cheek beneath the flap, which is lateral and inferior to the oral commissure. Reconstruction of the lower lip is classically achieved with excision of three triangles (Fig. 18-47). One of these is removed on each side, from a region that is lateral and superior to the oral commissure, while a larger triangle is made extending down to the chin from the lip in the midline.

Figure 18-44 *A, B,* **A method of performing a commissuroplasty. A horizontal incision is made through the blunted portion of the commissure. This may be made in one or two steps (as shown here). In some patients, very little tissue is resected.** *C,* **Mucosa is advanced forward onto the upper lip, lateral commissure, and lower lip as necessary to restore the vermilion.**

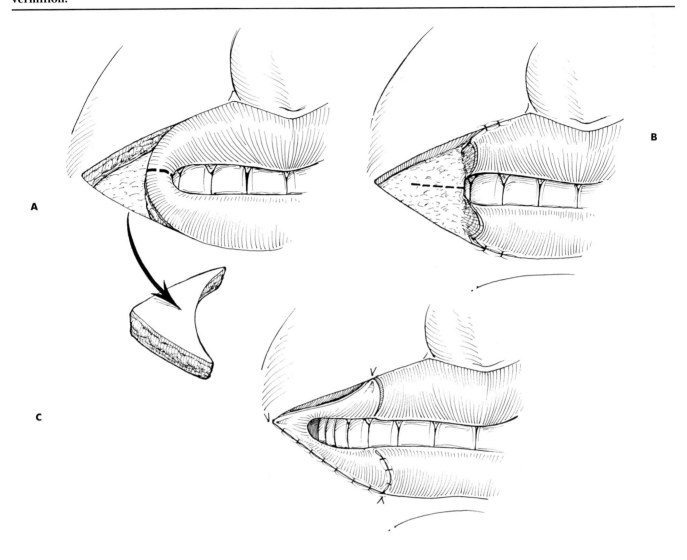

Significant modifications of the Bernard–von Burow repair have been described by several later authors.[2,9,25] These changes range from the use of full-thickness advancement flaps to the use of flaps that are cutaneous only, preserving the underlying facial musculature and sensory innervation. In a modified design for lower lip reconstruction proposed by Webster, resection of the tumor is performed in a rectangular-shaped excision and without violation of the chin (Fig. 18-48).[26,27] A total of four triangular excisions is used, one on each side in the melolabial sulcus and one on each side extending downward along the lateral side of the chin. This technique allows the scars to be in or parallel to the natural lines of the face.

Most surgeons today prefer to design these cheek advancement flaps as cutaneous flaps only and then devise some other method of replacing buccal and vermilion surfaces (Fig. 18-49). All forms of reconstruction using cheek advancement flaps fail to restore a fully functioning orbicularis muscle. The need for a muscle sphincter is offset partially by the inherent tightness of the lip that is reconstructed in this manner. Because the face is rounded in the axial plane, the reconstructed lip commonly appears tight or sunken, in contrast to the unviolated opposing lip or chin, especially in the edentulous patient. Even with the use of cutaneous flaps, the expressive motor functions of the involved lip will be altered to some degree.

Figure 18-45 *A,* A method of performing a commissuroplasty. Plan for skin excision is made. A vermilion flap from the blunted commissure is also planned for reconstruction of the upper lip. *B,* The vermilion flap is raised and a horizontal incision is planned through the blunted commissure. This incision is carried upward lateral to the muscle to obtain a mucosal flap that is used for resurfacing of the vermilion of the lower lip. *C,* Vermilion repair is accomplished by advancing flaps. *D,* The completed commissure revision.

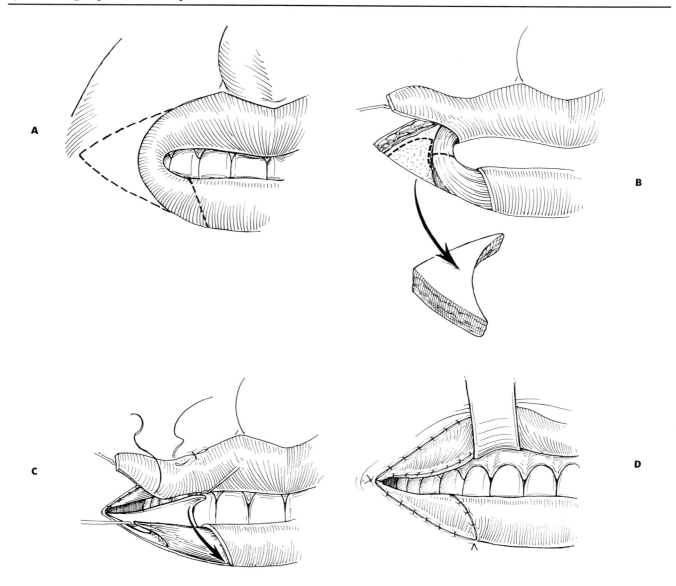

Figure 18-46   Bernard–von Burow reconstruction of the upper lip with use of four triangular excisions.

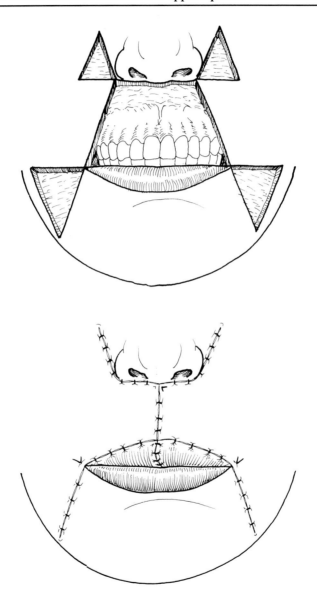

Figure 18-47 Bernard–von Burow reconstruction of the lower lip with use of three triangular excisions.

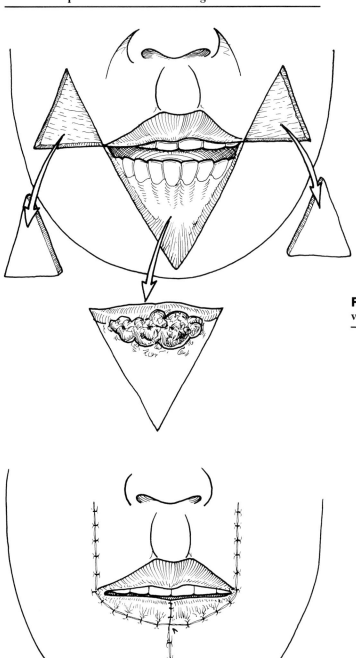

Figure 18-48 Webster modification of the Bernard–von Burow method of lip reconstruction with cheek flaps.

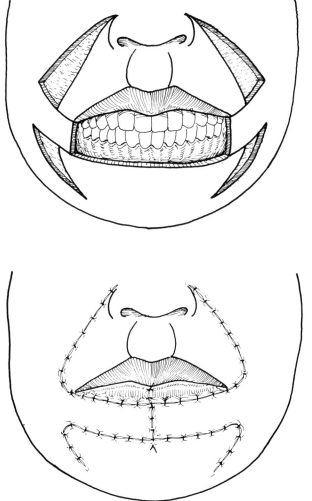

Figure 18-49   *A,* Plan for modified reconstruction of the lower lip with use of two triangular excisions for advancement of cheek flaps and a large *W*-shaped excision for a wide tumor. It should be noted that this patient had a previous *V*-shaped excision for malignancy of the lower lip, which has already made the lower lip much smaller than the upper lip. *B,* Alternate plan for excision and repair is considered. This design avoids violation of the chin unit and is similar to the modification described by Webster. *C, W*-shaped excision is chosen for this case and plans made for advancement flap closure. The Bernard–von Burow design would make the triangular excision in the cheek extend to the commissure instead of following the melolabial sulcus. In this case the deeper incision is taken only through the orbicularis muscle, to a point approximately in line with the melolabial sulcus. The mucosal incision is made horizontally at a level slightly higher than the cutaneous incision so that the mucosa does not have to be stretched tight as it is used to restore the vermilion. *D,* Completed surgical result. There is relative redundancy of the lateral portion of the upper lip.

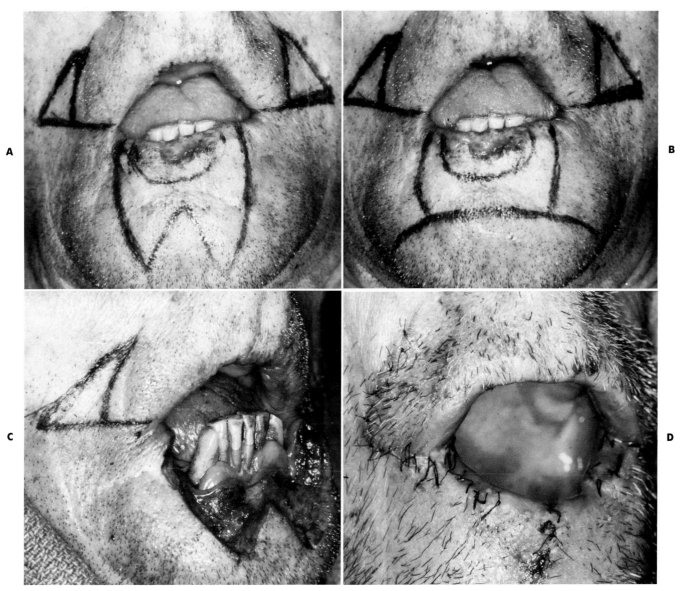

A

B

C

D

Continued.

Figure 18-49, cont'd   *E*, Surgical result at 2 months. In this view the reconstructed lip looks reasonably natural in appearance. *F*, Result at 2 months with the lips open. There is now relative tightness of the lower lip and cheek. The tightness helps compensate for lack of orbicularis muscle in the reconstruction. *G*, The patient cannot smile at this point without opening the lips. *H*, As he tries to purse the lips to simulate kissing or whistling, the lips cannot be kept closed.

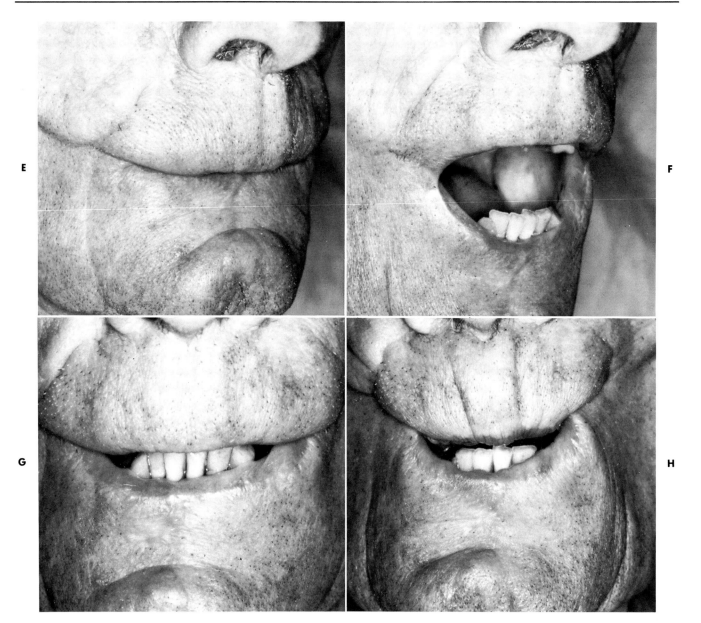

SUMMARY

The lips are a very well-defined anatomic unit and serve many functions. The melolabial and mental creases are favorable sites for placement of surgical scars and can be used in a variety of ways for flap design. The vermilion and labial rhytid lines also tend to be well-defined and favored sites for scar placement.

Since the lips have no direct skeletal parts, they have considerable capability for stretch. As much as possible, reconstruction of the lip should be done with plans that optimize motor and sensory functions. Many lip reconstructions appear reasonably good while the lips are relaxed and held closed, but problems can become much more apparent when the lips attempt to perform various functions.

In general the most preferred tissue for lip reconstruction comes from within the lip unit itself. Only when this would result in significant microstomia or distortion should flap tissue from adjacent or distant regions be used. Since the lips are a major structure of the face, it is very important to apply good aesthetic surgical principles and technique in reconstructions of this site.

REFERENCES

1. Mazzola RF, Lupo G: Evolving concepts in lip reconstruction, *Clin Plast Surg* 11:583, 1984.

2. Zide BM: Deformities of the lips and cheeks. In McCarthy JG, editor: *Plastic surgery*, vol 3, Philadelphia, 1990, WB Saunders.

3. Renner G, Zitsch R: Reconstruction of the lip, *Otolaryngol Clin North Am* 23:975, 1990.

4. Converse JM: Reconstructive plastic surgery, vol 3, Philadelphia, 1977, WB Saunders.

5. McGregor IA: The tongue flap in lip surgery, *Br J Plast Surg* 19:253, 1966.

6. Goldstein MH: A tissue-expanding vermilion myocutaneous flap for lip repair, *Plast Reconstr Surg* 73:768, 1984.

7. Renner GJ: Cancer of the lip. In Gates G: *Current therapy in otolaryngology—head and neck surgery*, vol 4, Trenton, NJ, 1989, F C Decker.

8. Panje WR: Lip reconstruction, *Otolaryngol Clin North Am* 15:169, 1982.

9. Webster JP: Cresuntis Pin-ader cheek excision for upper lip flap advancement with a short history of upper lip repair, *Plast Reconstr Surg* 16:434, 1955.

10. Calhoun KH, Stiernberg CM: *Surgery of the lip*, New York, 1992, Thieme Medical Publishers.

11. Pelly AD, Tau EP: Lower lip reconstruction, *Br J Plast Surg* 34:83, 1981.

12. Rea JL, Davis WE, Rittenhouse LK: Reinnervation of an Abbé-Estlander and a Gilles fan flap of the lower lip, *Arch Otolaryngol* 104:294, 1978.

13. Jabaley ME, Clement RL, Orcutt TW: Myocutaneous flaps in lip reconstruction: application of the Karapandzic principle, *Plast Reconstr Surg* 59:680.

14. Jackson IT: Local flaps in head and neck reconstruction, St Louis, 1985, The CV Mosby Co.

15. Karapandzic M: Reconstruction of lip defects by local arterial flaps, *Br J Plast Surg* 27:93, 1974.

16. Abbe RA: A new plastic operation for the relief of deformity due to double harelip, *Medical Record* 53:477, 1898.

17. Kinnebrew MC: Use of the Abbe flap in revision of the bilateral cleft lip-nose deformity, *Oral Surg* 56:12, 1983.

18. Franchebois P: Improved surgical treatment of cancer of the lower lip, *Int Surg* 60:204, 1975.

19. Templer J, Renner G, Davis WE, Thomas JR: A modification of the Abbé-Estlander flap for defects of the lower lip, *Laryngoscope* 91:153, 1981.

20. Flanagin WS: True composite graft from lower to upper lip, *Plast Reconstr Surg* 17:376, 1956.

21. Millard DR: Composite lip flaps and grafts in secondary cleft deformities, *Br J Plast Surg* 22.

22. DePalma AT, Leavitt LA, Hardy SB: Electromyography in full thickness flaps rotated between upper and lower lips, *Plast Reconstr Surg* 21:448, 1958.

23. Smith JW: The anatomized and physiologic acclimatization of tissue transplanted by the lip switch technique, *Plast Reconstr Surg* 26:40, 1960.

24. Estlander JA: Ene Methods Aus der Einen Lippe Substanzverluste der Anderen Zu Ersetzen, *Archiv für Klinische Chirurgie* 14:622, 1872, reprinted in English translation in *Plast Reconstr Surg* 42:361, 1968.

25. Freeman BS: Myoplastic modification of the Bernard cheiloplasty, *Plast Reconstr Surg* 21:453, 1958.

26. Walker AW, Schewe JE: Nasolabial flap reconstruction for carcinoma of the lower lip, *Am J Surg* 113:783, 1967.

27. Webster RE, Coffey RJ, Kellcher RE: Total and partial reconstruction of the lower lip with innervated muscle-bearing flaps, *Plast Reconstr Surg* 25:360, 1960.

EDITORIAL COMMENTS

Shan R. Baker

The lips play a key role in deglutition, formation of speech, and facial expressions. Their reconstruction offers a unique challenge to the surgeon. Few other sites require attention to such precise details of form and function. Dr. Renner has provided the reader with a large number of surgical alternatives and an in-depth discussion of their indications for repair of defects of the lips.

Surgical procedures utilized to reconstitute the lip following tumor ablation may be classified as follows[1]:

(1) those that use remaining lip tissue, (2) those that borrow tissue from the opposite lip, (3) those that use adjacent cheek tissue, and (4) those that use distant flaps.

The algorithms displayed in Figures 18-50 and 18-51 may be helpful in the cognitive process of managing the problem of lip reconstruction.[2] This method categorizes the size of lip defects into those less than one-half the width of the lip, those between one-half and two-thirds of the lip, and defects greater than two-thirds of the entire lip width.

Figure 18-50 Algorithm for reconstruction of lower lip defects.

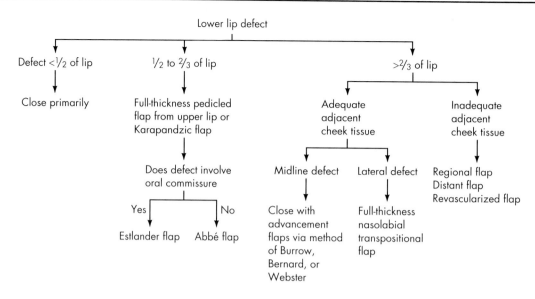

Figure 18-51 Algorithm for reconstruction of upper lip defects.

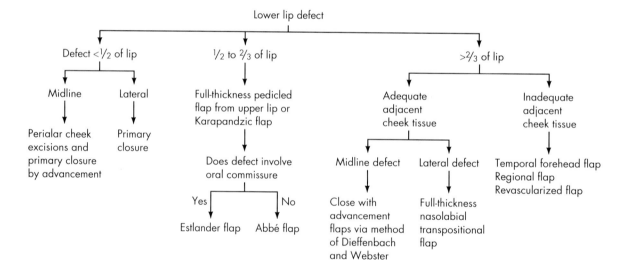

Defects of less than one-half of the lip width can usually be managed by primary wound closure. In the lower lip, conversion of the defect into a *W*-shaped configuration may be preferred and in its simplest form is usually adequate for primary closure, though modification to include lateral advancement flaps may be required when the defect base is broad. The *W*-shaped configuration maximizes conservation of tissue and prevents an unsightly pointed chin when it is necessary to extend the incision beyond the mental crease. Primary closure should be in three layers; that is, mucosa, muscle, and skin. Care is taken to perform a precise approximation of the "white line" at the vermilion border on either side of the defect. When extensive leukoplakia is present along the entire lip, vermilionectomy is indicated. A new vermilion is reconstructed by advancing the mucosal lining of the lip outward. In instances when leukoplakia is present in association with a small invasive carcinoma, a wedge excision can be combined with vermilionectomy. A more contemporary method of performing a vermilionectomy is to vaporize the upper layers of the vermilion with a carbon dioxide laser and allow the wound to heal by second intention.

Primary wound closure of defects in the midline of the upper lip can be facilitated by excising a crescent of cheek skin in the perialar region. This method is similar to that described by Webster.[3] Perialar skin excision allows advancement of the remaining lip segments medially and lessens wound-closure tension after primary wound repair.

Vermilion mucosal defects may be reconstructed with simple mucosal advancement flaps from inside the mouth. When vermilion substance has been lost in addition to mucosa, a flap of muscle and mucosa from the anterior tongue may be used, as discussed by Dr. Renner. A mucosal flap from the ventral surface of the tongue is initially attached to the skin at the vermilion-cutaneous border. From 14 to 20 days later, the pedicle is transected, releasing the tongue and retaining muscle for bulk and mucosa for vermilion reconstruction. Although this technique does not result in discernable limitation of tongue mobility, the newly created vermilion mucosa retains a somewhat pebbled surface, reminiscent of the tongue surface.

Reconstruction of defects consisting of from one-half to two-thirds of the lip width usually requires lip augmentation procedures. Closure can be most readily achieved by a full-thickness pedicle flap from the opposite lip (lip-switch flap) or from the adjacent cheek. The Karapandzic flap[4] may also be effective in closing medium-sized defects of the lip and in some instances may provide better functional results than other uninnervated or denervated flaps. This technique consists of circumoral incisions through the skin and subcutaneous tissue, encompassing the remaining portions of upper and lower lips.[5] The orbicularis oris is mobilized and remains pedicled bilaterally on the superior and inferior labial arteries. Adequate mobilization enables primary closure of the defect by rotating portions of the unoperated lip into the defect. The advantage of the Karapandzic flap is that it restores a continuous circle of functioning orbicularis oris muscle, which maintains oral competence. However, since no new tissue is recruited to aid in reconstruction of the lip, microstomia may be a problem. Patients in the sixth decade of life or older will often develop laxity of the oral stoma following a Karapandzic flap and not require bilateral commissuroplasties to correct microstomia (Fig. 18-52).

Local flaps are preferable to regional flaps for closing defects of less than two-thirds of the lip width because of their close skin color and texture match and the availability of mucous membrane for internal lining. Defects located away from the commissure are best closed with an Abbé flap consisting of a full-thickness flap from the opposite lip pedicled on the vermilion border and containing the labial artery.[6] Estlander's original operation was devised for closure of lower lip defects near the commissure of the mouth.[7] Since the original description of the Abbé and Estlander flaps, the operations have been modified in many ways to accommodate surgical defects located anywhere in the lower or upper lip (Fig. 18-53).

The Abbé and Estlander flaps should be constructed so that the height of the flap equals the height of the defect. The width of the flap should be approximately one-half that of the defect to be reconstructed, so that the two lips are reduced in width proportionately. If portions of the nasal base or nasal sil are missing, the flap should be designed to completely replace this tissue so as to restore the nasal base with a full complement of skin and soft tissue. The pedicle should be made narrow to facilitate transposition, but care must be taken not to injure the labial artery. The secondary defect should be closed in three layers. Accurate approximation of the vermilion border of the flap with that of the remaining lip segment prevents a notched appearance.

The superiorly based Estlander flap may be modified from its original description by designing the flap so that it lies within the melolabial sulcus.[8] This provides better scar camouflage of the donor site and at the

Figure 18-52 *A,* A 10 × 6 cm skin and muscle defect of upper lip following resection of a squamous cell carcinoma. The patient had a total rhinectomy for skin cancer several years earlier. *B,* Karapandzic flap designed to reconstruct upper lip defect. *C,* Defect repaired. Note marked microstomia causing remaining lower lip to pout. *D,* One year postoperative. Lip tissue has stretched sufficiently to correct microstomia. Commissuroplasty was not necessary.

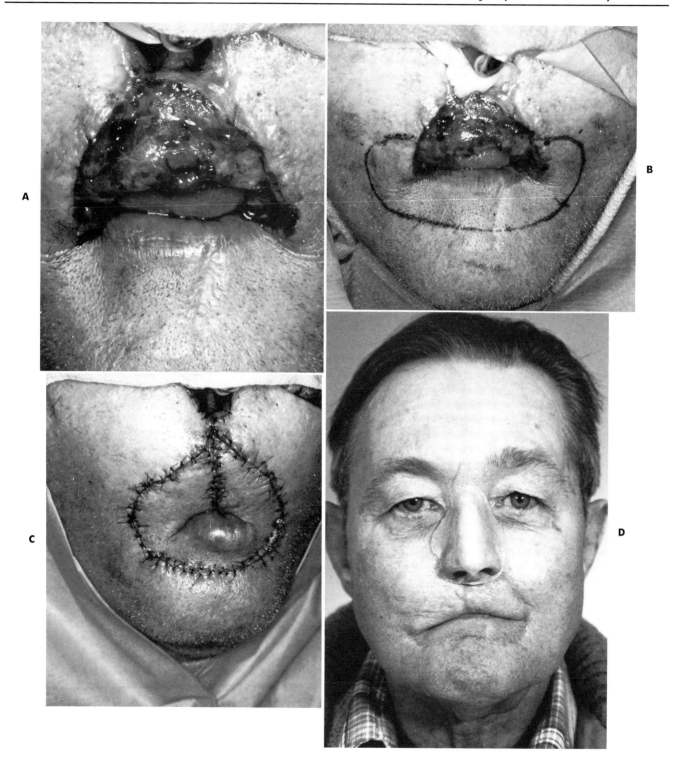

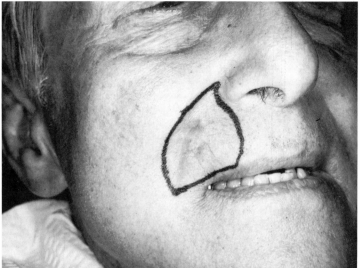

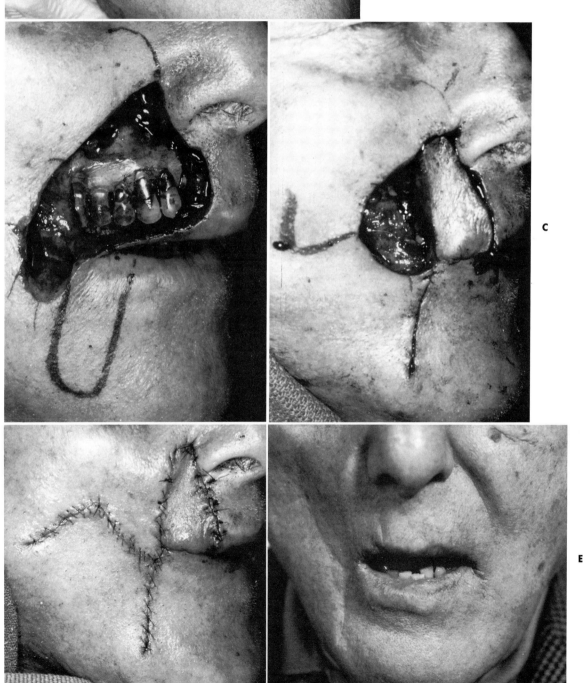

Figure 18-53 *A,* Extensive carcinoma of the upper lip. Marking indicates proposed surgical resection. *B,* Following resection, there is a 6 × 5.5 cm full-thickness defect of lateral upper lip with extension into the medial cheek. Extended Estlander flap is designed to repair the lip component of the defect. *C,* Estlander flap transposed and donor site wound closed primarily. Vertical length of the flap is such that it provides tissue for repair of the alar-facial sulcus. A separate transposition flap is designed to reconstruct the medial cheek component of the defect. *D,* Cheek flap transposed and donor site wound closed primarily. *E,* Seven months postoperative.

same time allows easy rotation of the flap into the lower lip defect. Oral commissure distortion is caused by the Estlander flap. This distortion, or microstomia, may be corrected with a secondary commissuroplasty when desired.

The pedicle of the Abbé flap crosses the oral stoma and may be severed in 2 or 3 weeks. During the interval between transfer of the flap and division of the pedicle, the patient is maintained on a liquid or soft diet that does not require excessive chewing. It is essential that precise approximation of the vermilion border be ensured at the time of pedicle severance.

Defects greater than two-thirds of the entire lip, and some smaller lateral defects, are best reconstructed by using adjacent cheek flaps in the form of advancement or transposition flaps (Fig. 18-54). Massive or total lip defects are best reconstructed by using regional or distant flaps or vascularized free flaps.

Figure 18-54   *A,* A 3 × 3 cm skin defect of upper lip is seen following removal of a recurrent basal cell carcinoma. Superiorly based transposition flap is designed to repair defect. *B,* Flap transposed and donor site wound closed primarily. *C,* Six months postoperative. No revision surgery was performed.

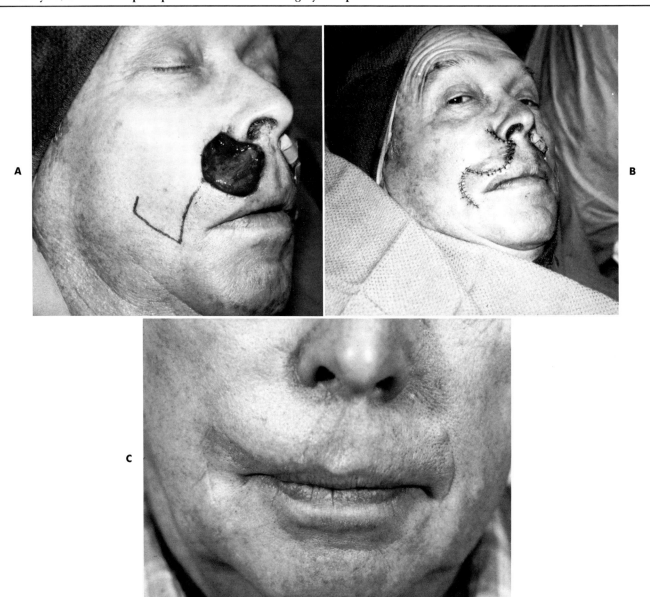

Large defects of the upper lip may be reconstructed by excising crescent-shaped perialar cheek tissue and advancing flaps medially. If wound-closure tension is excessive, an Abbé flap may be added in the midline.[8]

Similarly, midline lower lip defects may be closed by full-thickness advancement flaps, as described by Dr. Renner. These techniques require excisions of additional triangles in the melolabial region to allow advancement of the cheek flaps. The triangular excision should follow the lines of the melolabial sulcus and should include only skin and subcutaneous tissues. The underlying muscle is mobilized to form a new commissure. The mucous membrane is separated from the muscle and advanced outward to provide a vermilion border. Incisions are made in the gingival buccal sulcus, as far back as the last molar tooth if necessary, to allow proper approximation of the remaining lip segments without tension.

Melolabial transposition flaps consisting of skin and subcutaneous tissues only or full-thickness consisting of skin, subcutaneous tissues, and mucosa can be useful in reconstructing lip defects as large as three-fourths of the width of the lip.[9] Matched full-thickness flaps can be created in the area of the melolabial folds of each cheek with a Z-plasty at their base to enhance the ease of transposition. The flaps are transposed into the lip defect and sutured in three layers. Mucosa from the flaps can be advanced to create a new vermilion, or a tongue flap may be required.

Adjacent cheek tissue may not be applicable or sufficient for reconstruction of near total defects of the lip. In such cases, regional flaps may be used for reconstruction. Excisions of the lower lip, chin, and anterior section of the mandible for carcinoma often require such flaps for reconstruction. This book does not deal with regional or distant flaps, but for completeness, a brief discussion follows.

The temporal forehead flap designed as a bipedicled advancement or unipedicled interpolation flap may be used for total upper lip reconstruction, but the unsightly secondary deformity precludes its common use. The flap may be lined with a split-thickness skin or mucosa graft. In males, hair-bearing scalp may be incorporated to provide hair growth for scar camouflage.

In the past, the medially based deltopectoral or Bakamjian[10] flap has been the most commonly used regional flap for reconstruction of the upper and lower lip.[9] The deltopectoral flap may be lined with a skin or mucosal graft. The flap may be turned on itself to supply the inner lining of the reconstructed lip. A deltopectoral flap may also be used for an inner lining of the lower lip combined with a melolabial transposition flap to reconstruct the external portion of the lip.[7] The melolabial flap provides a superior color and texture match with the remaining lip, while the deltopectoral flap provides tissue bulk and coverage for exposed mandible and missing lip lining.

More recently, the pectoralis major musculocutaneous flap has been used for lip reconstruction following extensive ablative surgery for malignancy of the anterior floor of the mouth involving large portions of the lip or skin of the chin. Ariyan and Krizek were the first to describe the pectoralis major musculocutaneous flap and reported its use in the reconstruction of large facial defects.[11] Since the introduction of this flap, it has gained popularity among head and neck reconstructive surgeons. It has the advantage of being an axial flap that can be elevated as a strip of muscle and an attached segment of overlying skin for a one-stage reconstruction of the lip. A portion of the flap may be turned on itself to provide tissue for the inner aspect of the lips or the anterior floor of the mouth. The flap has sufficient bulk to provide structural support when a mandibulectomy is necessary for tumor exenteration.

When large segments of the lower lip have been resected, oral competence requires adequate support for the reconstructed lip. Whenever possible, orbicularis oris muscle flaps should be included in the tissues used for reconstruction, with or without overlying skin and mucosa. If this is not possible, it may be necessary to sling the lower lip with a fascia lata graft from the upper lip muscle on either side.

When the anterior mandibular arch has been resected or destroyed, oral competence requires support of the lower lip. This is best accomplished by reconstructing the mandibular arch; rarely will the mass of soft tissue alone provide sufficient rigidity to allow oral competence. I prefer to use an iliac crest bone graft to restore the mandibular arch, in a separate stage after achieving soft tissue healing of the oral cavity. Stabilization of the mandibular segments is provided by an acrylic biphase appliance and the graft itself, using miniplate fixation.

The development of microvascular surgical techniques has allowed one-stage reconstruction of the lip, chin, and anterior manibular arch by transferring free composite osteomusculocutaneous and osteocutaneous flaps, providing vascularized bone grafts for mandibular reconstruction and soft tissue for restoration of the lip and chin. Revascularized bone is advantageous because it heals more readily and has an overall better success rate than conventional nonvascularized bone grafts. In addition, the simultaneous reconstruction of soft tissue deficits provides a superior rehabilitation technique for patients with massive defects of the lip and jaw.

REFERENCES

1. Kazanjian H, Converse JM: *The surgical treatment of facial injuries*, ed 2, Baltimore, 1959, Williams & Wilkins.

2. Baker SR: Lip reconstruction. In Holt GR, Gates GA, Mattox DE, editors: *Decision making in otolaryngology*, Burlington, Ontario, 1983, BC Decker.

3. Webster JP: Crescentic peri-alar cheek excision for upper flap advancement with a short history of upper lip repair, *Plast Reconstr Surg* 16:434, 1955.

4. Karapandzic M: Reconstruction of lip defects by local arterial flaps, *Br J Plast Surg* 27:93, 1974.

5. Baker SR: Options for reconstruction in head and neck surgery. In Cummings CW, Frederickson JM, Harker LA, et al, editors: *Otolaryngology: head and neck surgery, update I*, St Louis, 1986, The CV Mosby Co.

6. Baker SR: Malignancy of the lip. In Gluckman J, editor: *Otolaryngology*, ed 3, Philadelphia, 1988, WB Saunders.

7. Estlander JA: Eine Methods aus der einen Lippe Substanzverluste der Anderen zu Ersetzen, *Arch Klin Chir* 14:622, 1872.

8. Baker SR, Krause CJ: Cancer of the lip. In Suen JY, Myers EN, editors: *Cancer of the head and neck*, New York, 1981, Churchill Livingstone.

9. Baker SR, Krause CJ: Pedicle flaps in reconstruction of the lip, *Facial Plast Surg* 1:61, 1983.

10. Bakamjian VY: A two-staged method for pharyngoesophageal reconstruction with a primary pectoral skin flap, *Plast Reconstr Surg* 36:173, 1965.

11. Ariyan S, Krizek TJ: Reconstruction after resection of head and neck cancer, Cine Clinics, Clinical Congress of the American College of Surgeons, Dallas, Texas, 1977.

19

RECONSTRUCTION OF THE CHEEK

Dennis R. Banducci

Ernest Kelvin Manders

INTRODUCTION

The cheeks on profile view are directly in the center of the face and blend in with the surrounding structures. *Dorland's Medical Dictionary* defines cheek as "a fleshy protruberance, especially the fleshy portion of the side of the face."[1] Zide[2] divides the cheek into three units: suborbital, preauricular, and buccomandibular. These areas overlap somewhat, but they extend along the lower border of the mandible to include the preauricular area to the lateral and inferior orbital rims, down along the melolabial fold to the horizontal line of the mandible. If one considers the cheek as an esthetic unit, the boundaries would be the same as in the above description but would include most of the lower eyelids and the lateral part of the nose and exclude the chin and the lower lip areas.[3]

In reconstruction of the cheek, form and function along with esthetics are the most important planning considerations. Much of the planning has to do with the cause of the defect. For example, the defect caused by the extirpation of a malignant tumor may be best reconstructed with a simple skin graft followed by observation to ensure that the tumor does not recur. The defect can be reconstructed with a more suitable method at a later date. If the defect is due to trauma, reconstruction can often proceed more expeditiously in certain cases, such as in the case of severe avulsion injuries.

Burns pose special problems for cheek reconstruction. For full-thickness skin loss due to burn wounds of the face, it is appropriate to reconstruct the defect initially with split-thickness skin grafts to allow healing of the wound. Revisions or more formal reconstruction can proceed at a later time. Generally, for more superficial injuries, it is best to wait 1 year or longer after a patient has been burned before attempts at reconstruction. A process of scar maturation and contracture stabilization first needs to take place. As Feldman[3] points out, "Contracture release or facial resurfacing that takes place within an area that is still contracting will undoubtedly yield results that are compromised by some degree of recontracture." However, in some cases if one knows that a scar will eventually need to be removed in its entirety despite its improvement with time, there is little point in waiting for it to improve before excision.

Rohrich and Sheffield[4] classified cheek defects into three categories: superficial, full-thickness, and subcutaneous contour defects. They emphasize that superficial defects may often be repaired with local skin flaps for small defects, and various types of cervicofacial or cervicopectoral flaps or soft-tissue expansion for larger defects. For full-thickness defects a variety of flaps may be used, but the important principles of provision of adequate lining, support, and cover are emphasized.[5] Local flaps may be used as lining flaps, with external coverage provided for by more distant flaps. For instance, one may use a pectoralis major flap with two separate skin paddles for cover and lining. Hurtwitz et al[6] and Coleman et al[7] described platysmal flap closure of various facial defects. Bunkis et al[8] and Skow[9] describe the use of combinations of flaps for reconstruction of full-thickness defects of the cheeks. Harii et al[10] described the use of combined myocutaneous free flaps to reconstruct total cheek defects.

The correction of contour defects of the cheeks remains a most difficult challenge. In general, if there are many ways to do a reconstructive surgical technique, none of those ways will solve all problems. This proves to be the case in attempts to correct contour deformities of the cheek. As Rohrich and Sheffield[4] have written, "To date there is no one form of treatment to provide consistent, long-term correction of cheek deformities." There are many techniques to augment contour deficiencies in the face. Dermis and dermis-fat grafts are two of the ways; however, there is a high resorption rate of the fat component of the graft. Fat injections have been tried, but clinical and experimental observations have shown that much of the graft is lost over time. We have been successful in the correction of small contour defects of the cheek and other parts of the face with minced autologous dermis grafts and strips of autologous dermis. This is very good to correct deep wrinkles and acne scars.

The use of silicone injections into the face to improve contour defects has largely been discontinued due to reports of serious long-term complications in a minority of patients. Problems include chronic inflammation, sinus tracts, contour deformities, and induration.[11,12]

Local flaps may be used to fill small to moderate-sized contour deformities. Platysmal flaps and superficial temporal fascial flaps are the most widely used local flaps. For larger contour defects, as in Romberg's hemifacial atrophy, microsurgical flaps are a good choice. Scapular, parascapular, groin flaps, and omentum have been used. Buried microsurgical muscle flaps give initially good results; however, they always atrophy and, unless one initially overcorrects the defect substantially, the contour deformity will persist. Unfor-

tunately, most flaps have a tendency to sag with time and, if skin is transferred with the muscle, it may have a poor color match with the facial skin. Several methods have been attempted to correct the eventual sagging of the flaps. These include deepithelialization of the flaps and sewing of the dermis to the fascia over the facial muscles as well as placement of many sutures in various places to attach the omentum to the face.[13] Evaluation of the long-term success of these procedures is still pending.

RECONSTRUCTIVE TECHNIQUES AND PROCEDURES

Reconstructive techniques may be simple or complex. Simple techniques include primary closure of defects by advancement of the wound margin, healing by second intention, and application of a skin graft. In order of increasing complexity and time required, other alternatives include local flaps, distant flaps,[14-16]

Figure 19-1 *A,* **Squamous cell carcinoma of cheek in 55-year-old woman. Tumor was excised as elliptical excision parallel to relaxed skin tension lines** *(dotted line). B,* **Appearance 1 year postoperatively. (B courtesy Shan R. Baker, M.D.)**

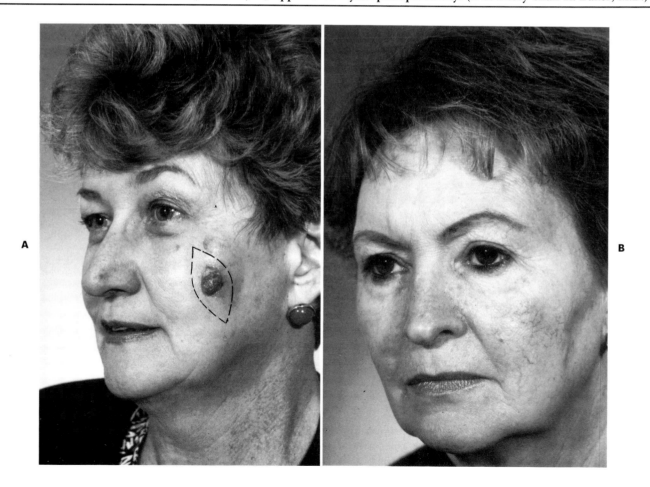

microsurgical flaps, and soft-tissue expansion. Only procedures that use local tissues will be discussed here.

Skin Undermining and Primary Closure

Skin undermining combined with primary closure of defects of the cheek is one of the most simple and straightforward ways to handle a small cheek deformity. It should be considered the treatment of choice for closure of most small defects. In determination of whether the defect will close primarily, the surgeon must consider the size of the defect and the laxity of the skin. As a person ages, skin mobility increases. In elderly patients who have more redundant skin, larger defects may often be closed primarily without excessive wound-closure tension. This is advantageous in the elderly, since most skin cancers appear in this patient population.

When planning an excision of a skin lesion, the surgeon should take into account where the final scar will lie. Scars should lie in or parallel to adjacent skin lines such as Langer's lines (Fig. 19-1). There are many different types of skin lines, which are well described by Borges.[17] Scars are least noticeable if they are placed in existing skin lines. Many elderly patients heal with

minimal scarring because of the many skin lines that are present and the laxity of facial skin. Sometimes it is not apparent that the patient has been operated on unless one looks very closely. In areas without skin lines (for example, the cheek area of a young patient), it is best to place the scar parallel to a wrinkle line one would expect to find in an older person. Even then the scar may be quite noticeable[18] (Fig. 19-2).

Wound Healing by Second Intention

Letting the wound heal by second intention is often a perfectly acceptable means of closure of an open wound of the cheek and is perhaps the easiest way to repair a large defect. Indications for this are limited, such as in certain operations in which only superficial tissue has been excised. Healing by second intention has been used with great success in selected patients after Mohs surgery. It does not work with every defect because there may be unwanted contractures that cause distortions of the eyelids or lips. All that is needed is to dress the wound with some type of occlusive gauze dressing or cover the wound with an ointment and wait until it heals. Bacitracin ointment can be used; however, this has a tendency to promote

Figure 19-2   *A,* **Hairy nevus of cheek in young man.** *B,* **Excision is planned so that final scar is in or parallel to melolabial fold.** *C,* **One year postoperatively scar is still noticeable.**

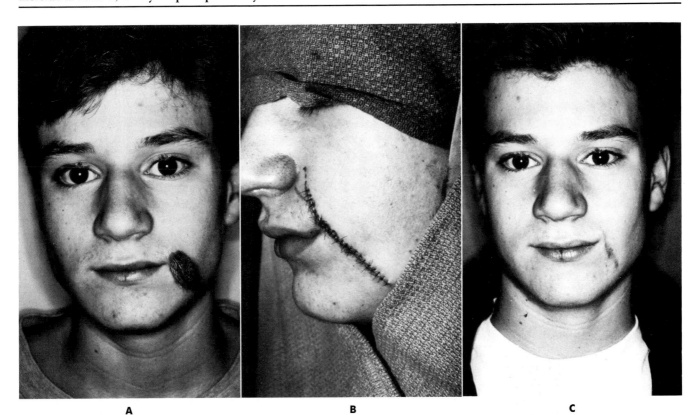

A   B   C

Figure 19-3   *A*, Angiosarcoma of cheek measuring 6 × 7.5 cm in 70-year-old man. Peripheral marking denotes proposed surgical margin. *B*, Defect covered with split-thickness skin graft. *C*, Appearance 1 year after surgery and postoperative radiotherapy. **(Courtesy Shan R. Baker, M.D.)**

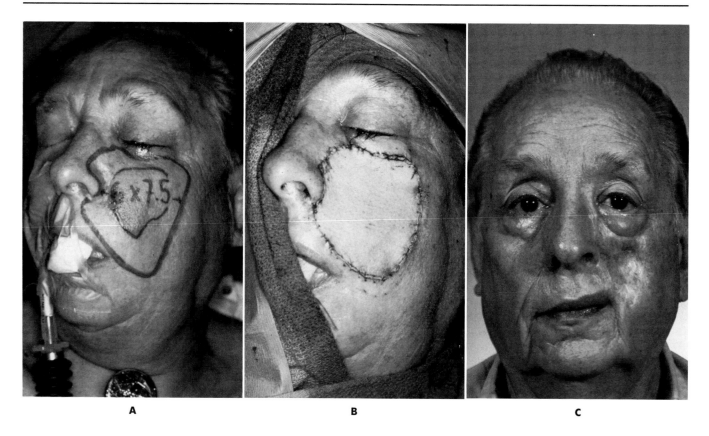

A   B   C

the formation of excessive granulation tissue. In our hands, the best method is to dress the wound with wet or dry gauze dressings moistened with saline and changed three to four times a day. The cosmetic result can be surprisingly good from this type of wound management.

Skin Grafting

Skin grafting of defects is a simple and efficient way to initially reconstruct a defect of the cheek. This is especially true of large defects that result from extensive tumor resections (Fig. 19-3). McGregor[19] advocates skin grafting after resection of malignant tumors of the cheeks. He then waits for approximately 1 year and, if there is no tumor recurrence, he will then reconstruct the defect with a local or distant flap. Another advantage is that the skin graft will shrink and make the defect somewhat smaller.

One of the problems with skin grafting is color match of the graft with the remaining skin of the cheek. Grafts should be taken from the postauricular or preauricular areas or the supraclavicular area to obtain the best color match. Another problem is that if a split-thickness skin graft is used near the eyelid, it has a tendency to contract and pull down the lower eyelid, causing an ectropion. Therefore, split-thickness grafts should be used in the lower cheek area or lateral to the eye. Full-thickness skin grafts do not contract as much as split-thickness skin grafts but, unless their borders are placed in the natural skin lines of esthetic units, they have a tendency to appear like a patch.

We like to use a bolster type of dressing to fix the skin graft to the defect (Fig. 19-4). First the skin graft is harvested from the preauricular, postauricular, or supraclavicular area and then defatted. The skin graft is then sewn to the edges of the wound with long silk or nylon sutures. A running 6-0 chromic gut suture is used to approximate the skin graft to the edge of the defect. Petroleum jelly (Vaseline) or bismuth tribromphenate-impregnated gauze covered by polyester fiber or moist cotton is used for the overlying stent. The dressing is allowed to remain in place for 5 to 7 days. Often initially there is a craterlike deformity; however, this has a tendency to fill in, flattening the contour deformity with time.

Figure 19-4   *A,* Wide local excision of melanoma of temple and upper cheek is planned. *B,* Full-thickness skin graft was harvested from supraclavicular area. Bolster dressing of medicated gauze and cotton is used to hold graft in place. *C,* Appearance 4 months postoperatively.

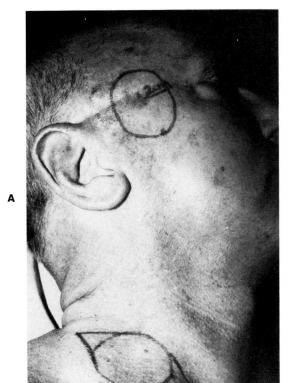

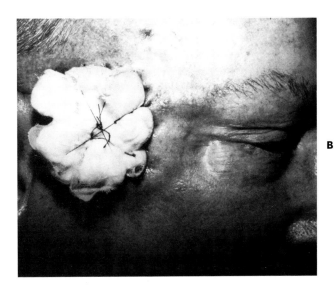

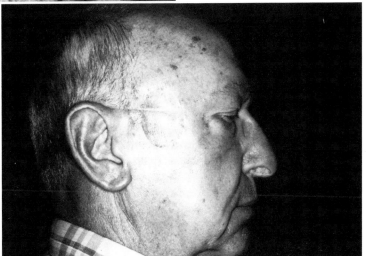

Transposition Flaps

Rhombic and other transposition flaps are very versatile. They can be used anywhere on the face for small to moderate-sized defects and are especially good for coverage of areas around the eyes. If oriented correctly, the pull on the skin will not cause ectropion. One must take into account the laxity of the surrounding skin and the orientation of the final scars in the design of these flaps. Occasionally the repair will result in a "trapdoor" deformity.

Transposition involves moving a square, rectangular, or triangular flap from a site adjacent to the defect into the defect (Fig. 19-5). There are many types of transposition flaps, including rhombic or Limberg flaps, bilobe flaps, Dufourmental flaps, and Z-plasties.

Figure 19-5   *A*, A 10 × 9 cm skin defect of lower posterior cheek after removal of basal cell carcinoma in 71-year-old woman. *B*, Inferiorly based transposition flap designed to recruit lax upper cervical skin. *C*, Appearance 6 months postoperatively. (*C*, from Baker SR: Local cutaneous flaps, *Otolaryngol Clin North Am* **27:**139, **1994.**)

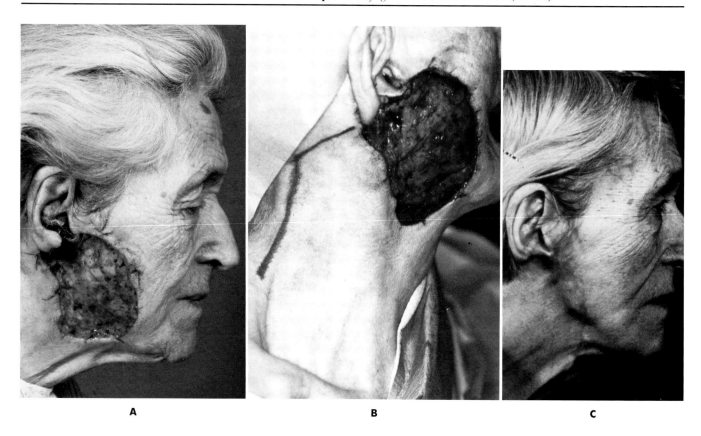

A   B   C

A transposition flap is a pivotal flap. According to Jackson[20] the angle of transposition of a flap can be a maximum of 90° from its original position. Others disagree and say that the flaps can be designed up to 180° away from the linear axis of the defect. However, the greater the angle, the greater the standing cutaneous deformity. Transposition flaps are usually random-pattern flaps.

In the design of a transposition flap, one must make the flap longer than the defect due to the fact that, when transposed, the flap becomes relatively shorter, because the edge of the base farthest from the defect effectively acts as a tether. The surgeon should try moving a template shaped like the required flap, with its base fixed at the same point as the edge of the base of the flap that is located farthest from the defect. Although skin flaps have some inherent elasticity, if the template does not adequately cover the defect, it is unlikely that the flap will. One of the problems encountered with transposition flaps is the possibility of the development of a trapdoor deformity. It may become necessary to defat the flap at a second stage, either in the conventional way or with suction lipec-

tomy, although this does not always completely correct the deformity.

Rhombic Flaps

Rhombic flaps are a type of transposition flap. The area to be removed is excised in the shape of a rhombus with 120° and 60° angles. The flap depends on adjacent areas of loose skin (Fig. 19-6). These areas should lie lateral to the 120° angle of the rhombus. The flap is designed by drawing a straight line out from the point of the 120° angle of the rhombus. The length of this line should equal the length of the side of the rhombus. At the end of this line, a second line is drawn parallel to the side of the rhombic defect and is of the same length. The flap is elevated in a subcutaneous plane, transposed, and sewn into position. The donor site is closed primarily. Four different rhombic flaps may be created next to a defect. Rhombic flaps are especially useful for closure of defects in the cheek and eyelid areas. If the flap is positioned properly, it will not create an ectropion.

Figure 19-6   *A,* Basal cell carcinoma of cheek (outlined by *circle*). Rhombic excision of tumor is planned. Rhombic flap is designed for repair. *B,* Tumor excised. Dotted line denotes extent of skin undermining necessary for wound closure. *C,* Wound repaired. Standing cutaneous deformity was excised at superior aspect of defect. *D,* Appearance 6 months postoperatively. (*D,* courtesy Shan R. Baker, M.D.)

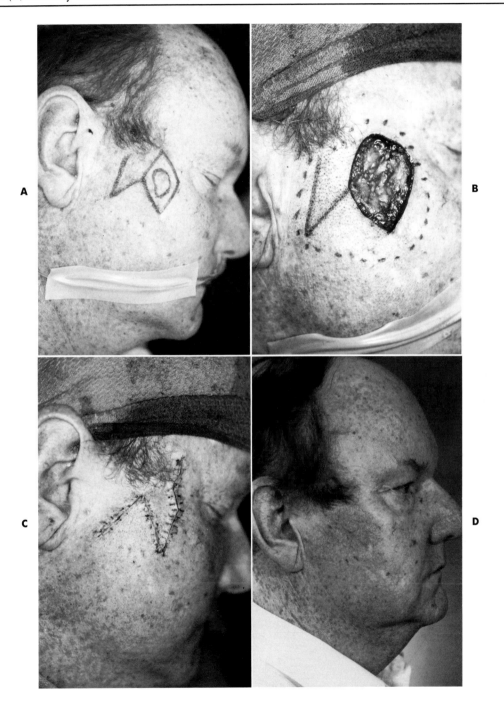

Bilobed Flaps

Similar to rhombic flaps, bilobed flaps are transposition flaps and take advantage of adjacent lax skin to close the donor defects. The flap is designed to resemble a mitten. The primary flap adjacent to the defect is designed slightly smaller than the defect, and the secondary flap adjacent to the primary flap is designed to be even smaller. The flap is raised in the subcutaneous plane and transposed into position. The trick is to make sure the donor defect of the secondary flap can be closed primarily. This is determined by the pinch test to see if the skin in this area is loose enough to permit primary closure. Bilobed flaps may be used anywhere on the cheek; however, care should be taken in the use of this flap, due to the fact that the incisions for the flaps may not fit into the natural lines of the face, and the esthetic result could be disappointing. It is probably best used for moderate-sized to large central defects in which the remaining lateral preauricular skin is used as the primary flap and the posterior auricular or cervical skin is the source of the secondary flap (Fig. 19-7).

Melolabial Flaps

Melolabial flaps can be designed as transposition flaps, advancement flaps, and subcutaneously based pedicle flaps.[21] They are very versatile but may be prone to developing a trapdoor deformity when designed as a transposition flap. Melolabial flaps can be used for small to moderate-sized defects of the upper, middle, or lower medial aspects of the cheek and can be superiorly or inferiorly based. They can be based on branches of the facial artery or can be random-pattern flaps. Ohtsuka[22] advocates the placement of the base of

Figure 19-7 Bilobed flap used to repair medial cheek defect. Standing cutaneous deformity is excised from inferior aspect of defect.

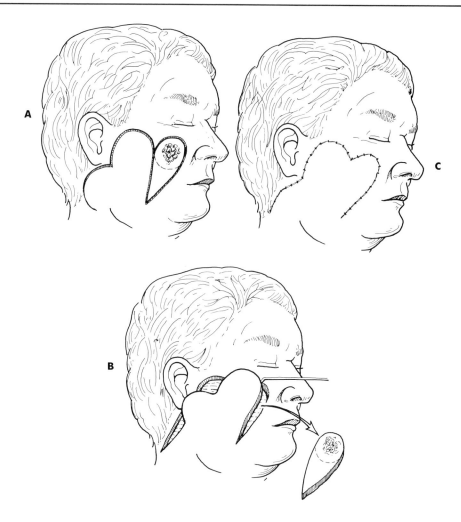

Figure 19-8   *A,* A 8 × 8 cm skin defect of medial cheek after removal of basal cell carcinoma in 57-year-old patient. *B,* Melolabial transposition flap designed for repair of wound. *C,* Flap transposed and sutured in place. Donor site is closed primarily. Standing cutaneous deformities are resected parallel to melolabial sulcus and infraorbital rim. *D,* and *E,* Appearance 3 months postoperatively. (*D* and *E* from Baker, SR: Local cutaneous flaps, *Otolaryngol Clin North Am* **27:139,** 1994.)

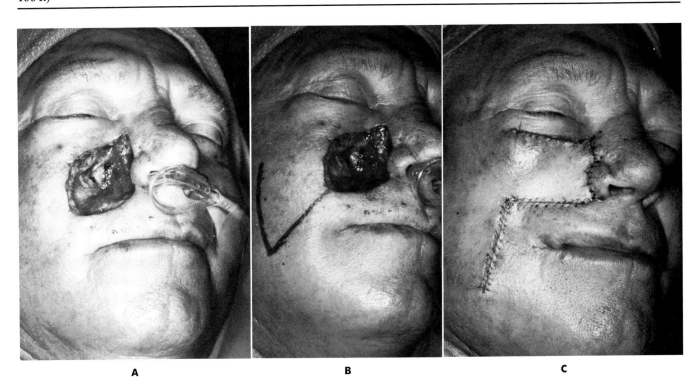

A   B   C

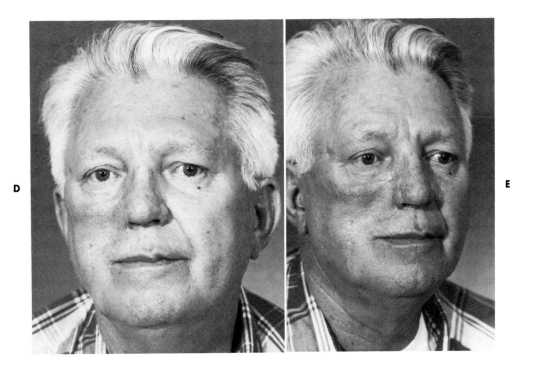

D   E

the pedicle adjacent to the alar base to obtain better blood supply. These flaps are excellent for repair of defects of the medial aspect of the cheek (Fig. 19-8). Unfortunately, if they are used for repair of more laterally located defects, they have a tendency to look like a patch. The flap is elevated, with its medial border in the melolabial sulcus. The maximum width of the flap is approximately 3 cm. The flap is then either transposed or tunneled into the defect on a subcutaneous pedicle and sewn into position. Long nonaxial pattern flaps may benefit from a delay procedure.

Forehead Flaps

Median and paramedian forehead flaps are mostly used for nasal reconstruction; however, they can be used for reconstruction of a limited area of the medial cheek (Fig. 19-9). The flap is based on the supraorbital or supratrochlear arteries. In design of the flap it is best to use a Doppler Probe to determine which set of arteries is dominant. If a large flap is required, it is best to delay the flap before its transfer or to use skin expansion. If a tissue expander is used, a rectangular one can be placed either under the skin in the subcutaneous plane or under the frontalis muscle. The increase in skin surface area gained by skin expansion allows repair of the donor site, which otherwise could not be closed primarily. An alternative to forehead expansion in cases in which a large flap is required and in which it is anticipated that the donor site cannot be closed primarily is to repair the donor site with a skin graft or allow it to heal by second intention. It is preferable, however, to close the donor site primarily. The flap is allowed to reside in its new location for a minimum of 2 weeks, and then the base of the flap is transected and the proximal portion of the flap is inset into the area between the eyebrows. One advantage of the forehead flap is the excellent color match with the rest of the face. Marchac has described transposition of large expanded forehead flaps to the face, with gratifying results.

Laterally based forehead flaps supplied by the superficial temporal vessels may also be used for reconstruction of the cheek. They are probably best used to close large superficial defects and small to moderate-sized full-thickness defects of the cheek. If this type of flap is to be used for a full-thickness cheek defect, it can be folded on itself and a portion deepithelialized. A disadvantage of a laterally based forehead flap is the necessity to repair the donor defect with a skin graft. It also leaves a contour deformity at the donor site, which gives the illusion that the patient has a sloping forehead. When used as an interpolation flap, the pedicle of the laterally based forehead flap can be partially tubed. Once the distal portion of the flap

has developed collateral circulation at the recipient site, the pedicle may be amputated and the proximal portion of the flap replaced. Conversely, the pedicle may be deepithelialized and tunneled under facial skin that intervenes between the defect and the base of the flap. If all of the skin of the forehead is harvested as a flap, it may be helpful to delay the flap. The forehead should be reconstructed with a single-sheet skin graft.

In situations in which reconstruction of a cheek defect does not require all of the forehead skin, a scalping flap is an alternative choice. This flap is more reliable from the standpoint of vascularity than the distal portion of a laterally based total forehead flap. Lateral forehead skin based superiorly on the scalp is elevated by incisions that cross over to encompass the superficial temporal vessels on the opposite side of the head (Fig. 19-10). The flap is raised full thickness including the galea, transposed to the cheek defect, and sewn in place. The exposed area of the scalp donor site is dressed with a medicated gauze dressing with a tie-over stent while the scalp is serving as a carrier. One problem with this flap is that it will typically temporarily obstruct vision in one eye. The flap is allowed to remain in place for several weeks (2 to 3) and is then released. A majority of the flap is returned to the scalp and sewn into position. The donor defect is reconstructed with a split-thickness skin graft at the time of the initial flap transposition. The skin graft may subsequently be removed and replaced with adjacent forehead skin by the technique of skin expansion.

Platysmal Flaps

Platysmal musculocutaneous flaps can be used for small to moderate-sized defects of the lower cheek. This flap should not be considered in patients who have had a radical neck dissection or have received radiation therapy to the neck. Potential problems that could arise are damage to the 11th cranial nerve and the cervical or marginal mandibular branches of the facial nerve. Platysmal musculocutaneous flaps provide better color match with the skin of the face than more distantly located flap donor sites. In men it also has the benefit of providing hair-bearing skin to replace the beard. The blood supply to the muscle and skin comes from submental branches of the facial artery and a small branch of the transverse cervical artery inferiorly (Fig. 19-11**A**).

The skin paddle is designed, and a generous portion of the skin and subcutaneous tissue is elevated off the platysma surrounding the flap. The flap is harvested with a 1-cm margin of platysma muscle surrounding the distal free edge of the skin paddle. The platysma, which serves as the superiorly based pedicle of the flap, is elevated off the underlying strap, sternocleidomas-

Figure 19-9   *A*, Temple defect and 12 × 12 cm defect of cheek and lateral nasal skin after Mohs surgical excision of two basal cell carcinomas in 70-year-old man. *B* and *C*, Midline forehead flap and cheek transposition flaps are designed. *D*, Forehead flap is used to repair lateral nasal defect. It also assists transposition flap in repair of upper lip and cheek defect. Temple defect is covered by skin graft. *E*, Appearance 9 months postoperatively. No revisional surgery was performed. (Courtesy Shan R. Baker, M.D.)

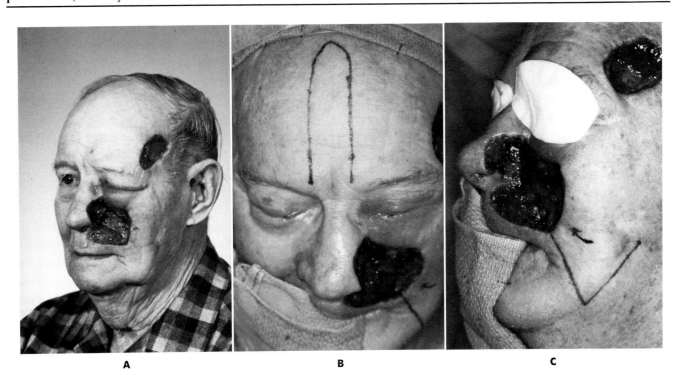

A   B   C

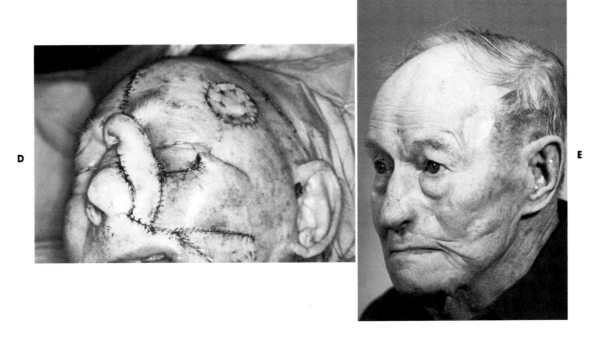

D   E

Figure 19-10 Scalping forehead flap used to reconstruct medial cheek defect. *A*, Tumor is removed from cheek, and scalping flap is incised. *B*, Full-thickness lateral forehead skin flap is pedicled on the anterior scalp and remaining forehead skin. *C*, Flap is transposed and sutured into cheek defect. Split-thickness skin graft is placed over lateral forehead donor site. *D*, Gauze bolster dressing covers graft and donor site. *E* and *F*, Pedicle is divided and returned 2 to 3 weeks after initial flap transfer.

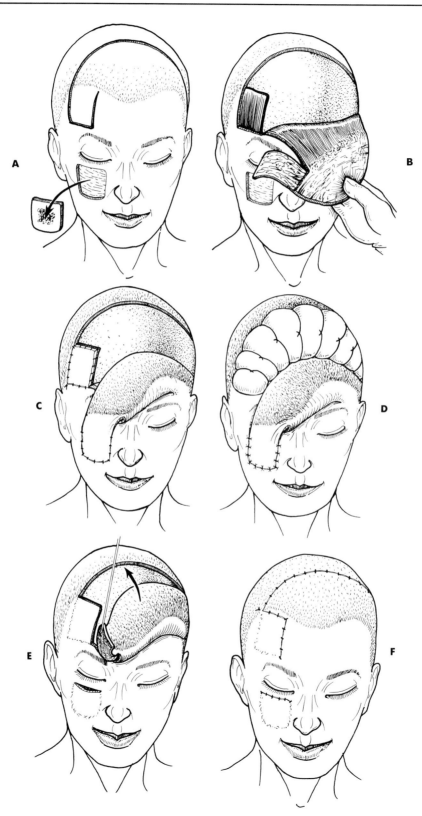

Figure 19-11   Platysmal musculocutaneous transposition flap used to repair defect of lower part of cheek. Pedicle is tunneled under intervening cervical skin to enable transfer of flap. Flap is nourished by submental branches of facial artery.

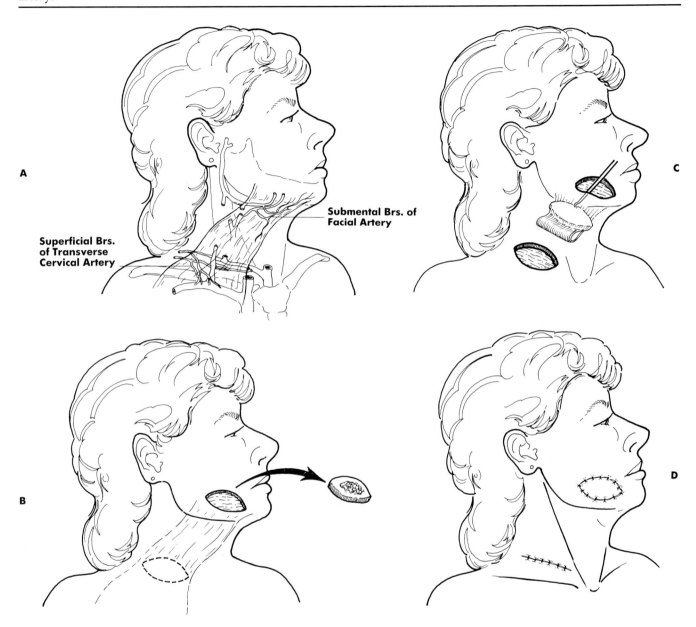

toid, and trapezius muscles. Care is taken not to sever the accessory or marginal mandibular nerves during dissection. Care is also taken not to buttonhole the platysmal muscle, as this could compromise the blood supply to the overlying skin paddle. The muscle should not be dissected off the mandibular border, as this could also compromise the vascular supply. The skin paddle with its muscular pedicle may then be transposed or tunneled into position to repair a defect of the lower cheek area. The donor defect may need to be skin grafted (Fig. 19-11).

Advancement Flaps

Advancement flaps take advantage of the elasticity of the skin to enable the flap to slide into a particular defect. Advancement flaps are moved forward without rotation or lateral movement. They have the disadvantage of being able to cover only relatively small defects and thus are best suited for use in older individuals who have greater skin laxity.[18]

Advancement flaps are best designed so that the incisions fall into the natural lines of the face. Two

Figure 19-12 *A,* Superficial spreading melanoma of cheek. *B,* A 18 × 12 cm skin defect after tumor removal. Advancement flap designed for repair with bilateral Z-plasties at base of flap to facilitate flap movement and reduce standing cutaneous deformity. *C,* Flap is advanced and sutured. Despite Z-plasties, it was necessary to excise small standing cutaneous deformity anteriorly along inferior mandibular margin. *D* and *E,* Appearance 1 year postoperatively. (*D* and *E* from Baker SR: Local cutaneous flaps, *Otolaryngol Clin North Am* **27:139, 1994.**)

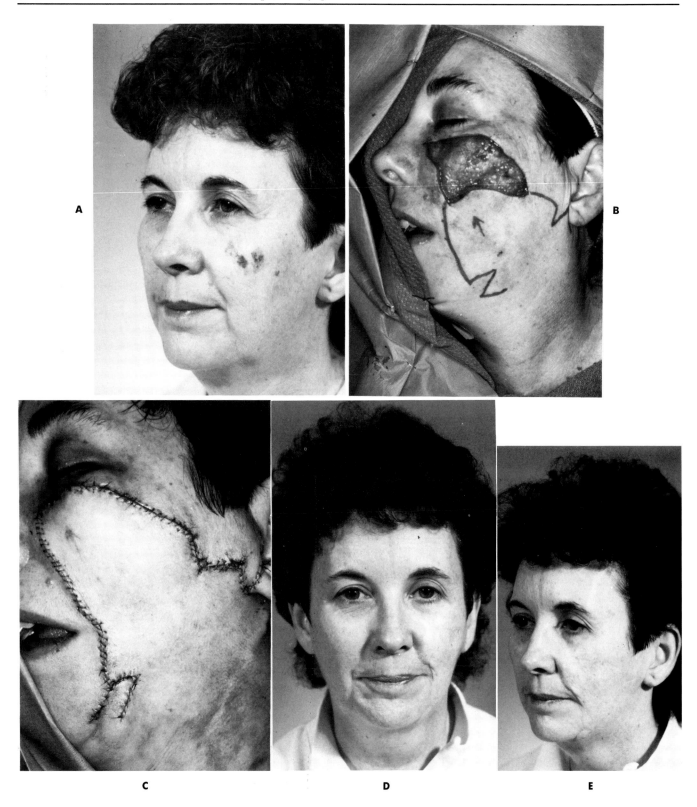

parallel incisions are made adjacent to the defect, and the flap is elevated and advanced over the defect. If the flap does not stretch sufficiently, one may need to create Burow's triangles at the lateral base of the flap. These triangular excisions help equalize the distances between the sides of the flap and the wound margins. Another approach is to perform bilateral Z-plasties of the base of the flap to reduce or eliminate the standing cutaneous deformity (Fig. 19-12).

V-Y Subcutaneous-Based Advancement Flaps

V-Y advancement flaps can be based on a cutaneous or subcutaneous pedicle. When based on a subcutaneous pedicle, the blood supply to the skin of the flap comes from subcutaneous and muscular perforating vessels. V-Y advancement flaps can be used to reconstruct numerous small defects about the lateral, central, and medial portions of the cheek. If a defect is too large for

Figure 19-13 *A,* Squamous cell carcinoma of right cheek in elderly woman. *B,* Margins of excision are drawn, and V-Y advancement flaps are designed. *C* and *D,* Lesion is excised, flaps are advanced, and wound is closed. *E,* Appearance 2 months postoperatively.

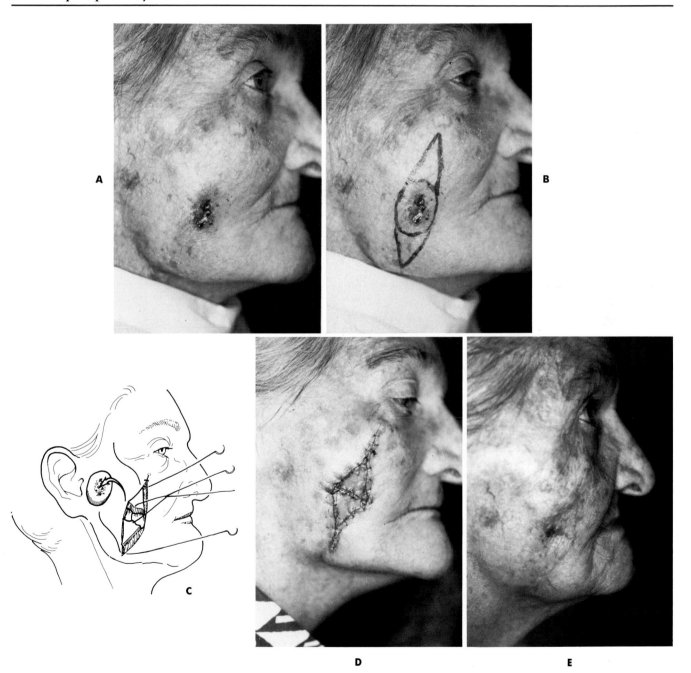

one V-Y advancement flap, a similar flap may be created on the opposite side of the defect and the two flaps are advanced toward each other (Fig. 19-13). One disadvantage to this is that scarring will result and may be objectionable, especially in the younger patient. A V-shaped flap is drawn next to the defect, with the widest part of the V the same width as the defect. The skin is incised down to and including a portion of the subcutaneous tissue, and the flap is advanced into the defect. The donor site is then closed primarily, and the resulting scar assumes the configuration of a Y.

Rotation Flaps

Rotation flaps are usually semicircular and are designed adjacent to the defect. The flap is rotated about a fixed pivotal point into the defect. The line of greatest tension is from the pivotal point out toward the defect. Most flaps are random in their vascularity. These flaps can be used anywhere on the face; however, they look best when designed so that the resulting scars approximate relaxed skin tension lines of the face or lie along borders of facial esthetic units (Fig. 19-14).

Figure 19-14   *A* and *B,* A 4 × 3 cm skin defect in 56-year-old patient after excision of basal skin carcinoma. *C,* Rotation flap is designed with border of flap coinciding with border of facial esthetic units (eyelid and cheek). *D* and *E,* Standing cutaneous deformity is excised in melolabial sulcus. *F,* One year postoperatively some standing cutaneous deformity persists at inferior aspect of melolabial sulcus. (Courtesy Shan R. Baker, M.D.)

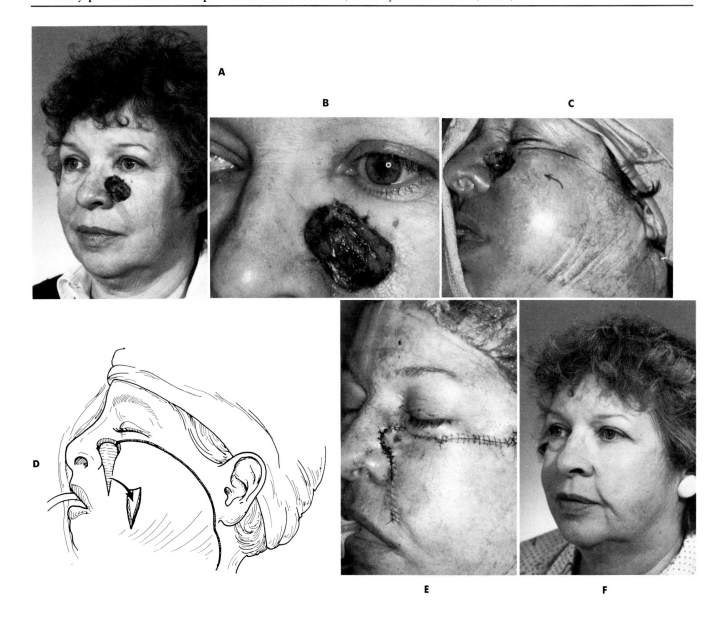

Figure 19-15   *A*, Melanoma of lower eyelid and upper cheek. Triangle beneath eye represents planned tissue resection. Cervicofacial rotation advancement flap is designed for reconstruction of lower eyelid and medial cheek. *B*, Lesion is excised and flap is raised. *C* and *D*, Flap is sutured into position. (*C* and *D* courtesy R. Bruce Shack, M.D.)

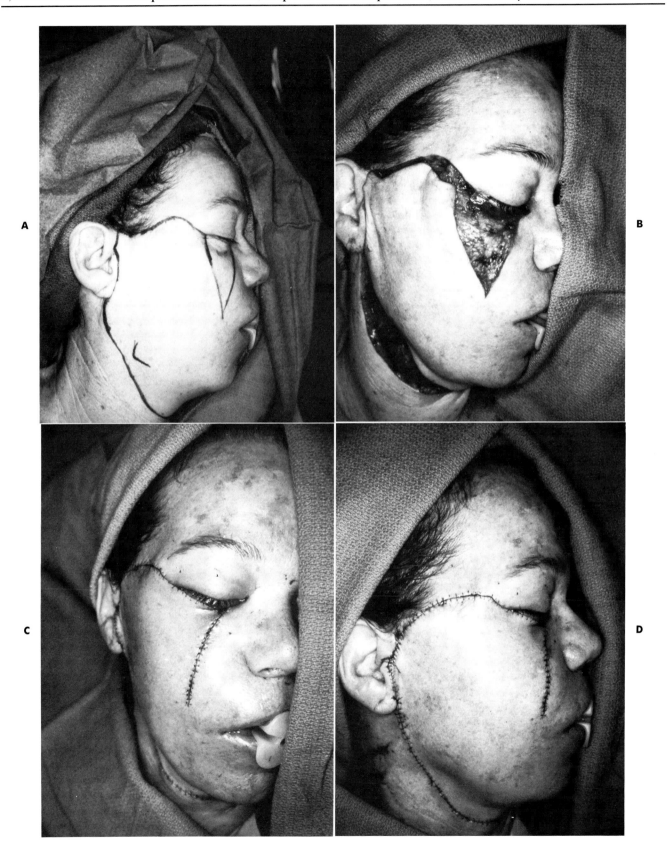

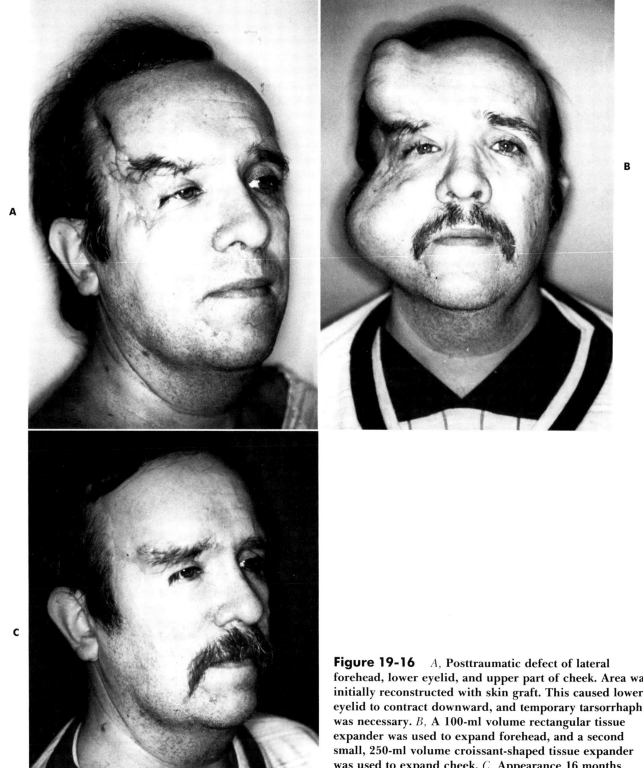

Figure 19-16   *A*, Posttraumatic defect of lateral
forehead, lower eyelid, and upper part of cheek. Area was
initially reconstructed with skin graft. This caused lower
eyelid to contract downward, and temporary tarsorrhaphy
was necessary. *B*, A 100-ml volume rectangular tissue
expander was used to expand forehead, and a second
small, 250-ml volume croissant-shaped tissue expander
was used to expand cheek. *C*, Appearance 16 months
postoperatively. Expansion provided sufficient skin to
develop advancement flaps from cheek and forehead,
allowing removal of previously placed skin graft and
take-down of tarsorrhaphy.

Cervicopectoral and Cervicofacial Flaps

The cervicopectoral flap is a large cutaneous rotation advancement flap that uses the remaining skin of the face, neck, and upper part of the trunk. The flap can be based medially or laterally. As described by Becker,[23] the cervicopectoral flap can be used for large full-thickness defects of the cheek (6 × 10 cm). When the flap is medially based, it derives its blood supply from the internal thoracic artery perforators and from musculocutaneous perforators of the platysmal muscle.[24] The flap should be designed to extend from the base of the defect to below the clavicle, and it is elevated in the subcutaneous plane. Under ideal circumstances (a patient with a short neck and broad chest), the flap can be designed so that it will reach to the zygomatic arch.

Similar to the cervicopectoral flap, the cervicofacial flap is a cutaneous rotation advancement flap. It is used to repair moderate-sized defects of the cheek (Fig. 19-15). It has been described as being either medially or laterally based. In young patients, portions of the secondary defect that result from movement of the flap may require skin grafting; however, this is not usually necessary in older patients with more laxity of the neck skin.

Soft-Tissue Expansion

Soft-tissue expansion is one of the most versatile methods of cheek reconstruction. Skin adjacent to the defect is expanded, which provides skin that closely matches the color and texture of the missing skin. Defects of the flap donor site are avoided by advancement of expanded skin directly over the defect. One disadvantage is that immediate reconstruction is usually not possible. A temporary wound repair is usually accomplished with a split-thickness skin graft. A tissue expander can be placed at this time or after the skin graft has healed. In planning reconstruction with use of an expander, we believe that a croissant-shaped expander works best for a circular defect. For more linear defects a rectangular expander is preferred.

For insertion of an expander, an incision is made and a suitable recipient pocket is created. This can be either in a subcutaneous, subfascial, or submuscular plane, depending on the type of flap planned. After the pocket has been created, hemostasis is controlled and the expander is inserted. If a remote port is used, a separate subcutaneous pocket for the port is created. This pocket should be located superficially to facilitate location of the port later. After the expander is inserted and the edges are smoothed out, the wound is closed. A drain may or may not be used.

Expansion is begun several days later. After expansion is completed, the expander is removed through the same incision in which it was placed, the defect is prepared, and the flap is advanced (Fig. 19-16). The capsule around the expander need not be excised.

SUMMARY

There is a myriad of methods to reconstruct defects of the cheek. The best color match is achieved when surrounding tissue is used for the reconstruction, that is, local flaps or grafts. A variety of local flaps can be used, including rhombic or other types of transposition flaps, V-Y advancement flaps, melolabial flaps, forehead flaps, cervicofacial and cervicopectoral flaps, and platysmal flaps. Soft-tissue expansion is also a good alternative for reconstruction of larger cheek defects because it uses local skin and leaves minimal scarring.

REFERENCES

1. *Dorland's Illustrated Medical Dictionary*, ed 25, Philadelphia, 1974, WB Saunders.
2. Zide BM: Deformities of the lips and cheeks. In McCarthy JG, editor: *Plastic surgery*, 8 vols, Philadelphia, 1990, WB Saunders.
3. Feldman JJ: Facial burns. In McCarthy JG, editor: *Plastic Surgery*, 8 vols, Philadelphia, 1990, WB Saunders.
4. Rohrich RJ, Sheffield RW: Lip and cheek reconstruction. In: *Selected readings in plastic surgery* 17:11, 1987.
5. Millard DR Jr: *Principalization of plastic surgery*, Boston, 1986, Little, Brown.
6. Hurwitz DJ, Rabson JA, Futrell JW: The anatomic basis for the platysma skin flap, *Plast Reconstr Surg* 723:302, 1983.
7. Coleman JJ III et al: The platysma musculocutaneous flap: experience with 24 cases, *Plast Reconstr Surg* 72:302, 1983.
8. Bunkis J et al: The evolution of techniques for reconstruction of full-thickness cheek defects, *Plast Reconstr Surg* 70:319, 1982.
9. Skow J: One-stage reconstruction of full-thickness cheek defects, *Plast Reconstr Surg* 71:855, 1983.
10. Harii K, Ono I, Ebihara S: Closure of total cheek defects with two combined myocutaneous free flaps, *Arch Otolaryngol* 108:303, 1982.
11. Achauer BM: A Serious complication following medical-grade silicone injection of the face, *Plast Reconstr Surg* 71:251, 1983.
12. Jurkiewicz MJ, Nahai F: The use of free revascularized grafts in the amelioration of hemifacial atrophy, *Plast Reconstr Surg* 76:44, 1985.

13. Walkinshaw M, Caffee HH, Wolfe SA: Vascularized omentum for facial contour restoration, *Ann Plast Surg* 10:293, 1983.

14. Bakamjian VY: Deltopectoral skin flap. In Strauch B, Vasconez LO, Hall-Findlay EJ, editors: *Grabb's encyclopedia of flaps*, Boston, 1990, Little, Brown.

15. Bakamjian VY, Long M, Rigg B: Experience with the medially based deltopectoral flap in reconstructive surgery of the head and neck, *Br J Plast Surg* 24:174, 1971.

16. Russell RC et al: The extended pectoralis major myocutaneous flap: uses and indications, *Plast Reconstr Surg* 88:814, 1991.

17. Borges AF: *Elective incisions and scar revision*, Boston, 1973, Little, Brown.

18. Jankauskas S, Cohen IK, Grabb WC: Basic technique of plastic surgery. In Smith JW, Aston SJ, editors: *Grabb and Smith's plastic surgery*, Boston, 1991, Little, Brown.

19. McGregor I: Personal communication.

20. Jackson IT: *Local flaps in head and neck reconstruction*, St Louis, 1985, CV Mosby.

21. Barron JN, Saad MN: Subcutaneous pedicle flaps. In Strauch B, Vasconez LO, Hall-Findlay EJ, editors: *Grabb's encyclopedia of flaps*, Boston, 1990, Little, Brown.

22. Ohtsuka H: Nasolabial skin flaps to the cheek. In Smith JW, Aston JA, editors: *Grabb's encyclopedia of flaps*, Boston, 1990, Little, Brown.

23. Becker DW Jr: A cervicopectoral rotation flap for cheek closure, *Plast Reconstr Surg* 61:868, 1978.

24. Becker DW Jr: Cervicopectoral skin flap to the cheek, In Strauch B, Vasconez LO, Hall-Findlay EJ, editors: *Grabb's encyclopedia of flaps*, Boston, 1990, Little, Brown.

EDITORIAL COMMENTS

Shan R. Baker

The authors have outlined a number of methods of reconstruction of cheek defects with use of local flaps. They also mention wound healing by second intention. Although healing by second intention often produces a satisfactory scar in areas of concavity, such as the medial canthal and lateral temple regions, it does not produce satisfactory scars on the cheek. An exception to this statement is in the preauricular area. This phenomenon is probably due to the relative immobility of preauricular skin compared with the more medially located cheek skin, which is subjected to constant motion as a result of talking, eating, and facial animation.

I have not commonly experienced the trapdoor deformity that the authors discuss in relationship to use of transposition flaps for reconstruction of cheek defects. I have also not found it necessary to delay either midforehead flaps or laterally based total forehead flaps when using them to reconstruct various defects of the head and neck.

I agree with the authors concerning the limited usefulness of advancement flaps for reconstruction of the cheek. In my experience most skin defects of the cheek can be repaired with either transposition or rotation flaps. Transposition flaps are usually harvested from adjacent cheek skin, as discussed by the authors, but can be developed in the upper neck to resurface larger cheek defects (Fig. 19-17). Rotation flaps are useful in repairing medial cheek defects located near the nasalfacial sulcus. The curvilinear border of the flap can often be positioned along the infraorbital rim, which

Figure 19-17 *A*, A 16 × 15 cm defect of central cheek after removal of extensive basal cell carcinoma. Tumor extirpation required sacrifice of facial nerve and removal of zygomatic arch. *B*, Large inferiorly based cervical transposition flap designed to resurface cheek defect. *C*, Appearance 6 months postoperatively. Flap donor site was in part closed with skin graft, and 1 cm of distal edge of flap necrosed and healed by second intention.

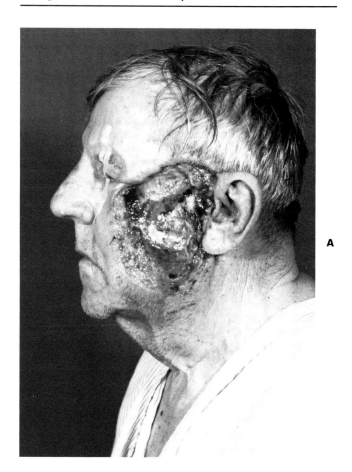

A

Figure 19-17, cont'd.   For legend see opposite page.

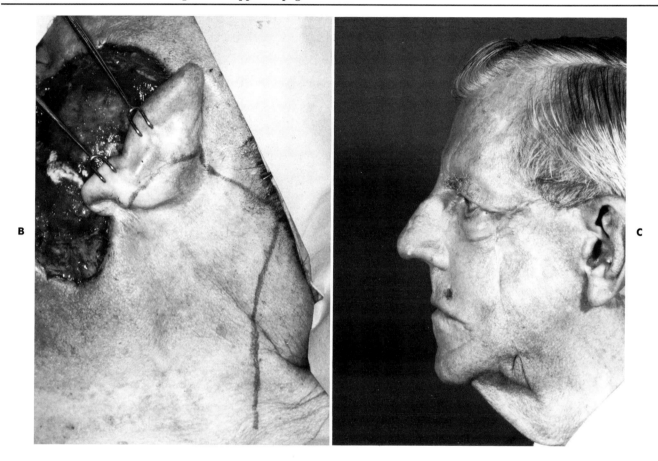

Figure 19-18 *A,* Squamous cell carcinoma of medial cheek skin in 74-year-old man. Outer circle marks proposed surgical margin around tumor. *B,* Rotation flap is designed along border of facial esthetic units (eyelid and cheek). Margin of flap is extended above level of lateral canthus. Planned excision of standing cutaneous deformity is designed to occur in melolabial sulcus. *C,* Tumor is removed, and defect is reconstructed with flap. Flap is suspended to periosteum of lateral orbital rim to assist in prevention of ectropion. *D,* Appearance 3 months postoperatively and following postoperative radiotherapy. Lower lid ectropion has developed in part due to minimal necrosis of medial border of flap and subsequent scar contracture.

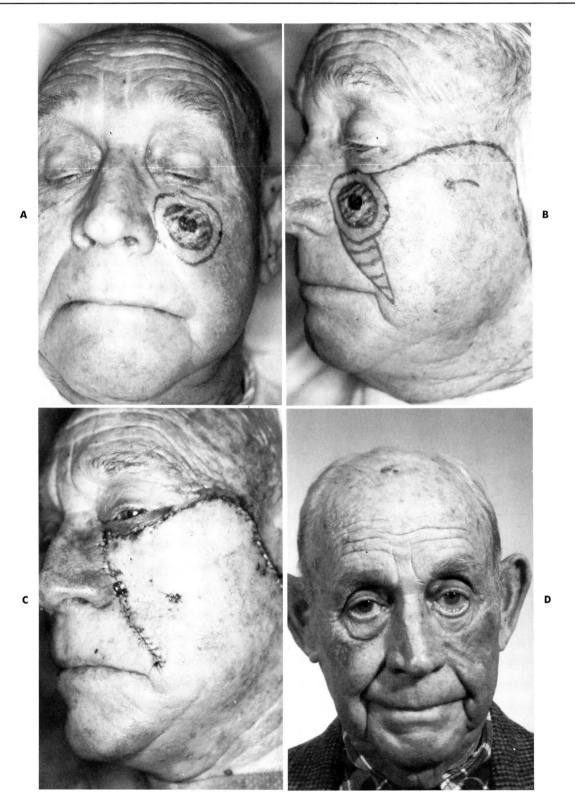

represents an important border of esthetic units (eyelid and cheek). By positioning the incision for the flap along this border, the surgeon can enhance scar camouflage. When possible, the margin of the rotation flap should extend above the level of the lateral canthus to assist in the prevention of lower lid retraction. It may also be helpful to suspend the flap to the periosteum of the lateral orbital rim. Despite these precautions, lower lid ectropion is not an uncommon sequela when large rotation flaps are used in this region to reconstruct medial cheek defects in elderly patients with lax lower eyelids (Fig. 19-18).

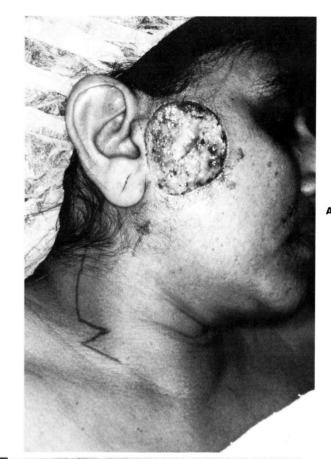

Figure 19-19   *A,* A 6 × 5 cm skin defect of posterior cheek after removal of squamous cell carcinoma. Cervical facial rotation flap is designed for reconstruction of defect. *B,* Flap is transferred into defect. Z-plasty at base of flap facilitates closure of donor site. Large standing cutaneous deformity is excised from inferior aspect of defect. *C,* Appearance 1 year postoperatively. (*C,* from Baker SR: Local cutaneous flaps, *Otolaryngol Clin North Am* 27:139, 1994.)

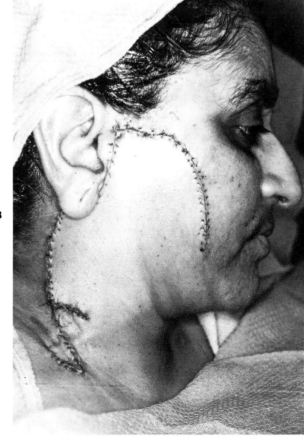

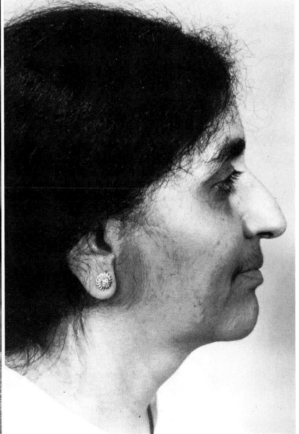

Large rotation flaps are particularly useful for reconstruction of sizable defects of the posterior cheek and upper part of the neck. Large medial inferiorly based rotation flaps provide a flexible means for transfer of large amounts of skin from the remaining cheek and upper cervical skin. Incisions for the flap are placed in a preauricular crease and can extend for some distance along the anterior border of the trapezius muscle to facilitate rotation of upper cervical skin toward the posterior cheek area. A Z-plasty at the base of the flap facilitates closure of the secondary defect (Fig. 19-19).[1]

Reference

1. Baker SR: Local cutaneous flaps, *Otolaryngol Clin North Am* 27:139, 1994.

EDITORIAL COMMENTS

Neil A. Swanson

There is a good basic discussion of correction of contour defects in the beginning of this comprehensive chapter. My success with autologous fat grafting may be slightly better than that of the authors. The cheek is one area where success has occurred, although often with the necessity for repeat autologous grafting. From my experience, if one is able to get the autologous fat graft to vascularize, it will last for a long time. It is unfortunate that we do not still have silicone in our armamentarium because the use of highly purified medical-grade silicone was safe and reliable to correct contour defects.

My results with healing by second intention and skin grafting on the cheeks have not been outstanding. These techniques will work better over the medial cheek than laterally toward the preauricular area. Wound contracture with healing by second intention can cause ectropion and often an unsightly depressed contour defect in the resulting scar. I disagree with the dressing used for healing by second intention. I think that most experienced Mohs surgeons find that moist occlusive healing will allow a wound to granulate more quickly and with a filling of the depth of the wound. My favorite form of moist occlusion is still debridement with peroxide followed by the use of polymyxin B-bacitracin (Polysporin) or a related ointment and an occlusive dressing. Skin grafts on the cheek are used as either a temporizing fashion or for a very large defect in an elderly patient. The reader is referred to Chapter 8, Dr. Glogau's excellent discussion of skin grafting, and my editorial comments. In general, I use the following differences in technique: (1) a rapidly absorbing gut suture is used to anchor the skin graft; (2) for grafts of large areas, such as would be necessary on the cheek, the graft is fenestrated, allowing for ooze of serosanguinous fluid so that it does not build up under the graft; (3) the graft is basted in place in several areas; (4) if a tie-over dressing is used, the tie-over sutures are placed away from the edge of the graft so as to put less trauma on the graft-skin junction; (5) whatever multilayered dressing is used whether tie-over or taped in place, the first layer that I use is N-terface, which is a nonadherent material.

I completely agree with the authors that when primary closure cannot be performed, local flaps are the best option. Rhombic flaps can be used on the cheeks, especially the lateral cheek and approaching the eyelid. In the latter case it is important to cut an oversized rhombic flap so as to push up on the free margin of the eyelid and prevent ectropion from secondary tissue movement. The trapdoor deformity with transposition flaps is real. It can be prevented by complete undermining around the edges of the defect before transposition of the flap, by squaring the angles of the defect and flap instead of having them round, and by defatting the flap at the time of transposition. If the flap needs to be defatted as a secondary revision, it needs to be done surgically because the tissue removed is fibrofatty tissue. The ability to remove this tissue by liposuction is minimal.

My favorite flaps in cheek reconstruction are usually sliding flaps. This is particularly true with medial cheek defects. These take the form of advancement and rotation, with a degree of each tissue movement dependent on the nature of the defect and recruitment of tissue. This can be done as a Burow's triangle advancement flap, as discussed by Drs. Banducci and Manders, or as a large rotational cheek flap. Both of these flaps have elements of advancement and rotation. One of the keys to the design of the latter is to make the incisions in the eyelid blepharoplasty (subciliary) line, and as one extends the incision laterally, the flap must be arced above the lateral canthus. When rotated, the flap is then anchored to lateral orbital rim periosteum and is large enough to not cause gravitational or a secondary movement ectropion.

I've used island pedicle flaps on the cheek but prefer them on the lateral portion of the cheek. When used over the medial and malar portions, unattractive suture lines and a central "pooching" can occur. This is especially true if the skin quality in this area is porous or sebaceous.

20

RECONSTRUCTION OF THE FOREHEAD

Ronald J. Siegle

INTRODUCTION

A paralyzed and ptotic eyebrow, an oblique midforehead scar, focal alopecia in a brow, an asymmetric hairline—for the skilled reconstructive surgeon these would be considered complications of forehead reconstruction. For the unskilled and unknowledgeable surgeon these are more likely to simply be written off as common sequelae of reconstruction.

Reconstructive surgery on the forehead may be simple or complex. Several goals must be considered: (1) preservation of motor function (frontalis branch of facial nerve) and, if possible, sensory nerve function; (2) maintenance of the normal boundaries of this esthetic unit, including position and symmetry of the brow and the frontal and temporal hairlines; and (3) optimal scar camouflage by placement of scars in or adjacent to the hairline, brow, and relaxed skin tension lines whenever possible. In this chapter we will review the anatomy of the forehead and the principles of reconstruction of this esthetic unit.

The reader also is referred to a number of well-written review articles on forehead reconstruction, many of which I have learned from and thus improved my own expertise in reconstruction of this facial unit.[1-5]

ANATOMY

The skin of the forehead varies not only from person to person but also changes notably with aging and exposure to the sun. Beginning in the suprabrow area and moving toward the hairlines, the dermal thickness and sebaceous gland concentration decrease. This decrease is seen and palpated as a decreasing skin thickness and a less porous, less oily skin. In youth the forehead skin is taut and smooth, with a shiny appearance. In contrast, older or sun-damaged skin shows an increased mobility, a dull appearance, and rhytids. Although esthetically compromising, these latter fea-

tures all facilitate reconstructive procedures, as will be discussed.

The predominant muscle of the forehead esthetic unit is the frontal belly of the occipitofrontalis muscle. The vertical orientation of the skeletal muscle fibers is responsible for the transversely oriented relaxed skin tension lines. Often quite prominent in younger individuals, the muscle thickness diminishes substantially with age. Extensive cutting of these muscle bundles during reconstructive procedures may cause local palsies that have a prolonged recovery. Also of note is the often present anterior extension of the galeal median raphe. This fascial extension in the midforehead is devoid of muscular fibers and accounts for the often excellent cosmetic result that is attainable with vertical midline closures on the forehead. The other muscles in the forehead region include the orbicularis oculi, procerus, and corrugator supercilii. As a rule, transection of portions of these muscles is without major consequence.

The forehead is a richly vascularized region. Centrally it is supplied by the right and left supratrochlear and supraorbital arteries and laterally by the bilateral anterior branch of the temporal artery. These vessels are located in the subcutaneous tissue and are very predictable in their location. Transection of these vessels should not be of any major consequence during the elevation of random-pattern forehead flaps.

Loss of nerve function, whether motor or sensory, has great consequence on the forehead. The major motor nerve is the temporalis branch of the seventh cranial nerve (Fig. 20-1). This nerve innervates the entire frontalis muscle and is most at risk not on the forehead itself but rather over the zygomatic arch. The thin skin and subcutaneous tissue here make the nerve very close to the skin surface, particularly in thin or aged individuals. Development of flaps in this region may transect the nerve if not cautiously elevated. Upon reaching the forehead, the nerve enters the frontalis muscle from its deep side, and inadvertent transection is much less likely. So that the motor nerve function of

Figure 20-1   Pathway of temporalis branch of seventh cranial nerve in relationship to subcutis, fascia, and muscle. Area C is at highest risk because of proximity of nerve to overlying skin.

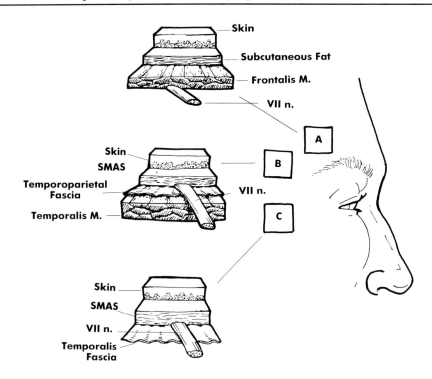

the forehead is not compromised, flap development, either in the subcutaneous tissue or below the frontalis muscle above the periosteum, is recommended.

The major sensory nerves of the forehead are the supraorbital and supratrochlear nerves, which run with their named arteries. After exiting their foramina in the subbrow area, they pierce the overlying muscle and extend cephalad in the subcutaneous tissue. Transection of these nerves yields anesthesia distal to the point of injury back to the level of the parietal scalp. The numbness perceived by the patient is not only annoying but also potentially harmful due to loss of the normal sensory feedback. To prevent sensory nerve damage when developing forehead cutaneous flaps, it is essential that the surgeon carefully undermine in the midsubcutaneous tissue plane. For larger flaps developed below the muscle, consideration should be given to placement of incisions peripheral to the path taken by these nerves.

FUNCTIONAL AND ESTHETIC CONSIDERATIONS

The first goal in forehead reconstruction is to maintain motor and sensory nerve function. Knowledge of forehead anatomy and proper flap selection will help accomplish this goal most of the time. At times, sensory

nerves will require transection, particularly with reconstruction of larger defects, but this should be done only if no other effective reconstructive alternative is available. The reconstructive surgeon should not burden the patient with a motor or sensory deficit just because an easy flap was available that also required cutting of a nerve. Compromised function of a nerve, particularly motor, should never be considered a routine consequence of reconstructive procedures of the forehead. With sensory defects regrowth of the nerve can be anticipated, but for complete transection of the supratrochlear or supraorbital nerves, anesthesia of the distal forehead and scalp commonly lasts for 1 or more years.

Often the surgeon is confronted with reconstructions in situations in which the facial nerve branch to the frontalis muscle has been cut, yielding a ptotic brow, facial asymmetry, and occasionally visual field limitation on upward gaze. Not all individuals are functionally compromised by this brow ptosis. If individuals wear glasses, they may adequately cover up the ptosis and not require surgical repair. However, for those situations with functional or significant esthetic alteration, there are several techniques available for unilateral brow elevation. I most commonly do a direct brow lift in which an exaggerated ellipse of skin is resected from the suprabrow area to elevate the brow approximately 4 to 8 mm higher than the opposite

Figure 20-2   Forehead unit is defined by junction lines with frontal scalp superiorly, temporal scalp and temple laterally, and eyebrows and glabella inferiorly. Reconstruction of forehead is facilitated by consideration of midline *(M)*, paramedian *(P)*, and lateral *(LT)* units as independent subunits. Tissue sources for forehead reconstruction include local *(L)*, glabella *(G)*, and temple *(T)*.

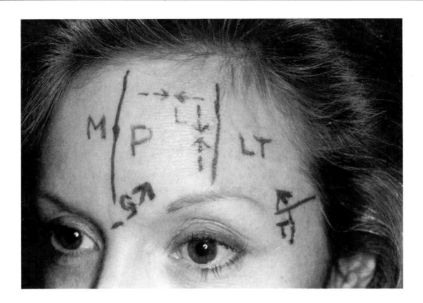

brow. The more lax the forehead skin, the higher will be the need for elevation. The inferior edge of the skin ellipse is incised along the superior margin of the brow parallel to the angle of the hair shafts. Deep horizontal mattress suspension sutures are placed from the deep subbrow dermis to the forehead periosteum approximately 1 cm above the desired point of brow elevation. I prefer 5-0 clear nylon for this suture. Skin repair then follows with a layered closure, preferably with intracuticular suturing hidden in the brow. A second alternative for correction of brow ptosis is to perform a procedure similar to the direct brow lift but in the midforehead, thereby camouflaging the incisions in the skin tension lines. Coronal forehead lifts for correction of unilateral brow ptosis are not indicated.

The concept of esthetic units has greatly simplified and, more importantly, improved the outcome of facial reconstructive procedures in the last decade. Esthetic units have borders which must be respected to maintain facial symmetry and, as a rule, contain skin that is relatively similar in quality throughout. If "neighborhood skin" can be recruited to repair a skin defect, optimal cosmesis may be obtained. Specific to the forehead, the unit is defined peripherally by the juncture lines with the frontal scalp superiorly, the temporal scalp and temple laterally, and the eyebrows and glabella inferiorly (Fig. 20-2). The forehead is somewhat different from other facial esthetic units in that is has both an actual and a perceived unit. Hairstyling can play a major role in forehead visibility

whether bangs or a sweeping hairstyle is used to cover all or part of the forehead. Thus hairstyling may be used to cover a large area of forehead scarring and/or disfigurement.

In planning the reconstruction of a forehead defect, the surgeon must first ask what the esthetic goals are. The specific esthetic goals for forehead reconstruction include: (1) maintenance of brow symmetry; (2) maintenance of natural-appearing temporal and frontal hairlines; (3) hiding of scars when possible (into hairlines or eyebrows); and (4) creation of transverse instead of vertical scars whenever possible (except in the midline forehead) and avoidance of diagonal scars.

RECONSTRUCTIVE PRINCIPLES

In cases of skin cancer of the forehead, a forehead flap that is beautifully designed and has healed perfectly at a 1-week follow-up visit is worthless if pathologic results show that tumor still is present in the margins of resection. As a Mohs surgeon, I am fortunate to be able to remove skin cancers with immediate feedback concerning tumor margins and can obtain tumor-free fields before I proceed with reconstruction. There are other means to obtain improved margin control such as traditional frozen sections. In addition, one can delay reconstruction several days until permanent pathologic reports are available. The message here is that local tissue rearrangement should not be performed until successful tumor removal has been confirmed. Priorities in order of importance are to completely remove tumor, maintain function, and maintain or reestablish appearance.

Local anesthesia for surgery on the forehead is usually well tolerated. One percent lidocaine with epinephrine at a 1:100,000 concentration is the anesthetic that I use most often. Many surgeons now add sodium bicarbonate to this solution with a final concentration of 0.1 mEq/ml to further minimize the pain of injection. There are several steps that can be taken to minimize the discomfort of infiltrative anesthesia. Complete forehead anesthesia may result from bilateral brow blocks. Anesthesia is injected bilaterally beneath the brow along the bone from midline to a point approximately two thirds of the length of the brow. Approximately 2 ml per side yields an anesthetic field back to the parietal scalp. Singular nerve blocks may be accomplished by injection adjacent to the foramen of the supratrochlear or supraorbital nerves. Field blocks with injections placed just proximal to the surgical site will often yield distal anesthesia within a minute and allow painless injection of the remaining portion of the anesthetic. An important point to remember is that local anesthetics affect motor nerves. Thus a lateral forehead nerve block may cause frontalis paresis, which in the intraoperative setting cannot be differentiated as surgery or anesthesia induced. This paresis may last several hours, and therefore no corrective procedures for brow ptosis are indicated until the cause of the ptosis is known.

Options for repair of forehead defects include healing by second intention, primary closure, a skin graft, and a local or, uncommonly, distant flap. As a rule, the healing of the forehead by second intention, although adequate for tissue replacement, yields suboptimal scars. In contrast, extreme lateral forehead and temple sites may heal beautifully by second intention.

Primary repairs of forehead defects are often possible. There is great variability in the laxity and availability of excess tissue on the forehead. Redundant skin is more likely in older individuals and those with sun-damaged skin. The excess skin may be located in either the horizontal or vertical planes and can best be defined by pinching and spreading of the forehead skin. Deep forehead furrows may hold large amounts of redundant skin. If adjacent tissue is not adequate for primary repair, options include borrowing of skin from regional sites, including the temple, scalp, and glabella, or use of skin grafts. Although skin grafts are an easy source of skin to cover large forehead defects, they usually yield suboptimal results because of poor color and texture match with that of the remaining forehead skin. Split-thickness skin grafts are appropriate for

patients with skin cancer at high risk for possible recurrence, enabling better surveillance of the tumor site.

FLAPS FOR FOREHEAD RECONSTRUCTION

Flaps are an excellent means to reconstruct forehead defects that cannot be repaired primarily. In most cases they make use of skin from the same esthetic unit, thus maximizing esthetic outcome. Because there are multiple flaps available, one can usually be designed that has minimal consequences in terms of functional impairment, and therefore recovery is usually rapid and without motor or sensory deficit. In general, small flaps can be developed fully within the confines of the skin and subcutaneous tissue, with undermining carried out in the fat layer. Although this maintains the subdermal plexus, it creates more bleeding and is more surgically challenging because of the need to dissect around the neurovascular bundles.

Musculocutaneous flaps dissected beneath the frontalis muscle are required for larger defects and in situations in which a cutaneous forehead flap might result in excess wound-closure tension. Musculocutaneous forehead flaps can be broadly undermined below the inframuscular layer of the superficial temporal fascia in a relatively avascular plane. Careful design is necessary to prevent or limit transection of sensory nerves. Undermining at this deep level may provide only small amounts of tissue for direct advancement because of the constraints of the underlying fascia. Musculocutaneous flaps, in contrast to cutaneous forehead flaps, involve mobilization of tissue over a fixed infrastructure, specifically the bone. Thus for larger defects repaired with musculocutaneous forehead flaps, there may be moderate to extreme tension on the closure line. Despite this, most flaps heal well because of their significant vascularity.

Advancement flaps are the most common flaps used for forehead reconstruction. Among their main benefits are that they maintain good contours, allow optimal scar placement in the horizontal forehead creases, and usually provide an adequate source of tissue for reconstruction. The two major disadvantages of advancement flaps are the need for extensive undermining and the need for multiple incisions. Multiple types of advancement flaps can be used, including unilateral, bilateral, island pedicle, and Burow's wedge flaps.

Rotation flaps are excellent for forehead reconstruction because they take advantage of the curvature of the skull. They are usually designed as large flaps and thus offer good viability. The major disadvantage of forehead rotation flaps is the lengthy incision lines that

Figure 20-3   *A*, Midline forehead defect (1.8 × 1.5 × 0.04 cm) in 48-year-old man following Mohs surgery to remove skin cancer, with planned vertical closure. *B*, Appearance at suture removal 1 week postoperatively.

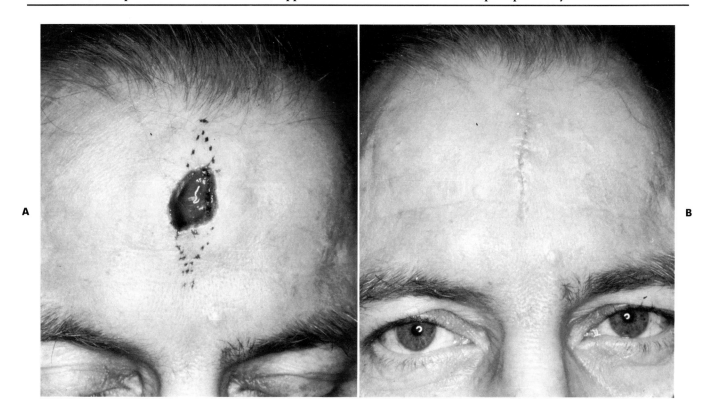

are often diagonal to the horizontal creases of the forehead. Multiple types are available, including unilateral and bilateral. Bilateral rotation flaps often take the form of an A-T, O-T, or O-Z closure.

Transposition flaps, the most common flaps used for repair of defects located in other areas of the face, play a lesser role in forehead repairs. They may be used in the glabellar and lateral forehead areas but often are suboptimal because of the multiple scars that result. As a consequence of the need to close the flap donor site, scars may be positioned in a less than ideal orientation. Transposition flaps also frequently cause a slight alteration to contour and are usually transferred under excess wound-closure tension. The types most commonly used include the rhombic and the 30° angle transposition flaps.

I have found that conceptualization of the forehead in three segments greatly simplifies the thought process and decision making used for flap selection. I will discuss these three areas separately. They include the midline forehead, the paramedian forehead extending over the convexity of the forehead from the midline to the midbrow, and the lateral forehead extending from the midbrow to the juncture with the temple (Fig. 20-2).

Midline Forehead Reconstruction

Midline or centrally located defects of the forehead can often be closed in a transverse orientation if their vertical height is not too great. Although tissue availability may be sufficient, the medial brows, functioning almost like a free margin, may be elevated to an unacceptable height. For vertically oriented midline or near-midline defects, primary closure along the long axis of the wound is often optimal (Fig. 20-3). Taking advantage of the anterior extension of the galea and the lack of midline frontalis muscle, the surgeon may perform closure in the midline. For large defects (near the midline) closed primarily, advancement of wound edges causes the development of standing cutaneous deformities, which may be excised with use of a W-plasty if feasible in the glabellar creases (Fig. 20-4). Although this form of repair optimally camouflages incisions, a noticeable drawback is the medial displacement of both brows. Depending on brow visibility, hair density, color, and esthetic concerns of the patient, this medial movement may or may not be acceptable and should be discussed with the patient preoperatively. This repair allows extensive undermining in the inframuscular plane without compromise of motor or

Figure 20-4   Planned excision of forehead tumor with asymmetric margins and inferior W-plasty to allow both midline closure and camouflage of scars in glabellar lines.

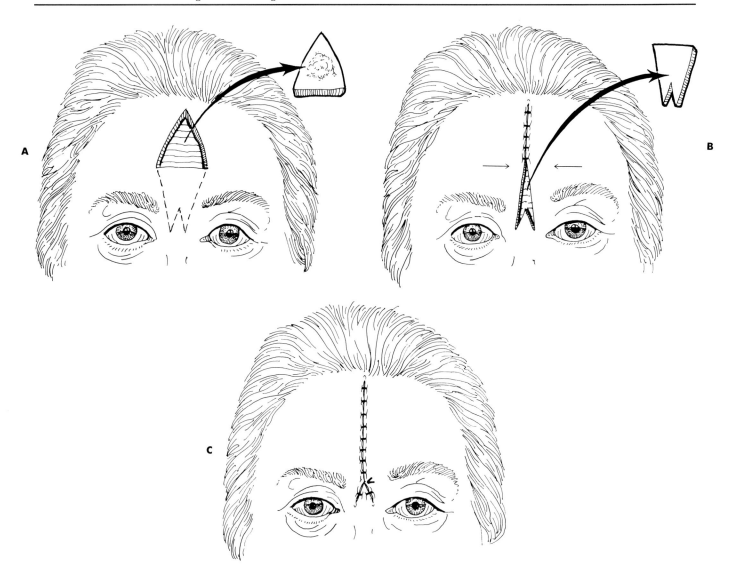

sensory function. For those defects slightly off center, when possible, sufficient tissue should be removed from the medial edge of the wound to create a symmetrical defect positioned directly over the midline so as to allow closure to occur exactly in the middle of the forehead.

Primary repair of large central forehead defects can be facilitated by intraoperative expansion of scalp and forehead skin (Fig. 20-5).[6] This technique has enabled me to recruit 1 to 2 cm of additional skin beyond that achievable by wide undermining. A 30-ml Foley catheter is tunneled below the frontalis muscle beyond the supraorbital nerve to the lateral forehead and temple region. The balloon of the catheter is inflated until the tissue blanches and is maintained at that volume for 3 minutes and then decompressed for 3 minutes. This

cycle is repeated two additional times, with each expansion yielding additional tissue stretch. The stretched tissue gained with intraoperative expansion is often sufficient to close midline defects, which otherwise could not be repaired by primary closure.

The use of intraoperative skin expansion has enabled the surgeon to close large defects of the central forehead, which in the past required the use of local flaps. When intraoperative skin expansion does not provide adequate tissue for primary repair, the use of bilateral rotation flaps is an excellent method of reconstructing sizable upper midforehead defects (Fig. 20-6). Created with an inferior lateral base, they allow rotation of large quantities of tissue toward the midline forehead. They often can be designed so that much of the incision for elevation of the flaps are adjacent to the

Figure 20-5   *A,* A 5 × 4 cm midline skin defect following Mohs surgery to remove skin cancer. *B,* Planned tunnel extending below frontalis muscle and beyond supraorbital nerve (SO) to allow tissue expansion of lateral forehead and temple. *C,* Foley catheter in place and balloon expanded. *D,* Closure of defect with W-plasty.

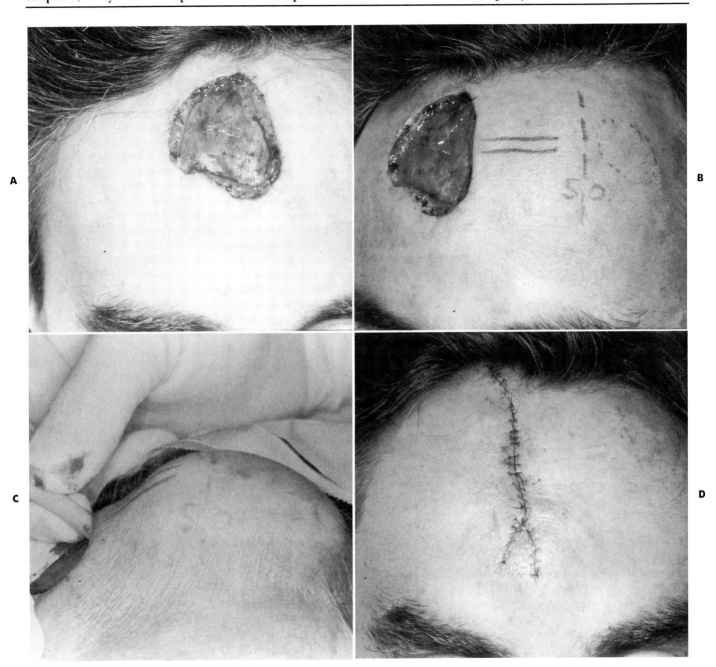

hair-bearing area of the frontal scalp and thus achieve excellent camouflage of the long incision. The use of rotation flaps for closure of central forehead defects may be unilateral or bilateral; however, due to lowering of the hairline, which tends to occur as a result of closure of the donor site, bilateral flaps are best to maintain symmetry. These flaps are large and developed in the submuscular plane and therefore require transection of the sensory nerves above the incision, with resultant numbness of the anterior scalp. The patient should be informed of this expected outcome preoperatively.

Paramedian Forehead Reconstruction

The degree of bossing of an individual's forehead is variable but, as a rule, the area from the midline to the midbrow of the forehead tends to be convex. I have

Figure 20-6   Midline forehead defect closed with two large rotation flaps with incisions hidden within frontal and temporal hairline.

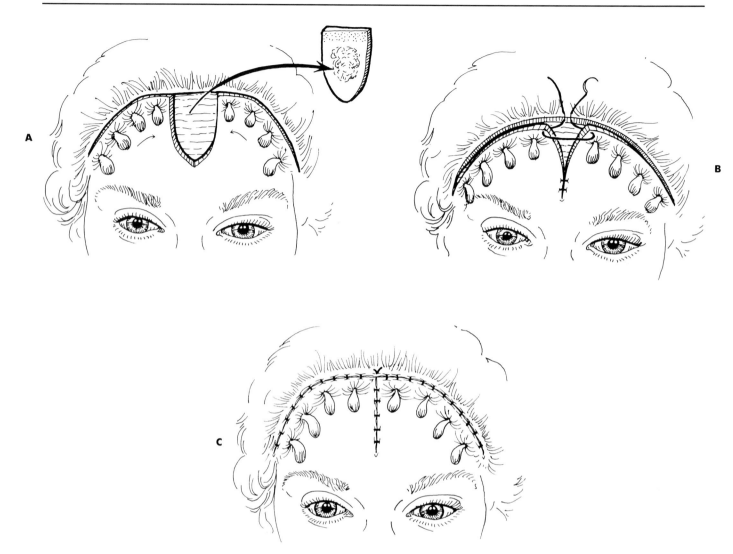

labeled this area the paramedian forehead (Fig. 20-2). There are fewer recommended methods of repair of defects in this portion of the forehead than in the central part of the forehead. The relaxed skin tension lines are horizontal in the forehead and they are the ideal location for placement of incisions. When possible, primary wound closure is best accomplished with a horizontal oriented layered repair to allow maximal scar camouflage. Horizontal oriented primary repair is restricted by the vertical height of the defect and hairline, degree of brow elevation resulting from wound closure, and lack of skin and scalp mobility on the upper part of the forehead. The mobility of this region of the forehead can be increased through percutaneous galeatomies, or more accurately described as the development of a bipedicle advancement

flap (Fig. 20-7). An incision is made 1 cm posterior and parallel to the hairline and is carried full thickness through the galea. The flap is undermined in all directions, which allows the flap to slide sideways into the initial defect and enable the primary repair. Depending on defect size, the gain in tissue movement may be 1 cm or more. The secondary defect created behind the frontal hairline is then closed by additional undermining posteriorly below the galea, allowing layered repair. This bipedicle advancement flap yields a very well-vascularized flap and a hidden donor site but does lower the hairline somewhat.

Brow elevation caused by primary layered repair of defects of the paramedian forehead region may or may not be disfiguring and must be individually assessed. Patients with lax and wrinkled forehead skin can often

Figure 20-7   *A,* **Excision of upper forehead tumor. Second incision full thickness to periosteum 1 cm behind hairline and parallel to long axis of defect.** *B* **and** *C,* **Advancement of bipedicle flap allowing closure of defect. Donor defect closed primarily after additional posterior undermining. Some lowering of the hairline may occur.**

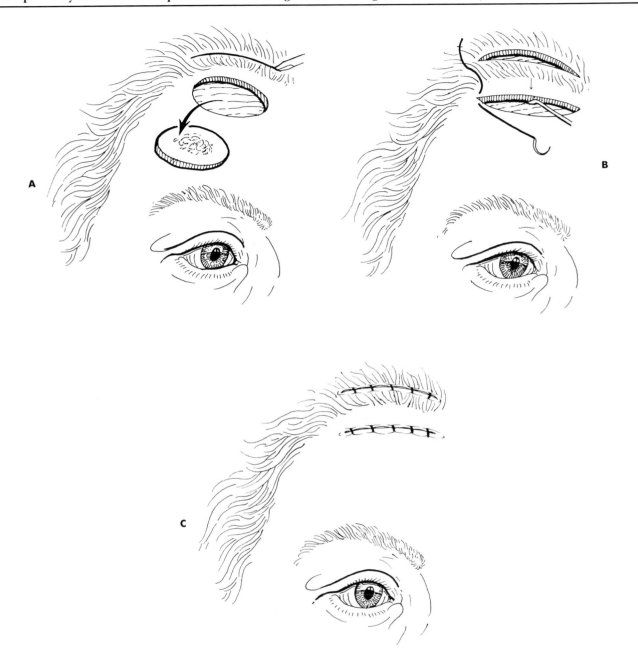

have brow elevation 1 cm above that of the opposite side, and within several weeks postoperatively the effects of gravity return the brow to a more symmetrical position. In contrast, in a younger individual, even a 3- or 4-mm brow elevation may persist because of the innate tissue elasticity. When primary closure of a forehead defect results in excessive brow elevation, this elevation can be restricted by suturing of the dermis of the brow and the underlying muscle to the periosteum

of the supraorbital rim. Secondary movement of the brow from primary repair or flap repair of a paramedian forehead defect is then minimized.

When defects of the paramedian forehead are too large for primary repair or have a lengthy vertical orientation, an advancement flap is usually the preferred method of closure. Incisions are made horizontally, extending laterally from the superior and inferior aspects of the defect. The incisions are limited in length

Figure 20-8 Forehead defect closed by direct advancement of lateral forehead tissue. Standing cutaneous deformities are excised by triangulation.

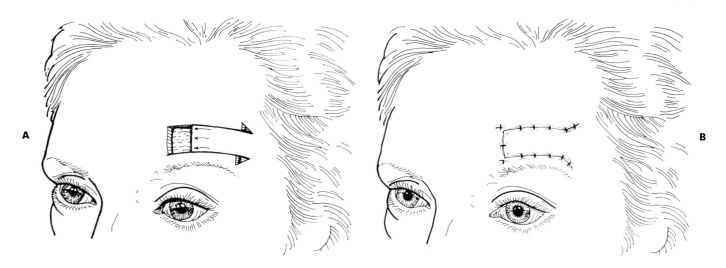

Figure 20-9 *A,* A 3 × 3 cm paramedian lower forehead defect in 55-year-old man after Mohs surgery to remove basal cell carcinoma. Unilateral advancement flap is planned. W-plasty within glabellar creases facilitates removal of standing cutaneous deformity. *B,* Three months postoperatively there is excellent scar camouflage by placement of incisions in natural horizontal and vertical creases of forehead.

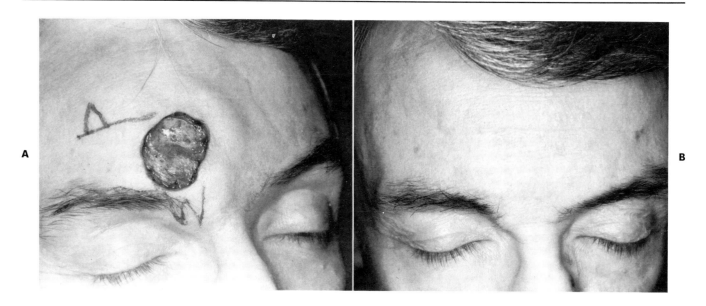

so as to create a flap with an approximate 4:1 ratio of length to width (Fig. 20-8). Most flaps are dissected in the midsubcutaneous plane. Dissection is superficial to the neurovascular bundles while avoiding excess thinning of the flap. The edges of the defect should be squared, and Burow's triangles should be removed laterally away from the flap's base (Fig. 20-8). The standing cutaneous deformity that develops with an advancement flap can be removed anywhere along the length of the flap. Thus the scar resulting from

excision can be placed in natural skin creases. A particularly good location for placement of the excision is in the glabellar creases (Fig. 20-9). Due to the elasticity of the lateral forehead and temple skin, where the flap is harvested, removal of standing cutaneous deformities is frequently not necessary if the rule of halves is used in closure of the donor site. Gathering of tissue occurs along the longer border of the wound. This is remedied by adjustment of the level of suture placement to essentially "bury" the long side of the

Figure 20-10   Suprabrow tumor excised and closed with bilateral advancement flaps (H-plasty). Note additional tissue resection below tumor to allow greater scar camouflage along border of brow.

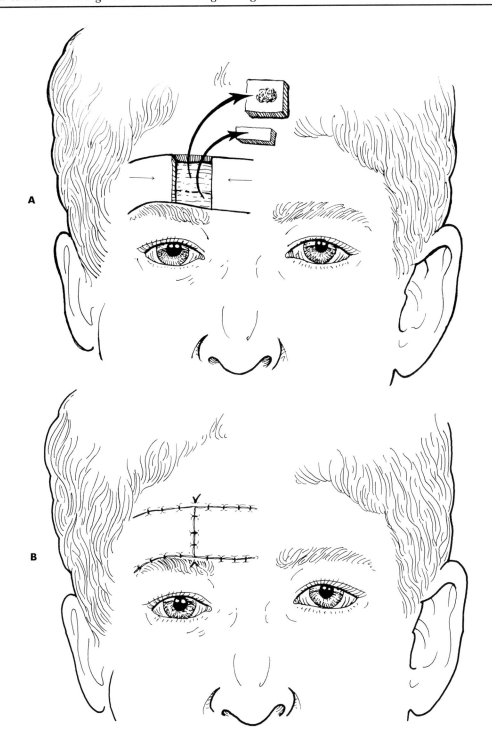

closure. Despite this adjustment in suturing, a significant step-off between the surface of the flap and the adjacent forehead skin is usually present. However, even at 1 week, this discrepancy is dramatically lessened. A helpful camouflage maneuver is to make the

flap slightly wider than necessary if there are nearby natural skin lines in which to hide the incisions.

For larger paramedian forehead defects, bilateral advancement flaps are useful for repair. Fig. 20-10 demonstrates the use of two advancement flaps to reconstruct a suprabrow defect. Note that residual skin just above the brow is removed to enable the development of a lateral flap, which has the inferior incision located along the brow. The lateral flap is longer than the medial flap because of the increased elasticity of lateral forehead skin, which facilitates a greater degree of advancement. Rectangular advancement flaps, whether single or bilateral, are perfect for paramedian forehead defects because of their ability to mobilize additional tissue, minimize vertical incisions, use relaxed skin tension lines for scar camouflage, and enable the removal of standing cutaneous deformities from a more lateral position.

Similar to the median forehead, reconstruction of the paramedian forehead area can be facilitated by the use of intraoperative tissue expansion. By expansion of lateral forehead and temple tissue, in a matter of minutes one is able to accomplish enhanced tissue mobility, often resulting in less wound-closure tension than if expansion were not used. Potential for vascular compromise of acutely expanded skin is theoretically possible but not likely, probably because the expansion is accomplished deep to the frontalis muscle and, in my experience, compromise of flap vascularity has not occurred. Intraoperative expansion can also be performed immediately adjacent to the defect, which will facilitate primary repair. Towel clamps or sutures are often necessary to prevent extrusion through the wound of the Foley catheter.

Most defects of the paramedian forehead can be repaired primarily, closed in horizontal orientation, or reconstructed with a unilateral or bilateral advancement flap. Attempts should be made to avoid vertical, curvilinear, and oblique incisions because their resulting scars are not in relaxed skin tension lines. Extrapolated to specific wound closures, this means that vertically oriented primary repairs, rotation flaps, and transposition flaps are to be avoided as a rule. However, these alternatives may be necessary when adjacent scarring from past surgical procedures has limited the ability to use traditional advancement flaps. Whenever possible, unfavorable scars should be positioned into the hairline or an eyebrow.

Lateral Forehead Reconstruction

The lateral forehead begins at the midbrow and extends to the lateral brow, where it joins with the upper temple (Fig. 20-2). Unique to this area is the transition in topography from the convexity of the paramedian forehead to a flat lateral forehead and then slightly concave temple. These surface features, along with the enhanced elasticity of lateral forehead and temple skin compared with the central part of the forehead, present a large number of reconstructive

alternatives. Primary wound closure is often possible with the orientation of the repair parallel to an individual's skin lines. On the lateral forehead the transverse forehead wrinkles become curvilinear, arch downward, and present excellent locations for placement of incisions. Some individuals have exaggerated transverse lines in this area, making them even better for scar camouflage. If lines are not apparent, the patient may better define the line location by squinting and brow elevation.

Because of the constraints of the position of the lateral brow, lateral upper eyelid, and temporal hairline, advancement, rotation, and transposition flaps can be used to resurface defects in this region when primary wound closure is not possible. The use of a flap for reconstruction is preferred to a skin graft and usually to healing by second intention. Those techniques, which make use of lateral temple skin, have the greatest potential for complications related to injury of the frontal branch of the facial nerve. It is here that the motor branch to the frontalis muscle is most accessible to injury as it runs in the superficial fascia over the zygomatic arch. Undermining in this area must be performed bluntly and with good visibility to minimize possible transection of the nerve. Even in thin individuals, there is usually sufficient subcutaneous tissue to allow a midsubcutaneous dissection plane, preserving the subdermal plexus and flap vascularity.

As already discussed, reconstructive options include single or bilateral rectangular advancement flaps. A variation of the true advancement flap that is effective both for lateral and paramedian forehead suprabrow defects is the O-T or A-T repair. This technique consists of making horizontal incisions on opposite sides of the base of the defect in relaxed skin tension lines or along the upper border of the brow (Fig. 20-11). This technique allows scar camouflage of all but the central vertical closure line. Burow's triangles can be resected from within the brow, or the standing cutaneous deformity can be eliminated by the rule of halves.

The Burow's wedge advancement flap is in reality a combined rotation and advancement flap. For this flap a curvilinear incision is made from the inferior aspect of the defect down onto the temple, and a Burow's triangle is removed at the lateral aspect of the brow or further down in a crow's-foot line (Figs. 20-12, 20-13). The Burow's wedge advancement flap allows good exposure for flap elevation and also advances easily into the defect. This is another situation when, if the defect is located near the brow, extension of the wound to the brow margin allows camouflage of the incision along the superior margin of the lateral brow.

Rotation flaps designed in a number of configurations are often effective in reconstruction of the lateral

Figure 20-11   A-T closure of lateral forehead defect using transverse forehead lines for scar camouflage.

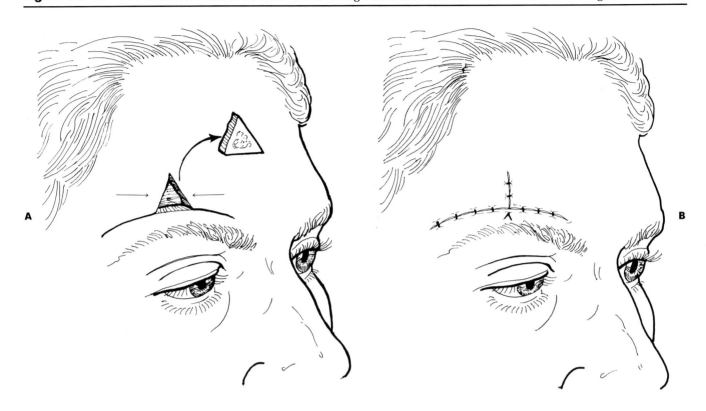

Figure 20-12   Burow's wedge advancement flap for repair of medial temple defect located just above eyebrow.

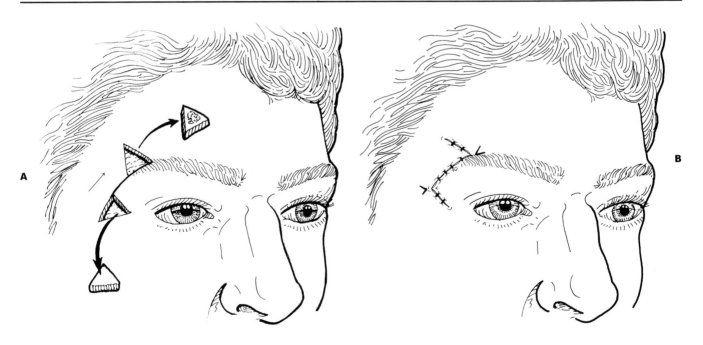

Figure 20-13 *A,* A 1.6 × 1.6 cm lateral forehead defect in 37-year-old man. Burow's wedge advancement flap is designed. Two triangles denote locations where standing cutaneous deformity can be removed with excellent scar camouflage. *B,* Closure hiding excision of Burow's triangle in lateral brow line and incision of flap in curvilinear lateral forehead line. *C,* Appearance 7 months postoperatively.

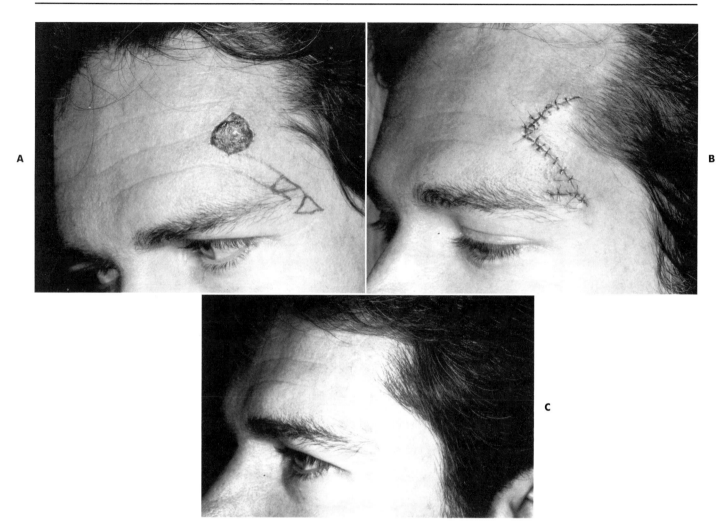

forehead. In particular, a unilateral rotation flap based inferiorly and laterally and designed so that its curvilinear incision is along the margin of the temporal hair tuft is an excellent method to reconstruct lateral forehead defects that are in close proximity to the hairline. Tissue excess on the long side of the flap can either be sewn out by the rule of halves, or a Burow's triangle can be removed in the hair-bearing skin, with resulting excellent scar camouflage. The curvilinear incision can be adjusted upward into the scalp as necessary to bring hair into the reconstructed area if some of the temporal hair tuft, for example, has been lost. The standing cutaneous deformity that forms medially and inferiorly at the pivotal point can be removed by excision of a triangle of skin in this area or at times by an M-plasty to prevent entering the brow or upper eyelid.

O-Z repair of a forehead defect consists of a combination of either two rotation flaps or one rotation flap and one advancement flap. The two flaps share in the closure of the defect, thus reducing the extent of wound coverage necessary by either flap alone (Fig. 20-14). This method to repair forehead defects is particularly effective for the lateral forehead. The oblique scar that results from wound repair may be an acceptable one in individuals who have prominent curvature to their lateral forehead creases. In contrast, this is not a good method of repair for paramedian forehead defects because the horizontal creases in this region of the forehead tend to be straight and not curvilinear.

Transposition flaps are commonly performed in the lateral forehead region to close skin defects, taking advantage of excess tissues of the temple. Suggested

Figure 20-14   Lateral forehead defect repaired with lateral rotation flap and medial advancement flap. Portion of scar resulting from repair has oblique orientation.

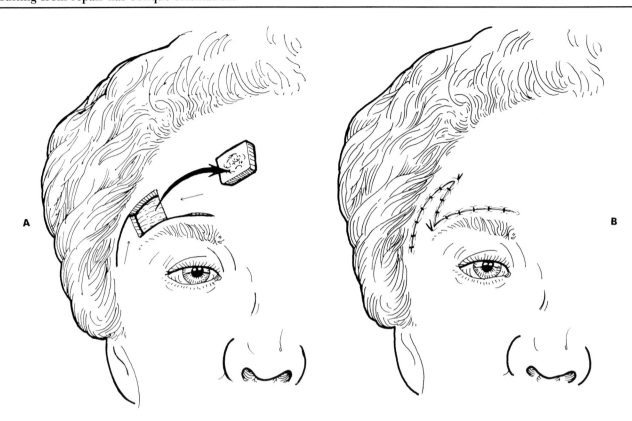

alternatives are traditional 60° or 30° angle flap with a superior or inferior base or two transposition flaps of similar or different angles participating in shared wound closure (Fig. 20-15). The scar that results from the multiple angulated incisions of these flaps tends to be well camouflaged on the concave surface of the lateral forehead.

EYEBROW RECONSTRUCTION

The challenges of eyebrow reconstruction are obvious. The goals are to maintain acceptable position and continuity of the eyebrow. Reconstructive considerations may vary somewhat between men and women, since a woman's pencil in of the eyebrow with makeup can negate the need for what otherwise might be a more advanced reconstruction, such as transfer of temporal scalp skin to the brow. Small tumors can often be resected from the eyebrow, and layered primary closure can be performed in a vertical orientation, maintaining brow continuity. Horizontal closure of brow wounds results in narrowing of the eyebrow, which often is quite noticeable and is not recommended. With vertically oriented primary closure, extension of the repair above and below the brow

results in scars that are perpendicular to relaxed skin tension lines and may produce suboptimal scars. This can be prevented by repair of intrabrow defects with bilateral rectangular advancement flaps similar to those described for defects located elsewhere on the forehead. The upper and lower incisions for these flaps are hidden in the suprabrow and infrabrow margins (Fig. 20-16). The only additional challenge is that incisions must be made parallel to the hair shafts (Fig. 20-16**A**). This will minimize transection of hair bulbs and subsequent problems with either alopecia or ingrown hairs.

COMPLICATIONS

All of the routine complications of cutaneous surgery exist for forehead reconstruction, and there are several that are more frequent in this region. Wound closures on the forehead are almost always tighter than those on other facial units because of the fixed bony infrastructure and the relative inelasticity of forehead skin. Thus pallor or a light blue cyanosis of the skin in the vicinity of the wound is more commonly seen in the early postoperative period than is noted elsewhere on the face. There is no single factor to determine how tight

Figure 20-15   *A*, A 2.5 × 2.1 cm lateral forehead defect in 74-year-old man with two alternative rhombic transposition flaps designed for repair. *B*, Same defect with 30° angle transposition flap and M-plasty drawn. *C*, Closure accomplished with 30° angle flap.

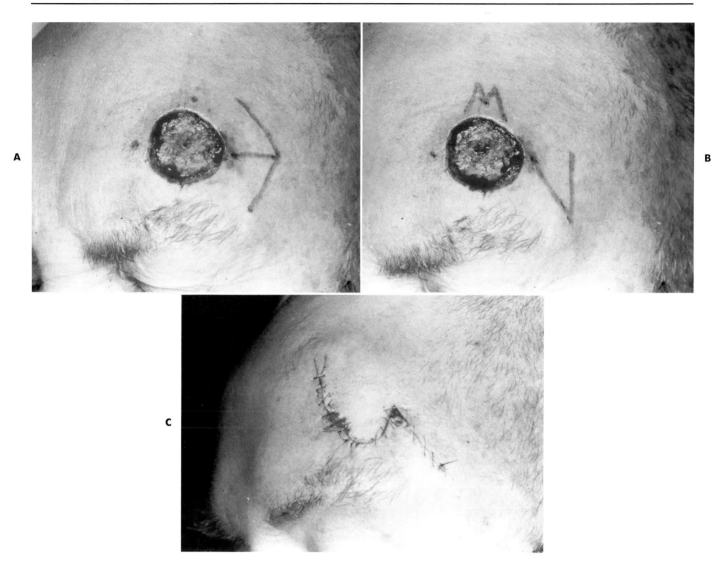

wound closure can be and still ensure skin viability. The surgeon must balance patient variables, such as a history of smoking or diabetes, with personal surgical experience to decide when excessive wound-closure tension is present. The consequence of misjudgment is a compromised blood supply to the skin with either superficial epidermal or deeper dermal tissue loss. As a rule these complications are quite uncommon, particularly when flaps are used for reconstruction because flaps are usually designed large to mobilize adequate tissue. However, many flaps used for forehead reconstruction are elevated in the subcutaneous plane, which increases the potential for bleeding and impaired vascularity. Inspection and then reinspection to ensure a dry field are indicated before wound closure. Despite

the reduced vascularity of some wound repairs and the potential for bleeding, wound infection appears to be no more frequent in reconstruction of the forehead than in other sites on the face.

Alopecia of the eyebrow or scalp hair can result from two causes. The first is improper angulation of incisions transecting the hair bulbs during flap elevation. The second is from undermining of hair-bearing skin in a plane that is too superficial. This results in injury of the hair bulbs and subsequent alopecia. Neither of these problems should occur in surgeries carried out by experienced surgeons. Ingrown hairs are often observed after reconstruction of the scalp and, to a lesser degree, of the brow. Despite proper surgical technique, the healing wound and resultant scar may entrap hairs

Figure 20-16   Bilateral advancement flaps used to repair intrabrow defect. *Inset,* Proper orientation of incision parallel to hair shafts to prevent permanent alopecia.

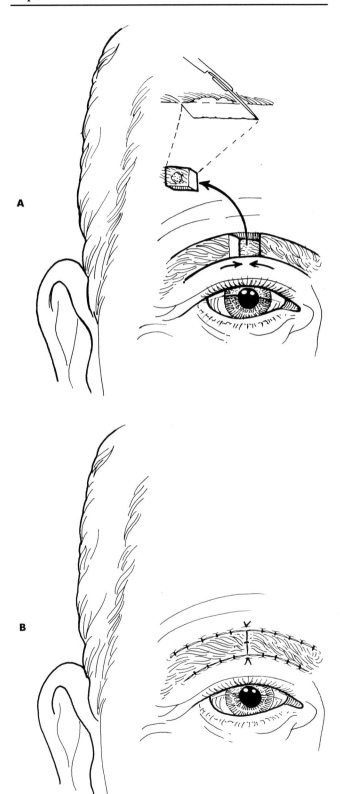

Figure 20-17   *A* and *B,* A 6 × 5 cm full-thickness skin defect of lateral temple and brow.

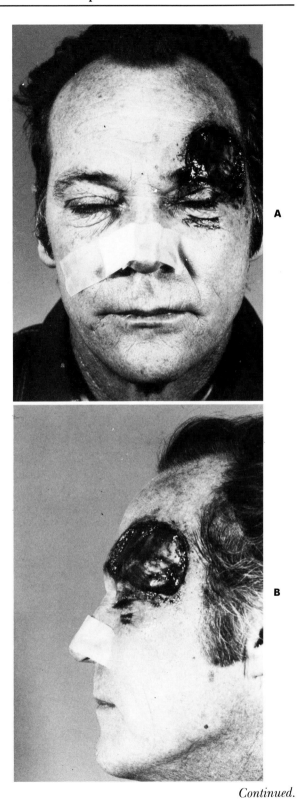

Continued.

Figure 20-17, cont'd *C,* Transposition flap designed to repair skin defect. Incisions for flap were made along anterior temple hairline. *D,* Large rotation scalp flap designed to close donor defect. *E* and *F,* Result of repair 9 months postoperatively.

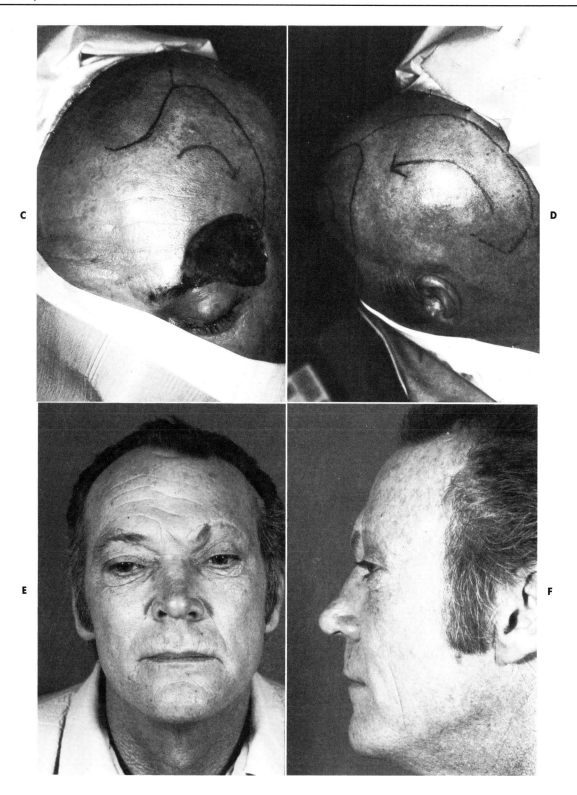

along the incision line and cause both ingrown hairs and milia. Sutures placed by chance into follicular structures may also lead to sinus tract formation and problems with small cysts in the incision line.

Edema is an expected consequence of any skin surgery. However, on the forehead, the tautness of repairs in combination with the immobile bone below reduces the degree of swelling that can be expected. However, it is routine for edema and bruising to appear in the periorbital region 1 to 3 days postoperatively. These consequences are often of great concern to patients, and they should be informed of the likely swelling to minimize their potential anxieties.

Two important complications of forehead reconstruction are injuries to the supratrochlear and supraorbital sensory nerves. The resultant anesthesia is not limited to a small area but rather extends for many centimeters onto the top of the scalp. These nerves should be spared whenever possible. Another serious complication is injury of the frontal branch of the facial nerve from transection or local infiltrative anesthesia. Transection will cause a permanent paralysis of the brow, whereas local infiltrative anesthesia will cause temporary paralysis. The difference is obviously a major one, and any corrective action should be deferred until the complete nature of the injury has been defined. Occasionally the nerve may be traumatized during dissection but not actually transected. In such situations prolonged temporary paralysis or paresis may be present for 3 to 6 months postoperatively. Nerve conduction and EMG studies may be helpful in distinction of the degree of nerve injury. In cases of permanent paralysis, brow-elevating procedures can return an adequate symmetry to the brows, in most cases leaving only the adynamic forehead as a marker for the paralyzed forehead.

SUMMARY

Reconstruction of defects of the forehead is not just a matter of wound closure. The reconstructive surgeon must maintain or reestablish the normal boundaries of this esthetic unit while preserving motor and sensory nerve function and maximally camouflaging surgical scars. The reconstructive surgeon must have a thorough knowledge of the anatomy and function of this region and must understand the principles of soft-tissue movement so that the optimal reconstructive procedure is designed and performed.

REFERENCES

1. Dzubow LM: Forehead. In Dzubow LM, editor: *Facial Flaps: biomechanics and regional application*, Norwalk, Conn, 1990, Appleton & Lange.

2. Jackson IT: Forehead reconstruction. In Jackson IT, editor: *Local flaps in head and neck reconstruction*, St Louis, 1985, CV Mosby.

3. Salasche SJ, Bernstein G, Senkarik M: Forehead and temple. In Salasche SJ, Bernstein G, Senkarik M, editors: *Surgical anatomy of the skin*, Norwalk, Conn, 1988, Appleton & Lange.

4. Siegle RJ: Forehead reconstruction, *J Dermatol Surg Oncol* 17:200, 1991.

5. Tromovitch TA, Stegman SJ, Glogau RG: Forehead. In Tromovitch TA, Stegman SJ, Glogau RG, editors: *Flaps and grafts in dermatologic surgery*, Chicago, 1989, Mosby–Year Book.

6. Greenbaum SS, Greenbaum GH: Intraoperative tissue expansion using a Foley catheter following excision of a basal cell carcinoma, *J Dermatol Surg Oncol* 16:45, 1990.

7. Zitelli JA: Wound healing by secondary intention: a cosmetic appraisal, *J Dermatol Surg Oncol*, 16:407, 1990.

EDITORIAL COMMENTS

Shan R. Baker, M.D.

The author has presented a detailed discussion concerning various alternative reconstructive techniques for repair of forehead defects. Dividing the forehead into three zones (median, paramedian, lateral) assists the author in planning reconstruction. In spite of a wound closure scar that is perpendicular to relaxed skin tension lines, defects of the central one-third of the forehead can be repaired in a vertically oriented axis with a predictably good esthetic result. This is probably due to the natural dehiscence and/or attenuation of the frontalis muscle in this portion of the forehead.

In contrast, defects located solely within the paramedian and lateral zones of the forehead are best repaired with primary closure oriented in a horizontal axis or with flaps that have a horizontal orientation to facilitate scar camouflage and to minimize any vertical component to the repair. Vertical scars in the paramedian and lateral zones of the forehead are often quite noticeable because they are perpendicular to relaxed skin tension lines, and their appearance is accentuated by movement of the frontalis muscle.

It is apparent that the most effective technique for reconstruction of the forehead usually involves one or more advancement flaps. In spite of the relative inelasticity of forehead skin, the use of the advance-

Figure 20-18 *A,* Split-thickness skin graft and area of radiation-induced alopecia after treatment of malignant fibrous histiocytoma. *B,* In anticipation of reconstruction of non–hair-bearing lateral temple and restoration of anterior temple hairline, two tissue expanders were used to expand non–hair-bearing forehead skin and hair-bearing parietal-occipital scalp *(arrows). C,* Three months postoperatively wound closure was achieved by advancement of forehead skin laterally and scalp anteriorly. (*C,* from Baker SR, Johnson TM, Nelson BR: Technical aspects of prolonged scalp expansion. *Arch Otolaryngol Head Neck Surg,* **[in press].**)

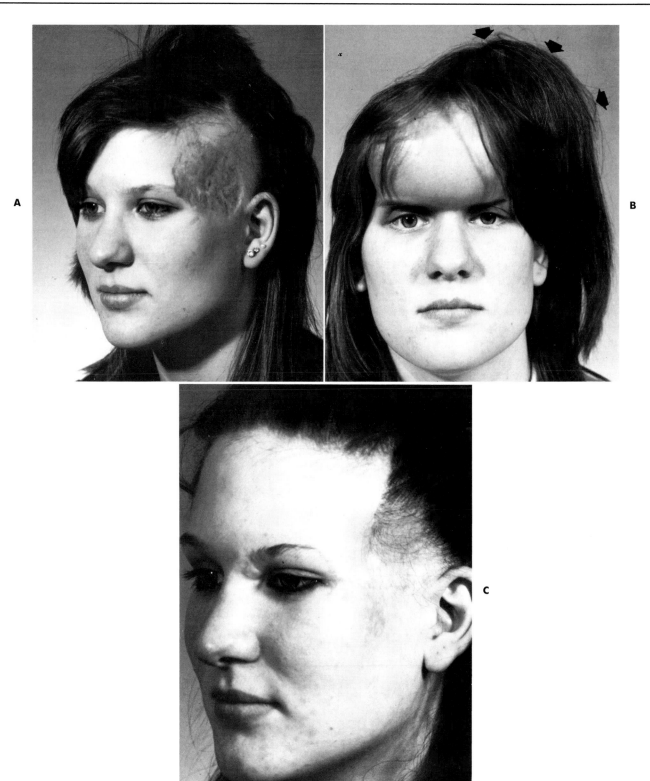

ment flaps versus pivotal flaps is preferred because they produce the most favorable cosmetic results. However, the surgon should be aware that many skin defects of the forehead can be successfully managed by not repairing the defect, but allowing the wound to heal by second intention. Healing by second intention often gives a cosmetic result that is comparable to flap repair when the appropriate forehead site is selected for this method of wound management. The most ideal location of wounds selected for second intention healing are located high on the forehead, well away from the brow, in the central and lateral one-third of the forehead. Second intention healing in these areas tends to produce a very acceptable scar. Topography (convex centrally, concave laterally), the rigid bony support under the wound, and the relative lack of skin movement in these areas probably account for the excellent result that can be obtained by second intention healing.

Although transposition flaps in general are not usually indicated for repair of most forehead defects, such flaps can be useful when transferring the entire remaining cosmetic subunit, especially in the lateral zone of the forehead. An example is seen in Figure 20-17 (*A-F*) in which the remaining lateral subunit of the forehead was transposed inferiorly to repair a 6 × 5 cm skin defect of the lower lateral forehead skin and brow. Incisions for the flap wrere made along the anterior temporal hairline. The secondary defect, located along the hairline, was repaired with a single large rotation scalp flap (see Fig. 20-17), which enabled a reasonable restoration of the temporal hairline and complete closure of the donor site.

The advent of tissue expansion now enables the surgeon to have the ability to reconstruct sizable forehead defects, which in the past could be repaired only with skin grafts. The author has discussed intraoperative tissue expansion to assist in wound repair by primary closure. Controlled prolonged tissue expansion can be used to reconstruct very large forehead defects by expansion of the remaining forehead skin over a 6- to 12-week interval. Reconstruction is achieved by direct advancement of the expanded skin by itself or in combination with other expanded or nonexpanded scalp or cheek and temple skin flaps (Fig. 20-18).[1] The disadvantages of tissue expansion in anticipation of reconstructing the forehead are that it is a two-stage procedure and there is considerable temporary deformity of the forehead during the expansion process. These disadvantages are far outweighed by the excellent results that can be achieved with tissue expansion in repair of very large defects of the forehead.

Reference

1. Baker SR, Johnson TM, Nelson BR: Technical aspects of prolonged scalp expansion, *Otolaryngol Head Neck Surg* (in press).

EDITORIAL COMMENTS

Neil A. Swanson

This is a very complete chapter, which discusses an anatomic site that I believe is difficult to reconstruct.

Discussion and diagrammatic representation of the temporal branch of the facial nerve and the sensory innervation of the forehead are excellent. Certainly in the lateral forehead and temple, the temporal branch of this facial nerve must be respected. There is a good discussion of brow lift and other "pexing" procedures if the nerve is cut and the patient has eyebrow and lid droop. In my experience lid droop is far more bothersome than brow droop. This often can be corrected with periosteal tacking sutures to bring the eyebrow and eyelid, particularly the lid, into position. This can be done at the time of reconstruction. I usually use a permanent clear nylon or polydiaxanone (PDS) suture.

There is also a good discussion of the priorities of reconstruction. As mentioned in the chapter, tumor removal must be of principal importance. The second principle, maintaining function, must also not be forgotten by the reconstructive surgeon. Both of these need to be taken into account as key elements of the reconstructive procedure itself. Remember, it is never any benefit, in particular to the patient, to have a beautiful reconstruction with tumor left behind or a functional defect.

Regarding reconstructive options, I agree completely that healing by second intention in the temple area can often yield excellent results. It is far superior to skin grafting and large multiple stage procedures. As one of the few Mohs surgeons old enough to remember chemosurgery "with zinc chloride paste" for which everything needed to granulate, I was always impressed by large temple defects that healed with excellent esthetic results.

The forehead is one of the few areas where pure advancement flaps can be used. The single and double advancement flaps (U-plasty and H-plasty) are examples and prove to be very useful on the forehead. As Dr. Siegle states, in the creation of these flaps it is often advisable to enlarge the defect so that the incision lines can be placed within existing forehead creases. This is a difficult concept for some Mohs surgeons who have spent time preserving normal tissue. However, it is often critical to an excellent esthetic outcome. The other advancement and rotation flaps described fit within the principles, discussed in Chapters 6 and 7, of the basics of tissue movement. I still believe that there are very few pure advancement and pure rotation flaps, and most of these are sliding flaps that combine advancement and rotational movement.

The forehead has limitations of tissue movement. This is partially because of the properties of the skin of the forehead but also because the galea extends over a good portion of the forehead. Therefore, as Dr. Siegle mentions, flaps need to be made longer than one might anticipate in reconstruction of forehead defects. My experience with intraoperative tissue expansion is similar to that of the author's. I find it useful on the forehead, usually using the Foley catheter technique described. The timing of the inflation and deflation cycles can vary. I personally use 5-minute cycling intervals. I place the balloon in the subgaleal plane and often will perform galeotomies before expansion. This helps give additional stretch, since the galea can expand in an accordionlike fashion.

A bipedicle flap in which an incision is placed in hair-bearing skin above a high forehead defect to allow primary closure of the defect is an excellent reconstructive option. As pointed out, it lowers the hairline slightly, but this is usually not a problem. This technique was taught to me by one of my mentors, the late Sam Stegman. He called this a *percutaneous galeotomy*, a term that I still use and believe represents this flap well.

Lastly, in consideration of hair in the forehead, particularly the eyebrows and frontal and temporal hairline, the author gives an excellent discussion of techniques to improve outcomes. One must always remember that a temporary telogen effluvium can occur from the trauma of moving tissue. Therefore, one should not assess hair regrowth until at least 8 to 9 months postoperatively.

21

RECONSTRUCTION OF THE AURICLE

Vito Quatela

Mack L. Cheney

Reconstruction of the auricle presents many challenges for the reconstructive surgeon. In order to reconstruct the intrinsic anatomy of the auricle, local and regional flaps need to be carefully chosen and executed. The ultimate goal of reconstruction of this appendage is normal appearance and position. The orientation, size, and shape of the reconstructed ear should have symmetry with the opposite ear. The relationship of the periauricular skin and scalp, and the posterior sulcus should be preserved. The high ratio of cartilage to skin coverage of the auricle is complicated by a limited and inconsistent blood supply. The complex three-dimensionality of the auricle's subtle topographic details increases the difficulty of reconstruction.

Paramount to the success of auricular reconstruction is thin, well-vascularized skin coverage. It is not uncommon that the complexity of auricular injuries involves both the skin and the underlying cartilage. In the presence of existing scar tissue, any poorly vascularized, noncompliant skin must be replaced to allow for an adequate three-dimensional reconstruction. Special consideration must be given to the reconstruction of auricular defects after oncologic surgery. Reconstructive plans are influenced by the location and size of the ablative defect, the vascularity of the portion of the auricle adjacent to the defect, and the extent to which it has been exposed to radiation.

In addition to applying established principles of plastic surgery as it relates to reconstruction, auricular reconstruction presents its own set of intrinsic requirements. Anatomic landmarks such as the vermilion border, eyebrow, nasal-alar margin, and ear represent free margins due to the discontinuity of skin borders surrounding them. Since such margins offer little or no resistance to the wound-closure tension created by surgical procedures in adjacent soft tissue, the immediate and delayed consequences of tissue manipulation of these areas must be anticipated by the surgeon. The helix of the ear is somewhat more resistent than the aforementioned areas because of the presence of cartilaginous structural support. However, auricular cartilage is very supple, and scar contraction will tend to distort the ear if attention is not paid to the method of primary wound repair and to wound-closure tension.

The presence of adjacent hair-bearing scalp must also be taken into consideration in order to avoid placing hair-bearing skin over the auricle. The hairline above the site of the proposed reconstruction is normally high enough not to interfere with accurate positioning of the ear. However, no compromise should be made in placing the ear in a position and orientation like that of the contralateral side, because hair-bearing skin can be eliminated at a secondary stage.

Along with its unique challenges, auricular reconstruction is not without its own set of frustrations and disappointments for both the physician and patient. Underestimation of the requirements of skin resurfacing and neglect in supplying cartilaginous structure will start the reconstructive surgeon on a journey of multiple revisional surgeries, with the inherent risk of increased scar tissue and decreased vascularity at each stage. However, if the surgeon adheres to well-established principles, the rewards of auricular reconstruction can surpass those obtained from all other types of restorative surgery.

ANATOMY AND EMBRYOLOGY

The morphologic uniqueness of the ear is unparalleled in the body except by its contralateral counterpart. The cutaneous cover of the lateral surface of the ear differs from the medial surface. The lateral surface is densely adherent to the perichondrium and is devoid of subcutaneous tissue. The fascial layer between the skin and perichondrium contains a subdermal plexus of vessels. The medial surface has loosely applied skin containing subcutaneous fat. The skin is not firmly adherent to the cartilaginous structure. As a result of the skin's relative abundance and its ability to slide easily, it provides an excellent donor site for grafts and flaps.

The skeletal structure of the ear is provided by the auricular cartilage, which occupies the upper two thirds of the auricle. The unique ability of this cartilage to be flexible and yet maintain form is unlike that of the more rigid cartilage of the septum or rib. Consequently, structural reconstruction utilizing rib or septal cartilage means losing this dimension of flexibility, yet currently this is the most acceptable of the alternatives.

Anatomic landmarks of the auricle are important when considering reconstructive options. Topographic landmarks of the auricle that correlate to cartilaginous structure are illustrated in Figure 21-1. The cartilaginous framework of the auricle can be thought of in terms of three-dimensional components. These components, starting medially, are the conchal complex, the antihelical and antitragal complex, and the helical and lobular complex.[1] These units are important in reconstructing defects that require cartilage segments as an element of the repair.[2]

The arterial supply to the auricle is derived from

Figure 21-1 *A,* **Cartilaginous landmarks of the auricular cartilage: lateral surface.** *B,* **Cartilaginous landmarks of the auricular cartilage: medial surface.** *C,* **Topographic landmarks of the auricle: lateral surface.**

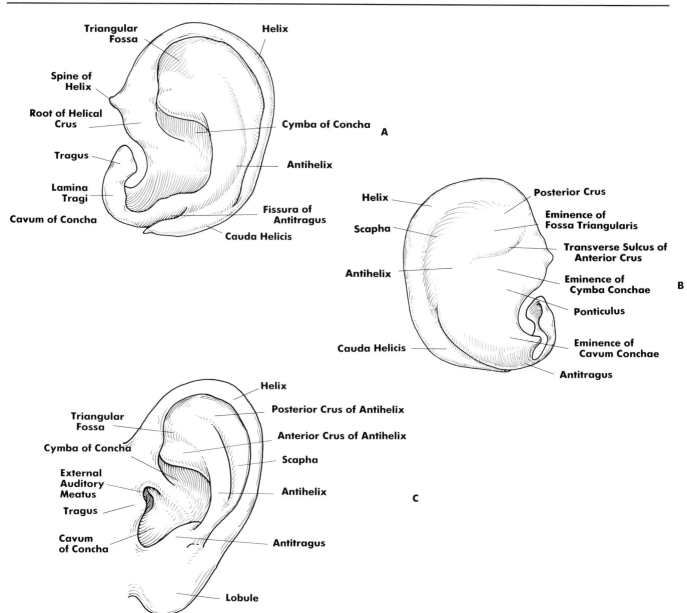

branches of the superficial temporal artery and the postauricular artery, the latter of which is a branch from the external carotid artery.[3] The cranial surface of the ear is supplied by the postauricular artery. The lateral surface is supplied by both the postauricular and superficial temporal arteries, creating two arterial networks.[4] The triangular-fossa-scapha network is supplied by the upper auricular branch of the superficial temporal artery. The conchal network is supplied from the posterior auricular artery, which gives several perforators to the conchal floor (Fig. 21-2). Flap planning and design should give due consideration to the arterial networks described. Venous drainage is via the postauricular vein, which drains into the external jugular system with supplemental venous drainage from the superficial temporal and retromandibular veins. Lymphatic drainage of the auricle is primarily to the preauricular, infraauricular, and mastoid lymph nodes.

The auricle is innervated by the greater auricular nerve (C2-3), the auricular-temporal nerve (V3), the lesser occipital nerve, and the greater branch of the vagus nerve (Arnold's nerve) (Fig. 21-3). The greater auricular nerve divides into an anterior and a posterior branch. The anterior branch supplies the lower half of the lateral aspect of the auricle. The posterior branch

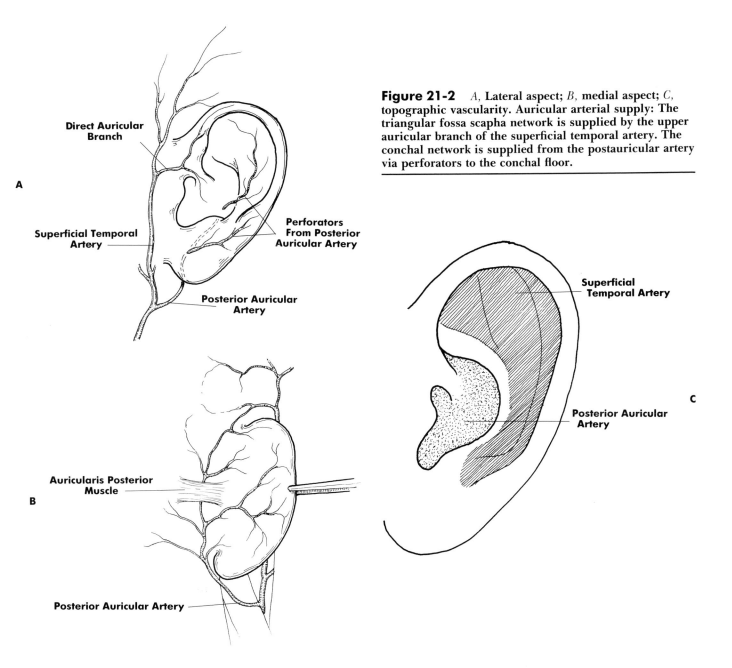

Figure 21-2   *A,* Lateral aspect; *B,* medial aspect; *C,* topographic vascularity. Auricular arterial supply: The triangular fossa scapha network is supplied by the upper auricular branch of the superficial temporal artery. The conchal network is supplied from the postauricular artery via perforators to the conchal floor.

Figure 21-3 *A*, Auricular innervation—lateral aspect. *B*, Auricular innervation—medial aspect.

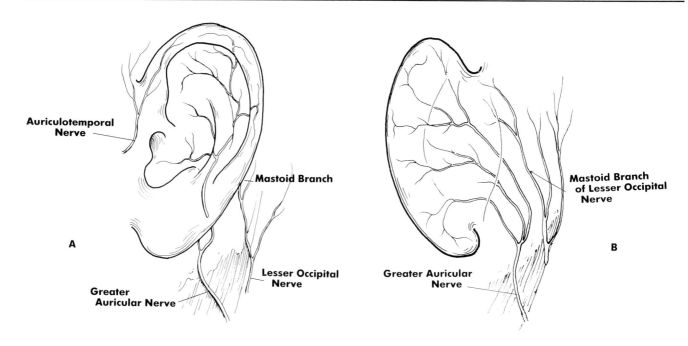

supplies a similar area on the cranial surface of the auricle. The superolateral surface is supplied by the auricular temporal nerve. The lesser occipital nerve supplies the superior aspect of the ear on the cranial side. The concha is supplied by Arnold's nerve, a branch of the tenth cranial nerve.

Embryologically, the auricle arises from the first (mandibular) and the second (hyoid) branchial arches.[5] The helix appears in these arches during the sixth week of gestation. The anterior hillock gives rise to the tragus, the root of the helix, and the superior helix, whereas the posterior hillock becomes the antihelix, tragus, and lobule. The first branchial groove forms the external auditory meatus and concha.

AURICULAR ARCHITECTURE

Analysis of the dimensions and proportions of the external ear are important for planning reconstructive procedures.[6-9] The verticle height of the ear is approximately equal to the distance between the lateral orbital rim and the root of the helix at the level of the brow. Ear width is approximately 55% of its length (Fig. 21-4), the helical rim protrudes 1 to 2.5 cm from the skull, and the angle of the protrusion from the skull averages 25 to 30 degrees. The vertical axis of the ear is inclined posteriorly at an angle of approximately 15 to 20 degrees[10-11] and not parallel to the dorsum of the nose, as originally thought. Excessive posterior inclination gives the ear a low-set appearance and should be

avoided. The superior level of the ear is set by the lateral brow. If the patient has brow ptosis, the upper eyelid is used as a landmark. When planning the reconstruction, it is most important to use the contralateral side as a template because individual variation in topographic features and positioning is the rule rather than the exception.[11] It must be remembered, however, that the size, location, and orientation of the ear are far more important than methodical attention to contour.[7] The necessary contour lines, which make an ear recognizable as such, are a helix with a root beginning in the concha, a tragus, and an antitragus and concha.[8-9]

GENERAL PRINCIPLES

The approach to repair of the auricle varies depending on the location and extent of the defect. Auricular defects can be divided into defects of cutaneous cover, with or without intact cartilagenous structure, and full-thickness defects. Skin defects of the densely adherent lateral cutis can rarely be closed primarily, whereas those of the more pliable medial surface can often be repaired by direct closure. This pliability permits the harvest of large postauricular skin grafts and primary closure of the donor site. Small cutaneous defects of the helical rim can be reconstructed with primary wound closure and may occasionally require slight contouring of the cartilage to avoid a mottled appearance.

Those lateral cutaneous defects where cartilaginous

Figure 21-4   **Proportions and inclinations of the normal ear.**

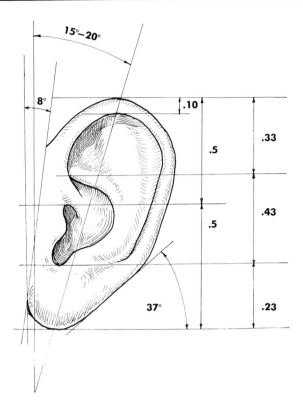

structure is intact are best treated by skin grafts, provided that there is intact perichondrium at the recipient site. The contralateral postauricular skin often serves as an excellent full-thickness skin graft for lateral resurfacing. Preauricular skin can also be used with minimum donor site morbidity. A small petrolatum-impregnated bolster provides satisfactory immobilization of the skin graft. In cases of reconstruction following Mohs surgery, the perichondrium is often absent, resulting in a poor recipient site for skin grafts. This problem can be circumvented by the removal of cartilage when it is not a determinant of auricular shape, thereby allowing the postauricular skin to become the recipient bed. The concavities of the lateral surface of the ear such as concha, triangularis fossa, and scapha are amenable to removal of cartilaginous structure and subsequent skin grafting. These repairs result in minimal distortions of the ear with good structural integrity.

When the loss of lateral cutis and supporting structure will result in a change in shape of the ear, or in the event of a full-thickness loss, then one must consider converting the defect into a full-thickness wedge-shaped excision or use of a composite graft or flap incorporating structural support. Size and location

of the defect dictate method of reconstruction. Small defects (less than 0.15 cm) of the helix or antihelix are best suited for conversion to a wedge-shaped excision and primary wound repair, with minimal resultant scar, the only disadvantage being an ear shorter in vertical height. When performing a wedge-shaped excision, one must be careful to alleviate circumferential tension by decreasing the central components of the concha to balance the helical defect; otherwise cupping and distortion will occur. Larger defects (up to 2 cm) in a similar location can be managed by composite grafting from the contralateral ear. Typically, a composite graft one-half the size of defect is transplanted from the opposite ear, thereby creating two ears of equal size (Fig. 21-5). Care is taken to approximate the cartilage edges with an absorbable suture. Graft immobilization is essential and can be accomplished by using bolster sutures to secure a splint over the ear, made of x-ray film. In addition, deepithelializing the medial aspect of the composite graft and implanting it into a subcutaneous recipient site increases survival. Transfer of composite grafts from the contralateral ear places both ears at risk for possible complications and is not always a first choice in reconstruction.

Many local flaps have been described for repair of full-thickness auricular loss.[12-21] Some flaps, such as chondrocutaneous composite advancement flaps, are better suited for the helical rim. These helical chondrocutaneous composite flaps take advantage of the available tissue along the helical rim, specifically the laxity of the lobule and the potential for V-Y advancement of the helical root, to achieve closure of helical rim defects (Fig. 21-6,A-D). Chondrocutaneous composite flaps can be designed keeping the medial skin intact or as a full-thickness flap, incising both medial and lateral skin. Although Antia originally described keeping the medial skin intact, we find greater ease of flap advancement with incision of the medial skin. The arterial network of the helical-scapha region allows for long chondrocutaneous composite flaps to be developed on a narrow pedicle. Depending on the size of the helical defect, appropriate wedges of cartilage and skin representing Burrows' triangles are appropriately excised to allow for the inset of flaps.[22] Chondrocutaneous flaps can also be used for nonhelical defects, usually designed as composite transposition flaps (Fig. 21-6,E-H).[23]

The retroauricular and preauricular skin serves as a good donor site for the creation of tubed flaps. These tubed flaps are suited for reconstruction of the helical rim. Initially the flap is elevated and tubed on itself (Fig. 21-7). Within 3 weeks the tube is attached at one edge of the helical rim defect. Three weeks later the tube is incised and inset in the other edge of the helical

Text continued on p. 454.

Figure 21-5 *A*, Congenital defect of the ear with more than 20 mm difference in vertical height compared to the contrilateral normal ear. *B*, Donor site composite graft harvested to equal one-half the size of the recipient defect, thereby reducing the disparity. The donor site is closed primarily, the only resultant deformity being shortened vertical height, which is desirable in this patient's ear. *C*, The donor ear is shortened by 1 cm but retains good form. *D*, Composite graft.

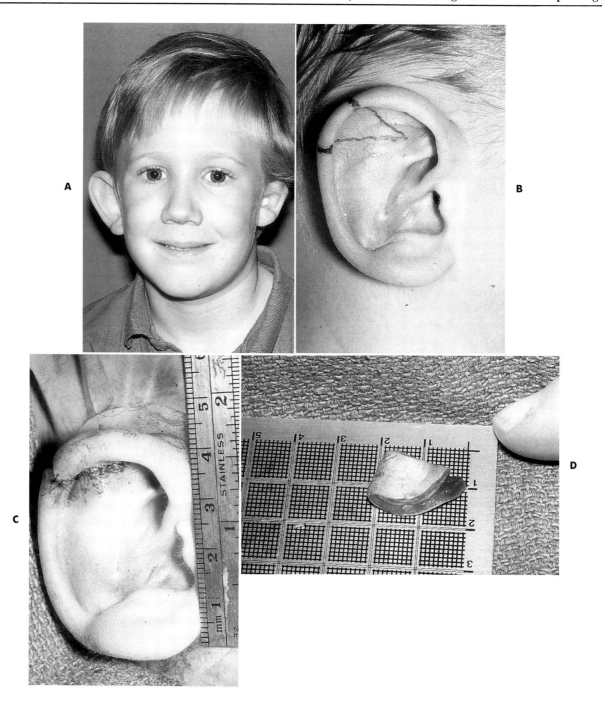

Figure 21-5, cont'd   *E,* Composite graft sutured into position. Vertical height increased by approximately 1 cm. *F,* Epithelium removed from medial aspect of composite graft and graft placed into postauricular subcutaneous pocket. The medial skin is still attached at the rim as a hinge flap. The medial perichondrium is in contact with retroauricular soft tissue. This will ensure maximum recipient contact for graft survival. Release is accomplished 2 weeks later, utilizing the hinge flap skin for medial resurfacing. *G,* Preoperative. *H,* Final result at 1 year.

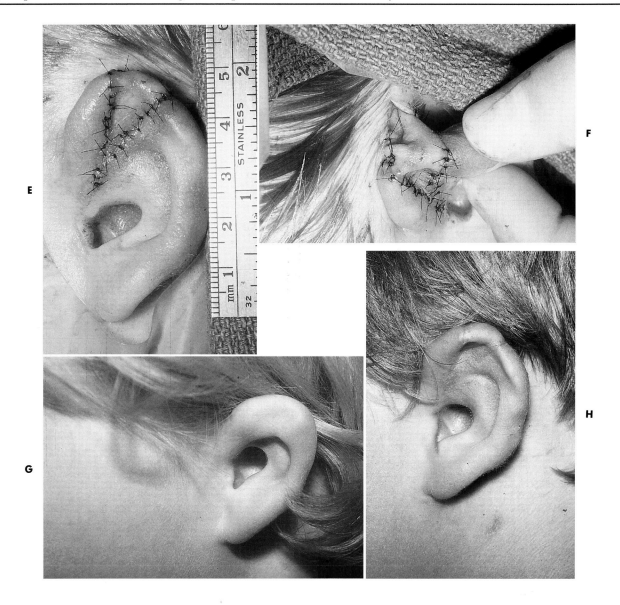

Figure 21-6   Chondrocutaneous composite flaps of the ear. *A,* Dotted lines indicate through skin and cartilage. *B,* Helical root is advanced on soft tissue pedicle. Helical rim is based on ear lobule. *C,* Flaps advanced. *D,* Final wound closure.

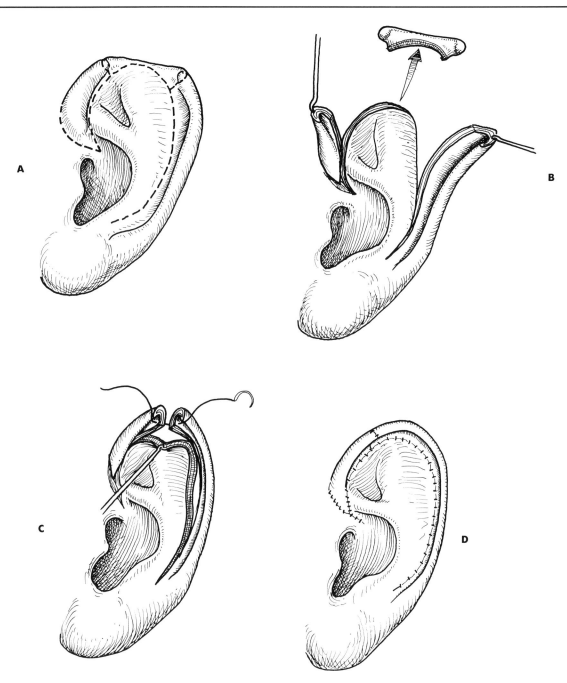

Figure 21-6, cont'd   *E*, Defect of upper ear. Chondrocutaneous composite transposition flap designed for repair. *F*, Flap transposed. *G*, Lateral skin advanced over edge of incised cartilage. *H*, Medial aspect of flap covered with a skin graft.

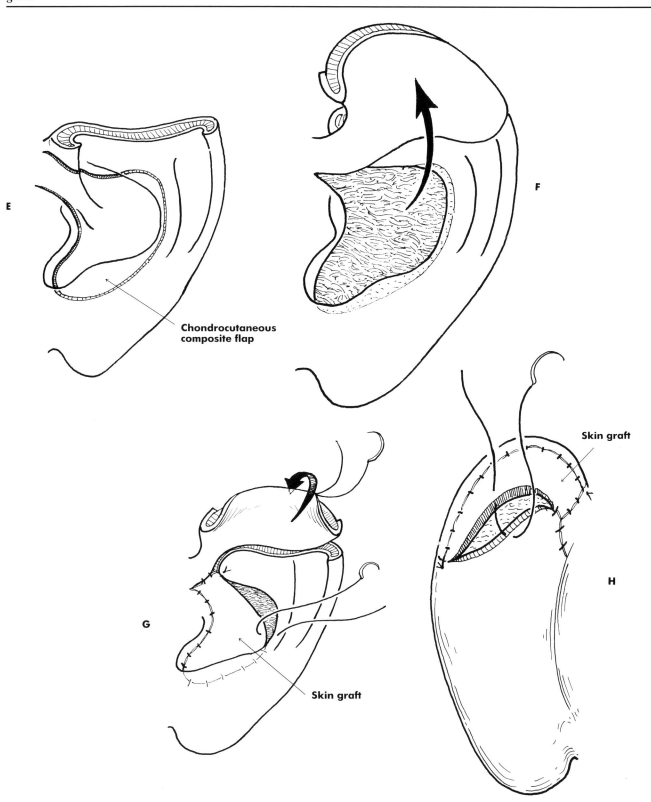

Figure 21-7 Preauricular tubed flap for repair of defects confined to the helical rim.

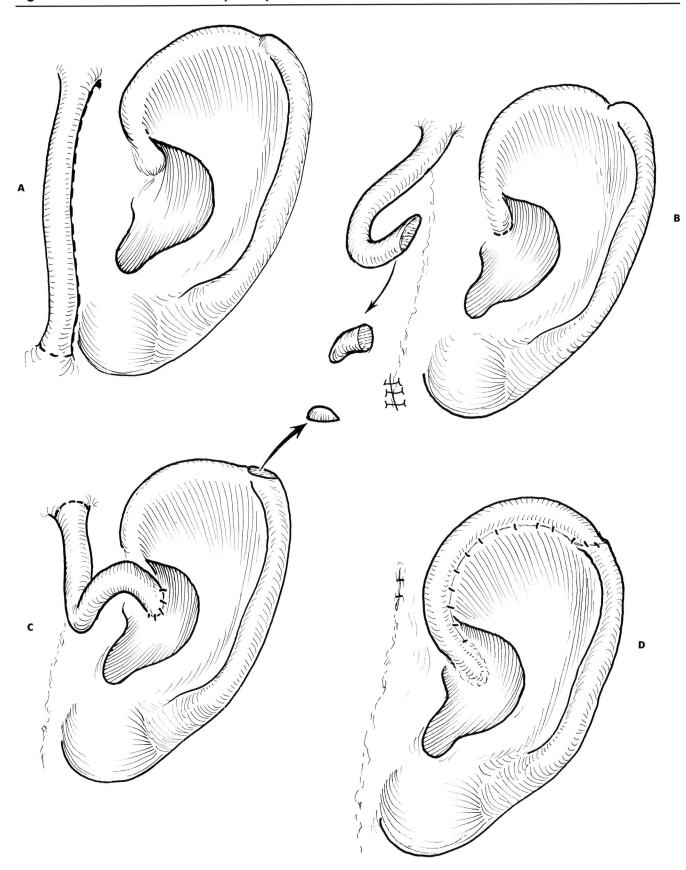

Figure 21-8   Retroauricular flap designed on postauricular skin transposed as an island flap into defect with primary closure of donor site. Flap is bivalved to provide medial and lateral resurfacing.

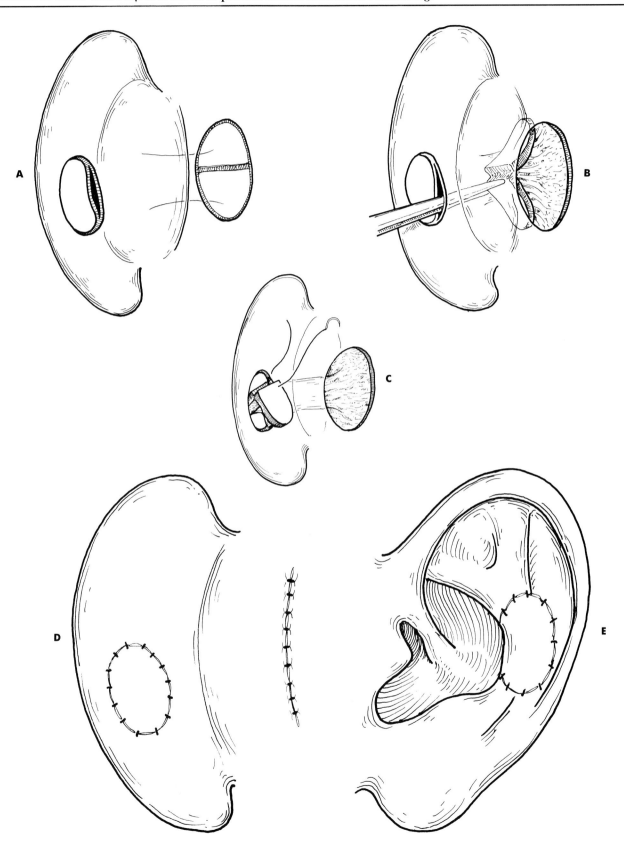

defect. Tubed flaps are most useful for those defects that are confined to the helical rim and are greater than 2.5 cm in length. For defects less than 2.5 cm, we prefer to use chondrocutaneous advancement flaps because the donor site morbidity is less.

Retroauricular island transposition flaps work well for conchal reconstruction and repair of full-thickness defects of the nonhelical portions of the ear.[24,25] The retroauricular flap is based on the auricular branch of the posterior auricular artery. It is harvested with a subcutaneous pedicle. The main advantage of the retroauricular island pedicle transposition flap is that it represents a single-stage repair with easy closure of the retroauricular donor site. When designed as an island flap, the skin island is outlined, and the flap is incised deeply to postauricular muscle. Posteriorly the mastoid periosteum is incised, and the elevation is performed in a superior anterior direction. Care is taken to preserve the vascular pedicle as it enters the flap inferiorly. With the subcutaneous pedicle intact, the flap can then be transposed into its respective conchal or nonmarginal auricular defect (Fig. 21-8). Retroauricular flaps can also be developed as interpolation flaps, requiring a two-stage procedure to include subsequent inset of the flap. Several authors have described interpolation retroauricular flaps as a single-stage procedure by deepithelializing the pedicle of the flap.[15,24] Similarly, other authors have described utilizing an interpolation flap harvested from the medial surface of the auricle for repair of lateral ear defects by deepithelializing a portion of the pedicle.[16]

All flaps used for auricular reconstruction must provide cutaneous cover and structure to maintain auricular form and size. When the vertical height of the ear will diminish by more than 20 mm using the option of local flaps, repair with a regional flap should be considered. The temporoparietal fascia flap combined with autologous cartilage framework has proven to be the most versatile regional flap for reconstruction of larger full-thickness defects, especially those of the upper half of the auricle.

The principles set forth by Tanzer and colleagues for microtia reconstruction are germane to reconstruction of larger acquired auricular defects.[26,27] The use of a three-dimensional autologous rib cartilage framework with adequate soft tissue coverage is the mainstay of microtia repair. Similarly, such a framework may be utilized in part for reconstruction of larger acquired defects. Success in microtia reconstruction as well as reconstruction following trauma or tumor ablation depends on supple, thin, and highly vascular skin coverage. Coverage of this nature allows for long-term survival of the cartilage graft as well as a full expression of its contours. When local skin is scarred or absent secondary to an acquired defect, the temporoparietal

fascia flap can provide the required thin, highly vascular recipient site for split-thickness skin grafting.

AURICULAR RECONSTRUCTION BASED ON ANATOMIC LOCATION

In planning auricular reconstruction one must consider the deformity and precisely what is missing. Our approach to acquired auricular deformities is to divide them into defects of cutaneous cover only, cutaneous cover and structure, and full-thickness defects where the medial and lateral skin surface and cartilaginous structure are absent. A discussion of these deformities is best presented by anatomic location because of the variable availability of local and regional tissue.

Defects of the Conchal Bowl and Root of the Helix

Conchal bowl defects offer several possibilities for reconstruction. Repair is frequently successful using skin grafts because they provide adequate aesthetic results and allow for careful postoperative monitoring of the area in cases where the defect has resulted from removal of skin cancer (Fig. 21-9). If the cartilage is devoid of perichondrium, it can be safely resected since conchal cartilage is not necessary for auricular form. The medial skin now becomes the nutrient bed for the skin graft. Flap immobilization can be satisfactorily achieved with Xeroform packing of the concha.

The retroauricular island transposition flap is well suited for conchal reconstruction because of its proximity to the defect. It is an excellent choice when lateral skin and cartilage of the concha are missing because it eliminates the necessity of a full-thickness skin graft and the inherent risks of secondary donor site morbidity. The flap is transferred from posterior to anterior toward the concha, followed by primary closure of the retroauricular donor site (see Fig. 21-8). Care must be taken to dissect this flap (off the mastoid cortex) in a posterior to anterior direction in order to maintain a thick subcutaneous pedicle incorporating the postauricular arterial branches and, if present, postauricular muscle. This flap can be bivalved, as shown, when there is a requirement for both medial and lateral skin coverage.

Seen either secondarily to resection of cutaneous lesions or after otologic surgery, defects of the root of the helix can be reconstructed with the use of a helical advancement flap. Patients suffering from such defects often present with a complaint of an unsightly external canal. Repair is accomplished by advancing the remaining root of the helix downward toward the defect. An incision is made in the lateral skin and cartilage along

Figure 21-9   *A*, Basal cell carcinoma limited to the conchal bowl. *B*, Extent of the defect after Mohs excision. *C*, One year following full-thickness skin graft.

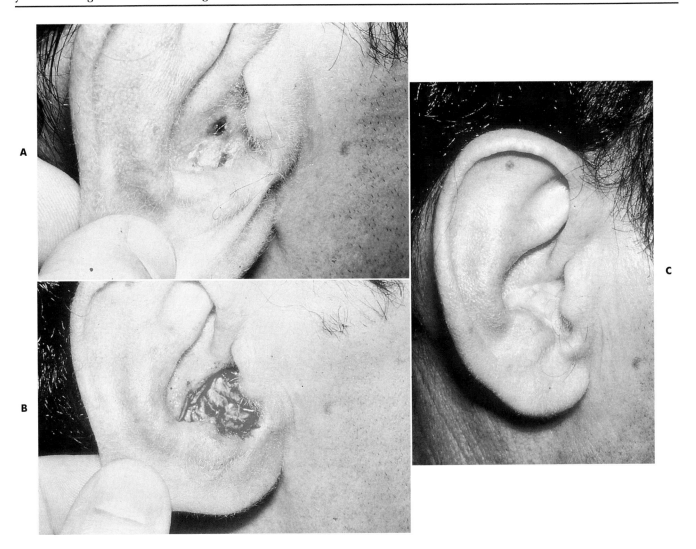

the helical rim, and the rim is advanced in a Y-to-V fashion to preserve one of the four basic contour lines of the ear. This flap consists of lateral skin and cartilage. It derives its blood supply randomly from medial soft tissue attachments. This technique is adequate for smaller defects (Fig. 21-10), but for larger defects a small Burrows' triangle of skin and cartilage must be removed from the scaphal area for adequate advancement.

Defects of the Upper One Third of the Auricle

Although the upper third of the auricle can be concealed by hair, it is of functional importance for many patients. Several surgical options are available for defects involving the upper third of the ear,

including primary wound closure, full-thickness skin grafts, helical advancement flaps, retroauricular and preauricular tubed flaps, and the use of an autogenous cartilaginous framework with temporoparietal fascia and split-thickness skin graft coverage. Both primary wound closure and helical advancement flaps are reserved for smaller, more limited auricular defects. Primary closure is used when the defect is less than 0.15 cm in width and extends from the helical rim into the body of the auricle. In such cases, repair is accomplished by converting the defect into a wedge-shaped resection, which is closed primarily without distortion (see Fig. 21-5). In some cases, small Burrows' triangles on either side of the wedge must be excised from the scapha or antihelix in order to allow for adequate closure without distortion or cupping.

Figure 21-10   *A*, Conchal bowl defect resulting from repeated otologic procedures that interrupted the spine of the concha. *B*, Root of helix mobilized to advance across the defect. *C*, Result at 6 months postoperatively.

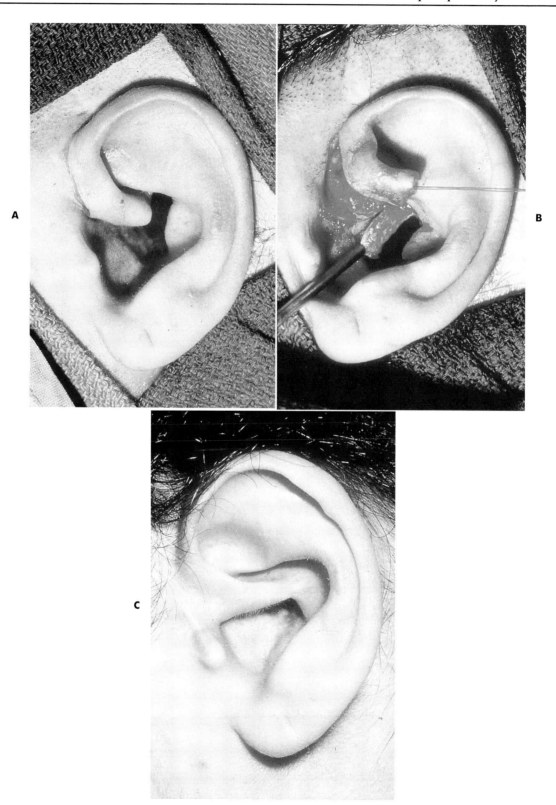

Helical chondrocutaneous advancement flaps as described by Antia are used in preference to primary wound closure when the defect is limited to the helix and is greater than 0.15 cm but less than 2.5 cm in width (Fig. 21-11).[22] This flap takes advantage of the movement of tissue that is achieved by advancement of the helix once it is released from the scapha. Additional opposing advancement can be achieved using V-Y advancement of the root of the helix. Although as originally described this procedure keeps the medial skin intact, we prefer to incise both lateral and medial skin to create a full-thickness flap that allows even greater flap mobility. The cartilage is approximated using absorbable sutures. It is important to minimize wound-closure tension of the cartilaginous approximation.

For defects larger than 2.5 cm in width and confined to the helical rim, consideration is given to a retroauricular or preauricular tubed flap (see Fig. 21-7).[28,29] This flap is randomly based, and the operation is a

Figure 21-11   *A,* Residual Breslow's I melanoma of the superior helical rim. *B,* Outline for resection and design of chondrocutaneous advancement flaps. *C,* Resultant defect, measuring approximately 2.5 cm, in preparation for full-thickness chondrocutaneous advancement flaps with complete incision through the medial auricular skin. *D,* Six months postoperative, with approximately 1 cm of vertical shortening. *E,* The contralateral, unoperated ear.

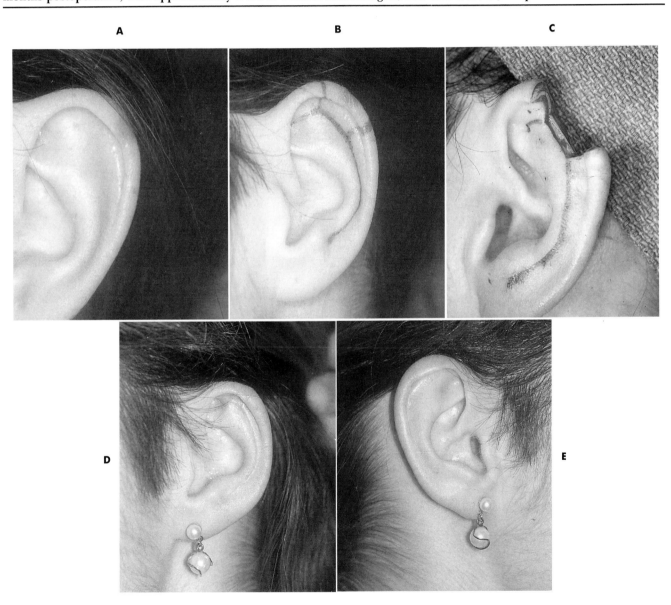

Figure 21-12 *A*, Centrally located full-thickness auricular defects after excision of basal cell carcinomas. *B*, A postauricular musculocutaneous flap pedicled on the postauricular artery and vein is designed and elevated. *C*, The skin island is folded to provide lateral and medial surface coverage. *D*, Results at 6 months postoperatively.

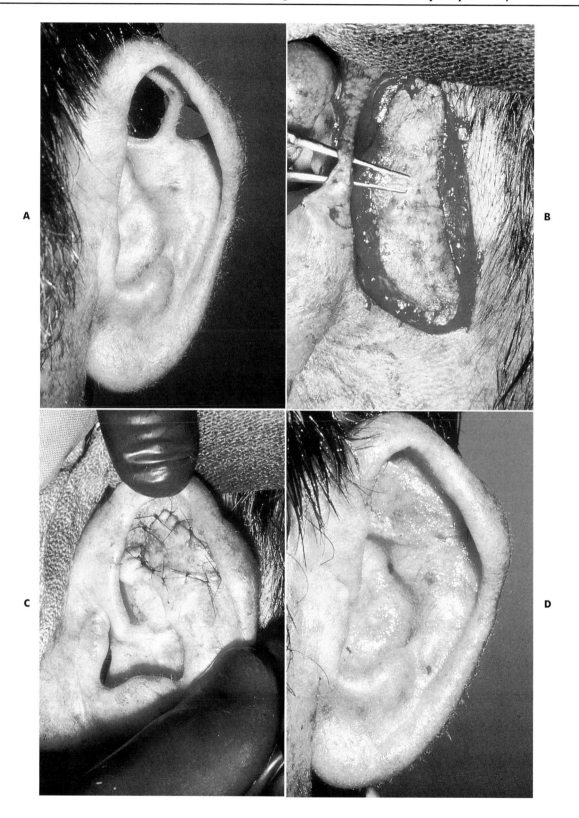

Figure 21-13   *A,* Basal cell carcinoma of the lateral auricle with rotational advancement skin flap designed to repair defect following resection of tumor. *B,* Immediate result. *C,* Postoperative result at 6 months. *D, E, F,* Rotation flap can also incorporate auricular cartilage as a composite flap for repair of full-thickness defects. Incisions are made through medial and lateral auricular skin.

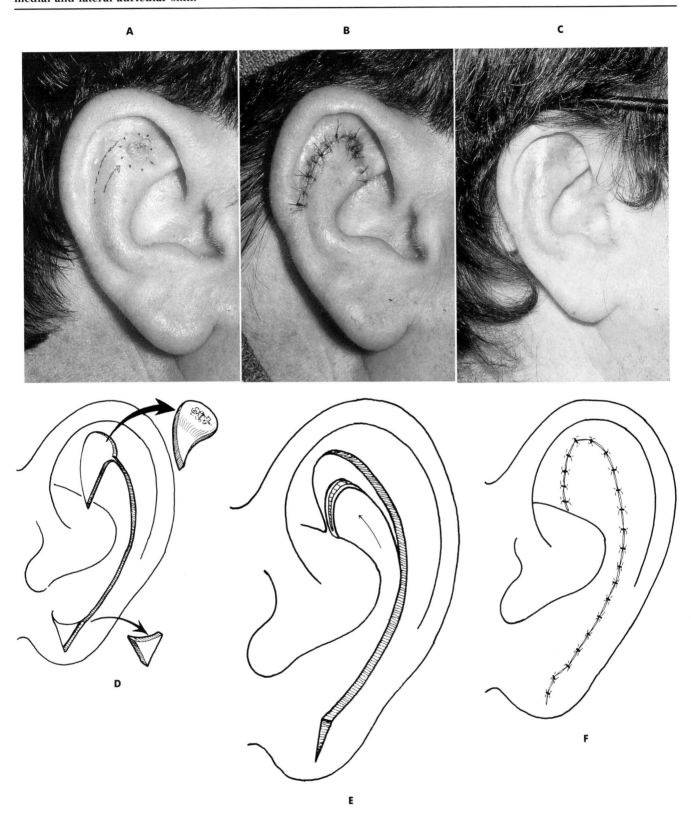

multistaged procedure. The preauricular area provides an excellent donor site for a tubed pedicle that can be used for the anterior helical rim. The first stage of this procedure requires formation of the skin tube leaving superior and inferior attachments. The second stage involves attachment of the tube to the auricle, and the third stage involves flap inset. Incorporating underlying soft tissue into the substance of the tube helps provide contour to the reconstructed helical rim, but the tube does not have an inherent structure. For this reason, its use should be confined to the helix only.

An unusual challenge occurs when a full-thickness defect of the upper auricle is present with an intact helical rim (Fig. 21-12A). Flaps used for repair of such defects must be well vascularized. This is particularly true in the repair of full-thickness auricular defects where the vascularity of the recipient site may be limited. The retroauricular island transposition flap allows the surgeon to transfer soft tissue into the body of the auricle with a reliable blood supply.[16] This flap has other advantages, including good skin color match, locally available tissue, and a well-hidden donor site scar. Based on the postauricular artery and vein, the flap incorporates postauricular skin and the postauricular muscle. It can be transferred, folded upon itself, and used to reconstruct full-thickness defects of the upper and middle auricle (see Figs. 21-8, 21-12). If the defect involves structurally important elements of the auricle, cartilage must be incorporated into the leaves of the flap.

Small lateral skin defects located in the upper and middle third of the auricle can be closed with rotation advancement flaps (Fig. 21-13) with consistent results.[30] An advantage of rotational flaps is that incisions can be hidden in the scapha to maximize scar camouflage. When the defect requires extensive soft tissue mobilization with the risk of free margin distortion, a full-thickness graft may give the best result, especially if the helical rim is intact (Fig. 21-14).

Reconstruction of large defects of the upper one third of the auricle in instances where portions of the helix, scapha, and triangular fossa are missing is best achieved by restoring the missing cartilage with a framework manufactured from autogenous rib cartilage. The framework is covered by a temporoparietal fascial flap, which in turn is resurfaced using a split-thickness skin graft (Fig. 21-15). The temporoparietal fascial flap is described in this chapter under the discussion dealing with reconstruction of microtia.

Defects of the Middle One Third of the Auricle

The absence of the middle third of the auricle is a very conspicuous deformity. Small defects (less than 1.5 cm) can be closed by converting the defect into a wedge-shaped excision with a direct impact on vertical height. Full-thickness helical defects (less than 2.5 cm) are amenable to helical chondrocutaneous advancement flaps. Defects that are larger than 2.5 cm in width and are confined to the helical rim can be repaired with a tubed flap, but we feel that its use is limited to soft tissue defects of the helix only.[31] Major defects of the middle third of the auricle involving the helix and antihelix require cartilage grafting to achieve the structural support necessary for satisfactory reconstruction.[32,33] Repair is accomplished by using a two-stage retroauricular composite flap to provide nonhairbearing soft tissue coverage and cartilage replacement (Fig. 21-16). The first stage involves creating a retroauricular advancement flap randomly based posteriorly on retroauricular scalp. The width of this flap is equal to the width of the defect, and it is used to cover the lateral aspect of the defect. The medial aspect of the remaining cartilage, from which the distal-most portion of the flap is harvested, is attached to the denuded retroauricular area. Often, septal or conchal cartilage is implanted beneath the advancement flap to replace the missing portion of the auricular cartilage during this first stage. Care should be taken to suture the cartilage graft to the remaining auricular cartilage. The second stage is performed 3 weeks later. The postauricular flap is detached from the scalp and used as a hinge flap to cover the medial aspect of the cartilage graft. Careful planning of the inset is important to ensure adequate skin coverage of the cartilage graft. A full-thickness skin graft can be used for repair of the retroauricular donor area. In most cases, however, the donor site can be closed primarily.

Defects of the Lower One Third of the Auricle

Relative pliability and laxity of auricular and periauricular skin in this area, especially in the older patient, makes the surgeon's task less difficult when reconstructing defects of the lower one third of the auricle. Half of the lobule can be removed by wedge-shaped excision and primary wound closure with only minimal resultant deformity. The lobule lends itself to small advancement flaps for repair of helical defects of the lower third of the ear. Loss of the entire lobule presents a more complex reconstructive challenge. When reconstructing the entire lower one-third of the ear and lobule, the repair must include cartilage grafting techniques to provide the support necessary to assure aesthetic results. Our preferred technique for reconstruction of the lobule utilizes a composite flap containing conchal cartilage in a two-stage procedure. The cartilage is embedded in a subcutaneous pocket below the auricle. Six weeks later, the cartilage and overlying skin are elevated as a composite flap based superiorly

Figure 21-14   *A,* Basal cell carcinoma of the lateral auricle. Dotted line outlines proposed surgical margin. *B,* Large defect with cartilage loss after Mohs excision. *C,* Full-thickness postauricular skin graft placed. Bolster sutures in place. *D,* Bolster applied to stabilize skin graft for 10 days. *E,* Result at 6 months postoperatively.

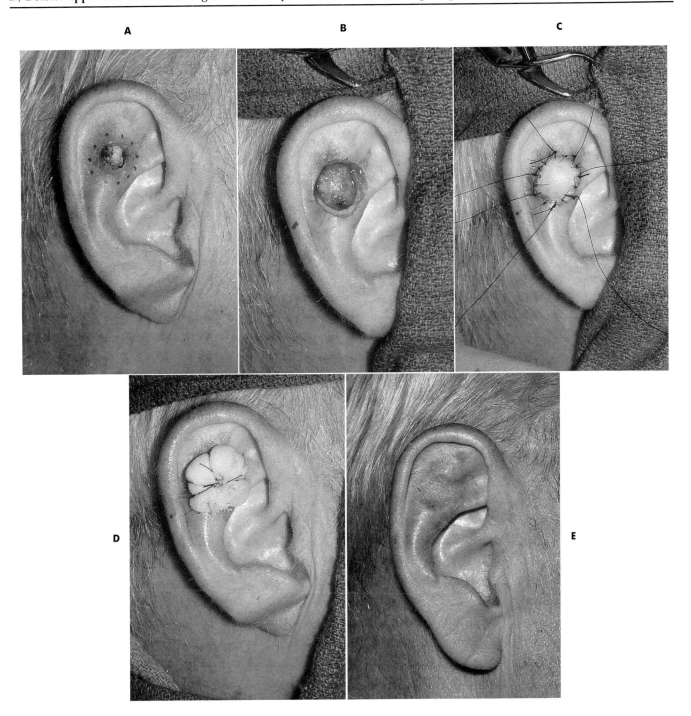

Figure 21-15 *A*, Extensive basal cell carcinoma of the superior auricle. *B*, Extent of the defect after Mohs excision. *C*, Appearance of auricle after 18 months following split-thickness skin graft applied to allow for careful postoperative monitoring.

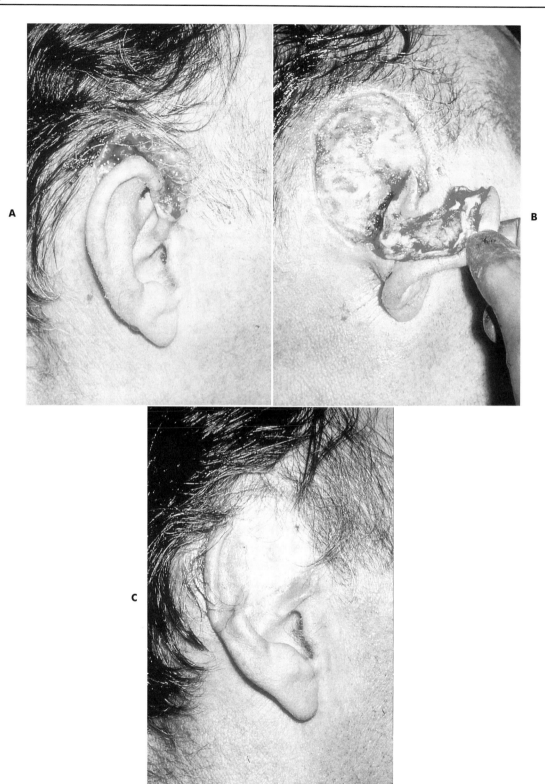

Figure 21-15, cont'd   *D*, Reconstruction utilizing autogenous rib cartilage framework. Temporoparietal fascial flap is dissected in preparation for coverage. *E*, Split-thickness skin graft placed over the cartilage/fascia composite. *F*, *G*, Appearance of auricle at 6 months postoperatively.

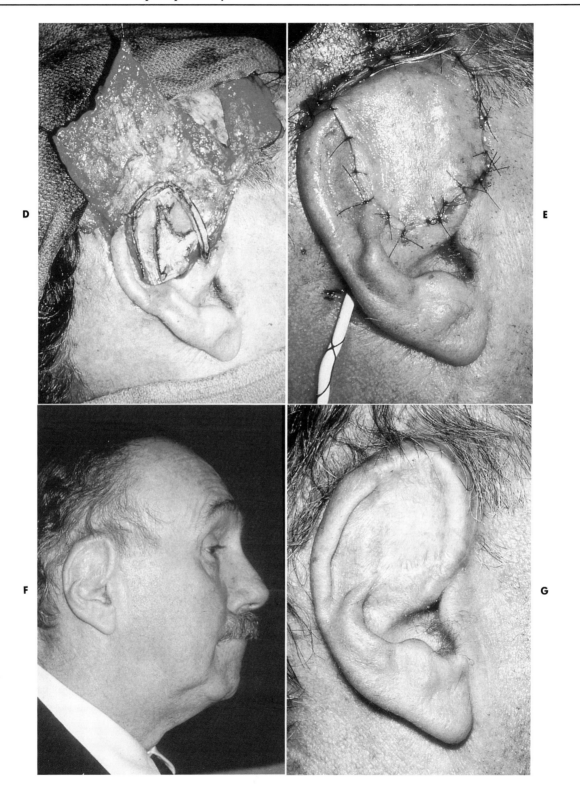

Figure 21-16 *A*, Helical rim defect following Mohs surgery. *B*, Elevation of a retroauricular flap. Septal cartilage in place to provide structural support. *C*, Retroauricular flap sutured in place. The flap is released 3 weeks later and the retroauricular donor area closed primarily. *D*, Result at 1 year postoperatively.

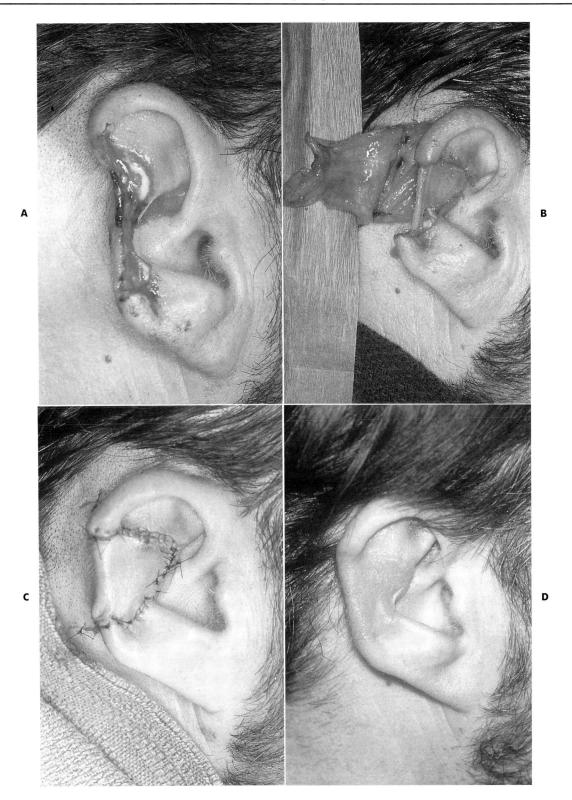

on the remaining auricle. The medial surface of the composite flap is skin-grafted (Fig. 21-17). This technique provides good skin color match, results in minimal local edema, produces a naturally shaped and textured ear lobe, and allows for proper lobule positioning.

Defects of the Preauricular Area

The most common preauricular defects occur secondary to excision of cutaneous lesions. The function of the facial nerve should be carefully examined before the removal of lesions in this location. Surgical options for the repair of preauricular defects include primary

Figure 21-17   *A*, Traumatic lobular defect. *B*, Lobular remnant excised and contralateral conchal cartilage harvested. *C*, Auricular pattern used to establish the vertical height required. *D, E*, Conchal cartilage placed in a subcutaneous pocket for 6 weeks. *F*, Eight weeks following second stage, which involves release of the skin/cartilage unit as a composite flap based superiorly on the auricle. A skin graft is placed on the medial surface of the reconstructed lobule.

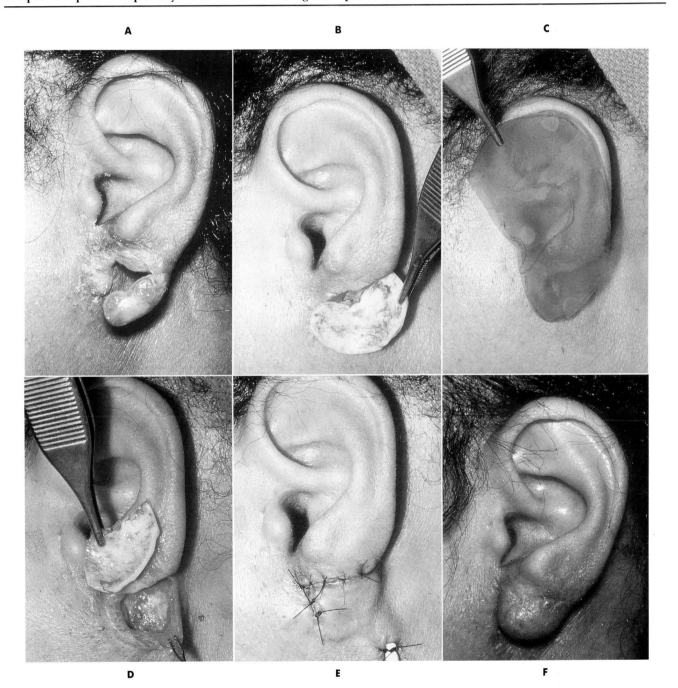

A   B   C

D   E   F

Figure 21-18   *A*, Basal cell carcinoma of the preauricular skin in patient with redundant facial skin. *B*, Six months following closure with advancement skin flap. Scar is camouflaged in preauricular crease.

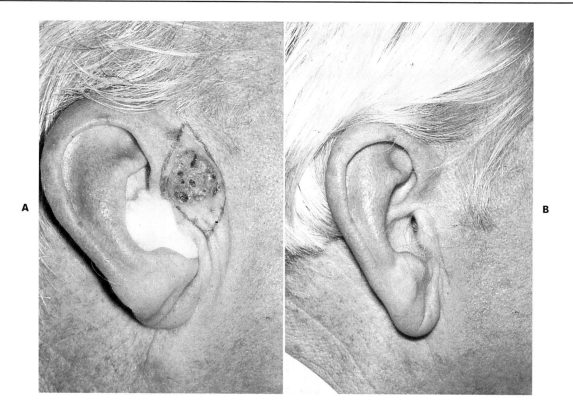

Figure 21-19   *A*, Defect following excision of recurrent basal cell carcinoma of the preauricular skin. *B*, Closure accomplished by opposing subcutaneous pedicled advancement flaps designed to avoid dissection in area of the frontal branch of the facial nerve and to maintain hair pattern. *C*, Result 6 months postoperatively.

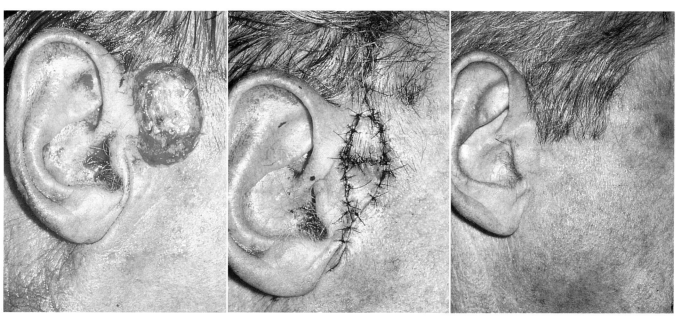

A   B   C

Figure 21-20   *A*, Large (3.5 cm) preauricular defect following resection of squamous cell carcinoma. Outline of bilobed flap. *B*, Bilobed flap transposed. *C*, Result at 1 year.

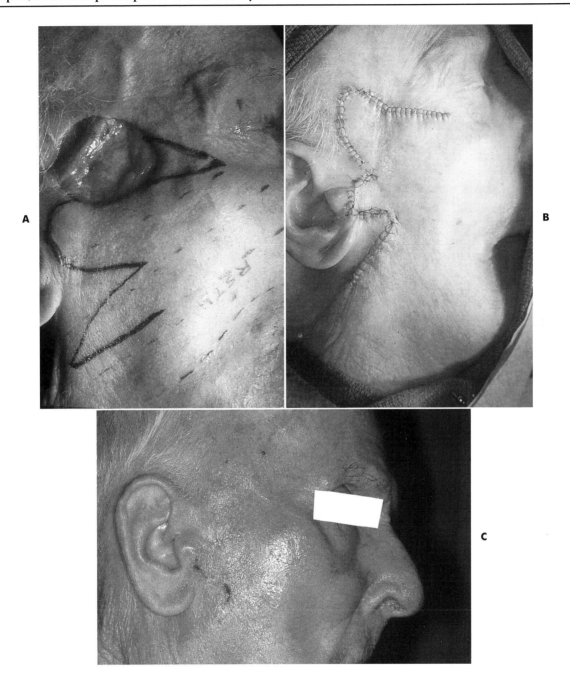

wound closure. With careful planning, the resultant scar can frequently be placed within the preauricular crease with minimal deformity. Cheek advancement flaps (Fig. 21-18), V-Y advancement flaps (Fig. 21-19), and transposition flaps (Fig. 21-20)[34] can also be used.

LARGE AURICULAR DEFORMITIES

Auricular defects encompassing one third or more of the entire auricle make greater demands on the reconstructive surgeon. The surgeon will be well served by incorporating both a fundamental knowledge of microtia reconstruction and an understanding of the temporoparietal fascia flap.

Unlike microtia repair, with larger auricular defects only a portion of the standard fabricated cartilaginous framework is utilized. Local skin may be adequate for coverage, but more often than not it is either absent or scarred, making it nonpliable and vascularly compromised. In these circumstances, coverage can be achieved utilizing a temporoparietal fascia flap and split-thickness skin grafts.[35] Combining the planning and execution of microtia repair with the anatomy and design of a temporoparietal fascia flap enables one to reconstruct defects beyond the compatibility of local flap repair.

Microtia Principles and the Temporoparietal Fascia Flap

By fashioning a new auricle or portions of it from autogenous cartilage, the surgeon can avoid the use of an auricular prosthesis or alloplastic implants.[36-37] Auricular prostheses pose problems with adherence to skin in the auricular area, and it has been our experience that patients adjust better, both physically and psychologically, to reconstruction of the auricle utilizing autogenous tissue. Some authors have demonstrated slight auricular growth in reconstructed ears.[6] We prefer autogenous cartilage for auricular reconstruction, as opposed to alloplastic implants, which have an unacceptably high extrusion and infection rate. However, because the ribs become more brittle and ossified with age, reconstruction utilizing costal cartilage must be carefully considered in patients over the age of 60. The cartilagenous components of the sixth, seventh, and eighth ribs provide the raw material for creation of the framework. The synchondrosis between the sixth and seventh ribs serves as the body of

the framework, and the helix is fashioned from the eighth rib. As with techniques employed in microtia repair, determination of the appropriate size and individual shape of the framework is obtained from a pattern of the contralateral auricle (Fig. 21-21). Contouring of the cartilaginous framework is achieved utilizing a basic framework of ribs six and seven. The concha, antitragus, and curve of the antihelix are derived from this. Creation of the helix is accomplished by removing the perichondrium from the medial side of the eighth rib and thinning the cartilage until bending of the cartilage toward the perichondrium occurs, thereby acquiring the curve of the helix. This is fixed to the basic framework with sutures using 5-0 stainless steel wire, taking care to allow that the root of the newly formed helix indents into the concha. Final contour is achieved utilizing 5-mm and 7-mm gouges to create the antihelix and form the triangularis respectively. The cartilaginous framework is stabilized and properly positioned based on preoperative measurements.[38,39]

Coverage of the cartilagenous framework requires that the tissue be thin, vascular, hairless, and capable of accepting skin grafts of a good color match with adjacent ear and periauricular skin. A pedicled temporoparietal fascial flap with skin graft satisfies this requirement and is frequently used to cover the cartilage framework.[40-43] The temporoparietal fascia flap also has the following advantages: (1) the anatomy

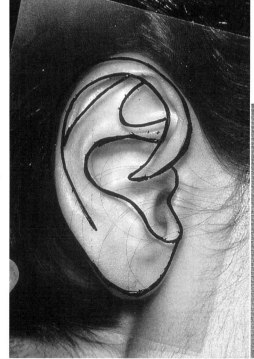

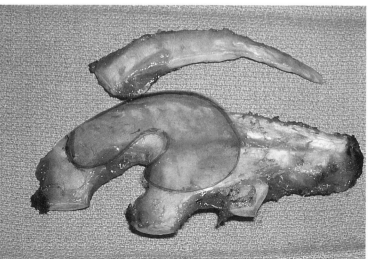

Figure 21-21 *A*, Pattern created from normal ear. *B*, Costal cartilage harvested for auricular framework.

Figure 21-21, cont'd   *C*, Helix and body of framework fashioned from costal cartilage. *D*, Scapha and fossa triangularis detailed. *E*, Vertical and horizontal height should match the template. *F*, Final costal cartilage framework.

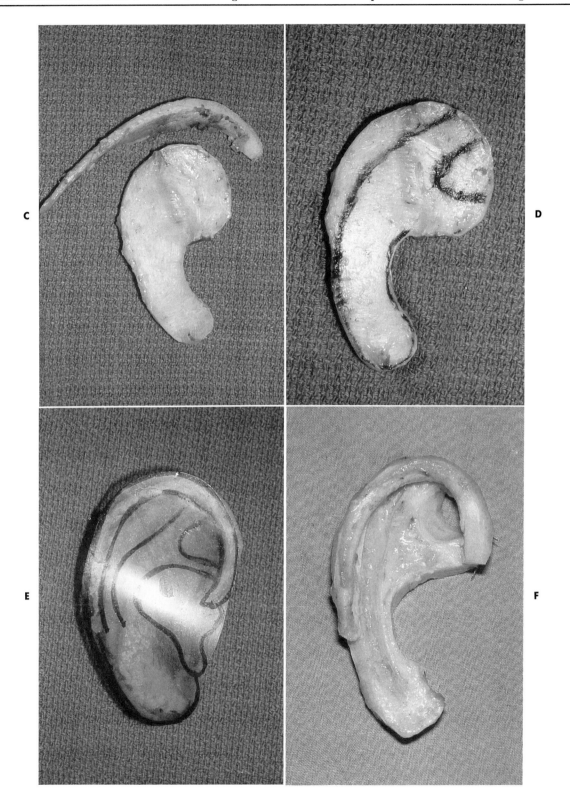

of the flap is well known to head and neck surgeons, (2) a large quantity of tissue (14 × 12 cm) can be harvested, (3) the flap can be rotated to cover a wide range of auricular defects, and (4) the fascia may be transferred to the contralateral auricular region if necessary, using microvascular techniques.[44-46]

The temporoparietal fascia, also known as the superficial temporal fascia, is continuous with the superficial musculoaponeurotic system, as well as the deep galea (Fig. 21-22). It lies deep to the skin and subcutaneous tissue to which it is firmly bound (particularly in the area of the temporal line.) This fascia should not be confused with the fascial layer surrounding the temporalis muscle. The temporoparietal fascia attaches to the zygomatic arch, whereas the temporalis muscular fascia is deeper, thicker, and divides to envelop the zygomatic arch. Measuring on average 2 to 3 mm in thickness over the parietal area, the temporoparietal fascia is highly vascular, with an abundant and consistent blood supply from the superficial temporal artery and vein.[3,47]

A 6-cm long verticle incision is made in the scalp immediately above the auricular defect, exposing the superficially located temporoparietal fascia. When harvesting the flap, care must be taken to keep the hair follicles and subcutaneous fat attached to the overlying scalp and under direct vision. Careful avoidance of the hair follicles prevents the iatrogenic complication of alopecia. The medial plane of flap elevation is over the temporalis muscular fascia in the loose connective tissue that separates the temporoparietal fascia from the muscular fascia. The vascular pedicle is identified and protected, and the anterior limit of the flap is determined. The frontal branch of the facial nerve is the limiting factor in flap elevation in this area. The posterior margin of the flap should capture the posterior branch of the superficial temporal artery and vein and can be back-cut to these vessels to facilitate flap transfer. The flap is rotated 180 degrees in an arc from superior to inferior such that the lateral surface of the flap becomes the medial surface adherent to the cartilage framework. The edges of the flap are tucked under the existing skin edges, similar to tucking a shirt in pants. Split-thickness skin grafts, obtained from the lateral buttock area, are used to provide external coverage of the fascial flap wound. Optimal drainage is provided by suction through a closed system that affixes to the patient's dressing, such as a red-topped vacuum tube or a bulb-system drain. The avoidance of wall suction promotes ambulation and prevents un-

Figure 21-22   Anatomy of the temporoparietal fascial flap.

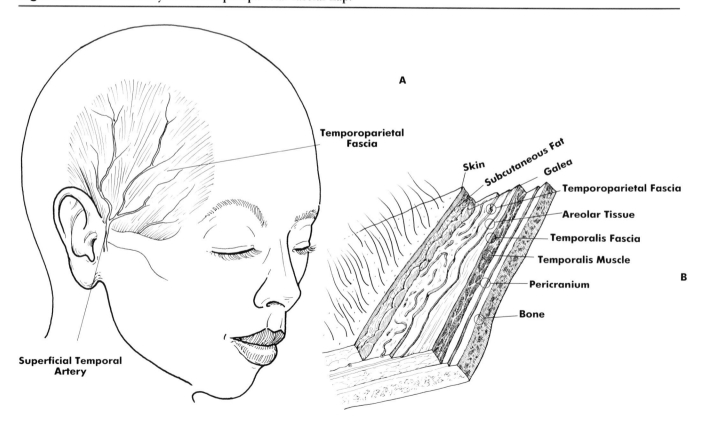

Figure 21-23   *A,* Angiolymphoid hyperplasia of the auricle; a benign lesion that does not affect the cartilage. *B,* Incision for exposure of the fascial flap. *C,* Appearance of the auricular cartilage after tumor excision. *D,* Temporoparietal fascial flap elevated.

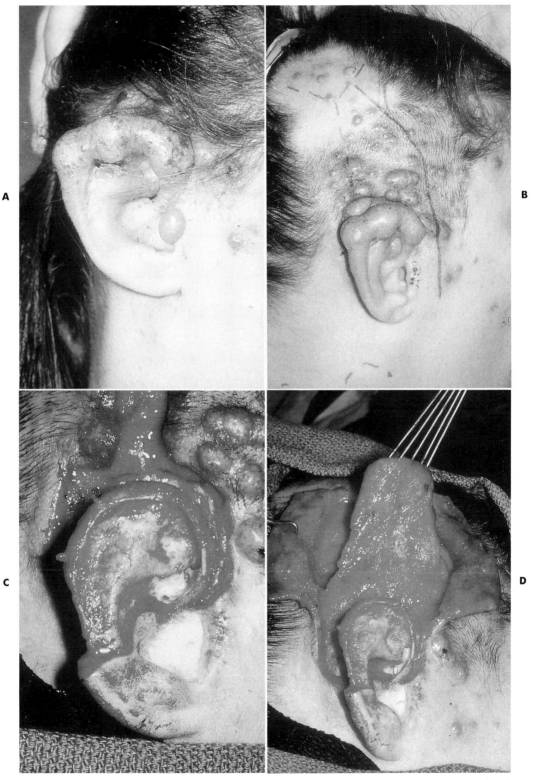

Continued.

Figure 21-23, cont'd *E*, Flap transposed over the auricular framework. *F*, Temporoparietal fascia stabilized under the adjacent periauricular skin. *G*, Split-thickness skin graft placed over the cartilage/fascia unit. *H*, Appearance after 1 year. Postauricular sulcus created at separate stage.

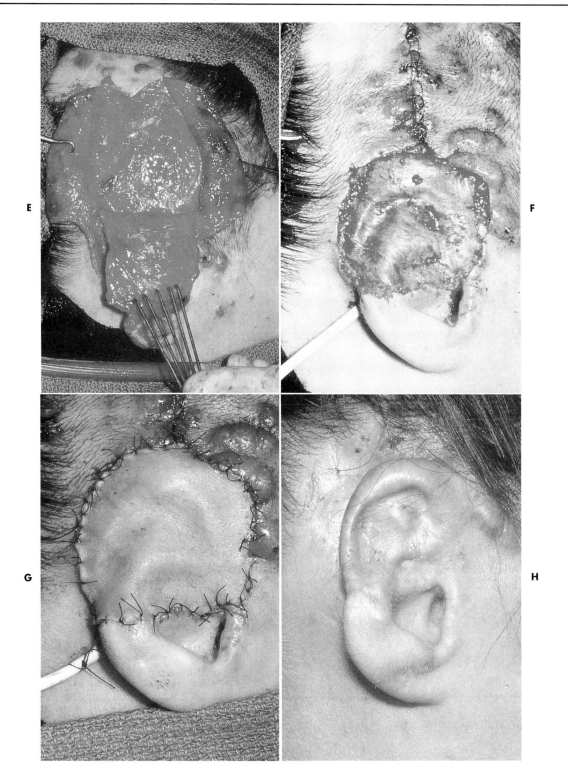

planned premature removal of the drain. Drains are removed after 3 days, and a light compression dressing is applied.

The temporoparietal fascial flap may also be used to cover autogenous auricular cartilage in instances where large areas of the cartilage is denuded of skin (Fig. 21-23), such as in total ear resurfacing.[48] Split-thickness skin grafts applied directly to auricular cartilage without its surface covering of perichondrium have a limited success rate. Incorporating a temporoparietal fascia flap to serve as a recipient bed for the split-thickness skin graft markedly enhances their successful healing.

Although the temporoparietal fascial flap can be tunneled under the supraauricular sulcus, it is frequently necessary to place the flap across the sulcus, thereby obliterating it. In such instances, it is necessary to reestablish the sulcus in a second surgical stage. This stage involves releasing the reconstructed auricle from its attachment superiorly and covering the medial aspect of the upper ear with a skin graft. This maneuver restores the supraauricular sulcus.

RESURFACING OF THE TEMPORAL CAVITY AFTER AURICULAR EXCISION

On occasion, large cancers of the auricle that do not involve the temporal bone necessitate complete removal of the ear. Several options are available for resurfacing of the exposed bone resulting from total auriculectomy, including the use of a bilobed cutaneous flap that can be transposed over the temporal bone and is designed to allow for the preservation of the external auditory canal (Fig. 21-24). Additional options for repair of such defects include cervical rotation flaps, regional chest and shoulder flaps and microvascular tissue transfer. Bulky musculocutaneous flaps have the disadvantage that the bulk of the flap often compromises the external auditory canal impeding hearing. In specific cases temporal bone defects can be covered with a temporoparietal fascial flap and skin grafted (Fig. 21-25). In these situations most cavities can be reliably lined with the temporoparietal fascia and skin-grafted. Subsequently the patient can be fitted for an auricular prosthesis (Fig. 21-25).

AURICULAR KELOIDS

Auricular keloids are a common sequelae of trauma to the lobule in susceptible individuals. The most common inciting event is ear piercing, but keloids can arise from a variety of causes, including elective procedures around the ear, such as otoplasty and facelift. A wide variety of techniques have been used in the management of keloids, including the use of lasers, injection of interferon, simple excision, and steroid injections.[48] Our recommended treatment begins with intralesional injections of Kenalog 40 (triamcinolone acetonide suspension 40 mg/ml) given 2 weeks apart for a total of four to five sessions.[49] The effect of the treatment is evaluated every 2 weeks, and when softening of the tissue is noted, surgical resection is scheduled. An

Figure 21-24 *A,* **Extensive basal cell carcinoma of the auricle.** *B,* **Bilobed flap designed for coverage of defect after total auriculectomy.**

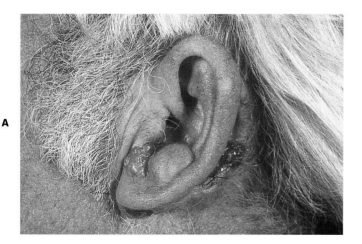

A

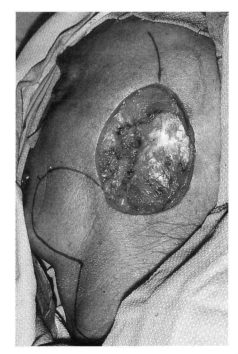

B

Continued.

Figure 21-24, cont'd *C*, Flap elevated and ready for transposition. *D*, Inset flap with external auditory canal preserved. *E*, *F*, Appearance at 6 months postoperatively.

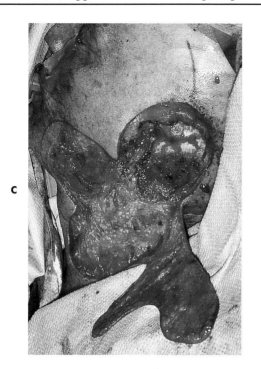

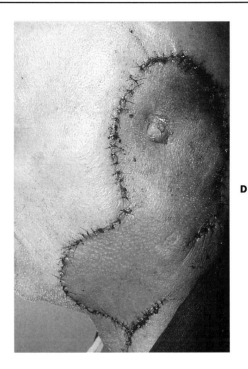

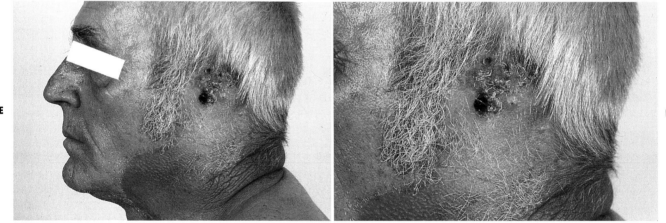

Figure 21-25   *A*, Squamous cell carcinoma limited to the conchal bowl. *B*, Incision used for resection and elevation of a temporoparietal fascial flap. *C*, Resection with exposed cartilage and mastoid cavity. Temporoparietal flap elevated. *D*, Temporoparietal flap transposed. *E*, Flap sutured into defect.

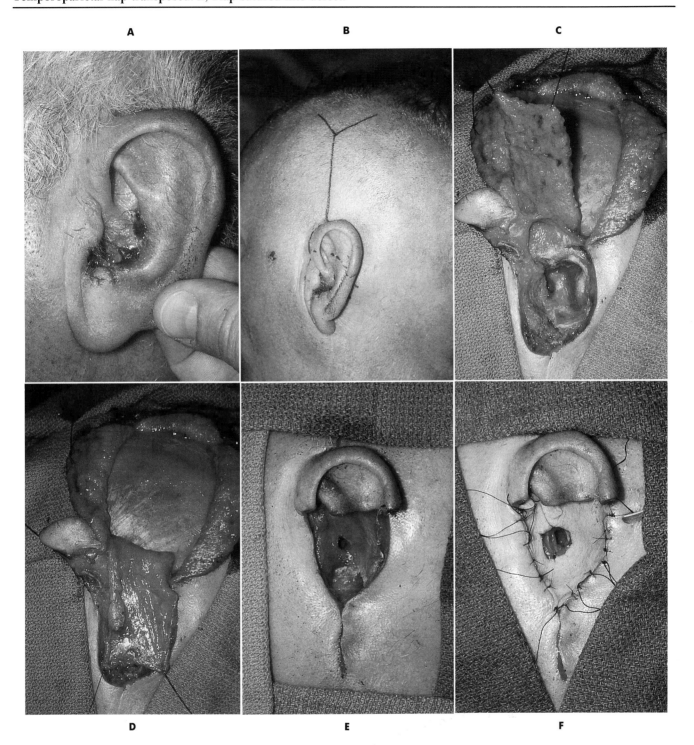

A   B   C

D   E   F

Figure 21-25, cont'd   *F,* Opening in flap allows exposure of the tympanic membrane to sound waves. Split-thickness skin graft placed over vascularized fascia. *G,* Result, with preservation of auditory function. *H,* Prosthesis fit for final result.

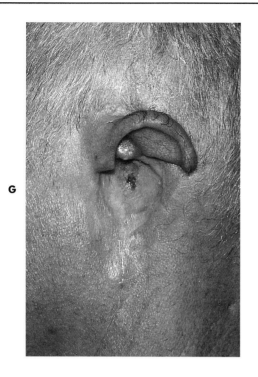

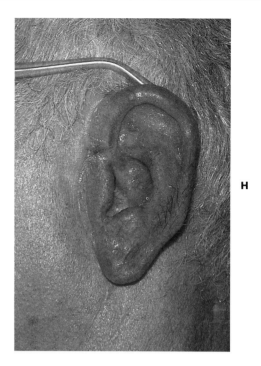

Figure 21-26   *A, B,* Large auricular keloids. *C, D,* Result at 1 year after excision preceded by Kenalog injections.

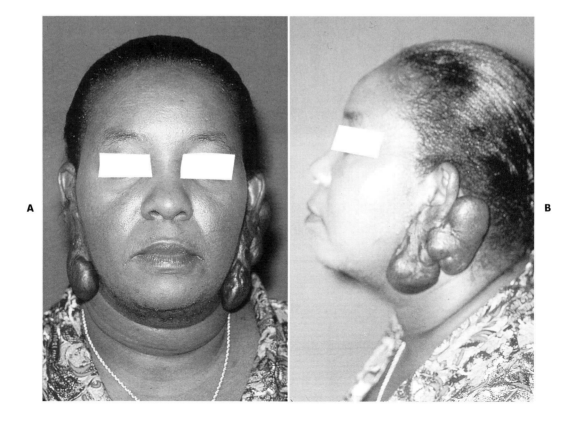

Figure 21-26, cont'd   For legend see facing page.

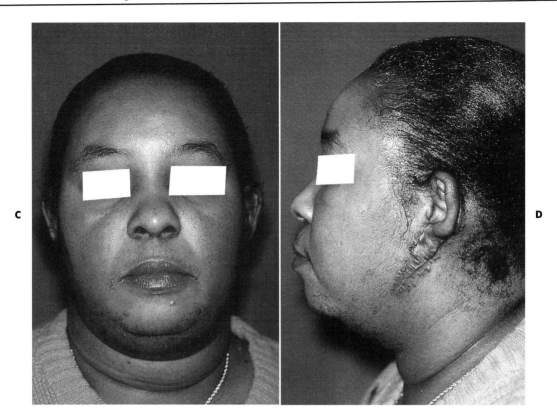

atraumatic surgical excision within the margins of the keloid tissue is performed followed by an intraoperative intralesional injection of Kenalog 40 (Fig. 21-26). Postoperatively, the patient is monitored carefully for any evidence of recurrence. If there is evidence of keloid reformation in the postoperative period, reinstitution of Kenalog 40 injections is initiated. Low-dose radiation therapy is reserved for intractable keloid formation.[50]

SUMMARY

When auricular reconstruction is approached systematically, successful results can be achieved. Its morphologic uniqueness of medial and lateral cutaneous cover over cartilage is a challenge to replace when partial or full-thickness defects are present. Constituent components of the defect need to be analyzed. Depending on the anatomic location of the defect, a variety of techniques for repair have been described, such as primary wound closure, skin grafting, and the use of local flaps. For larger full-thickness defects, facility with the principles of microtia reconstruction, utilizing an autogenous rib framework and a temporoparietal

fascia flap, is of paramount importance. The ultimate goal is a well-functioning appendage that is normal in position, size, and contour, in that order of importance.

REFERENCES

1. Allison G: Anatomy of the external ear, *Clin Plast Surg* 5:419, 1978.
2. Hayashi R, Matsuo K, Hirose T: Tension lines of the auricular cartilage, *Plast Reconstr Surg* 87:869, 1991.
3. Abul-Hassan HS, Drasek Ascher G Von, Acland RD: Surgical anatomy and blood supply of the fascial layers of the temporal region, *Plast Reconstr Surg* 77:17, 1986.
4. Park C, Lineaweaver WC, Rumly TO, Buncke HJ: Arterial supply of the anterior ear, *Plast Reconstr Surg* 90:38, 1992.
5. Adamson JE, Horton CE, Crawford HH: The growth pattern of the external ear, *Plast Reconstr Surg* 36:466-470, 1965.
6. Farkas LG: Growth of normal and reconstructed auricles. In Tanzer RC, Edgerton MT, editors: *Symposium on reconstruction of the auricle*, St Louis, 1974, The CV Mosby Co.
7. Thomson HG, Correa A: Unilateral microtia

reconstruction: is the position symmetrical? *Plast Reconstr Surg* 92:852, 1993.

8. Tolleth H: Artistic anatomy, dimensions and proportions of the external ear, *Clin Plast Surg* 36:466, 1978.

9. Tolleth H: A hierarchy of values in the design and constructin of the ear, *Clin Plast Surg* 36:466, 1978.

10. Postnick JC, Al-Qatta MM, Whitaker LA: Assessment of the preferred vertical position of the ear, *Plast Reconstr Surg* 91:1198, 1993.

11. Skiles MS, Randall P: The aesthetics of ear placement: an experimental study, *Plast Reconstr Surg* 72:133, 1983.

12. Brent B: Reconstruction of traumatic ear deformities, *Clin Plast Surg* 5:437, 1978.

13. Bumsted RM, Ceilley RI: Auricular malignant neoplasms, *Arch Otolaryngol* 108:225, 1982.

14. Cotlar SW: Reconstruction of the burned ear using a temporalis fascial flap, *Plast Reconstr Surg* 71:45, 1983.

15. Donelan MB: Conchal transposition flap for postburn ear deformities, *Plast Reconstr Surg* 83:641, 1989.

16. Elsahy NI: Ear reconstruction with a flap from the medial surface of the auricle, *Ann Plast Surg* 14:169, 1985.

17. Eriksson E, Vogt PM: Ear reconstruction, *Clin Plast Surg* 19:637, 1992.

18. Heberhold C: Reconstruction of the auriculum, *Facial Plastic Surgery Monograph* 5(5):385, 1988.

19. Rosenthal JS: The thermally injured ear: a systematic approach to reconstruction, *Clin Plast Surg* 19:645, 1992.

20. Song R, Chen Z, Yang P, Yue J: Reconstruction of the external ear, *Clin Plast Surg* 9:49, 1982.

21. Songharoen S, Smith RA, Jabaley ME: Tumors of the external ear and reconstruction of defects, *Clin Plast Surg* 5:447, 1978.

22. Antia NH, Buch VI: Chondrocutaneous advancement flap for the marginal defect of the ear, *Plast Reconstr Surg* 39:472, 1967.

23. Ramirez OM, Heckler FR: Reconstruction of nonmarginal defects of the ear with chondrocutaneous advancement flaps, *Plast Reconstr Surg* 84:32, 1989.

24. Gingrass RP, Pickrell KL: Techniques for closure of conchal and external auditory canal defects, *Plast Reconstr Surg* 14:568, 1968.

25. Krespi YP, Ries WR, Shugar JMA, Sisson GA: Auricular reconstruction with postauricular myocutaneous flap, *Otolaryngol Head Neck Surg* 91:191, 1983.

26. Tanzer RC, Bellucci RJ, Convers JM, Brent B: Deformities of the auricle. In Converse JM, editor: *Reconstructive plastic surgery*, Philadelphia, 1977, WB Saunders.

27. Tanzer RC: Total reconstruction of the external ear, *Plast Reconstr Surg* 23:1, 1959.

28. Renard A: Postauricular flaps based on a dermal pedicle for ear reconstruction, *Plast Reconstr Surg* 68:159, 1981.

29. Scott MJL, Klaassen MF: Immediate reconstruction of the helical rim after bite injury using the posterior auricular flap, *Injury* 23:333, 1992.

30. Elsahy NI: Ear reconstruction with rotation-advancement composite flap, *Plast Reconstruc Surg* 77:567, 1985.

31. Lawson VG: Reconstruction of the pinna using pre-auricular flaps, *J Otolaryngol* 13:191, 1984.

32. Millard DR: The chondrocutaneous flaps in partial auricular repair, *Plast Reconstr Surg* 37:523, 1966.

33. Millard DR: Reconstruction of one-third plus of the auricular circumference, *Plast Reconstruc Surg* 90:475, 1992.

34. Sutton AE, Quatela VC: Bilobed flap reconstruction of the temporal forehead, *Arch Otolaryngol Head Neck Surg* 118:978, 1992.

35. Bardsley AF: Primary reconstruction of a severed ear fragment using a flap of temporo-parietal fascia, *Br J Plast Surg* 39:524, 1986.

36. Brent B: Auricular repair with autogenous rib cartilage grafts: two decades of experience with 600 cases, *Plast Reconstr Surg* 90:355, 1992.

37. Nagata S: A new method of total reconstruction of the auricle for microtia, *Plast Reconstr Surg* 92:187, 1993.

38. Brent B: The acquired auricular deformity: a systematic approach to its analysis and reconstruction, *Plast Reconstr Surg* 59:475, 1977.

39. Brent B: The correction of microtia with autogenous cartilage grafts: I. The classic deformity. II Atypical and complex deformities, *Plast Reconstr Surg* 66:1, 1980.

40. Brent B, Byrd HS: Secondary ear reconstruction with cartilage grafts covered by axial, random, and free flaps of temporoparietal fascia, *Plast Reconstruc Surg* 72:141, 1983.

41. Brent B, Upton J, Acland RD, et al: Experience with the temporoparietal fascial free flap, *Plast Reconstr Surg* 76:177, 1985.

42. Jenkins AM, Finucan T: Primary nonmicrosurgical reconstrucion following ear avulsion using the temporoparietal fascial island flap, *Plast Reconstr Surg* 83:148, 1989.

43. Rose EH, Norris MS: The versatile temporoparietal fascial flap: adaptability to a variety of composite defects, *Plast Reconstr Surg* 85:224, 1990.

44. Tegtmeier RE, Gooding RA: The use of a fascial flap in ear reconstruction, *Plast Reconstr Surg* 60:406, 1977.

45. Smith RA: The free fascial scalp flap, *Plast Reconstr Surg* 66:204, 1980.

46. Cheney ML, Varvares M, Nadol JB: The temperoparietal fascia flap in head and neck reconstruction, *Arch Otolaryngol Head Neck Surg* 19:618, 1993.

47. Marty F, Montandon D, Gumener R, Zbrodowski A:

Subcutaneous tissue in the scalp: anatomical physiological and clinical study, *Ann Plast Surg* 60:406, 1977.

48. Cheney ML, Bhatt S, Googe P, Hibbard D: Angiolymphoid hyperplasia with eosinophilia, *Ann Otol Rhinol Laryngol* 102:303, 1993.

49. Farrior RT, Stambaugh KI: Keloids and hyperplastic scars. In Thomas JR, Holt GR, editors: *Facial scars*, St Louis, 1989, The CV Mosby Co.

50. Buchwald C, Nielsen LH, Rosborg J: Keloids of the external ear, ORL 54:108, 1992.

51. Lo TCM, Secckel BR, Salzman FA, Wright KA: Single-dose electron beam ear radiation in treatment and prevention of keloid and hypertrophic scars, *Radiother Oncol* 19:267, 1990.

EDITORIAL COMMENTS

Shan R. Baker

The auricle is perhaps the most difficult facial structure to restore to a natural appearance in cases where a significant portion of the ear has been lost from trauma or surgical resection. This is because of the complex topography of the external ear; a structure with multiple convolutions and convexities covered with extremely thin, tightly adherent skin. A number of methods for reconstructing defects of the auricle have been discussed, but a few comments should be made in support of healing by second intention. Skin or skin plus cartilaginous defects of the concha cymba and cavum heal very well by second intention without distortion of the auricle. This is because concave surfaces in general heal well by second intention and because the surrounding auricular cartilage giving shape to the helix, and the antihelix resists the forces of scar contracture, thus preventing deformation of the external ear. A note of caution is offered concerning defects that extend near to or involve the lateral aspects of the ear canal. Wounds left to heal by second intention in the area of the auditory meatus are very likely to result in stenosis of the ear canal. Skin defects involving the meatus should be skin-grafted or covered with a skin flap.

As in the area of the concha, defects of skin or skin and cartilage of the fossa triangularis heal very nicely by second intention if the medial auricular skin is still present. No deformation of the auricle occurs because of the relatively strong adjacent cartilage giving form to the posterior and anterior crus of the antihelix. All wounds that are allowed to heal by second intention should remain moist through the use of ointment or an occlusive dressing, which will promote rapid reepithelialization. The presence of perichondrium on exposed cartilage enhances reepithelialization but is not necessary for successful wound healing.

22

RECONSTRUCTION OF THE SCALP

William R. Panje and Lloyd B. Minor

The scalp has many anatomic features that give it unique reconstructive potential. Reconstruction of the scalp is required following resection of benign or malignant lesions, traumatic injuries, or for aesthetic correction of alopecia.[1] These conditions present two different categories of reconstructive challenges. Following excision of a scalp lesion or trauma, immediate decisions must be made concerning the method of repair. Local flaps in combination with free skin grafts will repair most scalp defects. Replacement of existing scar or areas of baldness with hair-bearing skin calls for a completely different reconstructive approach. In the latter category, the surgeon can plan reconstructive procedures with local flaps while preserving all or a portion of the existing scar or bald skin. Serial excision of the area of alopecia advances hair-bearing tissue as a replacement. Tissue expansion techniques can be valuable adjuncts in each of these reconstructive categories.

In cases involving a soft tissue defect of the scalp, the first reconstructive priority is to provide adequate coverage of exposed bone. Other goals include restoring symmetric contour of the head and providing an appropriate distribution of hair-bearing skin. The scalp's unique anatomy affects the surgical techniques employed in reconstruction. The scalp's rich vascular supply protected by a dense fibrous layer allows wound repair under more wound-closure tension than is safely possible with other tissues. Defects measuring up to 3 cm in greatest dimension may be closed primarily. Intermediate-sized defects may be repaired with local flaps, involving transposition, advancement, or rotation and used as single or multiple flaps. Expanded local flaps work well for defects that are larger than 30% of the hair-bearing area. Either skin grafts and/or regional (distant) flaps are best for massive scalp losses.

This chapter presents the senior author's (WRP) approach to various reconstructive problems of the scalp. Anatomic features of the scalp affect the selection of surgical technique and methodology for scalp reconstruction. In particular, the scalp's compartmentalization by the fascia and galea are important deter-minants of successful repair of scalp defects using local flaps.

ANATOMY

The scalp proper extends from the superior nuchal line posteriorly to the supraorbital rims anteriorly. Lateral extension of the scalp is into the temporal fossae and to the level of the zygomatic arches. Functionally and for reconstructive purposes, the scalp region includes the nonhair-bearing forehead and nape of neck areas (Fig. 22-1).[2] Five layers comprise the scalp (Fig. 22-2): skin, subcutaneous connective tissue, galea, subaponeurotic loose areolar tissue, and pericranium. Muscle and fibrous bands tether the skin to the subcutaneous connective tissue and the galea. Local flaps are usually designed to incorporate only the outer three layers of scalp. The pericranium adheres to the outer surface of the calvarium by connective tissue fibers. It has relatively poor osteogenic properties in adults, meaning that bony defects in the skull will not regenerate spontaneously.

The location and composition of the galea determine scalp mobility. The galea consists of a thick membranous tendon (galea aponeurotica) connecting and encasing the occipital and frontalis muscles. These scalp muscles each consist of two bellies joined in the midline by posterior and anterior extensions of the galea, respectively. The occipitalis muscle inserts into the superior nuchal line posteriorly and extends anteriorly into the galea. The frontalis muscle has no bony attachments. It extends from the anterior galea down to the eyebrows, attaching to the corrugator supercilii, procerus, and orbicularis oculi muscles. Clinical realization of the fascial extension is immediately evident in cases of total scalp avulsion. Three independently vascularized layers of temporalis fascia lie below the galea in the temporoparietal region. Areas of the scalp in which no muscle or fascia is present are relatively less distensible (are tight regions) in comparison to

Figure 22-1 Cutaneous limits of the scalp.

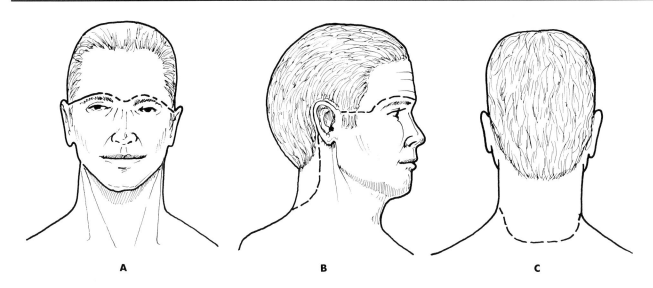

| A | B | C |

Figure 22-2 Scalp anatomy.

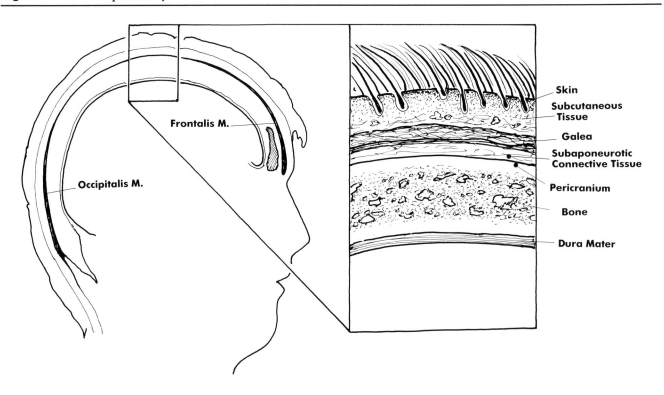

Figure 22-3   Tight and loose regions of the scalp. Tight region has a dense galeal layer, no underlying muscle, and poor distensibility. In the loose region the galea thins into a facial layer overlying muscle and is considerably more distensible. Understanding the concept of tight and loose regions is fundamental to successful reconstruction of the scalp with local flaps.

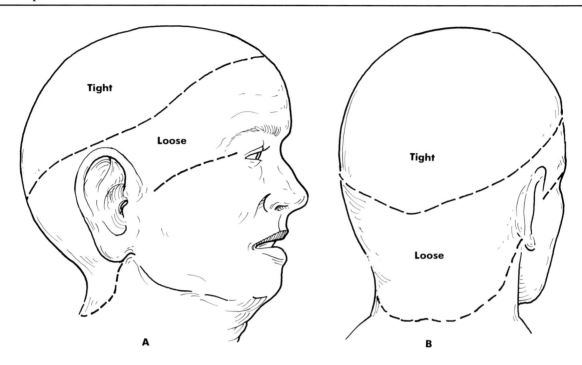

areas where they are a component of the scalp (Fig. 22-3). Utilization of scalp tissue composed in part of muscle (frontalis, occipitalis) or overlying muscle (temporalis) produces a more distensible flap.

Vessels and nerves enter the scalp in a centripetal direction and travel within the subcutaneous connective tissue layer. The abundant arterial supply comes from the internal carotid system anteriorly (supraorbital and supratrochlear arteries) and from the external carotid artery posteriorly (superficial temporal, postauricular, and occipital arteries) (Fig. 22-4). Extensive anastomoses between these vessels exist, such that a single superficial temporal artery is capable of supplying blood to virtually the entire scalp.[3] A relative watershed zone exists near the midline. Long, narrow flaps that cross the midline without an identifiable arterial supply require a delay.

The ophthalmic division of the fifth cranial nerve provides sensation to the anterior half of the scalp. The occipital nerve, a derivative of the second cervical nerve, innervates the posterior half of the scalp. The greater auricular nerve is responsible for sensation in the postauricular area. The auriculotemporal and maxillary nerves supply the area of the temple. Infiltration of an analgesic around the scalp's periphery can produce total scalp analgesia.[4]

The lymphatic system of the scalp is unique in that there are no lymph nodes in the scalp region and therefore no barriers to lymphatic flow. The lymph network is primarily subdermal and subcutaneous in location and interlaces with medium-sized blood vessels. Lymph from the scalp drains toward the parotid gland, the preauricular and postauricular areas, the upper neck, and the occiput.

The scalp's hair covering is an important aesthetic feature. Many patients will undergo any number of painful experiences as well as pay large sums of money to preserve or recover their hair. Functionally, hair acts as a sun shield to prevent skin cancer. Hair also provides a cushioning layer of protection against direct blows and abrasions.

The thickness of the epidermis and dermis of the scalp varies from 3 to 8 mm, making it the thickest skin of the body. This thickness makes the scalp an ideal donor site for split-thickness skin grafts. The subcutaneum is a dense layer of connective tissue and fat that binds the skin to the underlying galea. Just superficial to the galea, the subcutaneum contains adnexal tissues, nerves, lymphatics, and principal arteries and veins for the scalp. Typically a scalp flap includes the epidermis through the galea (7 to 14 mm in thickness).

The subgalea is a space made up of a thin, relatively

Figure 22-4 Vascular anatomy of the scalp.

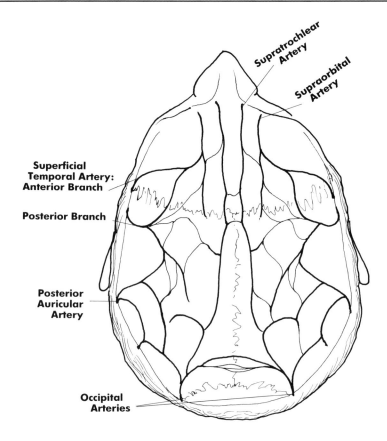

avascular connective tissue between the galea and the pericranium. The avascularity and scarcity of tissue within this anatomic plane provide for most of the slippage of the scalp. The character of the loose areolar tissue within the subgalea provides a cleavage plane for separation of the scalp from the pericranium. The deep dissection plane of most scalp flaps occurs within the subepicranial space.

RECONSTRUCTION

Reconstruction of the scalp, like that of the nose, dates back to the Egyptians in 3000 B.C. The chronology of scalp reconstruction has been described.[5] Wars and the industrial revolution resulted in many different types of scalp wounds. Total avulsion of the scalp, a hideous insult to the human body, frequently caused the patient to die from hemorrhage, chronic infections, and intracranial complications. During a high-speed mechanical avulsion, the scalp usually separates from the calvarium just deep to the galea, leaving periosteum attached to the skull (Fig. 22-5). Interestingly, the American Indian realized the scalp would readily and

Figure 22-5 Immediately following high-speed mechanical scalp avulsion. Note that scalp avulsion follows cutaneous limits of scalp and leaves periosteum intact. Patient has been intubated and placed in a neck brace.

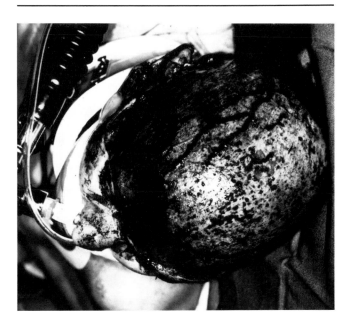

rapidly strip from the skull when the tomahawk or knife had cut through the galea, also leaving periosteum. Skin grafts, especially the split-thickness type, readily survive and grow on periosteum. In the early 1900s a number of reports described attempts to replace the avulsed scalp. Usually, restoration of the scalp as a simple full-thickness graft without restoration of the blood supply would subsequently mummify (Fig. 22-6). Experience in the management of these wounds indicates early closure with split or full-thickness skin grafts rather than replacement with full-thickness scalp.

SKIN GRAFTING (PARTIAL THICKNESS RESTORATION)

Split-thickness skin grafting of deficiencies of hair-bearing scalp regions is inferior to local flap reconstruction. Lack of hair and tissue thickness are the major

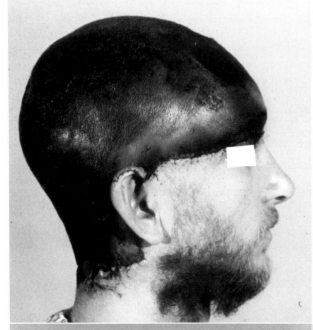

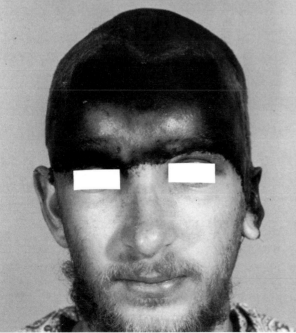

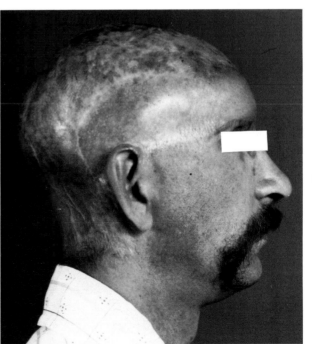

Figure 22-6   *A, B,* **Ten days following scalp avulsion and immediate replantation without microvascular anastomosis. The scalp has darkened and hardened (mummified). Note the typical limits of avulsion, and compare to Figure 22-1.** *C,* **One year following debridement and skin grafting.**

hindrances in using split-thickness skin grafts to reconstruct scalp defects. Hair-bearing scalp with its tissue thickness tends to protect the skull from injury. Traumatic scalp injuries, such as are sustained from clubbing, hitting the windshield in an auto accident, or avulsions, tend to dissipate through some slippage in the subaponeurotic connective tissue layer. Split-thickness skin when grafted onto either the pericranium or calvarial bone becomes fixed to the underlying tissue. The immobility of the graft, as well as lack of hair and thickness, provides little protection from an applied force (e.g., scraping and abrasion). A skin graft when placed on either the calvarium or periosteum can, on occasion, virtually dissolve from something as innocuous as friction produced by a hat band or by lying on a pillow. Thus, restoring the scalp with skin grafts following burns or avulsions often results in subsequent skin problems. Wearing a hat or toupee can often lead to skin graft ulceration. The location of a skin graft becomes of some significance when restoring a scalp deficiency. Skin grafting the parietal, vertex, and forehead areas has the best long-term success. If there is enough remaining scalp hair, especially if located on the occipital or parietal areas, it can hide and protect the skin from friction by being combed over the graft site (Fig. 22-7). Covering the graft with residual hair from the remaining scalp is usually not socially acceptable for forehead defects in males. The forehead, in contrast to the occipital location, is less vulnerable to trauma (e.g., from resting one's head on a pillow). Placing a muscle flap beneath a skin graft avoids ulceration and osteomyelitis.[6] The muscle provides additional thickness and vascularity.

Skin graft restoration of scalp defects does offer some distinct advantages over other reconstructive methods in that the procedure is simple and can be rapidly accomplished with minimal blood loss and with excellent graft healing. Split-thickness skin grafts, in

Figure 22-7   *A,* **Prior excision of melanoma of scalp with split-thickness skin grafting.** *B,* **Covering of graft site with longer hair.**

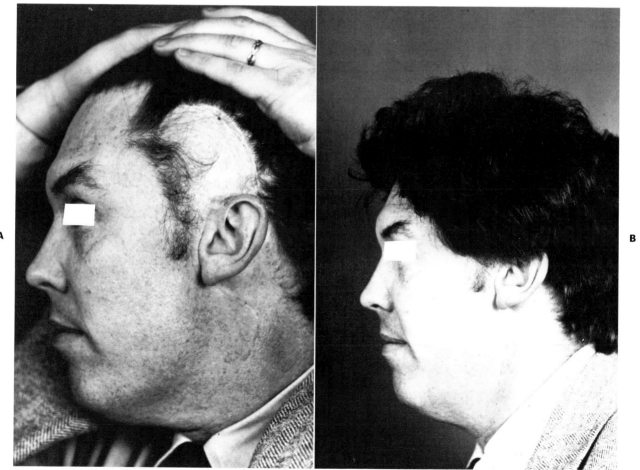

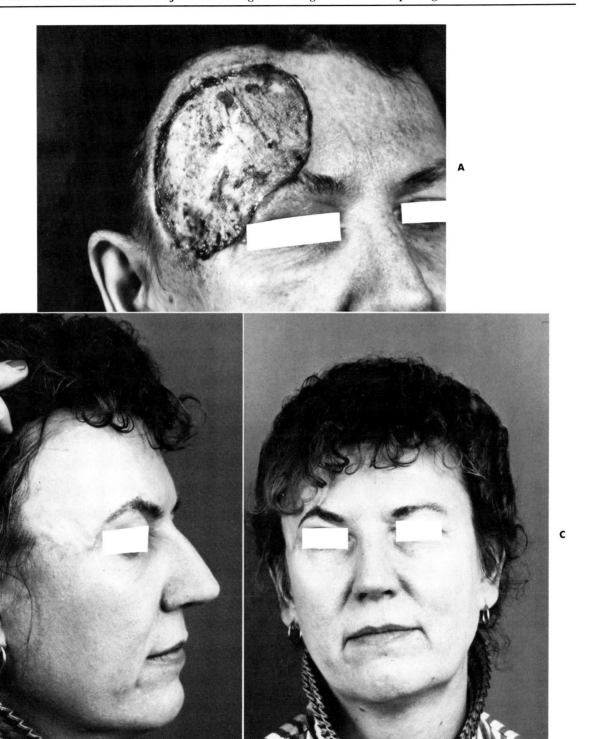

Figure 22-8   *A,* Following excision of epithelial cancer from temporal forehead. *B,* Appearance 8 months after partially meshed split-thickness skin grafting. *C,* Maintenance of eyebrow and combing hair over forehead helps to camouflage graft site. Color and texture are major disadvantages of skin grafts used in repairing forehead defects.

Figure 22-9   Appearance following forehead flap reconstruction of the oral cavity and split-thickness skin grafting of forehead. Note areas of skin graft necrosis and erosion with underlying osteomyelitis of the frontal bone. Unsightly appearance is evident.

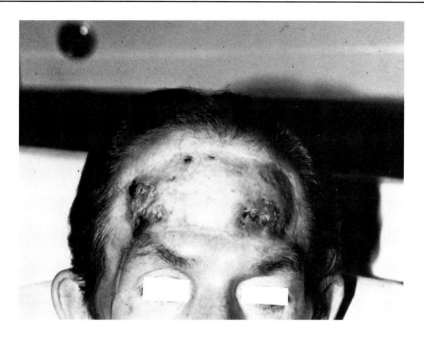

contradistinction to general thought, can survive on in situ calvarium denuded of periosteum. Some surgeons advocate decortication of the outer table of the calvarium to improve recipient site vascularity for subsequent skin grafting. The irregular surface produced from skull bone decortication usually predisposes the skin graft to subsequent injury and ulceration. Skin grafting of the nondecorticated skull bone is more prone to injury and ulceration than when the graft is placed over pericranium or galea.

Skin grafting of scalp defects appears best for covering forehead defects unamenable to primary closure; following skin cancer excisions, especially if aggressive and/or if there is uncertainty of tumor margins; or in medically unstable patients (Fig. 22-8). McGregor, in the 1960s, developed the forehead flap for the immediate reconstruction of oral cavity defects following cancer ablation.[7] Many patients had their forehead defects covered with split-thickness skin grafts. From this experience, it appeared that meshed grafts placed on a well-granulated tissue bed had the best survival rate and subsequent appearance. Skin grafting the whole forehead, from the eyebrows up to the hairline, was more aesthetically pleasing than grafting one side of the forehead. A meshed split-thickness skin graft is also useful to temporarily close a scalp defect in instances where tumor margins are being assessed or in cases where the donor site is covered for a vascular pedicle used to supply an interpolation flap.

Although skin grafting provides for a relatively simple and successful scalp reconstruction, a number of drawbacks exist. Esthetically, hair-bearing tissue is best for scalp replacement. Skin grafts tightly adhere to the calvarium and are subject to the slightest injury (e.g., from wearing a cap) (Fig. 22-9). The thickness of the scalp, the presence of hair, and the subaponeurotic layer of loose connective tissue are all elements that dissipate external forces applied to the head, and these features are not present with the use of skin grafts.

PRIMARY CLOSURE

The scalp, like other body integuments, is subject to developing benign and malignant neoplasms.[8] Optimal management emphasizes surgical ablation, which often results in a full-thickness scalp defect. Reconstructively speaking, the old plastic and reconstructive surgery dictum "for the best function and cosmesis, the surgeon should, if possible, replace tissue losses with like tissues" takes on a special emphasis with reference to the scalp. Thus, the best reconstructive method for full-thickness scalp loss is to utilize adjacent scalp for replacement. This maintains the physiologic and aesthetic integrity of the scalp.

Primary closure of scalp defects of up to 3 cm in greatest dimension is relatively achievable. If the scalp is exceptionally mobile, even larger defects are often amenable to primary closure. The rich vascular supply of the scalp and the presence of the galea make wound closure under tension possible. Larger defects (up to 30% of the surface area of the scalp) are repairable by either skin grafting or, preferably, local flaps. Experience and the ability to work with soft tissue and possibly tissue expansion are imperative when attempting to close defects with local flaps consisting of more than 30% of the hair-bearing scalp.

LOCAL FLAPS

Anatomic Considerations

Local flaps employed in scalp reconstruction involve transposition, advancement, and rotation flaps used individually or in combination. The scalp's unique anatomy imposes special considerations when attempting to use a local scalp flap to reconstruct a scalp defect. Unlike the rest of the body's integument, the scalp is densely hair-bearing, has an intervening layer of connective tissue (galea), and is spherical in shape. Direction of hair growth and potential for baldness can affect early as well as long-term aesthetic results.

The galea severely limits the distensibility of the scalp and produces a stiffness within the tissue. The scalp's thickness also retards tissue distention. These characteristics impede the twisting and stretching of tissue frequently required as part of local flap transfer. Closing a scalp defect without leaving a secondary defect is considerably more difficult than closing a similar defect on other parts of the body, except for the

palms and soles, which are similar to the scalp. To reduce or avoid a secondary defect, local flap tissue is harvested from the periphery or "loose" region of the scalp. Segregating the scalp's tissue into tight and loose regions has been helpful in determining where secondary defects are either more conducive to immediate closure or will readily heal by second intention. The scalp's "tight" region encompasses the vertex of the cranium. The scalp tissues within the tight area are thick and resist turning, twisting, or stretching. The "loose" region of the scalp encircles the cranium and tends to cover muscle (i.e., frontalis, temporalis, or occipitalis). The loose region is a transitional area in which the galea dissipates into a thin layer of fascia. The scalp tissue in the loose region is more malleable, taking on the tissue characteristics of neck and facial integument. Typically the surgeon mobilizes tissue from the loose region of the scalp as well as the adjacent neck, periauricular, and forehead regions when closing larger scalp defects. Utilizing tight scalp tissue only to close either a tight (central or vertex) or loose (peripheral) scalp defect requires extensive undermining of scalp tissue, the liberal use of releasing incisions (e.g., back cuts), incising galea, and often requires leaving a secondary defect.

The scalp's unique geometry is another important consideration in designing local flaps. The scalp, unlike the rest of the body's integument, covers a sphere. The scalp's thickness and tissue makeup causes the scalp to retain the shape of the cranium. Releasing incisions flatten the scalp and increase the relative length of a

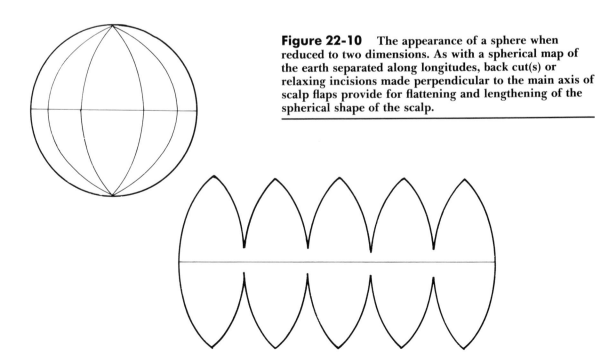

Figure 22-10   **The appearance of a sphere when reduced to two dimensions. As with a spherical map of the earth separated along longitudes, back cut(s) or relaxing incisions made perpendicular to the main axis of scalp flaps provide for flattening and lengthening of the spherical shape of the scalp.**

Figure 22-11 Example of flattening (extending) the scalp. *A*, Scalp widely elevated off of calvarium retains its spherical configuration because of the galea. *B*, Scalp dramatically extended by two relaxing incisions, similar to the techniques demonstrated in Figure 22-10.

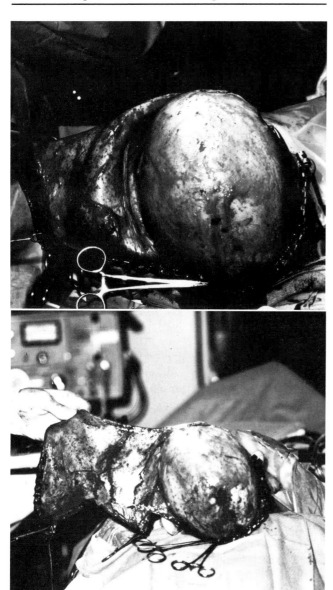

and provides more coverage than the more malleable long, narrow flap.

Transposition Flaps

Transposition flaps have many variations and have found wide applicability in scalp reconstruction. Examples of transposition flaps include the temporoparietal, temporoparietal-occipital (Juri flap), and the parietal temporal postauricular vertical flap (Fig. 22-12). These flaps have all been used with excellent success in reconstructing scalp deficiencies and baldness.[9-18]

Technically, the scalp transposition flap is most successful when the length/width ratio of the flap does not exceed 4:1 (length to base) unless the pedicle has a known vascular supply (e.g., superficial temporal ves-

Figure 22-12 Examples of transposition flaps used in scalp reconstruction.

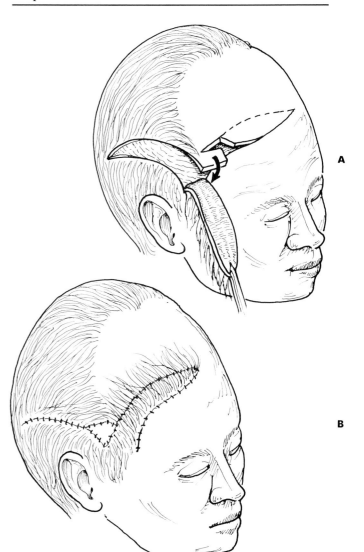

local flap by relaxing the skin of the scalp. Taking an example from map makers, a spherical map of the earth projects onto a flat surface by making a few cuts parallel to the longitudinal meridians starting at either the north and/or south axis of the globe (Fig. 22-10). Similarly, relocating scalp tissue across the dome of the cranium requires one to several relaxing incisions or the use of a long, narrow strip of scalp (Fig. 22-11). The former type of flap is usually more difficult to relocate into a new position but has a greater chance of survival

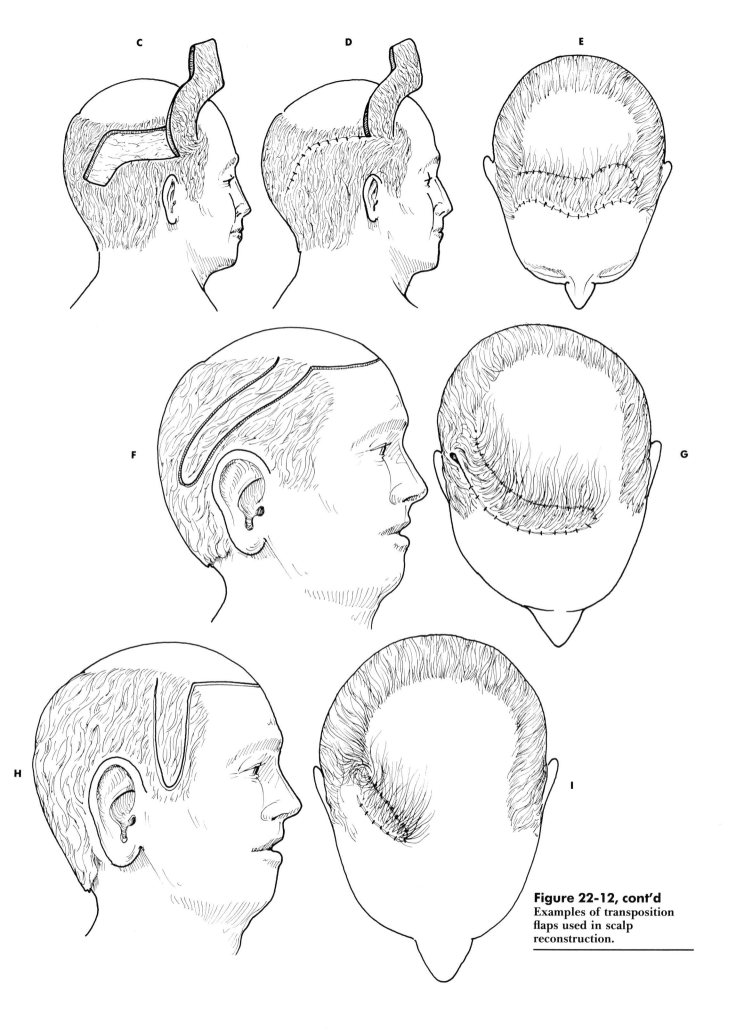

Figure 22-12, cont'd
Examples of transposition flaps used in scalp reconstruction.

Figure 22-13 As transposition flap pivots, the flap changes shape and shortens, wound-closure tension increases, and the standing cutaneous deformity increases. As flap pivots about point A, flap's effective length shortens along circumference B rather than C. Approximate percent of shortening as related to the flap's pivot is in parentheses. (Adapted from Gorney M: Tissue dynamics and surgical geometry. In Kernakian DA, Vistnes LM, editors: *Basic concepts of reconstructive surgery,* Boston, 1977, Little, Brown.)

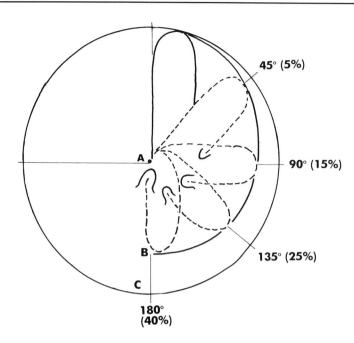

sels) or there has been adequate surgical delay. A transposition flap is a pivotal flap and involves some degree of torsion or twist at the base.

The greater the arc of pivot, the greater the standing cutaneous deformity that develops at the flap's base, and the less the effective length of the flap (arc of utilization).[19] Increasing the flap's pivot will change the flap's shape, shorten the effective length of the flap, increase the wound-closure tension, and deform the flap's base by development of a standing cutaneous deformity (Fig. 22-13). To reduce these restricting factors, the flap's arc of pivot should not exceed 90 degrees. Increasing the arc beyond 90 degrees will invariably produce flap and donor site management difficulties because it will usually require a secondary surgical procedure (Figs. 22-14–22-17). For scalp reconstruction, transposition flaps should be designed so that the base is within the loose scalp area, preferably over a known arterial and venous vascular supply. The area of desired coverage and donor site origin dictate the flap's proportions.

ADVANCEMENT FLAPS

An advancement flap is tissue partially dissected from its underlying attachments but maintaining its blood supply and a cutaneous base that is literally stretched along a single axis. There is no pivot or twisting of the flap. Closure of a simple fusiform defect after undermining and then approximation of the wound edges constitutes two opposing advancement flaps. Advancement flaps play a limited role in scalp reconstruction, although scalp reductions and donor site closure of transposition flaps rely on this method of wound repair.[20-23] Unlike the rest of the body's integument, the scalp, except for the forehead, does not exhibit relaxed skin tension lines. However, the scalp has its own characteristic lines of tension inherent in its galea. The galea produces lines of tension in a multidirectional fashion throughout the scalp. Unlike body integument defects, which become much wider when oriented perpendicular to relaxed skin tension lines than when oriented parallel to them, scalp defects

Figure 22-14   A short temporoparietal scalp flap has an excellent blood supply regardless of whether the pedicle includes the superficial temporal artery or not. Usual dimensions of this flap are 2 to 3.5 cm in width with a length no longer than 10 to 17.5 cm. *A,* Typical temporoparietal transposition scalp flap to correct male pattern baldness, *B,* Preoperative planning before second temporoparietal transposition scalp flap. Patient is shown with proposed placement of second scalp flap. Note importance of joining scalp flaps in the midline and maintaining a frontal and temporal hairline consistent with the patient's other maturing features. *C, D,* Postoperative appearance following the use of bilateral temporoparietal scalp flaps.

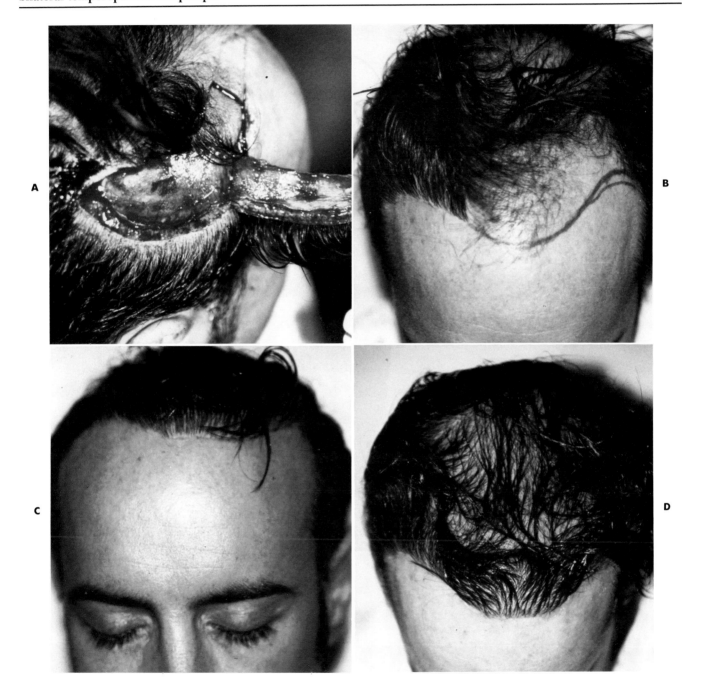

Figure 22-15   *A*, Young male with receding frontal and temporal hairline as well as hair thinning. *B*, Temporoparietal transposition flaps immediately improve hairline. Curly permanent helps to thicken hair and partially camouflage receding hairline.

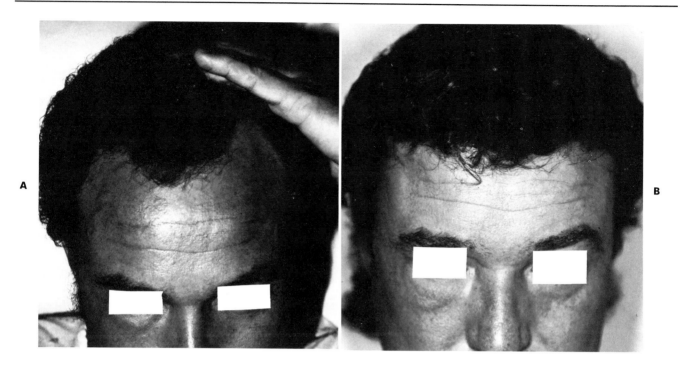

when located within the galea area will have limited retraction. What retraction does occur distributes equally about the circumference of the wound, regardless of wound geometry or orientation. The failure of scalp wounds to retract and conversely their inability to easily contract is why wound healing by second intention in galea-located scalp is slow without grafting (Fig. 22-18). Attempted primary closure by advancement of tissue when wounds exceed 4 cm in greatest dimension, especially in the tight zone, produces extreme wound-closure tension with potential development of infection and widened scars (Fig. 22-19). In contrast, larger defects of the scalp in the loose region are frequently amenable to repair by use of advancement flaps. However, wide undermining and significant wound-closure tension are usually necessary (Fig. 22-20).

The galea resists tissue distention or stretching and protects the scalp from ischemia while allowing for greater wound-closure tension. This is in contrast to wound closures over the rest of the body's integument, which are much easier to stretch but more likely to succumb to ischemia with less wound-closure tension. To produce a greater degree of scalp stretching, some surgeons advocate making parallel incisions through the galea perpendicular to the direction of desired

lengthening (Fig. 22-21).[24,25] This maneuver can increase scalp flap expansion by 5% to 15%. Incising the galea can jeopardize scalp/flap blood supply and increase the incidence of hematoma formation.

ROTATION FLAPS

The rotation flap is one of the most useful and successful methods of scalp or cranium reconstruction.[26-29] The scalp's unique anatomic characteristics (thickness, galea, spherical configuration, hair-bearing, centripetal blood supply) require the surgeon to adhere to the following key points when designing and dissecting rotation flaps. The length of the arcing incision should be no less than four times the greatest dimension of the defect measured along the arcing incision (Fig. 22-22). The scalp's inelasticity, especially within the tight region, will prevent adequate tissue movement and result in a secondary defect unless the arcing incision is either long enough or extends into the loose scalp zone. As the flap rotates through its radius, a line of tension develops diagonally from the leading tip of the flap to the base (see Fig. 22-22). The larger the flap, the more diffuse the distribution

Text continued on p. 500.

Figure 22-16 *A,* Norwood-Hamilton class VI baldness. *B,* Temporoparietal-occipital (Juri) transposition scalp flap is delayed by incising along the length of the flap, creating a bipedicle flap. *C,* Appearance 3 months after transfer of the flap to the anterior hairline. *D,* Head tilted with hair combed forward reveals drawbacks evident when attempting to overcome class VI male pattern baldness with a single long transposition scalp flap: (1) uneven hair distribution, (2) need for long hair to camouflage bald areas, and (3) unnatural hairline.

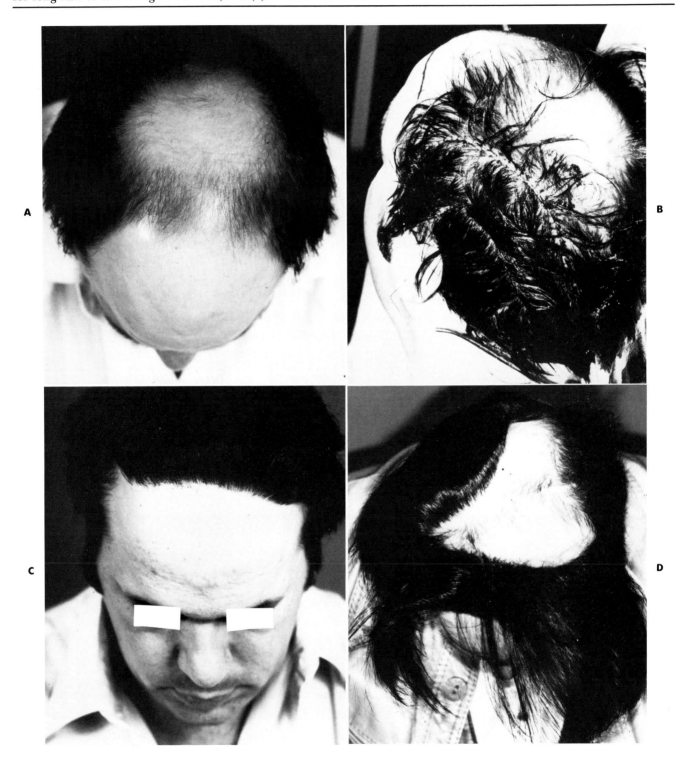

Figure 22-17   *A, B, C,* Illustrations showing use of a long temporoparieto-parietal interpolation scalp flap to reconstruct the total upper lip. A Doppler is utilized in developing such a long flap (34 cm) to ensure a discernible arterial supply. The flap is 4 cm wide, crosses the midvertex into the opposite parietal scalp, and is transferred without surgical delay. The undersurface of the distal flap (lip) is skin grafted. *D,* This patient underwent upper lip reconstruction using a temporoparieto-parietal interpolation flap. The flap is being "trained" by intermittently clamping a distal part of the flap proximal to the part of scalp flap that will remain as the upper lip. The proximal part of the scalp flap is returned to its donor site. *E,* Postoperative appearance. The nose was reconstructed with an extended trapezius musculocutaneous flap.

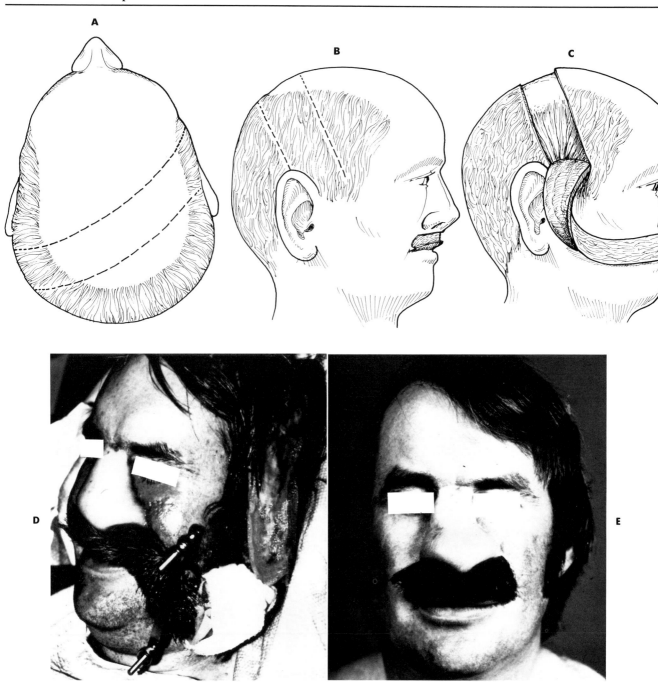

Figure 22-18   *A*, Circumferential full-thickness scalp defect following tumor excision. *B*, Defect located in "tight" region of scalp was allowed to granulate for 6 weeks. Little wound contraction or epithelialization has occurred. *C*, Secondary defect located over "loose" region of scalp. *D*, Excellent wound contraction and epithelialization has occurred within 3 months so that no further reconstruction is needed.

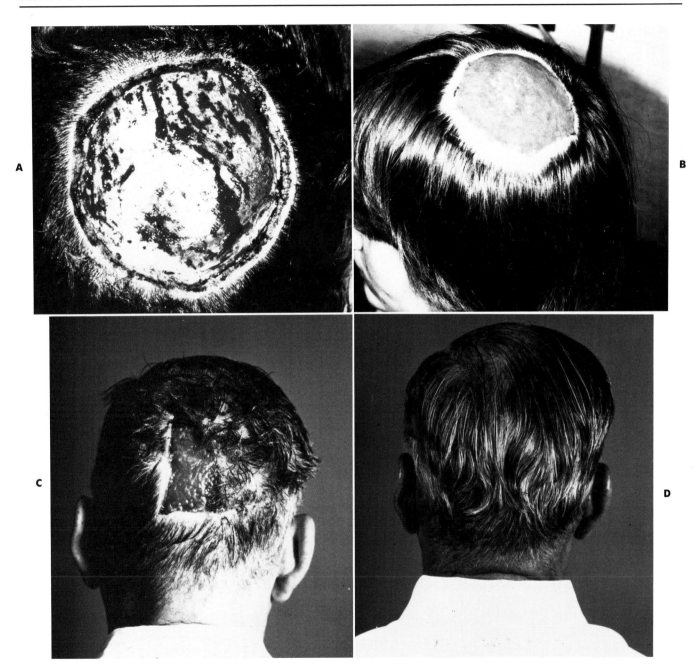

Figure 22-19 *A, B,* Advancement flap closure of circular defect at the junction between "tight" and "loose" scalp. Closure is difficult when advancement flaps are in tight area only. The cephalic part of the defect is the most difficult to repair. *C, D,* Same defect using one advancement flap placed in "loose" scalp. Wide inferior undermining of the base of the flap (*dotted line*) allows for a more successful closure of the defect.

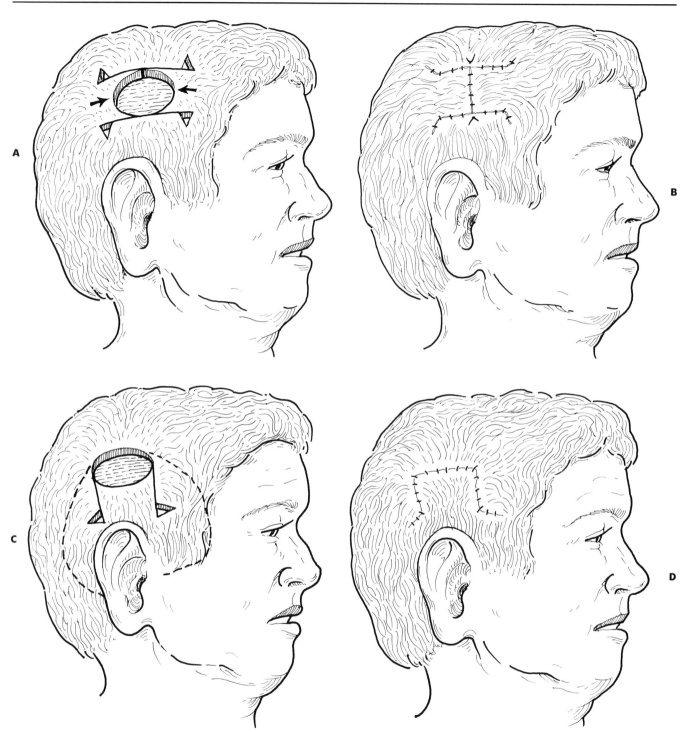

Figure 22-20   *A*, Large (14 × 7 cm) posterior scalp compound congenital nevus. *B*, Nevus completely removed at later age. *C*, Wound repaired with large advancement flap. Most of advancement is derived from the skin of the neck. *D, E,* One year following reconstruction.

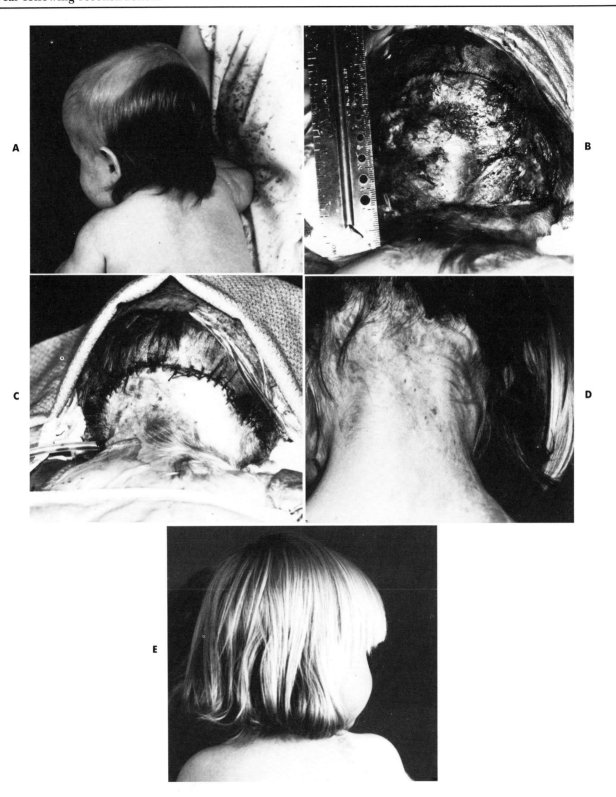

Figure 22-21   Multiple parallel incisions of the galea allow for greater flap expansion. These incisions can run parallel and/or perpendicular to the flap's blood supply. One must use caution in performing this technique since the flap's blood supply can be jeopardized.

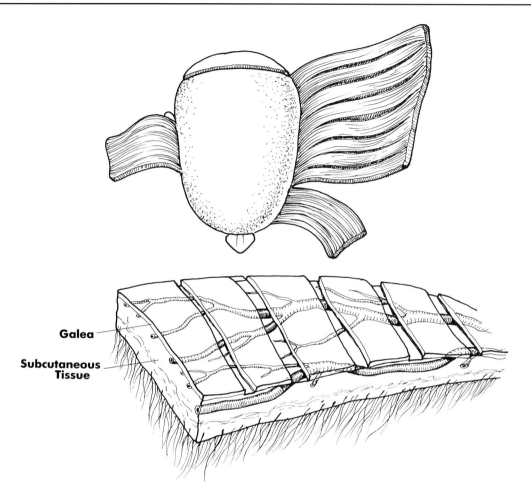

Galea

Subcutaneous
Tissue

of the wound-closure tension. If the arcing incision crosses the vertex of the cranium, greater wound-closure tension will occur than when closing a scalp defect of similar size located more peripherally. Rotation of the flap will shorten its useful length. This is more pronounced when using scalp tissue, especially from the tight region. Because of the scalp's inelasticity, back-cuts or relaxing incisions are necessary to allow for maximum stretching of tissue (see Fig. 22-22**C**). Likewise, persistent secondary defects are more common along the arcing incision than at the back-cut, especially when the latter incision is in the loose region (Fig. 22-23). In some cases multiple back-cuts made perpendicular to the arcing incision allow for flap lengthening and conformation of the

scalp to the skull. In this situation, back-cuts of the arcing incision frequently leave a secondary defect. *Standing cutaneous deformity* is the term applied to the bunching of tissue that occurs at the proximal (toward the closure) base of the flap. Usually, the larger the radius of the arc of rotation, the greater the standing cutaneous deformity. Attempting to reduce or flatten the deformity at the time of flap transfer is usually a hazardous undertaking because such a maneuver will reduce the blood supply to the base of the flap, especially after a back-cut. The standing cutaneous deformity tends to flatten over a 4- to 6-week interval. Usually after 6 weeks, any remaining deformity is removed because recipient site vascularity is sufficient to maintain flap viability.

Figure 22-22   Rotation scalp flaps. The length of the perimeter (arc) of the flap should be at least four times the width of the defect. The arcing incision should extend into the loose region of the scalp. Sometimes one or two back-cuts are helpful in reducing wound-closure tension. The secondary defect can be skin grafted or left to heal by second intention, as seen in Figure 22-18C.

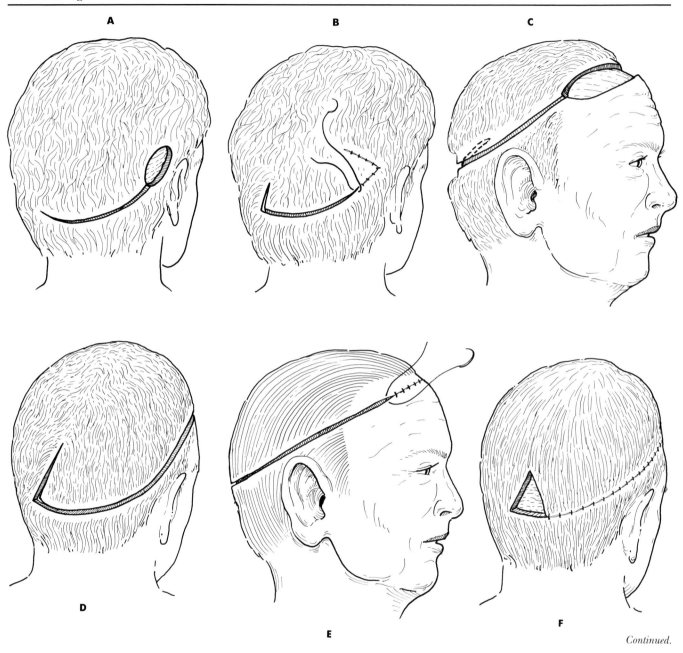

A

B

C

D

E

F

Continued.

Figure 22-22, cont'd   Rotation scalp flaps.

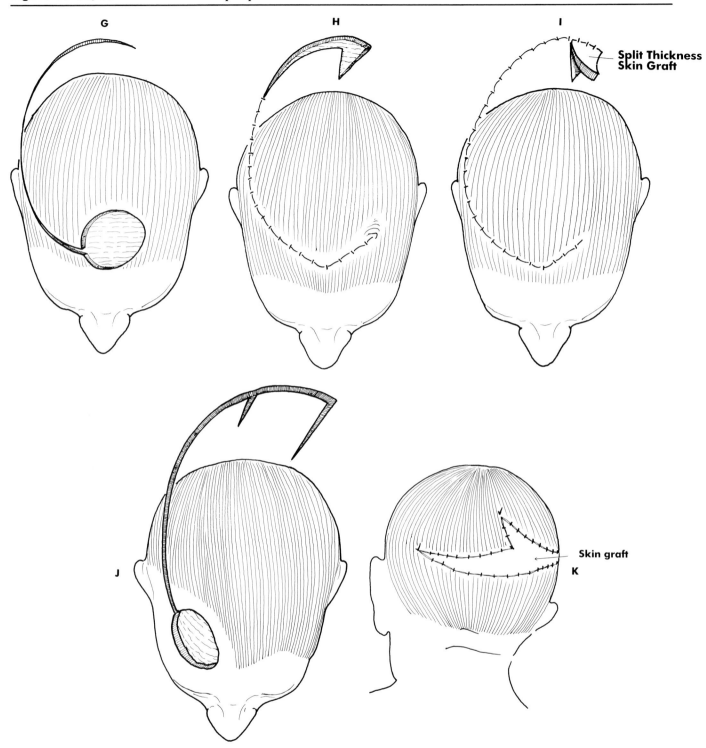

Figure 22-23   *A,* Single rotation flap designed to repair a large (120 cm²) scalp and cranial defect. *B, C,* Note that a split-thickness scalp graft (removed from anterior frontal scalp) is needed along the arcing incision. *D,* Even though a back-cut is made, it is closed primarily. Extensive undermining into the loose scalp region is necessary. *E, F,* Appearance 1 year following scalp reconstruction.

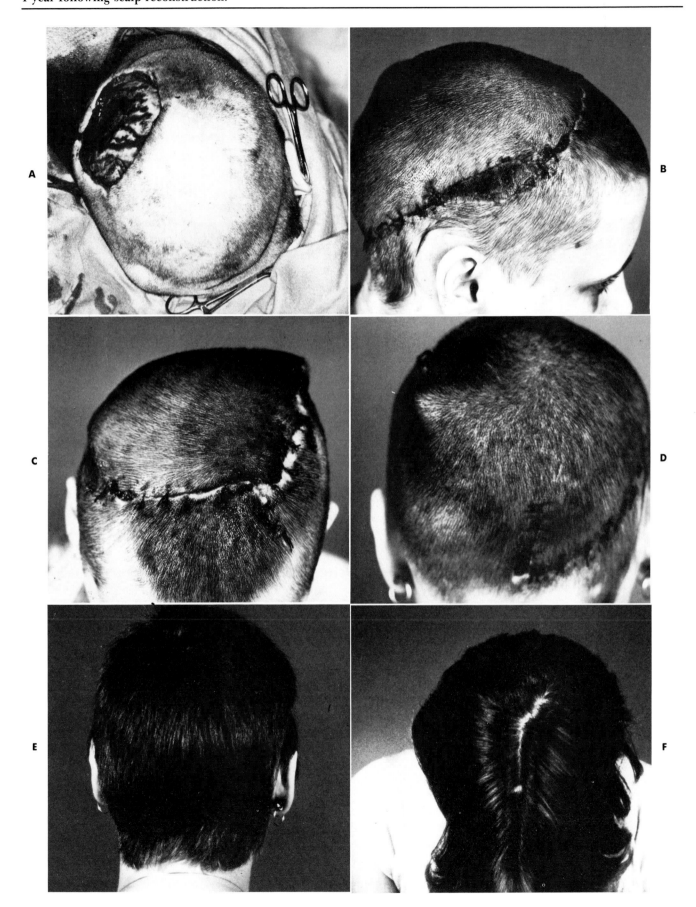

ISLAND FLAPS

Due to the dense network of collateral vascularity throughout the scalp, relatively narrow (3 cm) flaps with lengths of 12 to 15 cm that cross through the scalp's vertex can be transferred in one stage if a recognizable arterial and venous supply is within the pedicle. Rather long *island* or *peninsular scalp flaps* (pedicle less than 1 cm in width) are possible if the main vessels (i.e., superficial temporal artery or occipital artery) are contained within the long axis of the flap. To maximize flap viability, the base or pedicle is usually within the loose scalp region and over a known vascular supply. Use of a Doppler intraoperatively is helpful in assuring adequate flap pedicle vascularity. When using an island flap, special precautions are necessary to avoid pedicle strangulation as well as flap bleeding. The advantage of the narrow peninsular or island scalp flap is its extreme arc of utilization without producing a standing cutaneous deformity or an unnecessarily large secondary defect.

Z-PLASTY AND RHOMBOID FLAPS

Z-plasty and rhomboid flaps are essentially modified transposition flaps. Their use in scalp reconstruction is limited. The scalp's thickness and inelasticity and the shape of the cranium are deterrents to expected results achieved in other areas of the body. Since the z-plasty must decrease in one dimension (width) to increase in another (length), the greater the tissue elasticity, the more ideal the result. The scalp, with the palms and soles, has the least tissue elasticity of the human integument.

MANAGEMENT OF SECONDARY DEFECTS

The use of local scalp flaps for repair of scalp defects can often produce secondary defects as large as the primary defect. The importance of preoperative planning cannot be overemphasized. The patient needs to be aware of the potential for bald spots on other parts of the scalp, altered direction of hair growth, and the potential for subsequent scar widening. Most of these problems are correctable, but the patient must wait at least several months to a year to allow complete wound maturation.

The most dreaded complication of scalp reconstruction is flap necrosis.[30] Unnecessary wound-closure tension applied to the distal end of a scalp flap in an attempt to repair a defect can cause flap necrosis. It is better to be prudent, use less wound-closure tension, leave a residual primary or secondary defect, and

return in 3 or 4 months to complete the reconstruction. Proper patient education before the first operation leads to a more satisfied patient. Patients should understand that a second and sometimes a third operation may be necessary.

In reconstructing most scalp defects, design the flap to close the primary defect, with subsequent consideration given to managing the secondary defect. Transfer the flap with as little wound-closure tension as possible. In designing the scalp flap, create the secondary defect if possible within the loose zone. Wounds in the loose zone tend to close more easily because of diminution of the galea's density, reduction in the integument's thickness, and ability to undermine widely into the neck, mastoid, periauricular, and facial areas (Fig. 22-24). In addition, the nonhair-bearing skin located along the scalp's periphery is considerably more elastic than scalp tissue. An added advantage of placing the secondary defect within the loose zone is the ability to better camouflage with hair any skin grafts used to repair the defect.

Reconstruction of acute scalp deficiencies (i.e., trauma, burn, tumor ablation) with a local flap will often leave a secondary defect that needs repair. Attempting to develop secondary flaps to close the secondary defect usually produces more scarring and a persistent scalp defect. This is because the majority of the total scalp distensibility is utilized for repair of the primary defect, and there is little or no remaining tissue distensibility to assist in repair of the secondary defect. Thus, skin grafting is preferable for most secondary defects. The use of a split-thickness (0.012 in) meshed skin (one to one) graft secured by a tie-over bolster of sponge or a gauze dressing provides for excellent coverage. Previously placed skin grafts and redundant bald scalp can be useful for covering secondary defects without resorting to harvesting skin from another part of the body. Bald scalp must be thinned to the dermis before using as a free graft. Widened scars and skin grafts in secondary defects not amenable to reexcision, and primary closure can be camouflaged by punch grafting. The reduced blood supply of scarred tissue requires 2-mm or smaller punch scalp grafts in the areas of scar alopecia.

MULTIPLE LOCAL FLAPS

The location of the defect on the scalp is of great importance in determining the preferred method of reconstruction. A larger defect on the edge of the hair-bearing scalp is much more difficult to repair with similar tissue than a defect of the same size surrounded by hair-bearing skin. Bardach has concluded that a defect of hair-bearing skin of the scalp can be recon-

Figure 22-24   Closure of temporoparieto-occipital scalp flap donor site. Extensive undermining into the "loose" area *(dotted line)* is necessary to allow for primary closure.

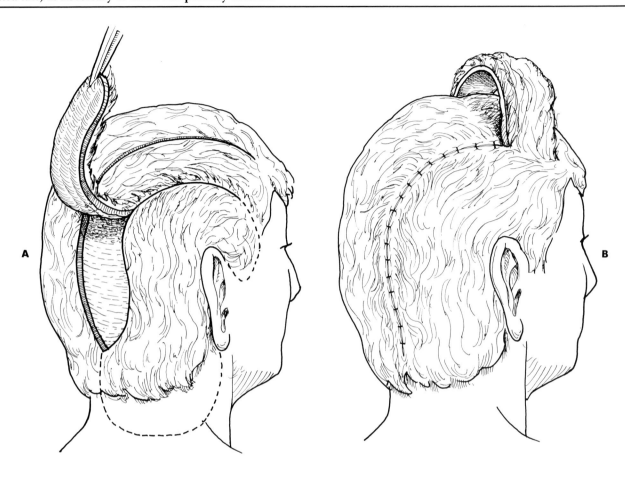

structed with a single rotation advancement flap if the surface area of the defect constitutes no more than 10% of the entire hair-bearing area. Although defects encompassing 10% to 15% of the surface area of the hair-bearing scalp are repairable with a single local flap for a centrally located defect, multiple local flaps and several separate procedures are necessary to reconstruct a defect of similar size located more peripherally. Defects larger than 30% of the hair-bearing area always require the use of multiple local flaps and, in some cases, tissue expansion.

Orticochea has reconstructed large scalp defects by utilizing multiple scalp flaps based on known vascular territories. Enhanced tissue distensibility of the flaps is achieved by making multiple longitudinal galea incisions parallel to the vascular axis of the flaps (Figs. 22-25, 22-26). The flaps are all based peripherally on a known vascular supply.[31,32] Extensive scalp flap elevation with wide undermining and preservation of principal blood vessels is necessary for a successful clo-sure.[33] Blood loss can easily exceed 1500 cc. Circulatory monitoring and possible blood replacement may be necessary. Several subsequent reports support the reliability of this method, at least in experienced hands. The surgeon must be cautious in incising the galea since the principal blood supply to the scalp tissues lies immediately above the galea. Liberal use of bipolar coagulation of bleeding points along the edges of the scalp flap and galea incisions is helpful in reducing blood loss. Incising the galea and applying tension allow for greater flap distensibility; however, stretching a scalp flap without the protection of an intact galea may narrow and limit flap circulation.

TISSUE EXPANSION

Tissue expansion techniques offer an alternative in scalp replacement. Neumann first used tissue expansion in 1957 to reconstruct an ear.[34] The concept

Figure 22-25   Three-flap technique of Orticochea for repair of forehead defect. This technique requires wide undermining, liberal use of galea-relaxing incisions, and considerable experience. I have found the use of rotation flaps and the introduction of tissue expanders more reliable in closing larger scalp defects (20% to 40% of the scalp's surface area). (Modified from Orticochea M: New three-flap scalp reconstruction technique, Br J Plast Surg 24:184, 1971; with permission.)

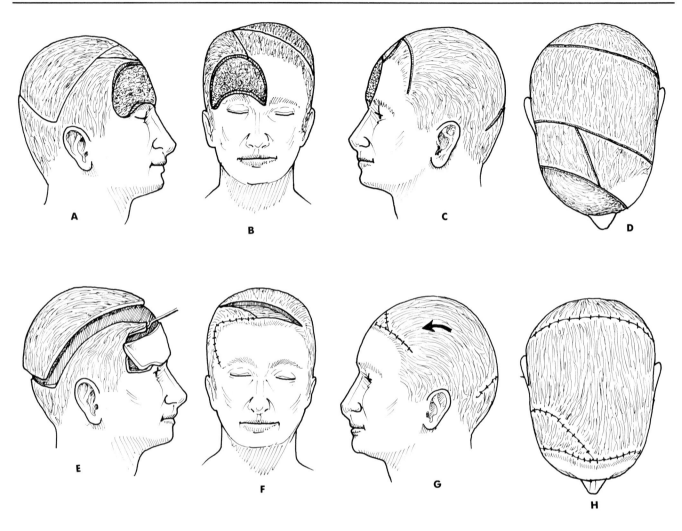

remained dormant for two decades but has since been employed for reconstruction of large skin defects in virtually all regions of the body.[35] The advantages of tissue expansion are particularly evident in scalp reconstruction.[36] Reconstruction of scalp ideally involves replacing hair-bearing skin with similar tissue. Expansion of adjacent hair-bearing skin provides such replacement tissue. The tissue expander is placed in a pocket created in the subgaleal plane, superficial to pericranium. After expansion, reconstruction can occur using simple advancement of expanded tissue or the development of other types of local flaps. Tissue expansion does require a staged operative approach, with implantation of the expansion device at least 6 to

8 weeks before the planned reconstruction (Fig. 22-27). Full-thickness erosion of the skull is possible, although it appears to be unusual. Expanders are particularly helpful in reconstruction of defects following resection of scalp carcinomas, in the treatment of alopecia, and in the closure of large defects resulting from the excision of giant congenital segmental nevi of the scalp in children (Fig. 22-28). Our experience with expanders in the head and neck has emphasized the importance of surgical technique and wound care to avoid complications. For example, I have encountered situations in which placement of the tissue expander transgressed cancer-bearing tissue. This is a very bad practice because of possible cancer dissemination.

Figure 22-26   Three-flap technique of Orticochea for repair of large posterior scalp defect.

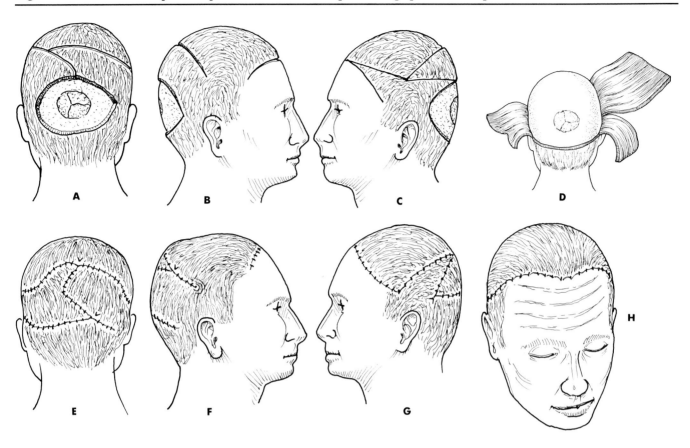

Figure 22-27   Tissue expansion has been successfully utilized in the correction of male pattern baldness and reconstruction of larger scalp defects. *A,* Appearance of scalp 4 weeks after insertion of two tissue expanders and progressive saline insufflation. *B and C,* Illustration of the technique of scalp reduction to correct male pattern baldness following tissue expansion.

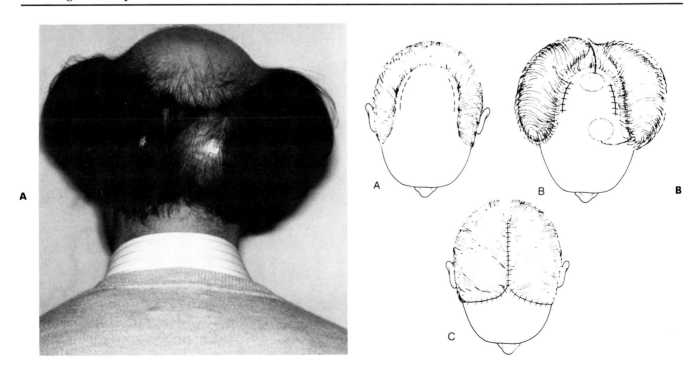

Figure 22-28 Use of tissue expansion and rotation flaps allowed for near total scalp reconstruction of this prior scalp burn. *A,* Preoperative appearance of scalp. *B,* Widened scar area was further reduced 3 months later. *C, D,* One year postoperative.

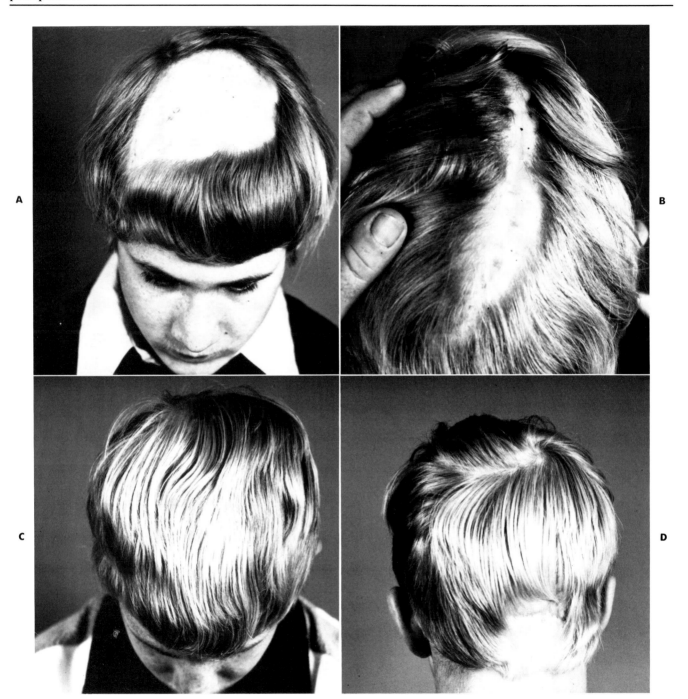

COMBINED CRANIAL DEFECTS

Defects of the cranial vault and overlying scalp frequently require multidisciplinary intervention by the neurosurgeon and the head and neck surgeon (Figs. 22-29, 22-30). Reconstruction of the dura protects the brain from dessication and contamination, minimizing intracranial complications and infection. The sequential repair of dura, skull, and scalp is the ideal management tactic. Each layer is composed of different tissue, which may be replaced with like tissue or a substitute material.

The dura is replaceable with a variety of different types of grafts (e.g., lyophilized dura, fascia lata, temporalis fascia, preserved dura). The brain can even be covered directly with a skin graft or a vascularized flap without replacement of the dura. Full-thickness vascularized tissue is preferable since there are inherent pulsations of the brain that can retard skin graft survival as well as produce brain herniation. In many cases of skull osteomyelitis and cerebrospinal fluid leaks, I have elected to avoid calvarial replacement or dural replacement and used a vascularized flap (i.e., local, regional, or distant) to reconstruct the composite cranial defect. Subsequent reconstruction of the calvarium requires separation of a portion of the flap away from the brain, leaving a deep layer (galea) in continuity with the brain and adjacent dura. A bone graft, methacrylate, or other hard substance is then inserted into the bony defect and covered by the superficial layer (supragaleal) of the flap.

Figure 22-29   Bitemporal bipedicle flap. A local bipedicle flap that in some cases may represent a transposition or an advancement flap has been useful for reconstruction of either the forehead, nose, or the chin. The flap's vascular supply is derived from the superficial temporal vessels. The flap is usually rectangular in shape and extends over the vertex of the calvarium with remaining attachments over the temporal area. To increase the flap's arc of utilization, the vertex part of the flap is extended posteriorly over the occiput. The bipedicle nature of the flap makes for an extremely hardy and successful flap.

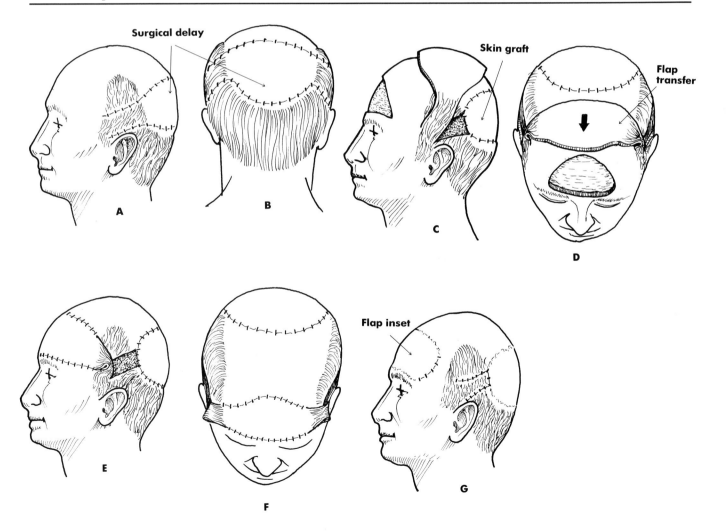

Figure 22-30 Repair of frontal cranial and scalp defect. *A*, Preoperative appearance of bald scalp vertex. *B*, Intraoperative appearance of frontal cranial defect. The dura has been repaired with lyophilized dura. *C*, Appearance 6 months postoperative. *D*, Temporal flaps are returned to the original donor site. The vertex is skin grafted. The frontal cranial defect healed uneventfully. This patient suffered from basal cell nevus syndrome and had multiple prior excisions and grafting.

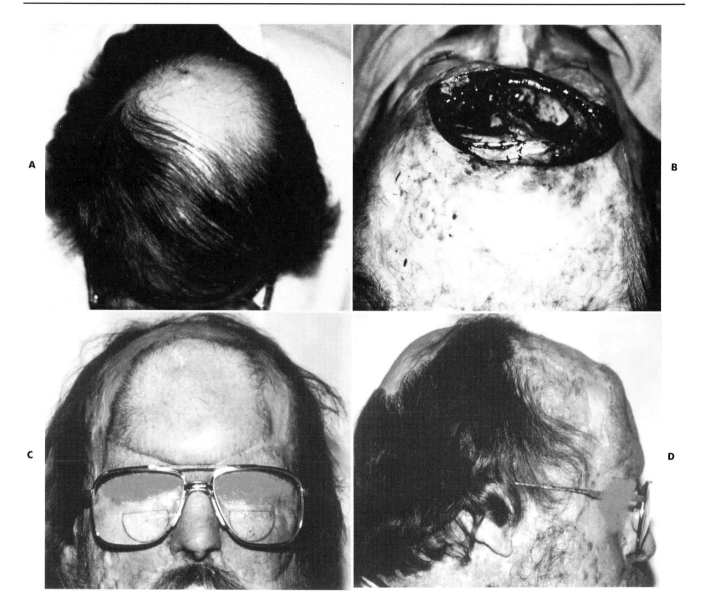

REFERENCES

1. Longacre JJ, Converse JM: Deformities of the forehead, scalp and calvarium. In Converse IM, editor: *Reconstructive plastic surgery,* vol 2, Philadelphia, 1977, WB Saunders.

2. Orticochea M: Flaps of the cutaneous covering of the skull. In Grabb WC, Myers MB, editors: *Skin flaps,* Boston, 1975, Little, Brown.

3. Alpert BS, Buncke JH, Mathes SJ: Surgical treatment of the totally avulsed scalp, *Clin Plast Surg* 9:145, 1982.

4. Panje WR: Nerve block anesthesia of the head and neck. In Epstein E, Epstein E, Jr, editor: *Skin surgery,* Philadelphia, 1987, WB Saunders.

5. Vallis CP: Symposium-scalp defects and injuries including hair transplantation, *Clin Plast Surg* 9:2, 1982.

6. Shagets FW, Panje WR, Shore JW: Use of temporalis flaps in complicated defects of the head and face, *Arch Otolaryngol* 112:60, 1986.

7. McGregor IA: The temporal flap in intraoral cancer: its use in repairing the postexcisional defect, *Br J Plast Surg* 16:318, 1963.

8. Minor LB, Panje WR: Malignant neoplasms of the scalp—etiology, resection and reconstruction, *Otolaryngol Clin North Am* 26:279, 1993.

9. Bouhanna P: The post-auricular vertical hair-bearing transposition flap, *J Dermatol Surg Oncol* 10:551, 1984.

10. Chajchir A, Benzaquen I, Arellano A: A new scalp flap for baldness, *Aesthetic Plast Surg* 15:271, 1991.

11. Dardour J-C: Treatment of male pattern baldness with a one-stage flap, *Aesthetic Plast Surg* 9:109, 1985.

12. Dardour J-C, Pugash E, Aziza R: The one-stage preauricular flap for male pattern baldness: long-term result and risk factors, *Plast Reconstr Surg* 81:907, 1988.

13. Elliott RA Jr: Lateral scalp flaps for instant results in male pattern baldness, *Plast Reconstr Surg* 60:699, 1977.

14. Fleming RW, Mayer TG: Short vs. long flaps in the treatment of male pattern baldness, *Arch Otolaryngol* 107:403, 1981.

15. Juri J: Use of parieto-occipital flaps in the surgical treatment of baldness, *Plast Reconstr Surg* 55:456, 1975.

16. Juri J, Juri C: Use of pedicle flaps in the surgical treatment of alopecia. In Unger WP, Nordstrom RE, editors: *Hair transplantation,* ed 2, New York, 1988, Marcell Dekker.

17. Mayer TG, Fleming RW: Short flaps: the use and abuse in the treatment of male pattern baldness, *Ann Plast Surg* 8:296, 1982.

18. Nataf J: Surgical treatment for frontal baldness: the long temporal vertical flap, *Plast Reconstr Surg* 74:628, 1984.

19. Gorney M: Tissue dynamics and surgical geometry. In Kernakan DA, Vistnes LM, editors: *Biological aspects of reconstructive surgery,* Boston, 1977, Little, Brown.

20. Alt TH: Scalp reduction as an adjunct to hair transplantation: review of relevant literature and presentation of an improved technique, *J Dermatol Surg Oncol* 6:1011, 1980.

21. Alt TH: History of scalp reductions and paramedial method. In Norwood OT, editor: *Hair transplant surgery,* ed 2, Springfield, Ill, 1984, Charles C. Thomas.

22. Bell ML: Role of scalp reduction in the treatment of male pattern baldness, *Plast Reconstr Surg* 69:272, 1982.

23. Unger MG, Unger WP: Management of alopecia of the scalp by a combination of excisions and transplantations, *J Dermatol Surg Oncol* 4:670, 1978.

24. Arnold PG, Randarathnman CS: Multiple-flap scalp reconstruction orticochea revisited, *Plast Reconstr Surg* 69:605, 1981.

25. Sasaki GH: Scalp repair by tissue expansion. In Brent B, editor: *The artistry of reconstructive surgery,* St Louis, 1987, The CV Mosby Co.

26. Heimburger RA: Single-stage rotation of arterialized scalp flaps for male pattern baldness, *Plast Reconstr Surg* 60:789, 1977.

27. Juri J, Juri C, Arufe H: Use of rotation scalp flaps for the treatment of occipital baldness, *Plast Reconstr Surg* 61:23, 1978.

28. Panje WR: Physiological aspects of wound healing. In Scott-Brown's *Otolaryngology,* ed 5, vol 1, London, 1987, Butterworths.

29. Rageer B, Ahuja MS: Geometric considerations in the design of rotation flaps in the scalp and forehead region, *Plast Reconstr Surg* 81:900, 1988.

30. Unger MG: Postoperative necrosis following bilateral lateral scalp reduction, *J Dermatol Surg Oncol* 14:541, 1988.

31. Orticochea M: Four-flap scalp reconstruction technique, *Br J Plast Surg* 20:159, 1967.

32. Orticochea M: New three-flap scalp reconstruction technique, *Br J Plast Surg* 24:184, 1971.

33. Jurkiewicz MJ: Scalp reconstruction with multiple flaps In Brent B, editor: *The artistry of reconstructive surgery,* St Louis, 1987, The CV Mosby Co.

34. Neumann CG: The expansion of an area of skin by progressive distention of a subcutaneous balloon, *Plast Reconstr Surg* 19:124, 1957.

35. Radovan C: Tissue expansion in soft tissue reconstruction, *Plast Reconstr Surg* 74:482, 1984.

36. Manders EK, Au VK, Wong RKM: Scalp expansion for male pattern baldness, *Clin Plast Surg* 14:469, 1987.

EDITORIAL COMMENTS

Shan R. Baker

Dr. Panje has described a number of different types of local flaps used for repair of scalp defects. In my opinion, the preferred method of reconstructing the majority of small to intermediate-sized defects (defined as those that can be repaired with the remaining scalp tissue utilizing local flap techniques) is the utilization of two or more rotation flaps. Rotation flaps are pivotal flaps, with curvilinear configurations. As such, they are ideally suited for use in repairing scalp defects because they depend for tissue movement primarily on a pivotal rotation rather than advancement. Because of the inelasticity of scalp tissue, advancement flaps are poorly suited to scalp surgery. The curvilinear configuration of rotation flaps conforms very well to the spherically shaped contour of the scalp. Normally, it is difficult to design curvilinear incisions that continue to parallel relaxed skin tension lines, but this is not an issue in the scalp, where such lines are not present.

In general, multiple rotation flaps are preferred to the use of a single flap for scalp reconstruction. Each flap is designed to pivot on an independent pivotal point. When using two rotation flaps, the flaps may be designed to pivot in opposite directions, as in an O to T configuration wound repair, or in the same direction, as in an O to Z repair (Fig. 22-31).[1] Using more than one rotation flap is advantageous because it recruits tissue for reconstruction from different locations on the scalp. Within limits, the greater the number of flaps used, the more diffuse is the tissue recruitment. Likewise, the burden of repair of the secondary defect is shared by the number of flaps utilized. I find two or three rotation flaps to work best for reconstructing most scalp defects. When utilizing three flaps, each flap is responsible for repairing one third of the surface area of the defect. Wound closure is accomplished by pivoting all three flaps in the same direction. Repair of the defect has the appearance of a pinwheel, and wound closure configuration resembles the closing of a camera lens (Fig. 22-32).[1]

Figure 22-31 Circular scalp and upper forehead skin defect 11 cm in diameter. Two rotation flaps were used to repair the defect *(dotted lines)* in an O to Z wound closure. The lateral flap recruited skin from the preauricular area. *B,* Six months postoperative.

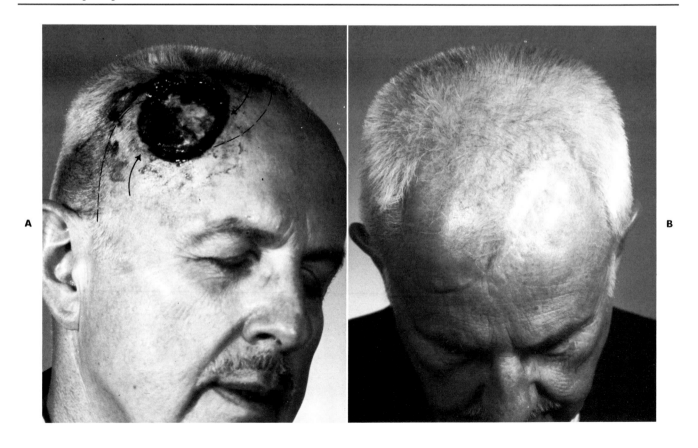

Figure 22-32   *A,* Circular defect 9 cm in diameter. Three rotation flaps are designed to repair defect. *B,* All three flaps pivot in the same direction to close defect. *C,* Two months postoperative.
(From Baker SR: Local cutaneous flaps, *Otolaryngol Clin North Am* 27:139-159, 1994.

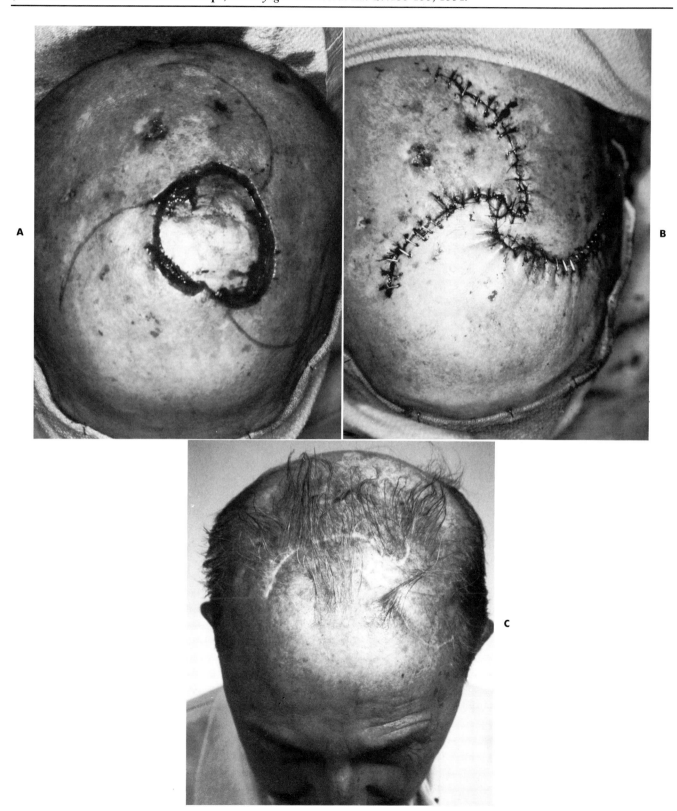

Tissue expansion is now the most appropriate method of scalp reconstruction in most instances where there is inadequate adjacent hair-bearing tissue to allow either primary closure or repair with local flaps. The obvious advantage of tissue expansion is that it provides the surgeon with ample hair-bearing scalp for covering large defects, providing excellent aesthetic results. Although compressed, the pattern of hair growth and the structure of the hair follicle during scalp expansion remain unchanged. Temporary telogen effluvium may occur from scalp expansion, but this is uncommon. Unfortunately, expansion does not stimulate growth of new hair, and thus, as expansion progresses, the hair follicles are separated further from each other. Depending on the preexpansion density, reduction in hair density is not usually noticeable until density has decreased more than 50%. Thus, given normal hair density, the scalp can be expanded to two or three times its original surface area before a change is evident. This advantage allows reconstruction of sizeable scalp defects using tissue expansion without a noticeable difference in the appearance of the scalp. The major disadvantage of scalp expansion is that the reconstruction requires two operations, the first to place the expander, and the second to perform the reconstruction. Other significant disadvantages are the prolonged interval required for expansion and the temporary deformity of the head that occurs toward the end of the expansive process.

Reference

1. Baker SR: Local cutaneous flaps, *Otolaryngol Clin North Am* 27:139, 1994.

EDITORIAL COMMENTS

Neil A. Swanson

The scalp can be one of the more frustrating areas to reconstruct. It would seem simple, but the galea aponeurotic severely limits tissue movement, making closure of small defects more difficult than expected. As a result, large arcs must be made with sliding flaps when closing defects on the scalp. Often galeotomies and/or relaxing incisions prove very useful. As Drs. Panje and Minor very aptly discuss, this makes an understanding of the concept of secondary defect and its placement critical when performing flap surgery on the scalp. The secondary defect can be handled in several ways, including closure, granulation, and skin grafting. I agree that, in general, skin grafting on the scalp as a sole means of reconstruction can be fraught with difficulty. However, it may be necessary to skin graft a secondary defect, realizing that alopecia will result. Once the flap has healed and the scalp loosened, the grafted and secondary defect can be excised.

In reference to the "Juri flap," the only real transposition flap utilized on the scalp, the authors did a very nice discussion of the concepts of movement about a pivotal point, with the effective shortening of the flap as well as the creation of the cutaneous standing deformity.

They also give a nice discussion of the use of multiple flaps to close scalp defects.

Section III

Adjunctive Surgery

23

CONTROLLED TISSUE EXPANSION IN FACIAL RECONSTRUCTION

Louis C. Argenta

INTRODUCTION

Over the past 20 years reconstructive surgery of the head and neck has advanced to the point that patients expect not only functional reconstruction but also maximal esthetic benefits. Among the many procedures, including myocutaneous flaps and microsurgical flaps, that have evolved, tissue expansion offers unique potential for functional and esthetic reconstruction of the facial area. An understanding of the basic technology and techniques of tissue expansion in the head and neck is now mandatory for any surgeon who wishes to excel in the reconstruction of this area.

There is no other part of the human body where there is a wider variety of skin color, texture, and hair-bearing qualities confined in a small area than the head and neck. Because the head and neck are always visible, the proper distribution of these specialized tissues is mandatory to achieve an optimal reconstruction. The use of tissue expansion to increase available tissue for use as a source for local flaps in the head and neck has distinctive advantages over the use of esthetically incompatible distant tissues.

Esthetically the head and neck can be divided into six zones in which local tissues have specific qualities (Fig. 23-1). The use of tissue expansion in these areas helps provide adequate skin for the development of advancement or rotation flaps, which in turn enables reconstruction with a maximal esthetic result.[1] Although massive defects of the head and neck may require the use of distant flaps, almost all defects can be reconstructed by tissue expansion, particularly in cases of congenital and traumatic deformities.

TOPOGRAPHIC ZONES OF THE HEAD AND NECK

Scalp (Zone 1)

The presence of a specific density and quality of hair in the human scalp makes the area distinctly different from any other skin on the human body. The use of hair-bearing tissue from other locations on the body for the purpose of scalp reconstruction usually results in esthetically unacceptable results. Tissue expansion has revolutionized reconstruction of the scalp.[2-5] Defects up to one half of the surface area of the scalp can be reconstructed by expansion of the remaining scalp, resulting in a relatively normal distribution of hair and with minimal donor site morbidity. Furthermore, reconstruction usually can be accomplished in a shorter time and with fewer operations than when scalp expansion is not employed. Scalp expansion is an adjunctive procedure that allows the development of larger and more reliable flaps, which can then be manipulated by usual plastic surgery procedures. New hair follicles are not created in the process of expansion, nor are they usually destroyed; therefore, remaining follicles can be distributed in a uniform pattern to cover areas of alopecia.

Reconstruction of the scalp must address two priorities: first, restoration or maintenance of a normal-appearing anterior hairline and second, even redistribution of remaining hair to minimize alopecia. Careful planning is necessary to achieve optimal results of reconstruction of large or irregular defects. The larger the defect, the more it becomes necessary to expand as much of the remaining normal hair-bearing scalp as possible to achieve a final homogeneous distribution of follicles (Fig. 23-2).

Figure 23-1   Zones of face are outlined as in diagram. By use of techniques described in chapter, defects of any size in various zones can be reconstructed with maximal esthetic results.

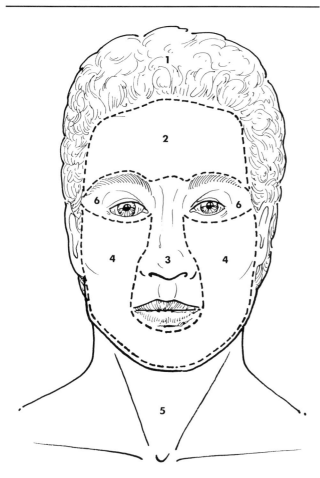

Figure 23-2   *A,* A 4.5 × 3 cm defect of frontal temporal scalp, which has been covered by split-thickness skin graft. Two 400-ml volume expanders are placed, one on either side of defect, and expanded over period of 8 weeks. *B,* At second procedure, expanders are removed and scalp extensively mobilized. Note that area of alopecia is not excised until it has been determined that there is adequate coverage available to allow removal of graft. *C,* Tension-free primary scalp repair is achieved.

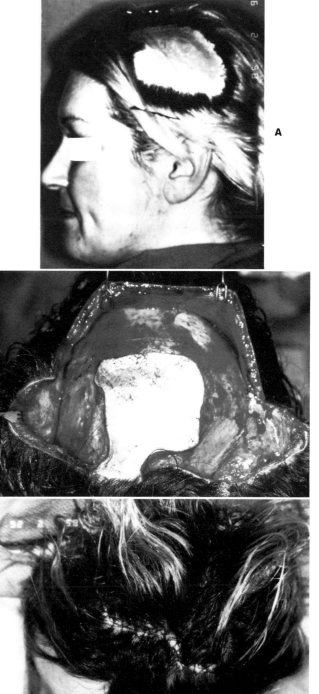

The vitality of hair depends on an adequate blood supply. Knowledge of the normal vascular anatomy of the scalp is necessary to ensure that the major vessels that supply the scalp are incorporated into the base of the flap which is to be expanded. Proper preoperative planning will minimize the risk of necrosis, scar widening, and loss of hair follicles. Careful planning becomes even more important when the surgeon is confronted with complex defects that require multiple irregular or thin flaps.

Restoration of a normal-appearing frontal and temporal hairline is a requirement in many cases of scalp reconstruction. Multiple serial scalp expansions can be performed, if properly planned and sequenced. When the anterior hairline needs to be adjusted or reconstructed, the usual plan is to expand normal hair-bearing scalp on the posterior skull and advance it anteriorly (Fig. 23-3). In cases in which the donor surface area is limited, such as in children, serial sequential expansions and advancements of the scalp

Figure 23-3   *A*, Extensive burns with loss of right anterior and temporal side of scalp sustained in 4-year-old child. *B* and *C*, Single 800-ml volume tissue expander is placed under all of remaining posterior scalp and expanded over period of 10 weeks. *D*, Normal anterior hairline is reconstructed with single advancement scalp flap from posterior to anterior direction. *E*, Appearance 3 months postoperatively. Patient declined reconstruction of temporal area.

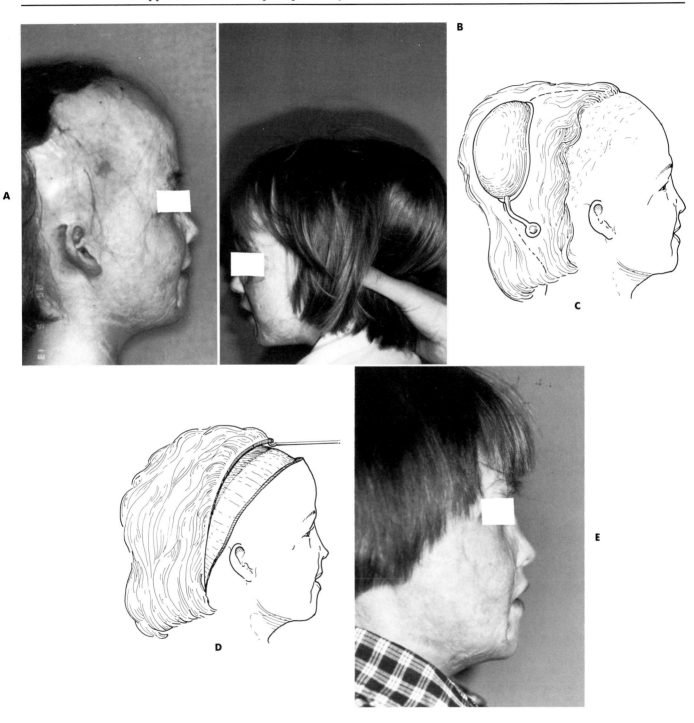

can be used to achieve a more normal-appearing hairline. When the temporal hairline needs to be reconstructed in addition to the frontal hairline, it is accomplished as a secondary procedure. The scalp that was advanced forward to restore the frontal hairline is reexpanded and a portion mobilized inferiorly to reconstruct the temple area.

Posterior occipital scalp defects are best managed by movement of temporal hair-bearing tissue posteriorly (Fig. 23-4).[6] Defects of the vertex can be reconstructed by expansion of scalp temporally or occipitally, then movement of tissue in a cephalad direction. Temporal defects are the most difficult to reconstruct and are best achieved by movement of expanded scalp from the vertex inferiorly and anteriorly into the temporal area.

It must be emphasized that meticulous planning in reconstruction of the scalp is important so that the primary reconstructive surgical procedure will not compromise the ability to perform subsequent procedures. This is particularly important in reconstructive surgery of the scalp because of the limited amount of hair-bearing skin available and the common need to reexpand the scalp. Overaggressive scalp expansion or mobilization can be disastrous and can result in loss of hair follicles. A conservative approach, even if it involves multiple expansion procedures, minimizes the risk to the patient and maximizes potential benefit. In children the scalp can be serially expanded two or three times before it becomes excessively attenuated. The adult scalp is more robust and can be expanded and mobilized three to four times without significant compromise. It is best to allow a period of 6 to 12 months for the scalp to normalize before reexpansion is attempted.

The choice of expanders depends on the size and contour of the defect. While a multitude of specialized expanders has been marketed, I prefer round or rectangular expanders without reenforced backing. As much of the normal hair-bearing scalp as is available is expanded, particularly in cases of large scalp defects. This will achieve maximum redistribution of hair follicles and allow the greatest number of potential reconstructive alternatives. Multiple smaller expanders are almost always preferable to a single large expander because they allow a more even scalp expansion and thus distribution of hair follicles (Fig. 23-5); in addition, expansion is achieved in a shorter interval and with less physical distortion of the patient's appearance. In fact, the use of multiple expanders can frequently enable reconstruction without obvious deformity to the patient, thus minimizing the amount of time lost from school and work.

Expanders are usually placed through incisions made at the margin of what will be the advancing edge of the scalp flap. Although some authors have advocated distant radial incisions, these usually make dissection more tedious and have the propensity to compromise later procedures. Dissection is carried out bluntly or sharply beneath the galea for a distance sufficient so that the expander can be placed in the evolved pocket, allowing the margin of the expander to be positioned at least 1 or 2 cm from the suture line. There is some benefit to scoring the galea at the time that expanders are inserted beneath the scalp. It has been my experience that scoring appears to hasten expansion and reduce the pain of the expansion process. However, excessive scoring can lead to subsequent extrusion of the expander or damage to the overlying hair follicles.[7]

Insertion of expanders is usually carried out with the use of general anesthesia, particularly in children, although it may be performed in cooperative adults under local anesthesia. Expanders with distant inflation reservoirs are usually used because incorporated reservoirs may be difficult to locate under the scalp and are frequently painful. Reservoirs can either be left externally or, as I prefer, placed at a distant site under normal scalp or adjacent tissue. Placement of inflation reservoirs under skin grafts in areas that have been previously irradiated and in other compromised areas is not recommended. It is my experience, when expansion is performed to excise a nevus, that reservoirs can be placed directly under the nevus because sensation in the area of the nevus is usually less than that of the adjoining skin.

Although children younger than 6 months of age may successfully undergo scalp expansion in critical situations, there are very few indications to expand the scalp in a child under 1 year of age. Usually some deformation of the skull occurs when infant scalp is expanded, resulting in the development of bony ridges at the margin of the expander. These ridges subside once the expander has been removed. I am unaware of any permanent skull deformities created by scalp expansion, even in the neonate.

The initial expansion of the scalp is tedious and causes discomfort to the patient, requiring frequent injections of small volumes of saline to overcome these impediments. Inflations are usually conducted at weekly intervals, with the expander inflated until the patient complains of discomfort. This discomfort is usually transitory and can be alleviated with mild analgesics for 24 hours after expansion.

The degree of expansion necessary is dependent on the number of expanders used and the size of the defect to be reconstructed. Although many formulas exist to determine the necessary extent of expansion to reconstruct a specific-sized scalp deformity, I have found few of them helpful. I prefer to measure the surface area over the expander to determine whether

Figure 23-4   *A,* Patient with giant cerebriform nevus of posterior scalp, measuring 13 cm in diameter. Two 400-ml volume rectangular expanders were placed in temporal area and expanded over 8 weeks *(arrows). B,* **Drawing showing location of expanders.** *C* and *D,* **Posterior view showing defect after excision of lesion. Scalp expansion enabled primary closure without wound-closure tension. Note location of laterally positioned expanders.** *E,* **Three years after surgery normal hair pattern is present.** (*E* from Argenta LC: Controlled tissue expansion in reconstructive surgery, *Br J Plast Surg* 37:520, 1984.)

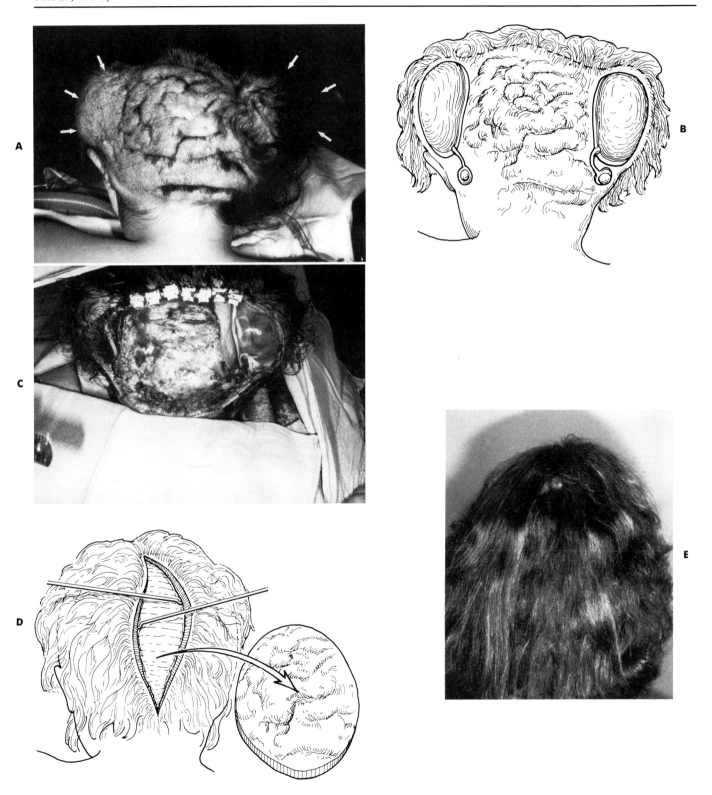

Figure 23-5   Use of multiple smaller tissue expanders is usually preferable to single large expander for reconstruction of scalp defects.

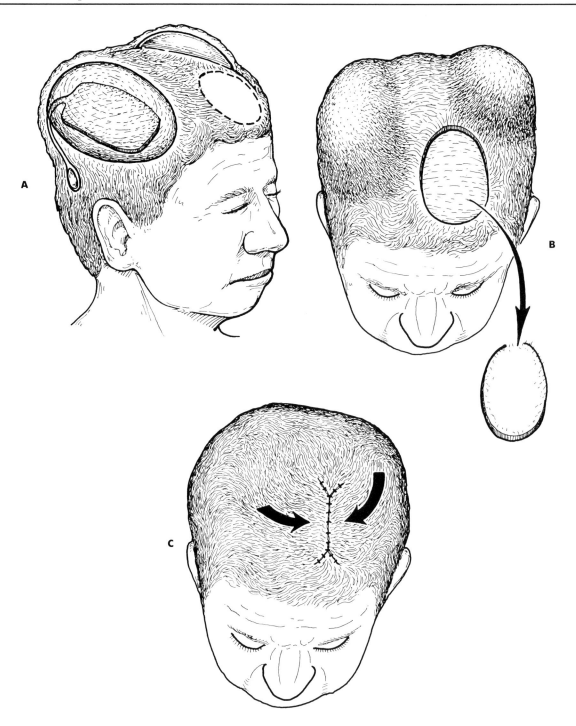

sufficient scalp is available to allow advancement over the area of alopecia or anticipated scalp defect. It is frustrating to have an inadequate amount of tissue available to cover all of the defect at the time of reconstruction. It is, however, a wiser surgeon who is willing to reexpand the scalp and perform an addi-tional surgical stage than one who attempts an overly aggressive procedure that may be catastrophic for the patient.

If exposure of the expander occurs late in the course of expansion, it is usually safe to continue slowly expanding to completion. If too great an exposure occurs early in the course of expansion or if there are any compromising factors, such as excess pain or infection, the expander is best removed.

A second procedure is necessary to remove the expander, usually through the same incision through which it was placed. Mobilization of the expanded scalp and as much of the adjacent scalp as is necessary to adequately reconstruct the defect is achieved by blunt and sharp dissection. It may occasionally be necessary to score the galea or the capsule surrounding the expander to achieve maximum tissue mobility. The capsule should not be removed because this is a bloody procedure and may compromise the viability of hair follicles.

Once maximum tissue mobilization has been achieved, the scalp flaps, usually in the form of advancement or rotation flaps, are secured in place using staples or towel clips. These devices allow the surgeon to evaluate multiple alternative methods to repair the defect with expanded scalp before being committed to a final solution. It is critical to create or maintain the normal position of the hairline and eyebrow in all cases of scalp reconstruction. Occasionally small amounts of excess tissue can be discarded. However, unless standing cutaneous deformities are particularly large, they are ignored, as they usually subside in time. Hemostasis should be achieved with limited use of electrocautery. Extensive electrocoagulation may result in alopecia or even necrosis of portions of the scalp flaps. The flaps are sutured in place using permanent 3-0 monofilament sutures. The sutures are left in place for 2 to 3 weeks. In infants, in whom suture removal may be difficult, I have found the use of 3-0 Maxon sutures, which last approximately 3 to 5 weeks, to be quite beneficial.

Forehead (Zone 2)

Anatomically and physiologically the forehead is a portion of the scalp. Aside from being hairless, the forehead has color and texture qualities almost identical to that of the scalp. The skin is thick and oily. There is great variation in the size and configuration of the forehead, and many defects of this area can be repaired with a variety of forehead and scalp flaps. In cases in which less than 20% of the surface area of the forehead requires reconstruction, particularly superiorly, the scalp can usually be advanced downward toward the brow without creation of a perceptible deformity. Defects in the central and lower parts of the forehead are more difficult to reconstruct.

Three important considerations should be addressed in the reconstruction of all forehead defects. First, the eyebrows must be positioned or maintained in a symmetrical position. Second, the junction of the forehead and scalp should be as symmetrical as possible. Third, the innervation of the frontalis muscle should be preserved to avoid later brow ptosis and cosmetic deformity.

If greater than 50% of normal forehead skin remains, this can be expanded usually with multiple expanders to achieve primary closure of a forehead defect (Fig. 23-6). When avulsions or extensive trauma have occurred to the forehead skin, several months should be allowed to pass before expansion so that tissue can be normalized. Skin grafts are used in the interim.

As much of the remaining forehead as possible should be expanded in the reconstruction of large forehead defects. Frequently the expander is placed under portions of the adjacent scalp or face (zone 4) as well so that maximum skin mobilization can be achieved without the development of excessive standing cutaneous deformities (Fig. 23-7). Expanders are placed beneath the frontalis muscle either through an incision at the margin of the defect or through a small incision in the scalp behind the hairline. Placement of expanders superficial to the frontalis muscle is technically much more difficult and results in greater blood loss. Complications, particularly extrusion of the expander, are also much higher than when expanders are placed beneath the frontalis muscle. A subgaleal plane is developed down to the level of the supraorbital rims, preserving the supraorbital vessels and nerves. Laterally, the dissection is carried into hair-bearing scalp.

The amount of deformity caused by progressive expansion of the forehead is minimized by placement of appropriate sized expanders on either side of a defect whenever possible. This also reduces the time required to achieve adequate skin expansion to enable reconstruction. Rectangular expanders with or without reenforcement backing are used. Most expansion of the forehead can be accomplished in approximately 6 to 8 weeks, although the process is frequently uncomfortable. The oral administration of analgesics for 12 to 48 hours after each expansion is frequently necessary. Discomfort can be minimized to a limited degree by scoring of the frontalis muscle in a vertical direction at the time that the expander is implanted.

On completion of sufficient forehead expansion, the expanders are removed, and the remaining forehead skin is advanced or rotated to cover the defect. It is important to preserve the anterior branch of the temporal artery when forehead flaps are based laterally and the supraorbital vessels when flaps are based at the orbital margin. Preservation of these vessels during reconstruction of forehead defects after skin expansion is particularly important when the defect is the result of

Figure 23-6 *A,* Patient who underwent resection of arteriovenous malformation down to pericranium. Defect measured 9 cm long and 8 cm wide. Catheter is inserted through lateral skin. Defect is covered with skin graft. *B,* Eight months later two 400-ml volume tissue expanders are placed under remaining forehead skin on each side of skin graft. *C,* Bilateral advancement flaps based on anterior branch of temporal artery were advanced medially to eliminate skin graft. Appearance 8 months postoperatively, after slight degree of brow asymmetry was corrected with secondary surgery.

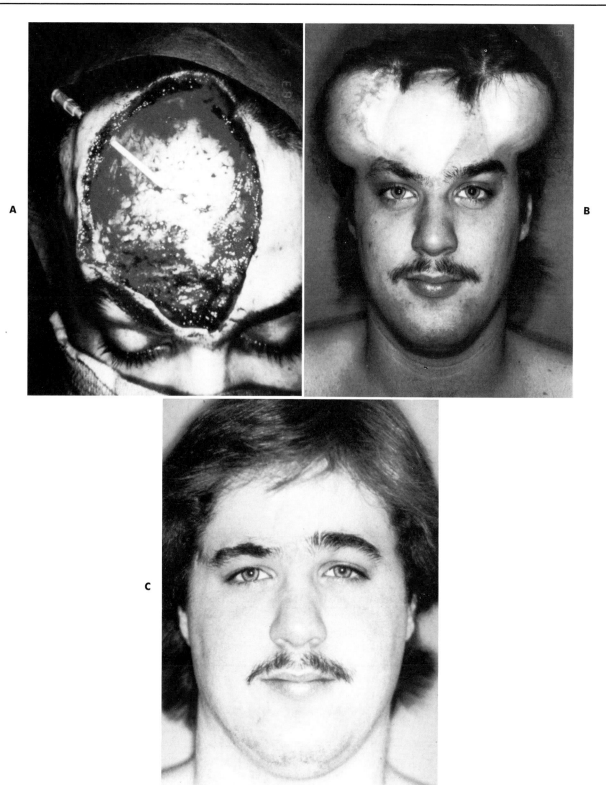

Figure 23-7   *A,* Giant hairy nevus measuring 7 × 6 cm above and lateral to left orbit of child. Two expanders were placed, one in preauricular area for purpose of expansion of facial skin, which could be advanced superiorly, and other expander in frontal area to allow mobilization of forehead skin laterally. *B,* Appearance 6 months after total excision of nevus and primary closure. Brow is elevated after surgery, but frontal branch of facial nerve functions normally. Brow is allowed to remain in this position for approximately 6 months before revision (if necessary) is undertaken.

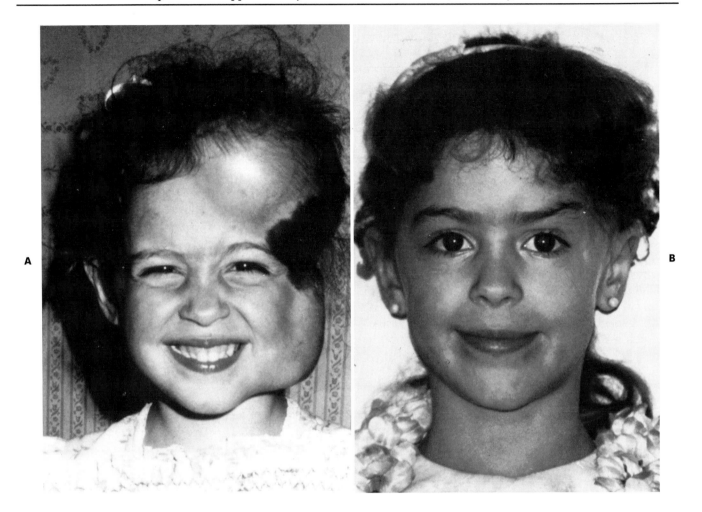

trauma or avulsion. In such circumstances considerable thought must be given to plans for the design of all flaps.

It is imperative in all reconstructions of the forehead that the brows be positioned so that they remain symmetrical and at a normal position. Once the defect has been closed, excess expanded tissue above the brow can be excised and the eyebrows positioned symmetrically. Wounds are closed in multiple layers, preferably with the use of clear permanent sutures for approximation of the muscle and subcuticular sutures for closure of the skin. The use of sterile bandages (Steri-strips) placed across suture lines to reduce wound-closure tension for several weeks may be useful in minimizing scar.

When greater than 50% of the entire surface of the

forehead must be reconstructed, skin expansion of the supraclavicular area is accomplished to create a source for a very large full-thickness skin graft, which can be used to resurface the entire forehead. This enables restoration of the entire esthetic unit. As long as some pericranium remains with a reasonable blood supply, an expanded skin graft can be used. This technique should not be used to cover an irradiated field or an area that is to receive irradiation.

The closer to the recipient site that a skin graft can be harvested, the better it will match the color and texture of that site. The site most readily expandable closest to the forehead is the supraclavicular area. It may be necessary to harvest such grafts from the medial side of the arm or lateral part of the chest below the axilla in particularly hirsute males. However, these sites are less optimal than the supraclavicular area because of possible delayed pigmentary changes in the grafted skin.

Large round expanders are placed in the subcutaneous tissue in any of the previously mentioned areas and expanded rapidly over a period of 3 to 4 weeks. Prolonged controlled expansion is accomplished until adequate tissue has been generated to cover the recipient site and allow concomitant primary closure of the donor site, preferably in a transverse orientation. The recipient site is prepared by removal of any remaining forehead skin so that the entire esthetic unit is resurfaced with the graft. Preservation of small patches of original forehead skin will frequently result in loss of homogeneity and compromise the results. If there is concern that the recipient site is not sufficiently vascularized, saline-moistened dressings are applied to the area, and the site is allowed to granulate until it will maintain a full-thickness graft. A template made of the forehead recipient site is placed directly over the expander to design the pattern of skin excision. A full-thickness graft is then harvested from the expanded donor site while the expander is in place. The graft is defatted so that only skin remains. Attempts at using thicker grafts, which incorporate the capsule, have met with uniform failure. The graft is sutured in place and immobilized appropriately. Drains are not used. The expander is removed, and the donor site is closed primarily.

In cases when postoperative inflammatory hyperpigmentation of the graft occurs, superficial chemical peels with dilute phenol have been helpful to reduce pigmentation. However, this should not be attempted for 6 to 12 months after the graft has been placed and allowed to mature.

Nose (Zone 3)

There is a wide variety of flaps available for reconstruction of small defects of the nose. Large defects often require the movement of tissue from an adjacent area, such as the forehead. Nonexpanded midline and paramedian forehead flaps are frequently used to repair large nasal defects; however, for repair of extensive midfacial defects and for total nasal reconstruction, the use of expanded forehead flaps may be helpful.[8]

Tissue expansion has several distinct advantages over standard methods of total nasal reconstruction. With expansion sufficient tissue is generated to close the donor site primarily; expanded skin is very thin and pliable, so it can be doubled on itself to reconstruct both the inner and outer surfaces of the nose; and the blood supply of expanded skin is enhanced so that a very reliable flap can be developed (Fig. 23-8).[9]

In many cases of total nasal reconstruction with use of nonexpanded forehead skin, the reconstructed nose is too small or is malpositioned. In females the external surface of the normal nose is approximately 35% of the total surface area of the forehead. If a flap is used to resurface the entire external surface of the nose and concomitantly create an adequate nasal vestibule, 50% to 60% of the surface area of the forehead must be used. Forehead expansion can provide the required skin to resurface the entire nose and nasal vestibule and allow primary closure of the donor site, resulting in minimal forehead deformity.

The first stage of nasal reconstruction in which expanded forehead skin is used is the insertion of a large rectangular expander, which encompasses as much of the surface of the forehead as possible. A small incision in the scalp is made, and the expander is inserted after the creation of an adequately sized recipient pocket beneath the frontalis muscle (Fig. 23-9). Pocket dissection is extended inferiorly to the brow, taking care not to injure the supraorbital vessels. The expander is then inflated at weekly intervals until a total volume of at least 400 to 600 ml of saline has been reached.

Nasal reconstruction may proceed as soon as adequate forehead expansion is accomplished. Missing skeletal support to the nose must be replaced with autologous tissue. Dorsal support is best reconstructed with a split cranial bone graft harvested from the frontotemporal region above the area of forehead expansion. The bone graft is trimmed to an appropriate size, shaped, and secured to the remaining nasal bones or cranium with miniature plates. Remaining nasal bone should be burred down to an appropriate level to accommodate the graft without creating a prominent hump deformity.

Support of the nasal tip is recreated with use of conchal auricular cartilage grafts, often harvested from both ears. The concha is exposed through an incision behind the ear, and sufficient cartilage is harvested to replace missing lower lateral cartilages. The cartilage grafts are contoured to an appropriate shape, mimicking the normal nasal cartilage, and sutured to the cantilever bone graft with fine wires. It is also important to secure the grafts to the lateral margin of the pyriform aperture. If this is not done, scar contracture can result in vestibular stenosis.

Sufficient skin may be available on the lateral margins of the remnant nose, to be used as turnover or hinged flaps to replace some or all of the missing nasal lining. However, these flaps may not be as effective as expanded forehead skin folded on itself. A template consisting of cloth or dental wax is used to design the size and shape of the flap required for reconstruction of the nose. The template is unfolded and placed over

Figure 23-8   *A*, An 80-year-old woman after total rhinectomy to remove extensive basal cell carcinoma. A 600-ml volume expander was placed beneath forehead skin through small incision in scalp. It was expanded over period of 5 weeks. *B* and *C*, At second procedure, expanded forehead flap is used to reconstruct both internal and external surface of nose. Note normal position and size of nose. Forehead scar is acceptable, and position of brow is normal. Nasal airway is patent bilaterally. No secondary procedures were performed.

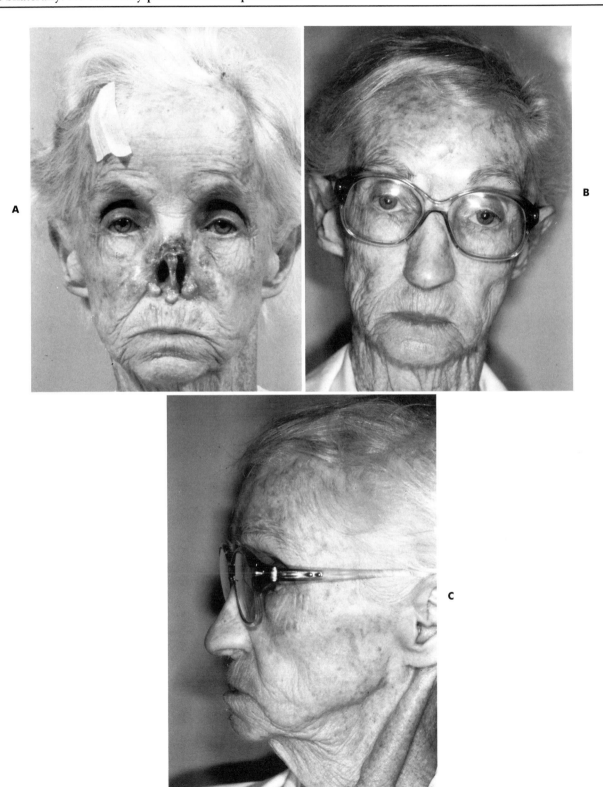

Figure 23-9 Large rectangular tissue expander is placed beneath frontalis muscle through small incision above hairline. Axis of expander should be horizontal.

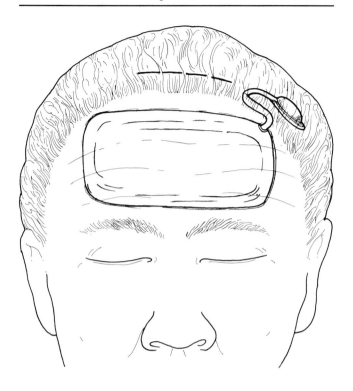

the expanded forehead. In cases in which the frontal hairline is low, the flap may extend into the hair to provide an adequate length to the flap. The hair follicles must be removed from the underside of the flap. The flap may be based on either the supraorbital or the supratrochlear artery, depending on which is found by Doppler examination to be dominant. The flap is incised, with the expander in place and fully expanded.

Dissection is carried out through the capsule of the expander, and the implant is removed. Approximately 2 cm above the superior orbital rim, the dissection is carried through the posterior wall of the capsule and pericranium. Dissection continues below the supraorbital rim in the subperiosteal plane, with care taken to preserve the nutrient artery and vein. Dissection in a subperiosteal plane facilitates the preservation of these vessels and allows the arc of pivot to be more inferiorly located, in contrast to keeping it at the level of the supraorbital rim. This movement increases the effective length of the flap.

The flap is transposed over the reconstructed nasal infrastructure, and the distal portion is folded on itself after the technique of Converse. Proper folding enables the creation of a columella and nasal vestibule on either side. The distal portion of the forehead flap that is to become the nasal lining is trimmed of its muscle

and subcutaneous fat to the level of the dermis. If hair follicles are present in the distal flap, these are removed from the deep aspect of the flap. The portion of the flap that will provide nasal lining is sutured to the mucoal margins of the defect. Care is taken to make sure that all of the bone and cartilage grafts are covered.

The external portion of the forehead flap is sutured to the remaining nasal or cheek skin margin while the flap is advanced inferiorly so that there is no cephalad tension on the flap. The flap is secured with deep dermal 4-0 polyglactin (Vicryl) sutures and 6-0 polypropylene (Prolene) sutures for approximation of the epidermis. The forehead wound is closed primarily side to side with permanent subcutaneous sutures of clear nylon and a subcuticular skin closure. The bridging pedicle is not tubed or covered on its deep surface with a skin graft. However, it is protected with gauze saturated with petroleum jelly (Vaseline).

At 2 or 3 weeks after the initial procedure, the flap is divided and inset. The flap attached to the nose is trimmed to an appropriate size and shape, trying to keep suture lines in the borders of esthetic units. The proximal portion of the flap is trimmed so that only the portion extending up to the medial margin of the brow is preserved. It is not necessary to retain the entire proximal flap, as this results in an inverted Y-shaped scar in the central part of the forehead above the natural glabellar crease, which is cosmetically less acceptable than if the trifurcated scar were kept within the glabellar region. No defatting or nasal revision is performed for 6 to 8 months, and most cases require very few revisions.

Lateral Part of the Face (Zone 4)

Zone 4 encompasses the soft tissues extending from the melolabial crease to the ear and from the infraorbital rim to the mandible. The color, texture, and hair-bearing quality of this skin varies with individuals but is relatively homogeneous in the same person. In children and young adults it is important to remember that this zone has hair-bearing potential in both males and females, and that there may be severe esthetic compromises if this area is not reconstructed as an entire esthetic unit.

Smaller defects in the lateral facial area can be reconstructed by mobilization of adjacent tissue. Incorporating postauricular skin into a flap for repair of defects anterior to the ear may be problematic in that this skin is non–hair-bearing, has a red hue, and is thinner than preauricular skin. Large defects of zone 4 that cannot be reconstructed by mobilization of adjacent skin of the cheek and neck are best repaired with use of tissue expansion as the first step in the reconstruction process. The remaining normal skin of the lateral part of the face and upper aspect of the neck is expanded, and a large inferior and medially based rotation advancement flap is created. This flap is well vascularized, reliable, and often enables the reconstruction of the entire zone 4 esthetic unit. By reconstruction of the unit in its entirety, suture lines are located along esthetic junction zones, which maximizes scar camouflage (Fig. 23-10).[10]

An incision is usually made in the preauricular area or, if a lesion is to be excised, on the lateral part of the face within the lesion itself. A subcutaneous plane similar to a facelift plane is developed over the superficial aponeurosis muscle. The dissection is extended inferiorly into the upper aspect of the neck, superficial to the platysma muscle. In the past I advocated placement of the expander below the platysma; however, I have found that this limits the freedom of movement of very large flaps. The surgical plane is developed sharply with use of Metzbaum scissors until an adequate pocket has been developed to allow the expander to easily fit under the area to be expanded. In a child it is particularly important that thin expanders without reenforcement be used; this will avoid folds developing in the expander, which increases the risk of extrusion. Reservoirs are placed beneath either the scalp or skin of the lateral part of the neck.

Expansion of the skin of the face and neck is relatively easy and does not elicit a great deal of discomfort. Expanders can be inflated to a volume of 600 to 800 ml within a 4- to 6-week interval. In children it is best to inflate frequently with small volumes of saline. This approach appears to minimize discomfort and reduce the risk of extrusion.

At a second operation a rotation flap is carefully planned over the expanded area so that the posterior margin of the flap is in the pretragal area. The flap is designed so that it extends in a cephalad direction anterior to the temporal hair and caudally into the postauricular and neck area as inferiorly as is necessary to provide sufficient tissue for reconstruction and to facilitate rotation of the expanded skin. If a large degree of rotation is required, the flap can be back-cut at a level near the clavicle, where the scar resulting from the back-cut can be hidden by clothing.

The flap is rotated in a fashion similar to the Mustarde cheek flap. The upper margin of the flap often extends from the lateral canthus to the medial canthus. In such circumstances the entire weight of the flap is supported at the medial canthus and at or above the lateral canthus (Fig. 23-11).[6] Suspension of the flap at these two locations ensures that the wound-closure tension is minimized along the junction of the flap with

the lower eyelid. In fact, it is best to leave redundant flap tissue along the length of the eyelid, which can be excised later so as to reduce the risk of development of an ectropion. Suturing of the flap to the periosteum of the infraorbital rim may also be useful in minimizing lid retraction. The standing cutaneous deformity that results from rotation of the flap is usually trimmed in such a way that the excision lies in the melolabial sulcus. It is best not to extend the flap onto the nose or upper lip, because these structures are separate esthetic units and are best reconstructed independent of the cheek.

The distal flap may be tenuous in its vascularity; thus compression dressings are avoided. Suction drains are useful to allow the flap to contour well. These are left in place for 7 days to ensure redefinition of the angle of the neck. The donor site is closed primarily by advancement of surrounding neck skin, which may involve undermining of skin in the supraclavicular area and the posterior part of the neck.

Hypertrophy of scars is not unusual in children. Scar compression may be helpful to minimize development of hypertrophic scarring. The revision of scars is best postponed until the child is fully grown, sometime between 12 and 15 years of age, because at this age patients are more cooperative and better tolerate scar revision surgery. The use of cosmetics to camouflage scars in children is not routinely recommended unless the patient develops psychological problems and wishes to try them. I usually wait until the patient asks about this, rather than recommending it prophylactically.

Neck and Lower Part of the Face (Zone 5)

The tissue of the neck itself is almost identical in color, texture, and hair-bearing qualities to the skin in zone 4. In most cases, however, it is unwise to compromise skin in the face to reconstruct the neck. In most circumstances there is adequate tissue in the neck so that uninvolved neck skin can be expanded to close defects. When adjacent neck skin is not sufficient for this purpose, a less than optimal reconstruction can be achieved by advancement of skin from the upper chest. This is preferable to the use of expanded skin from zone 4.

Less deformity and more rapid expansion and reconstruction of the neck can be accomplished if skin is moved in a horizontal rather than vertical direction. However, when defects involve the skin overlying the angle of the mandible, there is no alternative to moving skin in an inferior to superior direction. Neck skin of both males and females contains some hair-bearing skin. Most men have an area between the lower lip and

Figure 23-10 *A,* Defect that resulted from excision of facial soft-tissue sarcoma 5 years earlier. Patient had also received radiotherapy to affected region. There was no evidence of any recurrence. *B,* A 250-ml volume expander is placed beneath cheek skin of right side of face through pretragal incision and expanded over period of 12 weeks *(arrows).* Expander was inflated by patient's local physician. *C,* Results 2 years after reconstruction with use of nonexpanded forehead flap to reconstruct lateral nose, Estlander flap transferred from lower lip to upper lip to reconstruct commissure, and advancement flap of expanded skin to repair medial cheek defect. There is normal hair distribution of face. (*C* from Argenta LC, Watanabe MJ, Grabb WC: The use of tissue expansion in head and neck reconstruction, *Ann Plast Surg* 11:31, 1983.)

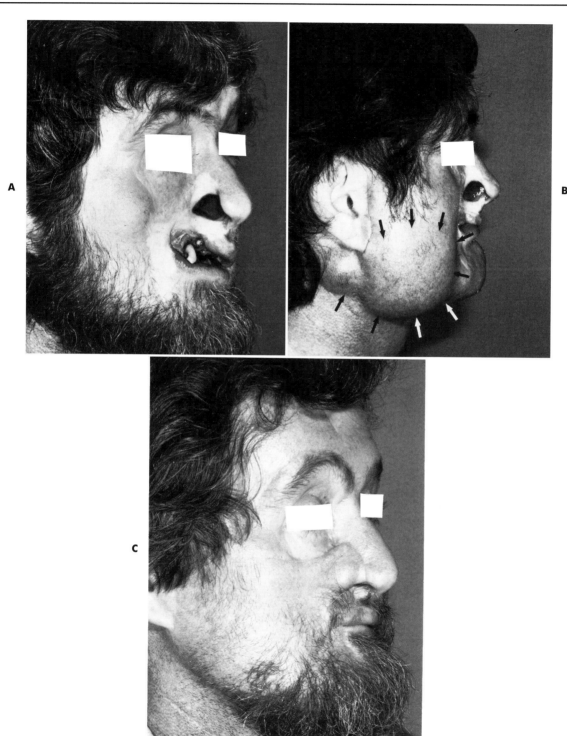

Figure 23-11   *A,* Giant hairy nevus of lateral face, extending onto nose and upper lip of child. A 500-ml volume expander was placed beneath neck skin through incision in nevus and expanded to total volume of 700 ml over 8-week interval. *B,* Large rotation cheek flap that used expanded tissue is mobilized from neck. *C,* Flap is suspended at lateral and medial canthi. *D,* Appearance 4 years after reconstruction. Upper lip was reconstructed with full-thickness skin graft from supraclavicular area. Note that there is no ectropion, although scars are still hypertrophic. (*D* from Argenta LC: Controlled tissue expansion in reconstructive surgery, *Br J Plast Surg* 37:520, 1984.)

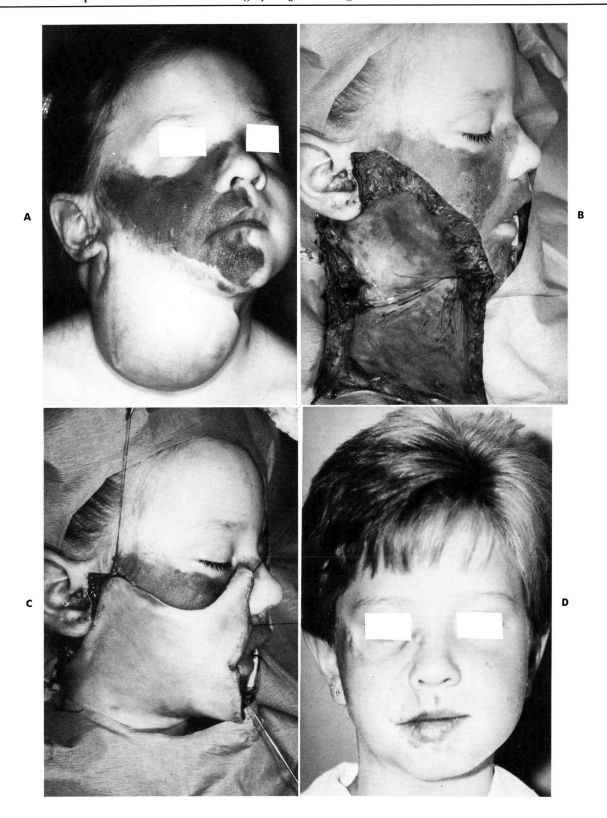

Figure 23-12 *A*, Burn scar extending from angle of mandible downward to anterior borders of both sternocleidomastoid muscles in a man. *B*, Two expanders are placed under remaining normal lateral neck skin and expanded over period of 7 weeks. *C* and *D*, Removal of entire scar and closure of wound with bilateral cervical advancement flaps. *E*, One week postoperatively there is poor definition of the angle and body of right mandible, but this improves over time.

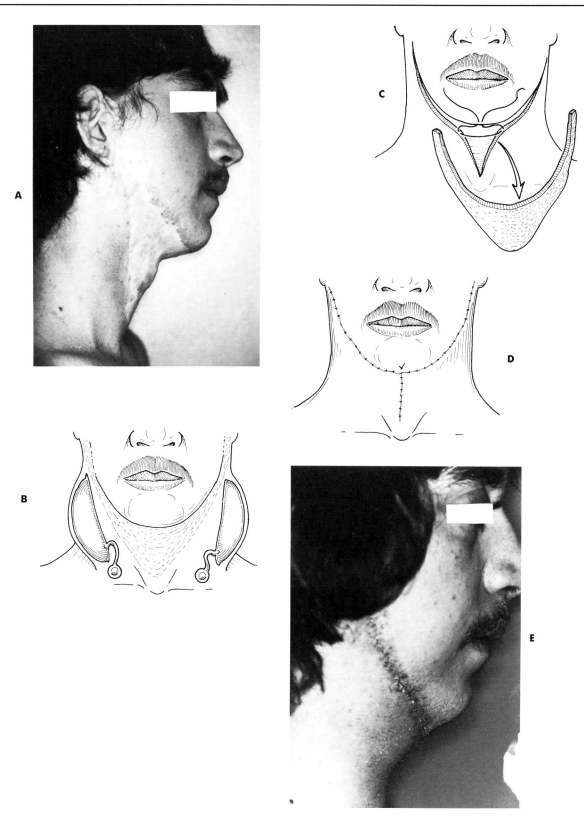

the chin in which there is minimal or no hair. This must be considered when flaps are advanced from the neck to reconstruct this region.

Two or more expanders on either side of a neck defect are recommended if sufficient skin for expansion remains. Central defects of the neck are most easily reconstructed by expansion laterally on each side of the neck and advancement of skin medially (Fig. 23-12).[11] Expansion of neck skin, overlying the major vessels, is well tolerated. A long straight vertical suture line in the midportion of the neck should be avoided, by the use of one or more Z-plasties in this area to reduce secondary scar contraction. If lengthy medial or lateral advancement of the expanded skin is required in the neck, an incision along the margin of the mandible may be necessary. In such cases, it is best to place the incision 2 cm above or below the margin of the mandible to reduce the risk of scar hypertrophy.

When reconstruction of defects located along the margin of the mandible and lower part of the face requires expansion of neck skin, several important points must be considered. Defects of the lower face, up to the commissure of the lip, can be reconstructed by expanding neck skin and moving it in a cephalad direction (Fig. 23-13). Hair-bearing tissue should not juxtapose the vermilion of the lower lip. The tension of wound closure should not cause eversion of the lip. This tension is in part avoided by suturing the flap to the mandibular periosteum and other underlying tissues lateral to the commissures. Flaps advanced from the neck over the mandible frequently tend to become somewhat tented over the angle of the mandible. When this happens, and the flap exhibits signs of vascular compromise, the neck can be placed in some flexion. This helps to reduce wound-closure tension. The neck is then gradually extended postoperatively after the suture line has had a chance to heal. The use of a neck splint while the patient is at rest or sleeping may help stretch the skin flap and create a better neckline postoperatively.

Periorbital Areas (Zone 6)

The skin of the periocular area, including both the upper and lower eyelids, and extending to the superior and inferior orbital rim, has very distinct properties. The skin is thin, pliable, nonsebaceous, nonhairy, and has no subcutaneous fat. For reconstruction of this area with maximum esthetic results, the use of full-thickness skin grafts is often required. The greatest problem is to obtain donor skin of similar likeness to that of eyelid skin without creating significant donor site morbidity. The nearer the donor site is to the periorbital area, the better the final tissue match will be. The use of skin from the lower portion of the neck immediately above

the clavicle affords an excellent color-texture match to that of the normal periocular skin (Fig. 23-14). Usually even in the most hirsute male, there is an area adjacent to the clavicle that has little or no hair. If this site is unavailable as a donor site for a full-thickness skin graft, the upper inner side of the arm or lateral part of the chest can be used but with less esthetically pleasing results.

A rectangular or round expander is inserted in the subcutaneous tissues of the neck immediately above the clavicle. Neck skin is quite easy to expand with minimal discomfort. Within 3 to 4 weeks, enough tissue can be generated to cover up to one half the surface area of the face.

Similar to reconstruction of other regions of the face, when it is necessary to skin graft most of an esthetic subunit, it is best to resurface the entire subunit with a single graft. This is true of both the upper and lower eyelids. When the entire eyelid must be skin grafted, it is usually best to harvest a single expanded full-thickness graft, which is used to cover both the upper and lower eyelids. The graft is sutured in place above and below, and a transverse incision is made in the graft to accommodate the palpebral fissure. Meticulous hemostasis of the recipient site must be obtained before grafting. If bleeding is problematic, it is best to cover the oozing area with a saline-moistened dressing for 24 hours and then graft it at a second procedure. Development of a hematoma beneath the graft will result in loss of the graft and will compromise the result.

A template is made of the recipient area with use of sterilized x-ray sheeting. The template is transposed directly over the expander, and a slightly larger area is outlined. The skin is then excised as a full-thickness graft with the expander in place and expanded. The graft is trimmed, removing all fat and subcutaneous tissue down to the level of the dermis. If there is any hair in the graft, the hair follicles are excised from below to minimize the chances of hair growth. The incision is then carried through the capsule surrounding the expander, and the expander is removed. The capsule is left intact but is abraded with gauze to facilitate adhesions and to minimize postoperative development of a seroma. The wound is then closed in a transverse direction above the clavicle, to maximize scar camouflage.

The expanded full-thickness graft is sutured to the recipient site with appropriate subcutaneous and fine monofilament sutures. If the entire periocular area is grafted, a tarsorrhaphy is performed. The portion of the graft placed in the periocular area should have a surface area that is 20% larger than the defect to compensate for contracture of the wound. A tie-over bolster dressing is used to secure the graft for 5 to 7

Figure 23-13 *A,* Extensive burns to face and eversion of lower lip, secondary to scar contracture, in a man. *B,* Two large rectangular expanders are placed beneath skin of neck and expanded over period of 9 weeks. *C* through *E,* Neck skin is then advanced superiorly to level of oral commissure, and entire scar is excised. *F,* Appearance 1 year after reconstruction. Patient has also had hair-bearing temporal interpolation flaps used to reconstruct upper lip. Note that there is no eversion of lower lip. (Patient was operated on by Malcolm W. Marks, M.D.)

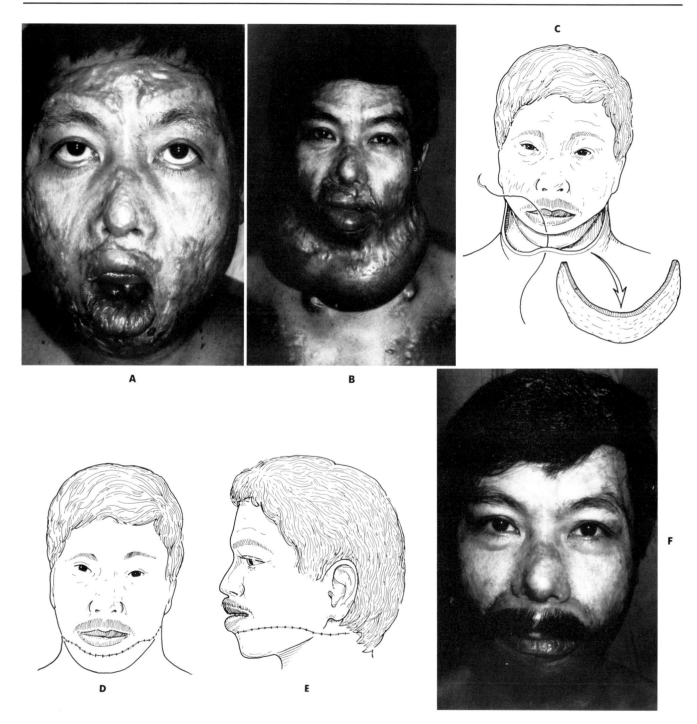

Figure 23-14   *A*, Giant hairy nevus of left side of face of a boy, who had previously undergone expansion of neck skin and subsequent rotation-advancement flap to reconstruct lower face. Left forehead area had been reconstructed with expanded full-thickness skin graft from upper inner part of left arm. *B*, Periocular nevus is excised. *C*, Expander is placed in supraclavicular area and expanded to total volume of 450 ml. Expanded full-thickness skin graft is harvested over inflated expander and used to cover cheek defect. *D*, Appearance 1 year after surgery. Eyebrow was excised at a later procedure and reconstructed with island scalp flap. Remaining nevus on lip will require serial excisions.

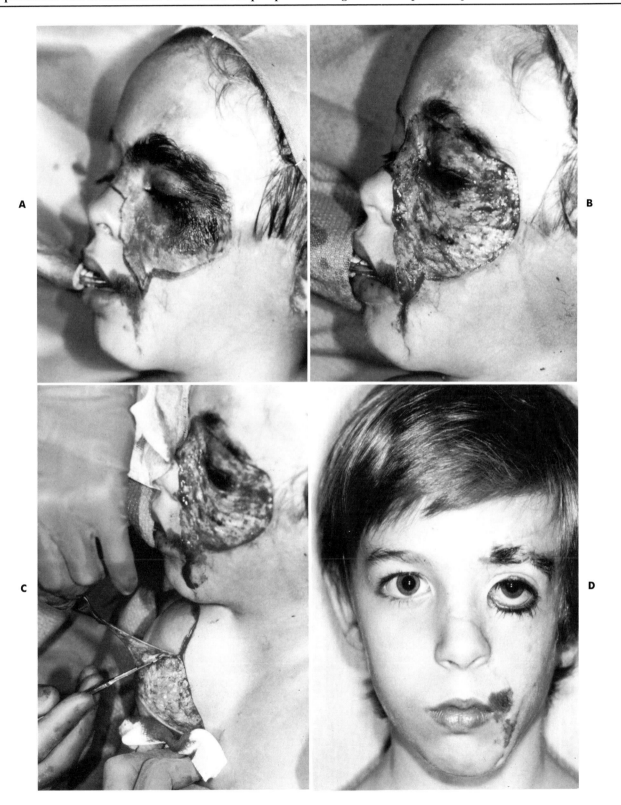

days. If bilateral eyelid grafting is necessary, it is best to stage the procedures and correct one eye at a time. This avoids the need to occlude both eyes simultaneously with bolster dressings, which is particularly distressful for children. Neonates should not have their eyes occluded until they are 6 to 10 months of age.

REFERENCES

1. Antonyshyn O, Gruss J, Zucker R, et al: Tissue expansion in head and neck reconstruction, *Plast Reconstr Surg* 82:58, 1988.
2. Leonard AG, Small JO: Tissue expansion in the treatment of alopecia, *Br J Plast Surg* 39:42, 1986.
3. Manders EK, Graham WP III, Schenden MJ et al: Skin expansion to eliminate large scalp defects, *Ann Plast Surg* 12:305, 1985.
4. Matthews R, Missotten F: Early tissue expansion to close a traumatic defect of scalp and pericranium, *Br J Plast Surg* 39:417, 1986.
5. Anderson R: Expansion-assisted treatment of male pattern baldness, *Clin Plast Surg* 14:477, 1987.
6. Argenta LC: Controlled tissue expansion in reconstructive surgery, *Br J Plast Surg* 37:520, 1984.
7. Antonyshyn O, Gruss J, Mackinnon S, et al: Complications of soft tissue expansion, *Br J Plast Surg* 41:239, 1988.
8. Bolton L, Chandrasekhar B, Gottleib M: Forehead expansion and total nasal reconstruction, *Ann Plast Surg* 21:210, 1988.
9. Mustoe T, Bartell T, Garner W: Physical, biomechanical, histological and biochemical effects of rapid vs. conventional tissue expansion, *Plast Reconstr Surg* 83:687, 1989.
10. Argenta LC, Watanabe MJ, Grabb WC: The use of tissue expansion in head and neck reconstruction, *Ann Plast Surg* 11:31, 1983.
11. Marks MW, Argenta LC, Thornton J: Burn management: the role of tissue expansion, *Clin Plast Surg* 14:543, 1989.

EDITORIAL COMMENTS

Shan R. Baker

Dr. Argenta has extensive experience in the use of tissue expansion for correction of congenital and traumatic deformities of the head and neck. The author discusses the application of tissue expansion by dividing the head and neck into six topographic zones based on the characteristics of the skin in these areas. He has described a number of clinical applications in each zone and has shown examples. In my opinion, some of the excellent esthetic results achieved by the author would not be possible without the use of tissue expansion. Although the author nicely demonstrates the versatility of tissue expansion, a detailed description of technical factors was not provided. Thus I would like to present a more in-depth discussion of the mechanical aspects of tissue expansion and explore the indications, advantages and disadvantages, and complications of tissue expansion of the head and neck.[1]

The relatively recent advent of tissue expansion for medical purposes precludes the availability of extensive knowledge concerning the physiologic and histologic changes that occur during prolonged controlled expansion of the skin. It can be concluded, however, that flaps harvested from skin that was previously expanded have an improved survival rate compared with similar flaps developed in nonexpanded skin. Increased vascularity to either the skin, the capsule that forms around the expander, or both, probably in some way accounts for the improved survival.

It can also be concluded that controlled expansion of skin results in the creation of additional new skin at the expense of thinning of the dermis and subcutaneous tissues. This thinning is associated with an overall decrease in tensile strength of the expanded skin. The increase in surface area gained from skin expansion probably varies according to the type of skin expanded and the underlying tissues that serve as a foundation for the expander. Discontinuation of expansion apparently results in a normalization of the skin, with the thickness of the dermis and subcutaneous tissue slowly returning to that of preexpanded tissue.[2]

Tissue expansion is indicated in the reconstruction of various defects of the head and neck in instances when there is inadequate adjacent tissue to allow either primary closure of the defect or repair with a local flap (Fig. 23-15).[3] Its use may also be indicated for reconstruction of a defect that can be repaired by a local, regional, or distant flap, but at the cost of severe deformity of the donor or recipient site. Tissue expansion offers the advantage of an increase in locally available tissue with preservation of sensation and adnexal structures. Thus the missing skin of the defect can be replaced with skin of identical color, thickness, and appendages (hair growth). This is unlike any other form of reconstruction because often there is no need for a secondary defect unless creation of a flap is necessary. Expanded skin can simply be advanced into the defect for primary closure. In cases that require the use of a flap, the secondary defect can be easily closed because of the additional skin created by the expansion

Figure 23-15   *A*, Giant pigmented nevus of scalp of a 1-year-old child. *B*, Fully expanded 100-ml volume rectangular tissue expander beneath right temporal scalp. *C*, Two weeks after total removal of nevus and reconstruction with rotation advancement scalp flap. (*C* from Baker SR, Johnson TM, Nelson BR: Tissue expansion of the scalp, *Arch Otolaryngol Head Neck Surg* **(in press).**

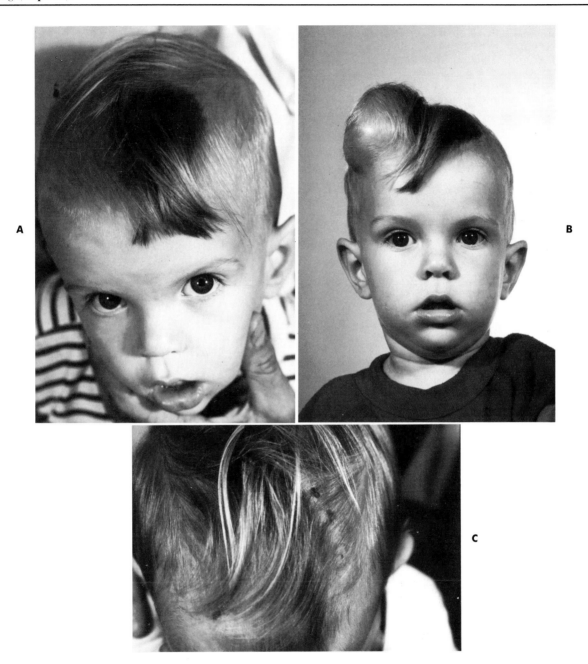

Figure 23-16 *A* and *B,* Extensive midfacial defect after excision of basal cell carcinoma. Majority of left nasal tip and ala was resected, as well as both upper lateral cartilages, leaving full-thickness tip and dorsal nasal defect measuring approximately 4 × 5 cm. *C,* A 250-ml volume rectangular expander is used to expand entire forehead. *D,* Ample skin is observed immediately after decompression of expander as preliminary step to reconstruction of nose. *E* and *F,* Appearance of forehead and reconstructed nose 1 year after surgery. (*E* and *F* from Baker SR, Johnson TM, Nelson BR: Reconstruction of midfacial defects following surgical management of skin cancer: the role of tissue expansion, *J Dermatol Surg Oncol* 20:133-140, Copyright 1994 by Elsevier Science, Inc.

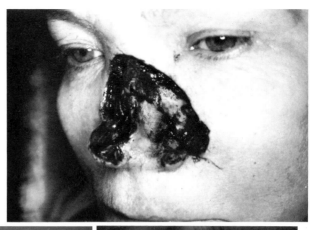

A

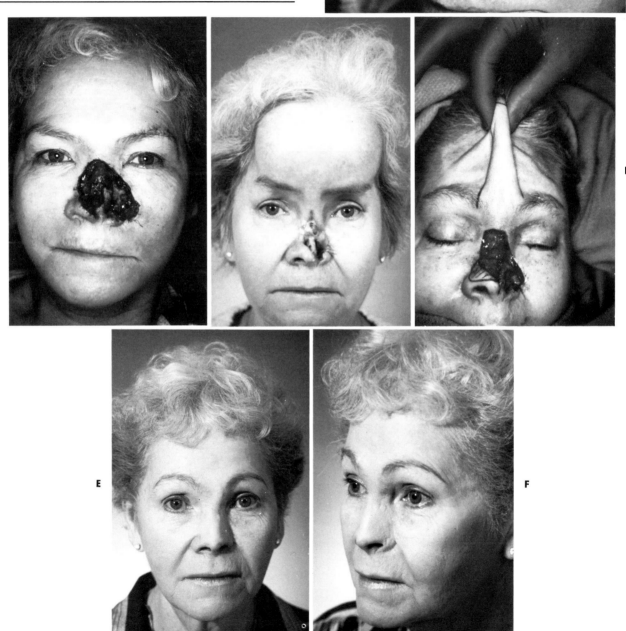

B, C

D

E

F

process; thus expansion obviates sacrifice of cosmesis of one area to improve that of another (Fig. 23-16).[4]

The use of skin expansion to close large defects of the head and neck usually obviates the need for multiple flaps or grafting procedures, thus reducing overall cost of reconstruction. Tissue expansion is tolerated well by most patients, can be performed in an outpatient setting, and can be accomplished before the ablative or reconstructive procedure so that additional tissue will be available at the time of excision and reconstruction. Tissue expanders can be placed in almost any area of the body. Functional disability imposed by the transfer of muscles such as the pectoralis major or latissimus dorsi in the form of musculocutaneous flaps for reconstruction of defects of the head and neck is not incurred with skin expansion.

Flaps harvested from expanded skin have increased vascularity; thus flaps that would fail as simple primary procedures can be harvested from expanded skin with relative impunity, significantly improving the surgeon's flexibility during reconstructive procedures. This flexibility is enhanced by the fact that expansion can be repeated. That is, the tissue can be reexpanded a second or third time if necessary to achieve the final goals in reconstruction.

The major disadvantage of tissue expansion in reconstruction of the head and neck is that it involves two surgical procedures, one to implant the expander and the other to remove the expander and perform the reconstruction. Fortunately, implantation of the expander can be accomplished as an outpatient procedure with the use of local anesthesia.

Tissue expansion is labor-intensive in that frequent visits to the surgeon's office are necessary for inflation of the implant. This is obviated in some circumstances by training paramedical personnel or a patient's family member to carry out the inflation.

Another major disadvantage of tissue expansion in the head and neck region is the temporary visible deformity that results from expansion, particularly toward the end of the expansion process. Its use may be precluded if the patient must interact with the public. Scalp expansion can be camouflaged by a large hat, and neck expansion can be concealed in part by a turtleneck sweater; however, expansion of the forehead and cheek areas cannot be easily hidden. It is important that the patient be properly informed concerning the substantial, but temporary, deformity that occurs in the area of expansion.

Tissue expanders are Silastic balloons with self-sealing valves or reservoirs that are completely implanted beneath the skin. They are available in many different sizes and shapes, such as round, rectangular, and elliptical. Expanders also are available in various volumes ranging from a few to several thousand milliliters. There are two basic types of expanders: one in which the injection port that receives the needle during inflation is attached by a stem of varying lengths to the expander, and one in which the expander and injection port are a single unit. The latter has been used in breast reconstruction but has the great disadvantage of possible inadvertent perforation of the balloon during attempted placement of the needle into the injection port during inflation. The advantage of the former type of expander is a decreased risk of perforation of the expander, since the injection port is removed from the balloon. This type of expander also permits placement of the injection port at a site far removed from the defect or area of expansion, or even allows external placement.[5]

Regardless of the type of expander selected, it must be of sufficient size to provide the required expansive forces necessary to achieve the desired tissue augmentation. One method of selecting the appropriate expander is based on the size of the base of the expander. Van Rappard et al[6] studied the increases in surface area of a number of expanders of different sizes and shapes and observed a clear difference. The authors recommended that in the clinical setting the appropriate size of expander would be one in which the surface area of the expander base is 2.5 times as large as the defect to be closed when rectangular or crescentic expanders are used. In the case of round expanders this correction factor of 2.5 holds true for the diameter of the expander base rather than the area of the base.

Another method of selection of an expander is based on the circumference of the inflatable balloon portion of the expander. The expander must be of sufficient volume so that the apical circumference of the dome of skin overlying the fully inflated expander is two to three times the width of the defect.[7] Generally this will allow coverage by the expanded skin of both the donor site and the defect.

There is a considerable margin of safety in selection of the proper volume, since expanders can be overinflated at least 15 times the vendors' stated maximum volume.[8] A disadvantage of overinflation, however, is increased leakage from the dome of the injection port. Nordstrom et al[9] found that the average pressure necessary for leakage from the injection port of an expander was 32 mm Hg, with a range of 8 to 110 mm Hg. Thus overinflation will predispose to leakage and may explain the partial disappearance of saline injected into some tissue expanders. These researchers also noted that when patients lay on their expander, which had been placed beneath the skin of the head and neck, intraluminal pressures in the expander increased up to 75 mm Hg, thus subjecting the patient to a higher risk of leakage from the expander. To circumvent the potential problem of leakage, it is prudent to select the largest expander that can reasonably be inserted beneath the region of expansion or to consider the concomitant use of two or more expanders placed in strategic locations. For most defects of the face, neck, and scalp, I have found a 250-ml rectangular expander to be optimal.

Tissue expansion is an extraordinarily simple technique. It allows the surgeon to undertake reconstructive procedures that would have been impossible to treat in the past. Although tissue expansion is simplistic in concept, it does require judgment and in-depth preoperative planning by the surgeon to ensure optimal results. An accurate analysis of the reconstructive requirements is necessary with respect to expected size of defect and the method of reconstruction. The surgeon must determine preoperatively if reconstruction can be achieved by simple advancement of expanded skin or whether some type of pivotal flap will be necessary. This decision will then dictate the location of incisions for implantation of the expander. In general, expanders should be located in positions that take advantage of simple advancement or transposition flaps; however, areas of scarring, atrophy, or previously irradiated skin should be avoided.

Incisions for placement of the expander are usually made at the junction of normal tissue and tissue to be replaced. An exception to this rule is at junctions of normal skin and skin grafts. Incisions should be avoided in such junctional zones because of the high risk of dehiscence of the incision during expansion. In such cases incisions for implantation should be located in skin of normal thickness that is far removed from the skin graft. Distant incisions allow for more rapid expansion of skin without the expander placing excessive forces on the incision. Detailed planning of proposed incisions is important so that the possibility of future flaps or other surgical procedures is not compromised or reconstructive alternatives limited.

Consideration should be given to the use of multiple expanders around the defect because it provides for more rapid development of sufficient tissue for reconstruction and at the same time minimizes the visible deformity created during expansion. Before implantation of the expander prophylactic antibiotics are administered, and the operative site is meticulously scrubbed with a bacteriostatic soap. Preoperatively I soak the expander in an antibiotic solution that consists of 500 ml of saline containing 1 g of cephalosporin. This solution is subsequently used to irrigate the subcutaneous pocket that is created to receive the implant before wound closure.

Tissue expanders used in the head and neck are implanted with the patient under local anesthesia following ringed block with use of 1% lidocaine and epinephrine (1:100,000) or with the patient under general anesthesia. In expansion of the scalp or forehead a recipient pocket is created between the periosteum and the galea (in scalp) or deep fascia of the frontalis muscle (in forehead). In the neck a recipient pocket is developed beneath the platysmal muscle or in the subcutaneous plane. The pocket should be of sufficient size to allow the base of the expander to lie flat without folding or distortion. The injection port should be placed through the same incision as that of the expander but situated in a separate pocket approximately 6 cm away from the balloon. Anchoring sutures to prevent migration of the expander are not necessary if the expander is placed beneath the scalp or forehead skin. Anchoring sutures are recommended to prevent migration of expanders placed beneath the skin of the cheek or neck due to gravitational forces. Meticulous hemostasis must be achieved, since drains are not used. The expander is partially expanded (approximately 50 ml for a 250-ml expander) with saline before wound closure to concomitantly obliterate dead space and assist with hemostasis. The incision is closed by layers using permanent sutures for approximation of both the subcutaneous and cutaneous tissue.

Inflation begins 2 weeks after implantation of the expander. Saline is infused by percutaneous puncture of the injection port with a 23-gauge scalp needle attached to a 50-ml volume syringe, after preparation of the injection site with an alcohol swab. Some children may require local anesthesia of the skin overlying the injection port before inflation. The volume of injection depends on the tensile strength and tension of the skin overlying the expander as well as on the amount of patient discomfort. If not precluded by discomfort, the tissue should be expanded until slight blanching is observed in the skin overlying the expander. Saline should then be withdrawn until the blanching disappears. Usually 25 to 50 ml of saline can be injected into a 250-ml volume expander on a weekly interval. Tightness or pain usually is the limiting factor in prevention of further expansion. This discomfort resolves within 24 to 48 hours, and the patient remains comfortable until the next inflation. Inflation is usually conducted as frequently as once or twice a week. More rapid expansion may be possible but is associated with a greater risk of extrusion of the expander.

The volume of injected saline is recorded. Measurement of the expanded skin is also noted. As mentioned, the patient or a family member can be taught the inflation technique. In-home expansion is facilitated by a written list of instructions and by marking of the injection site with indelible ink or a suture. A small amount of methylene blue dye may be initially injected into the expander. The person who performs the inflation may subsequently aspirate a small quantity of saline from the port before injection. If a blue solution is returned, proper placement of the needle has been achieved.

As expansion proceeds, the dermis becomes thinner and a capsule forms around the expander. This often results in a reversible blue or red discoloration of the expanded skin. Dilated subcutaneous veins are frequently observed, but this is not an indication of cyanosis or infection (Fig. 23-17).[4] Expansion continues until the circumference of the dome of the expanded skin measures two to three times the width of the proposed defect. This usually takes 6 to 8 weeks for the skin of the forehead and neck and up to 12 weeks for the scalp.

The second surgical stage involves removal of the expander, followed by reconstruction. The expander is deflated and removed either through the original incision used for implantation of the device or through one of the incisions used to create a flap. Usually a broad-base pivotal or advancement flap is designed and incised, depending on the size and shape of the defect to be reconstructed. The capsule surrounding the expander provides an excellent blood supply to the flap and therefore is usually not disturbed unless thinning of the flap is necessary to achieve optimal cosmetic results. A suction drain tube is employed at the donor site. Wound closure and postoperative care are similar to that used for standard flap surgery.

Complications of tissue expansion are high, but most are minor. Nearly all complications incurred can be managed without long-term sequelae. The complication rate is highest for tissue expansion in the head and neck[10] and is lowest for breast reconstruction. Manders and colleagues[11] studied 35 patients who underwent a total of 41 expansions for a wide spectrum of reconstructive needs. Of these patients 40% had a major or

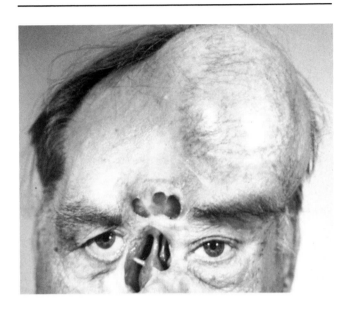

Figure 23-17   **Defect of midface after removal of extensive basal cell carcinoma. Note dilated vasculature of expanded skin over dome of expander. (From Baker SR, Johnson TM, Nelson BR: Reconstruction of midfacial defects following surgical management of skin cancer: the role of tissue expansion,** *J Dermatol Surg Oncol* **20:133-140, 1994.**

minor complication. Major complications, defined as those that required specific treatment and consequent alteration of the treatment plan, affected 25% of the patients in this series.[11] Antonyshyn et al[10] noted a 48% complication rate in 29 patients who underwent 33 tissue expansions in the head and neck area. Despite this high incidence of complications, sufficient tissue was generated to successfully complete the planned reconstruction in 70% of patients.

Complication rates of tissue expansion in the head and neck appear to be highest for expansion of the cheek and neck (69%) and forehead (50%).[10] Expansion of the scalp has the least risk of complications (17%).[10,12] Erosion of overlying tissue that results in exposure of the implant constitutes the most commonly observed major complication, occurring in 30% of cases.[10] There are two main causes for this phenomenon. The first is incisional dehiscence that can occur as a result of making the access incision for placement of the expander too close to the area of expansion. Also, if permanent sutures are not used to close the deeper layers of the incision, the expansive forces during inflation of the expander are sufficient to disrupt the incision even several weeks after implantation. A second cause for exposure of the expander is progressive thinning of the dermis and subsequent dissipation of the overlying skin and capsule. This occurs more frequently when there is inadequate tissue coverage of the expander during the initial implantation of the expander, or when expansion of previously irradiated skin is attempted.[11] A persistent fold in the silicone balloon of the expander that persists despite progressive inflation may also precipitate exposure. These folds can be brought into sharp relief beneath the skin and occasionally produce a discrete area of increased pressure on the overlying skin. Massage has not been useful in eliminating folds, nor has deflation and reinflation of the expander. The best option in such cases appears to be use of a slower rate of expansion than would normally be necessary.

Although an exposed expander may be left in position for a limited time while expansion continues,[11] I recommend removal and immediately proceeding with reconstruction if sufficient tissue is available. In instances in which marked thinning of the overlying skin has occurred with impending exposure, I recommend proceeding with surgery. Depending on the circumstances, a second expansion may be attempted after use of the available expanded soft tissue over the deflated expander. Fortunately, exposure of the expander usually does not occur until the expander is near maximal volumes of inflation. Thus exposure does not usually forecast a failure in the ultimate goal of reconstruction.

Mechanical failure of the expander is rare and is usually the result of physician error. The most common error is in faulty assembly of the connection device that joins the stem of the injection port with that of the silicone balloon. Most expanders are now available as a single unit, such as balloon, connection tube, and injection port. Although the surgeon can choose to shorten the connecting tube by cutting it and reconnecting the ends with use of a connector, it is probably prudent not to do so unless necessary. The other iatrogenic complication that results in failure of the system is leakage, which may result from inadvertent puncture of the balloon or the connecting tube during implantation of the expander or subsequent inflation. Care must be taken not to puncture the device during suturing of the access incision after implantation.

Infection of an implanted tissue expander is rare,[11] especially in the area of the head and neck because of the excellent blood supply this bodily region enjoys. The use of prophylactic antibiotics administered in the perioperative period is recommended. Infection is heralded by erythema, pain, and possibly fever. When infection is not severe, successful salvage with antibiot-

ics and drainage may be possible.[11,13,14] It is my opinion, however, that, once the pocket containing the expander becomes infected, removal of the device and draining or packing the pocket are required.

Hematomas and seromas may occasionally occur in the immediate postoperative period or may be delayed for several weeks.[11,15] There is a greater risk of these complications when tissue is expanded in the vicinity of hemangiomas. In these cases postoperative drainage at the time of expander implantation is necessary. In all other cases meticulous hemostasis at the time of implantation and partial inflation of the expander to "compress" the area of dissection appear to reduce the risk of hematomas and seromas. If they occur despite these precautions, treatment consists of judicial serial aspirations.

Bone resorption during scalp and forehead skin expansion has been observed on occasion.[12,16] This usually occurs from prolonged expansion with large-volume expanders (400 ml or greater). Bone resorption observed with expansion consists of thinning of the outer table of the calvarium. Thus expansion of the scalp in pediatric patients is not recommended until closure of the anterior and posterior fontanelles is complete.[16]

Intractable pain that prevents further expansion is a rare complication and occurs primarily with forehead expansion.[10] This probably results from compression of the supraorbital and supratrochlear nerves, which richly supply the forehead skin.

Despite the frequency of complications associated with tissue expansion, the intended reconstruction is successfully completed in almost all cases. Even when complications do arise, the final result obtained with tissue expansion is generally far superior to that seen with more conventional techniques. Because it minimizes deformity at both the donor and recipient sites, the benefits of tissue expansion far outweigh the risks; therefore tissue expansion should be used when anticipated results from other reconstructive techniques are not acceptable.

References

1. Baker SR, Swanson NA: Tissue expansion of the head and neck: indications, technique and complications, *Arch Otolaryngol Head Neck Surg* 116:1147, 1990.

2. Pasyk KA, Argenta LC, Hassett C: Quantitative analysis of the thickness of human skin and subcutaneous tissue following controlled expansion with a silicone implant, *Plast Reconstr Surg* 81:516, 1988.

3. Baker SR, Johnson TM, Nelson BR: Tissue expansion of the scalp, *Arch Otolaryngol* Head Neck Surg (in press).

4. Baker SR, Johnson TM, Nelson BR: Reconstruction of midfacial defects following surgical management of skin cancer: the role of tissue expansion, *J Dermatol Surg Oncol* (in press).

5. Jackson IT, Sharpe DT, Polley J et al: Use of external reservoirs in tissue expansion, *Plast Reconstr Surg* 80:266, 1987.

6. Van Rappard JHA, Molenaar J, Van Doorn K et al: Surface-area increase in tissue expansion, *Plast Reconstr Surg* 82:833, 1988.

7. Roenigk RK, Wheeland RG: Tissue expansion in cicatricial alopecia, *Arch Dermatol* 123:641, 1987.

8. Hallock GG: Maximum overinflation of tissue expanders, *Plast Reconstr Surg* 80:567, 1987.

9. Nordstrom REA, Pietila JP, Voutilainen PEJ et al: Tissue expander injection dome leakage, *Plast Reconstr Surg* 81:26, 1988.

10. Antonyshyn O, Gruss JS, Zuker R et al: Tissue expansion in head and neck reconstruction, *Plast Reconstr Surg* 82:58, 1988.

11. Manders EK, Schenden MJ, Furrey JA et al: Soft tissue expansion: concepts and complications, *Plast Reconstr Surg* 74:493, 1984.

12. Leighton WD, Johnson ML, Friedland JA: Use of the temporary soft-tissue expander in post-traumatic alopecia, *Plast Reconstr Surg* 77:737, 1986.

13. Geter RK, Puckett CL: Salvage of infected expanded scalp without loss of flap length, *Plast Reconstr Surg* 80:720, 1987.

14. Austad ED, Geter RK, Puckett CL: Salvage of infected expanded scalp without loss of flap length, *Plast Reconstr Surg* 80:724, 1987.

15. Ashall G, Quaba A: A hemorrhagic hazard of tissue expansion, *Plast Reconstr Surg* 79:627, 1987.

16. Maves MD, Lusk RP: Tissue expansion in the treatment of giant congenital melanocytic nevi, *Arch Otolaryngol Head Neck Surg* 113:987, 1987.

EDITORIAL COMMENTS

Neil A. Swanson

I had the pleasure and privilege of working closely with Dr. Argenta during our tenure at the University of Michigan. He truly is a pioneer in tissue expansion surgery, both in innovative patient care and in research. This chapter is a culmination of what probably represents more experience with tissue expansion than anyone. The author draws from his experience and gives his preferences for several of the details related to performing tissue expansion. The chapter is divided into facial units and expansion related to those units and therefore is very easy to read.

As stated in the chapter, there are multiple choices for tissue expanders. Dr. Argenta gives his preference, and the readers should experiment and use their own. After having consulted with Dr. Argenta on patients, I agree with his comment that multiple small expanders, especially on the scalp, often give a superior result to one large expander. He also believes that galeal incisions, performed conservatively and judiciously, can benefit stretch in areas limited by this facia.

The author discusses expansion of skin for skin grafting and harvesting. This gives a larger area for the graft and easier closure of the donor site. This is especially true for total eyelid reconstruction with expanded skin grafting. This apparently does not have enough stretch-back or contraction of the graft to be a

problem. His comment on using phenol for pigmentary problems on the grafts is interesting. I would use this very cautiously because phenol can cause complete bleaching. He mentioned "dilute phenol." The reader should remember that phenol, unlike trichloracetic and other acids, gets stronger in its ability to penetrate as the dilution decreases.

The discussion of nasal reconstruction is superb. It complements the chapter on the forehead flap very nicely. I've seen several of the author's total reconstructions of the nose, and his results are excellent.

The chapter does not mention rapid intraoperative tissue expansion. I realize that there is some debate, especially in the plastic surgery literature, as to the actual benefit of rapid expansion. In my hands I have seen benefit beyond what I believe would be tissue creep. It certainly is useful to harvest up to 1 cm of adjacent tissue intraoperatively when one has a very tight closure. Chapter 21 on forehead reconstruction mentions this usefulness. My technique for rapid intraoperative expansion is as follows: I use 15- to 75-ml Foley catheters, usually 30 ml. After testing of the balloon and cutting of the catheter tip, the catheter is slipped through a tunnel from the defect to be closed well into the adjacent skin that is to be used in reconstruction. If I'm doing this in skin that has galea, I often score the galea before insertion of the expander. I will then go through three to four inflation and deflation cycles of approximately 5 minutes. There has been no good study of the effect of inflation and deflation cycling times. In my experience this works as well as longer cycling times. The optimal cycling time may actually be less. The skin is then advanced and sutured in place with polyglactin (vicryl), polydiax-anone (PDS), or permanent nylon or polypropylene (Prolene) buried stitches, and the skin is closed. I sometimes also will suture the advancing edge of the flap approximately 1 to 1.5 cm back from the wound edge into the periosteum or deep structures to guide in the tissue movement and put less tension on the final wound closure. In my experience there has not been a huge amount of stretch-back of the scar. I've seen good results with use of rapid expansion in forehead flap surgery to gain just enough closure to widen the flap and still be able to close the forehead secondary defect. Therefore, although I realize there is controversy, rapid intraoperative expansion may have a role in reconstructive surgery.

24

COMPLICATIONS OF LOCAL FLAPS

Stuart J. Salasche

INTRODUCTION

Complications are a fact of surgery. They are feared, dreaded, and altogether too infrequently discussed.[1-3] Much of the energy that surgeons expend in preoperative evaluations and counseling patients, scrubbing, wearing surgical gloves and gown, and draping the patient becomes so routine we tend to forget that all this activity is aimed solely at the prevention of complications.[4-8] Despite all our precautions, complications can still occur. It is our responsibility to recognize, manage, and ultimately prevent their occurrence. This chapter will be devoted to these concerns.

Flaps are vulnerable to the same adverse conditions that jeopardize simpler wound closures, only more so. They are more precarious because, once elevated, survival of the isolated peninsula of tissue depends on the blood supply channeled through the pedicle. Accordingly the effects of excessive tension on the wound edges, blood under the flap, or contamination with bacteria become evident sooner and are more devastating than with simpler closures. Also, the stakes are higher because the best available skin is committed to the flap reconstruction. Any error or failure represents a loss of the repair of choice.

In addition to being concerned with the classic complications of necrosis, infection, hematoma, and dehiscence, the surgeon must also be concerned with flap design and the influence that tension vectors will generate on the free margins of the face. How will the intricate scar lines be camouflaged and how will they lie in relationship to the esthetic units and junction lines of the face? All these factors must be considered in the creation of a local flap.

What follows is a patient-oriented approach to the recognition and management of complications of local flaps. Although surgical complications may cause the surgeon stress, worry, guilt, a damaged ego, and even legal problems, it is ultimately the patient's well-being that matters most.

FLAP NECROSIS

The viability of any flap depends on its blood supply. It is almost axiomatic that acutely raised flaps, because of their sole dependence on the pedicle blood flow, are in an inherently vulnerable state.[9] This is especially applicable to the most distal portion of the flap.[3,10,11] Blood reaches the skin through musculocutaneous arteries or deep subcutaneous (septocutaneous or axial) vessels, which ultimately supply the critical subdermal plexus (Fig. 24-1). The deep subcutaneous vessels course just above and parallel to the musculofascial plane.[12-16] Examples are the superficial temporal or supraorbital vessels. On the other hand, the subdermal plexus resides in the upper subcutaneous fat just beneath the reticular dermis. During undermining on the face to raise a local flap, a thin layer of subcutaneous fat must be preserved to maintain the integrity of this plexus. These vessels represent the critical nutrient supply of the skin and likewise of any random flap. The distal portion of an axial flap trimmed of its subcutaneous fat is functionally random.

For each local flap there is a critical flap length beyond which the perfusion of the distal flap is compromised. This varies with the anatomic site, age of the patient, amount of actinic damage of the skin, status of the vasculature, and other factors. The temptation to widely undermine the pedicle to increase mobility and flexibility of the flap should be avoided because this increases the distance that blood must flow to the distal portion of the flap. On the other hand, widening of the pedicle will not always ensure the survival of a long flap.[12] A long flap with a widened base may have acquired only a parallel series of vessels, each of which still only reaches a finite distance along the linear axis of the flap and does not extend to the distal tip (Fig. 24-2). It may be more prudent to mobilize a thicker flap that contains the deeper subcutaneous vessels and, if needed, thin the flap later as a secondary revision.

Figure 24-1   Vascular anatomy of skin.

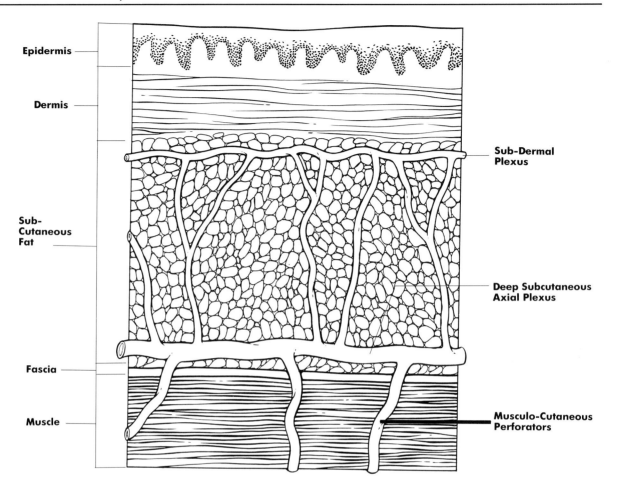

Epidermis

Dermis

Sub-Cutaneous Fat

Fascia

Muscle

Sub-Dermal Plexus

Deep Subcutaneous Axial Plexus

Musculo-Cutaneous Perforators

A newly created flap must overcome numerous perils over the first critical day or two. The flap must be designed to ensure sufficient perfusion pressure of the vessels in the most distal subdermal plexus.[17] This is especially critical during the vasoconstriction caused initially by local anesthesia with epinephrine and subsequently by a combination of factors.[18,19] These include the catecholamines (norepinephrine) released from the severed sympathetic nerves cut during incision of the flap. Thromboxane A, released from the platelet microthrombi, is another potent vasoconstrictor. The situation is compounded by other active mediators related to early wound healing events such as the quinines and prostaglandins. These may initiate edema that further compromises vascular flow by increasing vascular resistance as hemoconcentration occurs. Oxygen free radicals may damage endothelial surfaces, causing microthrombi and further vascular compromise.[20-22] Most flaps survive these treacherous first few days and become stabilized as neovascularization occurs from the undersurface of the flap. When this neovascularization takes place, the flap becomes less dependent on the pedicle's blood supply.[12,23-25]

On the other hand, not all flaps survive. Any one of a number of events may further compromise the already precarious blood supply to the distal flap, thus causing ischemia and cell death. The most critical of these factors is excessive tension on the wound edges.[9,26-28] Exaggerated tension may develop from tying the sutures too tightly, insufficient undermining and tissue mobilization, and expansion secondary to a hematoma or infection-related edema. The type of flap also determines the tension on the distal flap. Transposition flaps, on the whole, generate less distal tension than rotation or advancement flaps.[29] With transposition flaps, the secondary defect is closed first. Accordingly, most of the tension is diverted to this closure and thus the body of the flap is "pushed" into place under relatively little stress (Fig. 24-3). To the contrary, rotation and advancement flaps are "pulled" into place, and most of the tension is placed at the most distant segment of the flap. Because of this innate tension distribution, these latter types of flaps are at increased risk for necrosis. Multiple, strategically oriented subcuticular sutures along the secondary defect closure line can help alleviate distal tension on these flaps.

Figure 24-2   Widening pedicle does not increase distal flap perfusion, but increasing thickness of flap to include deeper, larger vessels does.

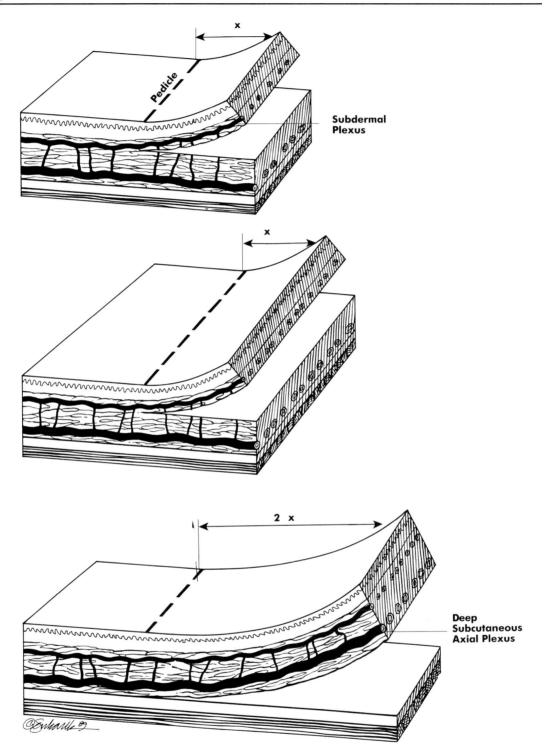

Figure 24-3   Transposition flap above is "pushed" into place when secondary defect is closed *(arrow)*, while rotation flap below tends to "pull" back to its original position. (Modified from Salasche SJ, Grabski WA: *Flaps of the central face,* New York, 1990, Churchill Livingstone.)

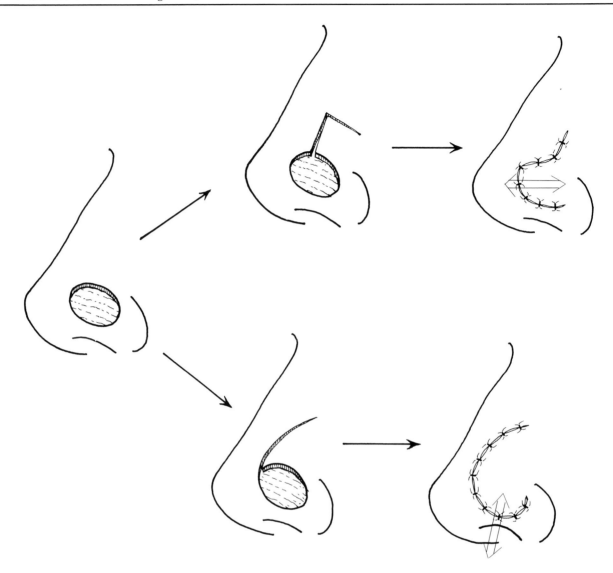

Blood supply to a local flap may also be jeopardized by a number of events. Examples are undermining too superficially, undermining too far under the pedicle, or design of a flap with an excessive length (Fig. 24-4). A large standing cutaneous deformity may kink the pedicle and strangulate the incoming vessels, cutting off blood supply. Care should be taken not to remove standing cutaneous deformities in a manner that will cut into the pedicle and compromise blood flow. Overzealous use of compression dressings may tip a precarious flap over the edge. Dressings should be constructed to compress and immobilize the wound, not strangulate it.[30] This is especially applicable to those flaps over convex surfaces with rigid understructures, such as the nasal tip or the helical rim of the ear.

The margins of the flap should bleed freely before being sewn into place. Hemostasis of these margins should be pinpoint and not heavy-handed. After final placement, the flap should remain pink and respond to digital compression with rapid blanching and subsequent immediate capillary refill and rapid return of color when pressure is released. If arterial insufficiency occurs, pallor of the flap supervenes. As varying depth and degree of cell death occur, mottled shades of gray, slate gray, and blue-gray occur until finally a black slough appears. During this sequence of events, blanching and refill become progressively prolonged until these maneuvers can no longer be elicited.[2,17]

Once it is evident that the flap is in danger of failure, there is an overwhelming desire on the part of the

Figure 24-4   *A*, Cheek advancement flap at limit of safe length-to-width ratio. Flap appears to be sutured under excessive wound-closure tension. *B*, Distal necrosis and dehiscence with poor healing of wound edges.

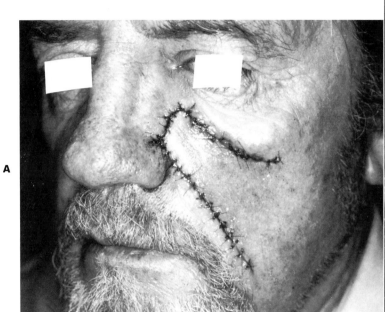
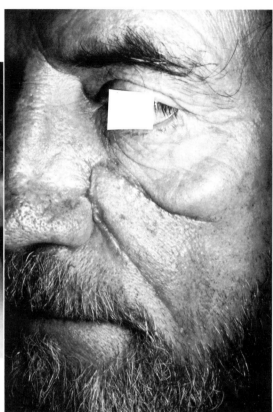

surgeon to do something to alter the declining course. Numerous approaches have been tried both experimentally and clinically with this aim in mind. Included are vasodilators, prostaglandins, calcium antagonists, endothelial cell growth factors, thromboxane blockade, hyperbaric oxygen, and free radical scavengers (allopurinol, superoxide dismutase), with only mixed to little effect on the eventual outcome.[20,31-40] It seems that the only consistently efficacious maneuver is to delay the flap. This is obviously helpful only in retrospect once the process of necrosis has been established. However, sometimes it is obvious during the actual surgical procedure that the chance of flap survival is marginal. A prudent approach would be to allow the flap to fall back into its original bed and delay the final closure for 1 or 2 weeks.

Flaps in the process of dying proceed through a sequence that includes ischemia, cell death, superficial or full-thickness eschar formation, separation of the eschar, and finally, healing by second intention.[2] The final result will depend on the anatomic location of the slough as well as its depth and extent. It is probably best to resist the temptation for active intervention and to just allow events to take their natural course.

Specifically, debridement should be delayed until after final demarcation has taken place and separation of the eschar has begun on its own. Otherwise, additional normal tissue may be injured. The eschar acts as a biologic dressing under which healing takes place. The time course of these events is variable, but may be prolonged, ranging from 2 to 3 weeks. Patients need ongoing support and assessment of their progress, prognosis, and timing of any subsequent surgical revisions. Depending on the depth and extent of the insult, scar revision may be required when healing is complete.

Smoking as a Cause of Flap Necrosis

It is imperative to know whether the patient smokes when a flap is being considered as a reconstructive modality. The risk of some degree of necrosis to the proposed flap is greatly increased with smoking, especially if the patient smokes a pack of cigarettes or more a day. Active high-level smokers develop necrosis three times more frequently than nonsmokers and low-level smokers (less than one pack a day). Furthermore, the extent and depth of the slough are more severe.[41]

Cigarette smoke deleteriously affects the cutaneous blood supply by at least two interrelated mechanisms.[41-45] The first mechanism involves nicotine, which causes systemic vasoconstriction through activation of the adrenergic nervous system. This vasoconstriction can be intense and subsequently may lower the tissue oxygenation pressure by more than 50%. The result is decreased tissue perfusion and oxygenation significant enough to threaten flap viability. The above occurs within 10 minutes of smoking a cigarette and lasts approximately 50 minutes. The second mechanism involves carbon monoxide, which causes systemic tissue hypoxia by competition with oxygen for hemoglobin-binding sites. This situation is compounded because carbon monoxide has a higher affinity for hemoglobin than oxygen, and therefore high levels of carboxyhemoglobin are produced. With nicotine and carbon monoxide present in the inhaled cigarette smoke, it is not difficult to understand why local tissue oxygenation can become compromised while a heavy smoker is awake.[44]

Once a history of heavy smoking is elicited, several choices become apparent. The surgeon may choose a less risky form of repair, such as side-to-side closure, healing by second intention, delayed closure, or a split thickness graft (full-thickness grafts share similar risk factors with flaps). Another option is to ensure that the patient has a 48-hour smoke-free period before surgery, which greatly improves the local tissue oxygenation. So if the patient reliably can stop smoking for 2 days before surgery and 7 days after surgery, flap reconstruction is much less hazardous.[41] Unfortunately, a high-stress situation such as an impending or just-completed surgery does not lend itself well to drastic behavior modification. Despite good intentions longtime heavy smokers are not always reliable about quitting smoking.

Case Examples

CASE 1

An otherwise healthy 42-year-old man underwent Mohs micrographic surgery for a morpheaform basal cell carcinoma of the tip of his nose. The tumor proved to be quite invasive and involved the perichondrium of the lower lateral cartilages. The tumor-free defect measured 14 × 13 mm and encompassed almost the entire esthetic subunit of the tip of the nose (Fig. 24-5**A**). A large expanse of denuded tip-defining cartilage was exposed, although the underlying cartilage itself was undisturbed.

A bilobe flap was transposed into the defect under seemingly little tension, but at the end of the procedure it was noted that the distal portion of the flap was pale (Fig. 24-5**B**). The remainder of the flap remained pink.

Figure 24-5 *A*, **Postoperative defect involving skin of entire nasal tip with exposure of cartilage.** *B*, **Note blanched appearance of distal flap.** *C*, **Flap 5 days after surgical repair.** *D*, **Flap at 6 months postoperative.**

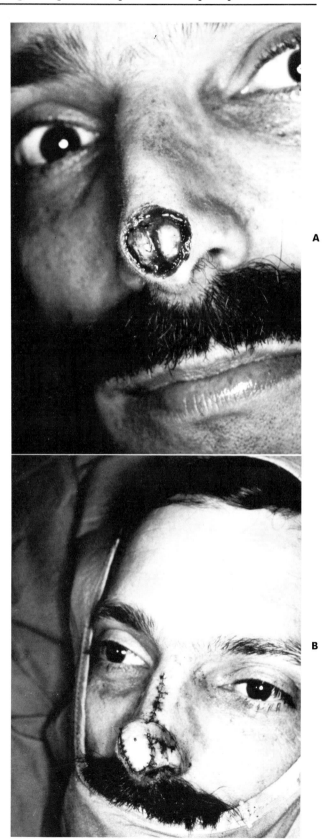

Figure 24-5, cont'd   For legend see opposite page.

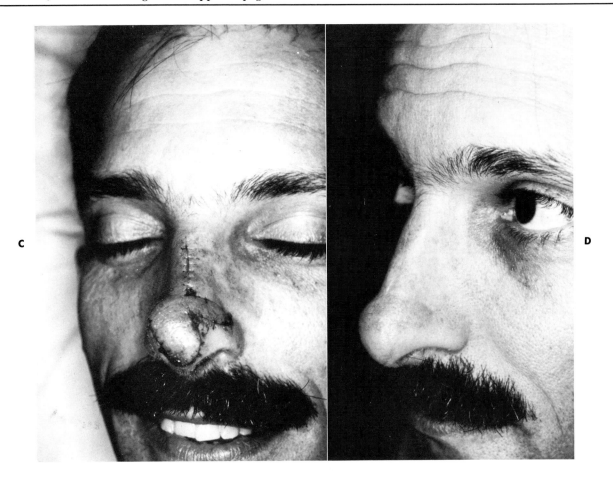

It was possible that the blanching was due to the effects of epinephrine or the local anesthesia, coupled with the effects of a thin flap draped over a convex, unyielding cartilage. The dilemma arose whether to consider the flap compromised and return it to its original position for delay or to just monitor it.

The latter approach was taken. No dressing other than an antibiotic ointment and a loosely draped nonadherent pad was placed over the repair. Later that evening the patient reported by phone that the flap not only had "pinked up" but also was bleeding slightly from the furthest suture line. At the time of suture removal, the entire flap was viable and somewhat edematous and responded well to compression with rapid blanching and refill (Fig. 24-5**C**). After several months edema improved, resulting in good contour and color and an overall pleasing result (Fig. 24-5**D**).

CASE 2

A 62-year-old woman with extensive actinic damage underwent microscopically controlled excision of a recurrent squamous cell carcinoma of the helix of the ear. She took no medications other than antacids. Portions of the underlying cartilage were sacrificed to obtain a tumor-free plane (Fig. 24-6**A**). The defect was repaired with an inferiorly based advancement flap that was mobilized by making a full-thickness incision in the scapha (Fig. 24-6**B**). A head-wrap compressive dressing was constructed and allowed to remain in place for 3 days. When the patient returned for a dressing change and wound check, the distal portion of the flap had an ominous gray-black color (Fig. 24-6**C**). While contemplating what had gone wrong and what to do next, the color spontaneously reverted to normal over a 15-minute period and actually became somewhat hyperemic (Fig. 24-6**D**). Healing then progressed normally, and the long-term result was excellent (Fig. 24-6**E**).

This case, as well as the previous one, points out how many factors relate to flap survival, even seemingly innocuous items such as wound dressings.

Figure 24-6   *A,* Postoperative defect of helical rim. *B,* Inferior based advancement flap. *C,* Apparent flap necrosis. *D,* Several minutes after removal of compression dressing. *E,* Healing 4 months postoperatively.

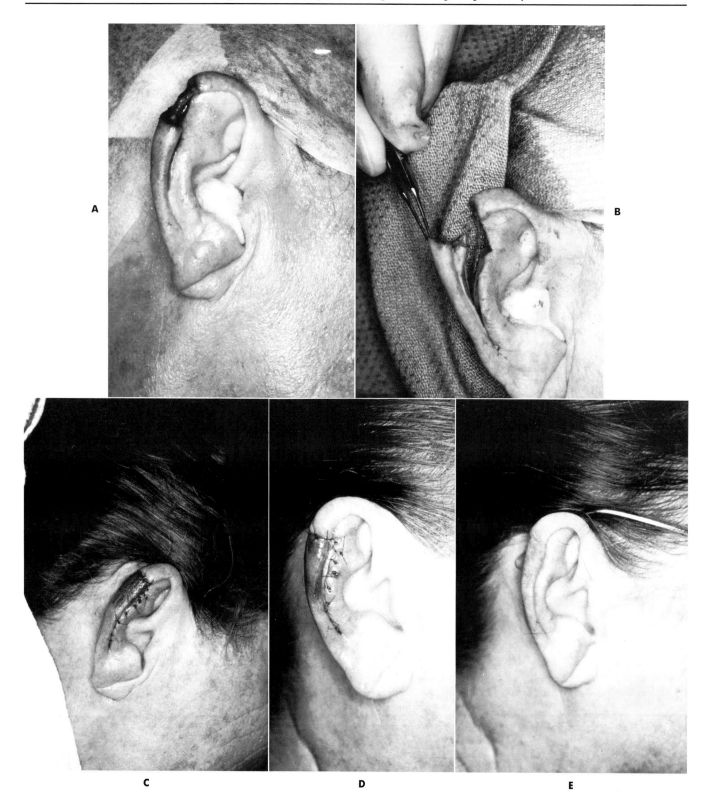

CASE 3

An 80-year-old woman with a history of several previous skin cancers underwent surgery to remove a skin cancer of the left cheek. The defect was repaired with a rhombic transposition flap (Fig. 24-7**A**). Two years later she developed a large recurrent basal cell carcinoma of the left cheek. Tumor margins were controlled with frozen sections, and the postoperative defect measured 53 × 38 mm (Fig. 24-7**B**). Undermining and attempts at primary closure resulted in distortion of the nostril as well as excessive wound-closure tension (Fig. 24-7**C**). An inferiorly based rotation flap was raised (Fig. 24-7**D**), but it soon became evident that this was ill-advised because of the prior rhombic flap, which appeared to compromise the vascularity of the

rotation flap. The scar from the rhombic flap and the wound-closure tension made movement of the flap extremely difficult. Rather than compound a bad situation, the flap was returned to its bed, and a full-thickness skin graft from the supraclavicular area was harvested and sewn into the surgical defect (Fig. 24-7**E**). The ultimate long-term outcome was satisfactory (Fig. 24-7**F**).

This case illustrates two points. The first is not to use a previously operated on, scarred site as donor tissue for a flap if it is possible to use other tissue. The other point is to resist the urge to try to fix everything at once. Placing a flap under excessive tension, extending the pedicle, or backcutting it to increase mobility may just aggravate an already precarious situation.

Figure 24-7   *A,* **Cheek defect and rhombic transposition flap designed to repair wound.** *B,* **Defect of cheek after removal of recurrent basal cell carcinoma.** *C,* **Attempt at primary closure distorts ala nasi.** *D,* **Rotation flap elevated.**

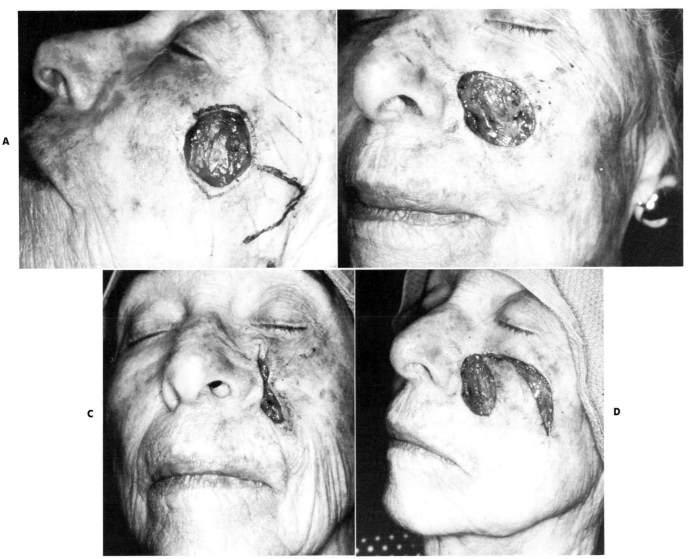

Continued.

Figure 24-7, cont'd *E,* Flap is returned to original bed, and defect is closed with full-thickness skin graft. *F,* Result 9 months after skin grafting.

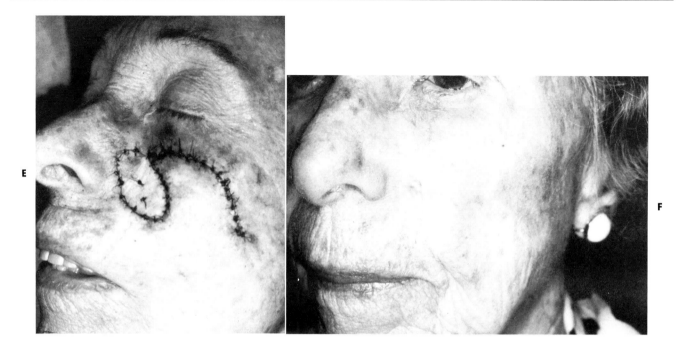

CASE 4

After removal of a recurrent basal cell carcinoma from the malar eminence of a 64-year-old man, the defect was closed with a rotation flap from the cheek (Fig. 24-8**A**). Three days after the operation he returned to the clinic expressing concern about the swelling and discoloration of his eyelid (Fig. 24-8**B**). He was reassured that the eyelid edema and ecchymosis were relatively common and harmless sequelae of the surgical procedure. However, the color changes to blue and gray within the flap indicated that all or a portion of the flap might be lost. After 1 week of conservative management consisting of observation and dressing changes, it became apparent that only a superficial slough of skin had occurred (Fig. 24-8**C**). Daily cleansing with hydrogen peroxide and application of an antibiotic ointment led to rapid reepithelialization of the wound. Fig. 24-8**D** shows the area of the wound 3 months postoperatively.

The lesson in this case is that it is not always possible to predict the extent and depth of necrosis of a flap once vascular compromise has occurred. The best approach is to share your concerns with the patient, see the patient in a supportive manner as often as required, and attend to the wound conservatively and cautiously. In this case the lack of active intervention was rewarded by limited death of the epidermis and papillary dermis. Both these entities regenerated completely, and the outcome was virtually as if the slough had not occurred.

Figure 24-8 *A,* Rotation flap of cheek.

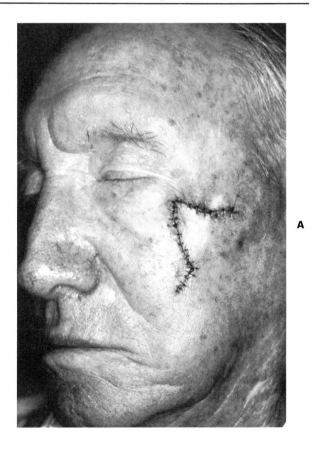

Figure 24-8, cont'd   *B,* Eyelid edema and ecchymosis with disky-colored flap. *C,* Superficial necrosis. *D,* Healing 3 months postoperatively.

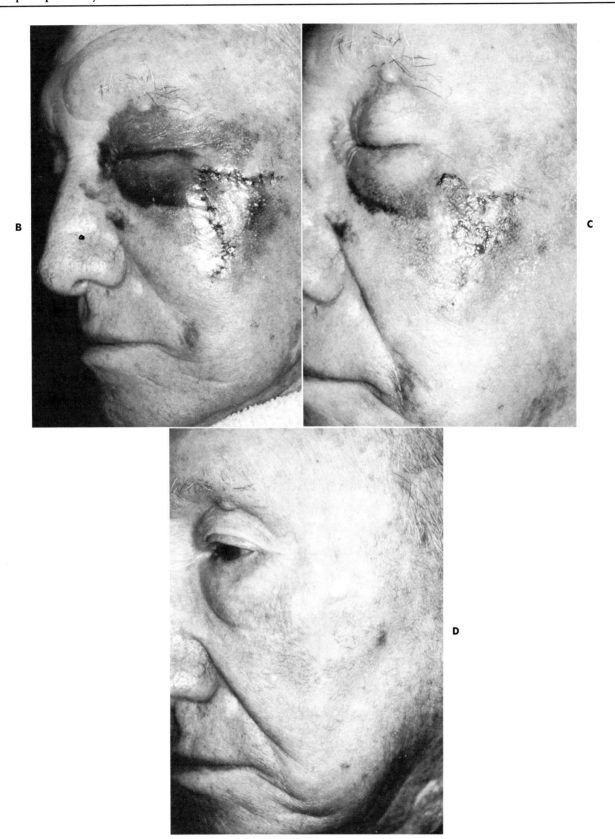

CASE 5

A 57-year-old woman underwent excision of a large primary morpheaform basal cell carcinoma of her forehead by Mohs micrographic surgical technique. The surgical defect was repaired with an inferiorly based rotation flap, which was intended to take advantage of the excess skin of the temple (Fig. 24-9**A**). The flap was rotated into place under some tension, as was evident from the distal pallor (Fig. 24-9**B**). At suture removal a slate gray area at the most distal flap tip indicated imminent necrosis of this area. Zones of superficial skin loss were already evident along the upper suture line (Fig. 24-9**C**). Two weeks postoperatively a thick eschar had formed, indicating full-thickness necrosis of the tip (Fig. 24-9**D**). Healing progressed slowly by second intention, ultimately forming an unsightly hypertrophic scar, which responded to intralesional injections of corticosteroids (Fig. 24-9**E** and **F**).

Figure 24-9   *A*, Rotation flap design to repair postoperative defect of lateral forehead. *B*, Distal pallor of flap. *C*, Impending necrosis of flap tip. *D*, Full-thickness necrosis. *E*, Thickened scar that healed by second intention. *F*, Outcome at 5 months. (*B* and *D* reprinted by permission of the publisher from Salasche SJ, Grabski WJ: Complications of flaps, *J Dermatol Surg Oncol* 17:132–40, copyright 1991 by Elsevier Science Publishing Co, Inc.)

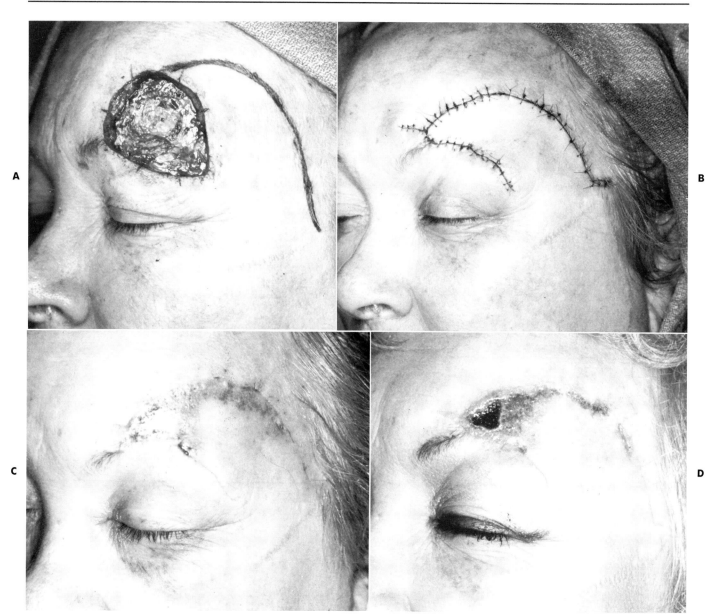

Figure 24-9, cont'd   For legend see opposite page.

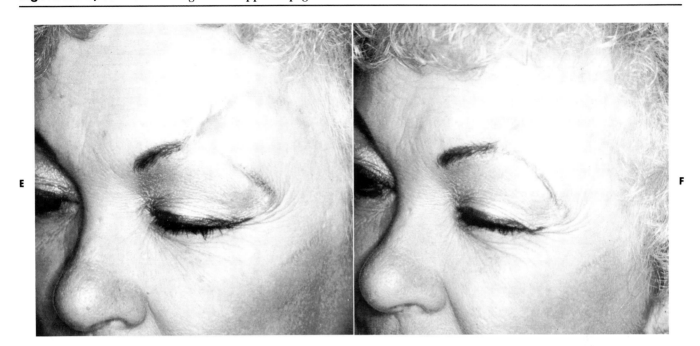

This case and the similarly fated transposition flap illustrated in Fig. 24-10 clearly demonstrate the need to drape the flap into the surgical defect with no tension on the wound edges and at the same time to ensure that there is sufficient intravascular pressure to nourish the most distal portion of the flap. It may take as long as a week to demarcate the portion of a flap that is vascularly compromised, although this is usually apparent within 48 hours. Healing beneath the escar, which forms in the area of flap necrosis, is a slow process that takes several weeks to be completed. During this time the patient must be constantly reassured and prepared for the subsequent stages of recovery until final resolution of the healing process is achieved. Following complete healing, it is often necessary to perform scar revisions and other refinements of the wound because of loss of portions of the flap.

Figure 24-10   *A,* Large transposition flap from neck. Note pallor of flap. *B,* Necrosis of flap 4 weeks postoperatively. (Courtesy Shan R. Baker, M.D.)

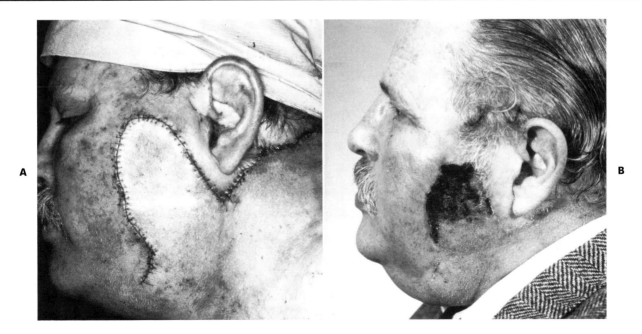

CASE 6

A 39-year-old man underwent Mohs micrographic surgery for a primary morpheaform basal cell carcinoma of his right cutaneous upper lip. The transversely oriented 18 × 10 mm defect extended from the melolabial fold to the right philtral crest (Fig. 24-11**A**). A superiorly based interpolation flap was designed, elevated, and transferred into the defect (Fig. 24-11**B**). It soon became evident that the distal portion of the flap that had been inset had necrosed (Fig. 24-11**C**). Subsequent scar revision was required (Fig. 24-11**D**).

There are no hard-and-fast rules when the surgeon considers the length of a random flap in relationship to the pedicle width. However, in this case, unless the angular artery had been included, it is apparent that the flap was too long for safe transfer without initial delay. The pedicle was also kinked, adding to the stress on the blood supply.

Figure 24-11 *A*, **Postoperative defect of upper lip and proposed interpolation flap.** *B*, **Long flap is transposed into place.** (*A* and *B* courtesy John Adnot, M.D.) *C*, **Necrosis of flap.** *D*, **Healing, with resultant hypertrophic scar and standing cutaneous deformity.** (*C* and *D* courtesy John Adnot, M.D.)

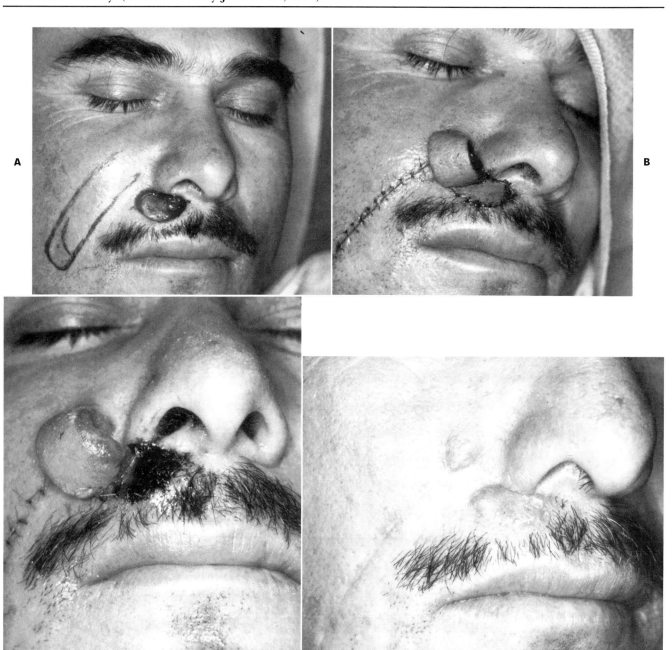

INFECTION

Fortunately, wound infections involving flaps of the head and neck are uncommon. Much of this has to do with a combined practice of aseptic and proper surgical techniques.[5-8] Equally important is the incredibly rich blood supply of the region. Well-vascularized tissue is very resistant to infection.[14,15,46,47] However, when infections do occur, they can have a devastating effect on the final outcome of the procedure. Necrosis of all or part of the flap may ensue. The flap may dehisce, or the final scar may widen or thicken. On occasion systemic dissemination of infection may supervene.

A wound infection exists when a sufficient number of microbial organisms are present in the wound to overcome the host's natural defenses. In the body's attempt to combat an incipient infection, an inflammatory reaction rich in white cells is created.[2,48,49] This inflammatory environment is toxic and is mitigated by the release of polymorphonuclear leukocyte–related proteolytic enzymes as well as by the production of oxygen free radicals. This toxic milieu interferes with normal wound healing so that collagen production and deposition are disrupted to such a degree that neither flap adhesion to the wound bed nor development of adequate wound tensile strength occurs. The absorbable dermal sutures are also subject to the same destructive enzymes. It is no wonder that dehiscence of the flap is a frequent sequela of wound infection.

Clinically the signs and symptoms of an early wound infection are exaggerated versions of those occurring with normal wound healing.[2,49-51] Most early wounds display mild edema and erythema, and the patient experiences discomfort. When these signs and symptoms become magnified or when variable degrees of tenderness, pain, or purulent exudate supervene, a diagnosis of wound infection should be made or suspected (Fig. 24-12). Before a systemic regimen of antibiotics is initiated, a culture and sensitivity should be obtained from the wound bed or any purulent drainage coming from the wound. Gram stain of the discharge may prove invaluable in selection of the proper class of antibiotic before the results of the culture are available. A recurring dilemma always arises as to the disposition of the still intact sutures. Should they be removed or not? Sutures do not initiate a wound infection, but they may potentiate it by interfering with normal host defenses. For example, infected tissue is already swollen and edematous. Unyielding sutures may further constrict and compromise the tissue gathered within its loops. This ischemic, devitalized tissue is less able to resist infection. In addition, as a foreign body, sutures add to the inflammatory response.

How to proceed depends on the timing of the initial

Figure 24-12   Erythema, edema, and exudate on fifth postoperative day. Pain also was present.

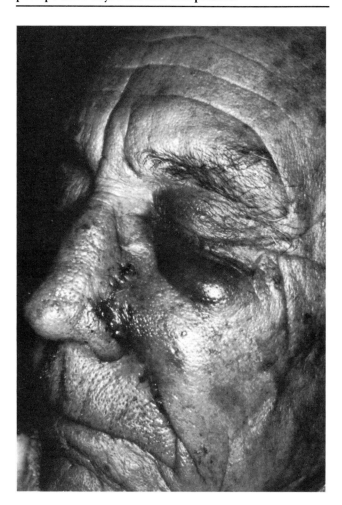

presentation and the magnitude of the signs and symptoms of the infection. Clinical symptoms of a wound infection usually appear between the third and sixth postoperative days. If, for example, the patient has increased tenderness and erythema at the surgical site on the third or fourth day, it may be wise to initiate antibiotic therapy (after culture of the suture line) and to allow the sutures to remain intact 1 or 2 days longer to observe the clinical course. If the diagnosis of infection is evident, however, the sutures should be removed and the incision site supported with surface antitension adhesive strips. If there is purulent discharge, the primary therapeutic approach is to address the drainage while initiating a systemic regimen of antibiotics.[52] A wick composed of plain or iodoform-impregnated gauze stripping should be inserted into the wound and subsequently replaced every day or every other day until the drainage has ceased (Fig. 24-13).[2] The area of dehiscence through which the wick is placed will need to heal by second intention but will probably require a scar revision. Surface antiten-

Figure 24-13   **Wick is changed daily until discharge ceases.**

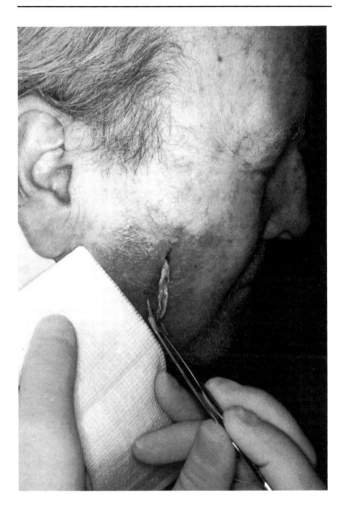

sion adhesive strips should be placed on any nonde-hisced portion of the flap to preserve what is left of flap fixation.

The best prophylaxis for wound infection is prevention. This is generally accomplished by a combination of practicing aseptic and proper surgical techniques. The former deters bacterial contamination through antiseptic preparation of the surgical site. This is accomplished by antiseptic solutions, scrubbing, wearing surgical gloves and gown, draping the patient, and use of sterile instruments. On the other hand, the proper operative technique helps protect the tissue and keep it vitalized. This is accomplished by gentle handling of tissue, attaining hemostasis with minimal char, undermining sufficiently at the proper level, and using appropriately chosen suture material tied without excess tension. There is no question that crushed, charred, poorly vascularized tissue is more prone to become infected.

The role of prophylactic antibiotics in the prevention of wound infection remains controversial and will likely remain so until a prospective, controlled study is done.[53,54] As a general rule, I reserve the use of prophylactic antibiotics to clinical situations where their use seems to make some empirical sense. Examples include use in immunocompromised and diabetic patients. Prophylactic antibiotics are also prescribed when an extremely long procedure is anticipated, such as Mohs micrographic surgery, or when reconstruction is to be delayed 1 or 2 days. Each surgeon must develop his or her own set of criteria. To be of any value, the antibiotic needs to be at the tissue level ahead of time, awaiting any bacteria that may be introduced during surgery. This means the antibiotic should be administered orally the day before surgery or parenterally a few hours before the inception of surgery. Otherwise, the bacteria are quickly sealed off from the antibiotic by wound coagulum.[51] Realistically, the antibiotic should be continued for 2 or 3 days postoperatively.

Case Examples

CASE 1

A 59-year-old man underwent excisional surgery of a primary basal cell carcinoma of the root and upper dorsum of his nose (Fig. 24-14**A**). A dorsal nasal flap was used to reconstruct the defect under virtually no wound-closure tension (Fig. 24-14**B**). When he returned for suture removal on the fifth postoperative day, the flap and the surrounding area were erythematous and tender to touch (Fig. 24-14**C**). Although not copious, pus was noted in the suture line as well as on the undersurface of the dressing. Gram stain of the exudate revealed many gram-positive cocci in clusters. A presumptive diagnosis of *Staphylococcus aureus* wound infection was made. The sutures were removed, and the patient was started on an oral regimen of full-dose dicloxacillin. Wound management consisted of daily wet compresses with hydrogen peroxide–soaked gauze sponges. This allowed for relatively pain-free debridement of the caked exudate and crusts, which formed from the infection (Fig. 24-14**D**).

A culture confirmed the presence of a staphylococcal infection as well as its sensitivity to the selected penicillin drug. The drug dose was doubled on the 10th postoperative day because the purulent exudate persisted and was having a deleterious effect on the flap surface (Fig. 24-14**E**). By the end of the second week both the discharge and the inflammation had abated completely. Subsequent healing was uneventful, and the eventual outcome bore no evidence of the infection (Fig. 24-14**F**).

On reflection, there was no evident break in aseptic technique or unusual handling of the tissue in this case. However, as infrequent as infections may be in surgical practice, each instance should generate a procedural reassessment. Are there new people on the surgical team who may be nasal carriers of pathogenic bacteria? Have any of the regular members of operative team developed a source of infection, such as an acute paronychia? Are aseptic precautions being strictly adhered to or becoming lax?

Figure 24-14 *A*, Postoperative defect. *B*, Transposition flap from glabella. *C*, Erythema on fifth postoperative day. Tenderness also was present. *D*, Purulent discharge and crusts.

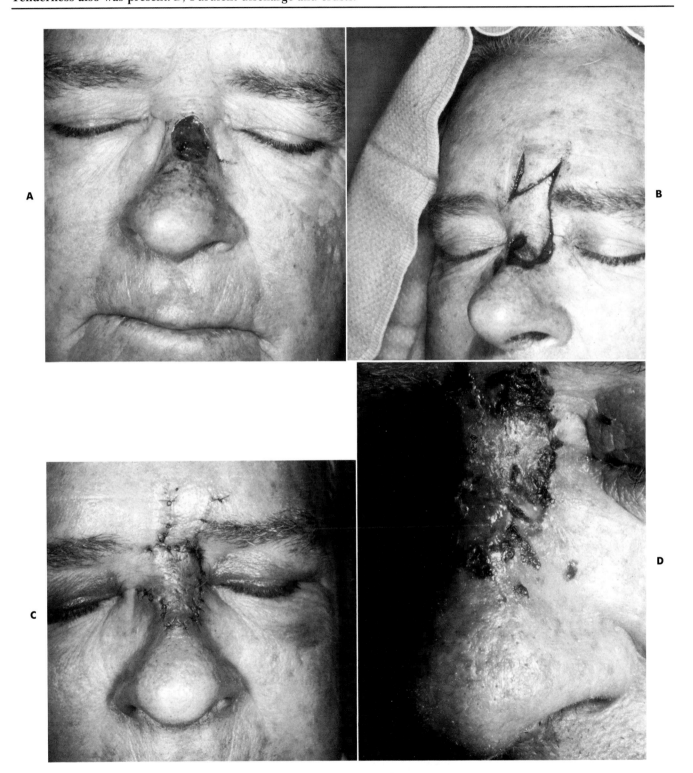

Figure 24-14, cont'd *E,* Severe infection. *F,* Eventual healing, with no apparent ill effects.

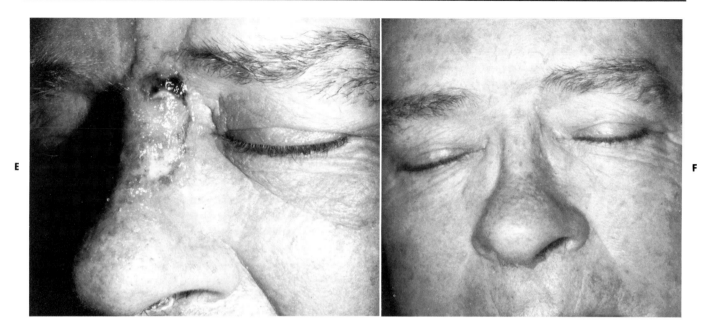

E   F

CASE 2

A 70-year-old man underwent multiple surgical procedures to remove skin cancers related to chronic solar damage. He was receiving antihypertensive medications as well as CAMA and dipyridamole (Persantine) for prevention of transient ischemic episodes. Use of the last two medications was temporarily discontinued 1 week before surgery.

A recurrent basal cell carcinoma of the left upper lip was treated with micrographically controlled surgery. The resulting 12 × 6 mm defect extended from the nasal sill to the vermilion-cutaneous border and involved the left philtral crest (Fig. 24-15**A**). The junction lines that outlined the anatomic subunits of the upper lip were drawn. A bilateral advancement flap was constructed by incision along these lines and undermining in the plane just above the orbicularis oris muscle (Fig. 24-15**B**). The final result was somewhat distorted, mostly due to postoperative edema and a previous surgical procedure that involved removal of most of the right ala nasi (Fig. 24-15**C**).

The patient returned to the clinic approximately 5 hours after surgery complaining of swelling, pressure under the dressing, and bleeding. The vermilion and upper lip were grossly swollen and tense, causing strain on the suture line (Fig. 24-15**D**). The area was immediately anesthetized and prepared. The sutures were removed, and the wound was opened to reveal a fresh blood clot and active bleeding from multiple sites (Fig.

24-15**E**). The offending vessels were cauterized, and the wound bed was flushed with sterile saline. After the flap was sewn back into place, the patient was started on a regimen of a broad-spectrum cephalosporin antibiotic (Fig. 24-15**F**).

On postoperative day 5, the patient complained of renewed tenderness and reported the onset of a purulent discharge that morning (Fig. 24-15**G**). Subsequently a single strain of penicillinase-resistant *S. aureus* was cultured. Unfortunately, the organism was not sensitive to the empirically selected cephalosporin he had been given earlier. Sutures were removed, and despite surface antitension adhesive strips the lower limb of the flap promptly dehisced (Fig. 24-15**H**). The infection responded promptly to methicillin, but the wound healed slowly by second intention. At 4 months the vermilion was retracted upward and a raised, thickened scar remained to mark the vertical portion of the flap (Fig. 24-15**I**).

This series of events underscores the need for meticulous intraoperative hemostasis. The sequence of postoperative bleeding with hematoma formation, infection, dehiscence, and poor cosmetic outcome was probably preventable by a more compulsive search for potential bleeding sites. Exposed, frayed orbicularis oris muscle fibers are particularly prone to become the site of delayed bleeding. It seems that the constricting effect of epinephrine is able to prevent active bleeding from cut muscle vessels for several hours. When the vasoconstrictive effect subsides several hours later, the vessels dilate and the newly formed platelet plugs are dislodged. This delayed bleeding is no doubt aided by the extreme mobility of the perioral region. Despite seemingly adequate dressings and instructions to the contrary, it is difficult for the patient to completely refrain from talking, smiling, and laughing.

In this case the blood in the wound, the unscheduled second operation, and the tissue manipulation that required a second set of sutures all no doubt cumulatively heightened the susceptibility to infection.

Figure 24-15   *A*, **Defect after removal of recurrent basal cell carcinoma.** *B*, **Bilateral advancement flaps.** *C*, **Flaps in place.** *D*, **Hematoma occurs under flap.**

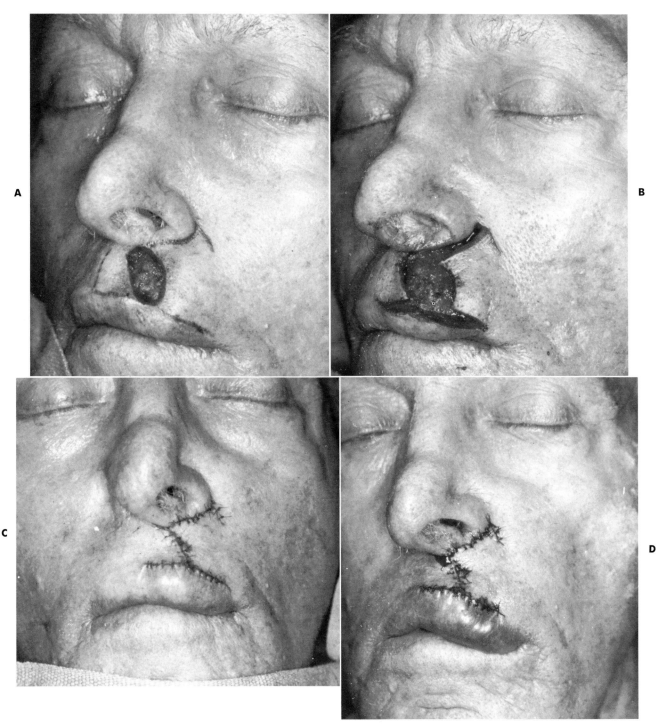

Continued.

Figure 24-15, cont'd   *E*, Sutures are removed, and hematoma is evacuated. *F*, Flaps are resutured into place. *G*, Signs of infection appear on fifith postoperative day.

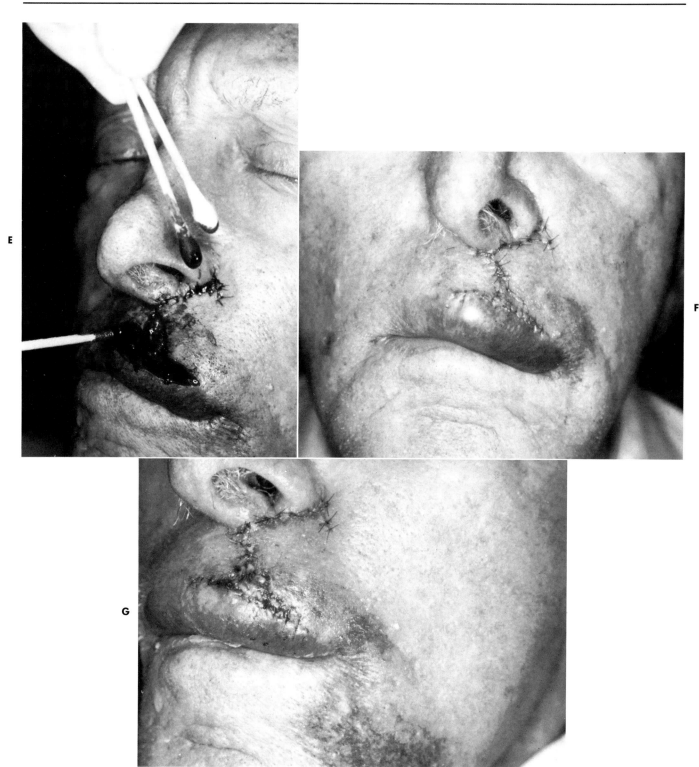

Figure 24-15, cont'd   *H,* **Dehiscence of lower portion of flaps after suture removal.** *I,* **Poor outcome, with thickened scar and ectropion of vermilion.**

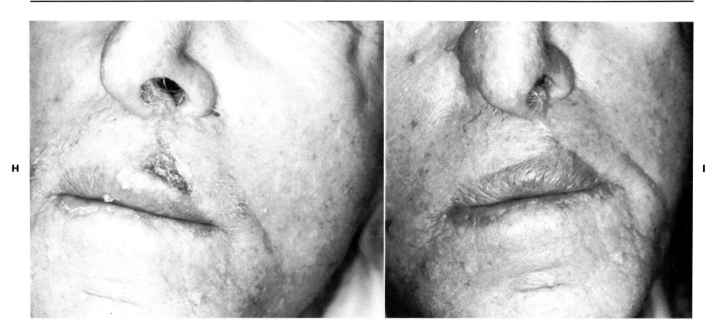

H   I

BLEEDING PROBLEMS

Bleeding-related problems are usually avoidable. When they occur, they can often be attributed to inattention to details such as inadequate intraoperative hemostasis, failure to illicit a history of medications that might interfere with clotting, or failure to ensure that the patient understood about limitations on postoperative activities. Generally patients will bring a genetic problem with bleeding to the physician's attention without provocation.[55] However, unless sought for and worked up with appropriate laboratory studies, more subtle clotting deficiencies might elude a casual history taking.[4] A bleeding dyscrasia is often attendant to many systemic diseases, especially renal failure, liver failure, collagen vascular diseases, and various cancers, particularly those of bone marrow origin.

Medications are the cause of many bleeding problems. It is often possible to discontinue use of anticoagulants several days before surgery with appropriate consultation and coordination with the patient's primary physician.[4,56] In other situations (for example, frequent transient ischemic episodes), this is not prudent and, if a skin cancer must be removed, a less risky repair or a delayed repair may be in order. In a busy clinical practice most drug-related coagulopathies involve the known or occult use of salicylates or nonsteroidal antiinflammatory drugs (NSAIDs).[57,58] Both types of compounds interfere with platelet function by blocking the cyclooxygenase pathway, which mediates the cascade that ultimately leads to platelet aggregation and thrombus formation. Salicylates have a more profound effect because they block the pathway irreversibly for the life span of the platelet. Use of salicylates and NSAIDs should be carefully elicited and, if possible, discontinued a week before surgery. Acetaminophen, which does not interfere with coagulation, is an excellent temporary substitute. As a cautionary note, salicylates are often a hidden component of many cold remedies, hay fever preparations, and other over-the-counter proprietary medications. Their usage may not be identified by a cursory history.

Bleeding and clotting are especially destructive to flap viability. A large potential space is created, encompassing the area beneath the flap as well as the undermined zone. A formidable volume of blood may accumulate within such a space. Similarly, there is a comparably large surface area from which bleeding may take place. The pooling of blood beneath a flap creates several problems. Toxic mediators, especially hemoglobin-derived oxygen free radicals, interfere with flap circulation.[21,59-61] The space-occupying mass may increase tension on the suture line. The mechanical separation of the flap undersurface and the wound bed prevents cohesion and normal wound healing events. A binding scar is thus prohibited from forming. Finally, blood in the wound acts as a culture media for bacteria and increases the risk of wound infection.

Bleeding-related problems take several forms. There may be persistent or difficult-to-control bleeding during surgery or, as more often is the case, bleeding that begins sometime in the postoperative period.

Postoperative ecchymoses and edema, especially of the eyelids or lips, while not a threat to flap survival, may be of such magnitude to greatly alarm the patient. Ecchymoses are caused by red blood cells dispersed in the tissue planes and are generally harmless. Routine undermining facilitates this dispersion. Hematomas or blood clots, on the other hand, are formed when blood collects within the wound bed as a space-occupying mass.

The clinical effects of a hematoma and the rationale for its management depend on the magnitude of the clot, the rapidity with which it develops, and the timeframe within the postoperative period that it is brought to the surgeon's attention.[2,3] Hematomas have a predictable life cycle. A fresh clot, within the first 1 or 2 days after surgery, consists of a watery, loosely aggregated gel, which is easily evacuated by manual compression and lavage with sterile saline. As it matures over the next several days, the clot becomes more organized, rubbery, and adherent to the wound bed. Evacuation is more difficult and requires mechanical debridement. Subsequently, after about 10 to 14 days, fibrinolysis begins, with ultimate liquefaction and reabsorption of the hematoma over the ensuing weeks. The uniqueness of each clinical situation will determine the nature and the timing of any intervention.

Case Examples

CASE 1

A 67-year-old woman underwent Mohs micrographic surgery to remove a recurrent basal cell carcinoma of the left ala nasi. She was in otherwise good health and was taking no medications except for vitamins and a daily children's aspirin, which she thought so unimportant as to think it was not worth mentioning. The surgical defect approached the rim of the nostril, but the underlying cartilage was undisturbed. A superiorly based transposition flap was elevated and sutured into place (Fig. 24-16**A**). The operation was, on the whole, rather routine and nothing unusual occurred during the surgery. The flap was transposed without tension and complete hemostasis was easily achieved. She called several hours later to report that bleeding had started about 3 hours after she had returned home. As per the written instructions she had been given, she had removed the soaked dressing and applied firm pressure for 10 minutes to no avail.

When she returned to the clinic, it was noted that the entire suture line was bleeding. Blood was oozing from between the sutures as well as from each suture puncture. The wound area was sterilely prepared and anesthetized, after which the sutures were removed and the flap was taken down. Bleeding was fairly

Figure 24-16 *A*, Transposition flap from cheek to nose. *B*, Persistent bleeding despite attempts to achieve hemostasis. Drain was left in overnight. (*B* reprinted by permission of the publisher from Salasche SJ, Grabski WJ: Complications of flaps, *J Dermatol Surg Oncol* **17**:132–40, copyright 1991 by Elsevier Science Publishing Co, Inc.)

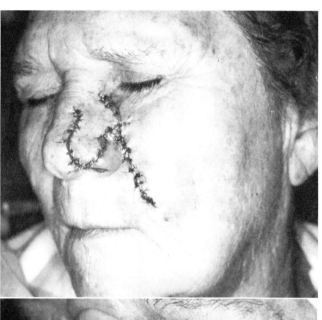

A

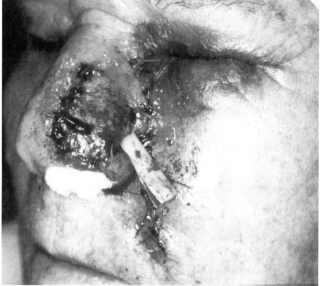

B

universal, coming from the wound bed as well as the undersurface of the flap. After several minutes the bleeding abated as the vasoconstrictive effect of the epinephrine took hold. However, despite good visualization, electrocautery did not seem to be effective in stemming the multiple bleeding sites. To the contrary, the tissue seemed friable with each touch of the electrode, causing new damage and bleeding. A decision was made to forego the possibility of causing any more tissue damage, and a sterile fenestrated Penrose drain was placed along the wound bed and secured inferiorly (Fig. 24-16**B**). The flap was loosely resutured and dressed with an intranasal pack and a multilayered, absorbent but firm outer dressing. By the next morning the hemorrhaging had stopped. The drain was removed, and events proceeded uneventfully. The flap survived the ordeal and healed satisfactorily.

This case underscores the need to accurately document all medications that may interfere with the coagulation cascade. Failure to do so may result in a situation similar to the events recorded here. On the rare occasions that oozing persists despite heroic electrocautery efforts, a prudent course is to insert a drain and leave the suture line porous enough to allow egress of blood. To allow the blood to accumulate as a hematoma puts the flap at higher risk for infection and necrosis.

Bleeding due to platelet dysfunction is usually diffuse. There are usually no specific large arteries or veins that are the main source of bleeding. Bleeding sites that are difficult to detect involve the small vessels that run parallel to the muscles of facial expression, especially those that are located superficial to the orbicularis oculi and oris muscles. Other trouble spots from bleeding are from vessels located deep in the valleys between subcutaneous fat globules and the vertically oriented vessels adjacent to the terminal hairs of the beard and mustache.

Drains within a wound act both as a foreign body that increases inflammation and as a possible conduit for bacterial contamination and subsequent infection. When used, drains should be sterile, be placed across the entire extent of the wound bed, and be fashioned to exit the wound dependently. Every effort should be made to remove the drain within 24 hours.

CASE 2

A postoperative defect of the cheek was repaired with an inferiorly based transposition flap in a 62-year-old man (Fig. 24-17**A**). The defect resulted from the removal of a recurrent basal cell carcinoma, treated initially with curettage and electrodesiccation. There was no pertinent medical history or use of medications to indicate a possible bleeding problem. Because intraoperative hemostasis had not been a problem, it was a surprise when he returned to the clinic after surgery complaining of bleeding and pain at the surgical site. When the dressing was removed, hemorrhage was noted in the suture line, and there was a diffuse, fluctuant swelling beneath the flap. After the wound area was prepared and anesthetized, the flap sutures were removed, revealing a mass that resembled currant jelly (Fig. 24-17**B** and **C**). This mass was

removed with a combination of manual compression and vigorous lavage with sterile saline. Although active bleeding was not evident initially, gentle manipulation of the wound bed and flap undersurface with a sterile gauze sponge revealed numerous bleeding points. Pinpoint cauterization easily stemmed this bleeding, and the flap was resutured into place (Fig. 24-17**D**). The patient was started on a regimen of antibiotics, which led to normal healing (Fig. 24-17**E**).

This case represents the fairly typical scenario of an early hematoma. Fortunately, the patient recognized that a combination of bleeding and progressive discomfort should be reported and attended to before the next day. The lack of active bleeding following evacuation of the hematoma is likewise not surprising because the expanding mass tends to tamponade the bleeding vessels. Stimulating the wound by gentle wiping with gauze will reveal incipient bleeding sites, which can be effectively sealed with pinpoint cautery. Otherwise they may become active and cause another hematoma. Within the first 2 postoperative days the clot is easily

Figure 24-17   *A*, **Transposition flap of cheek.** *B*, **Obvious bleeding and hematoma.** *C*, **Hematoma is exposed and evacuated.** *D*, **Cauterization of offending bleeding vessels.** *E*, **Suture removal 7 days postoperatively.** (*B* **Reprinted by permission of the publisher from Salasche SJ, Grabski WJ: Complications of flaps,** *J Dermatol Surg Oncol* **17:132–40, copyright 1991 by Elsevier Science Publishing Co, Inc.)**

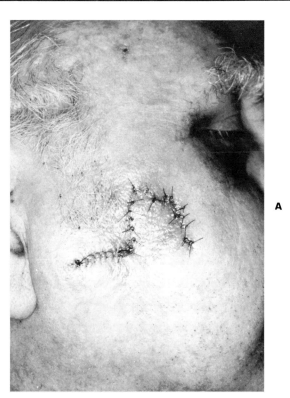

A

Continued.

and completely removed, allowing the flap to be resutured. On the other hand, if the clot is not discovered for several days, it becomes organized and adherent to the wound walls, precluding easy evacuation. In such an event, if the hematoma is sizable, management entails opening of the wound, removal of as much fibrous clot as possible, and treatment of the remaining wound debris with daily compresses or mechanical debridement and ultimately healing by second intention.

Figure 24-17, cont'd For legend see p. 567.

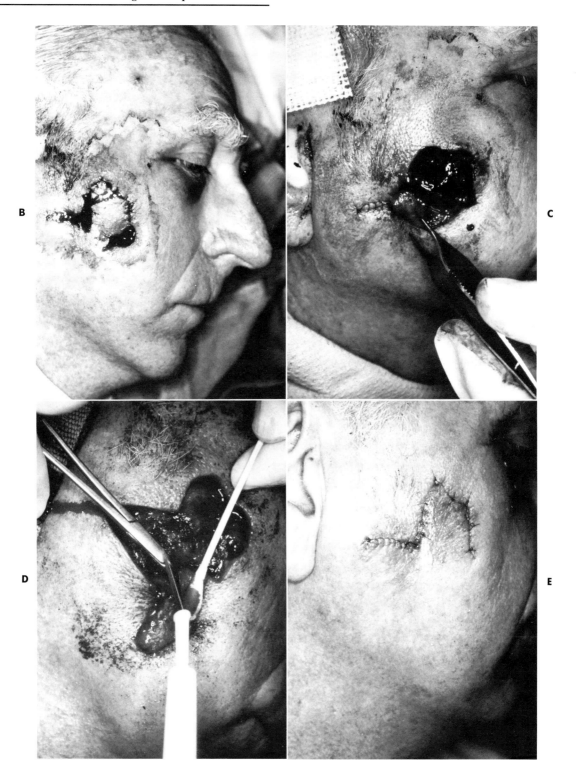

CASE 3

A 67-year-old man underwent excision of a 1.5-cm lentigo maligna from his right cheek. The defect was closed with a simple rotation flap. At the time of suture removal 5 days later, the area was noted to be indurated, but not fluctuant. There was no pain or tenderness. The patient returned to the clinic 2 weeks postoperatively because the flap remained bulky and had taken on a dark blue and black tinge (Fig. 24-18**A**). A fluid-filled space could be palpated beneath the flap. Again, there was no pain, tenderness, or inflammation. Aspiration with an 18-gauge needle yielded almost 2 ml of dark, thin, watery sanguineous fluid (Fig. 24-18**B**). Healing continued uneventfully without further evidence of bleeding or refilling with serum.

As this case demonstrates, occasionally a small hematoma will remain undetected until relatively late in the course of healing. These occult hematomas occur most frequently in the distensible cheek or neck, where they hide undetected or are initially thought to be routine postoperative edema or induration. The decision whether to drain the liquified hematoma or allow it to resorb naturally is not critical. The size and location often dictate the choice. Aspiration with a 16-

or 18-gauge needle is diagnostic as well as therapeutic. A compressive dressing the first postoperative day, to eliminate dead space and to protect the needle puncture site until it seals, is prudent.

WOUND DEHISCENCE

Usually wound separation or dehiscence of a flap is secondary to another major complication: the terminal event of an infection, a hematoma, or a full-thickness necrosis.[2] Examples of each have been documented earlier in this chapter. There are, however, other causes of wound separation. Less devastating wound separations occur from direct trauma or as a result of dynamic motion around the lips and eyes. Also, failure to use buried dermal (subcuticular) sutures or the early removal of sutures may lead to the wound splitting.

These types of wound dehiscence are all intimately associated with early wound healing events and the acquisition of tensile strength in the flap wound bed and scar line.[51,59] For the first week an inflammatory response takes place, highlighted by an influx of polymorphonuclear leukocytes and monocytes. Monocytes are especially important because they release

Figure 24-18   *A*, Discolored flap over fluid-filled space. *B*, Aspiration of liquified clot.

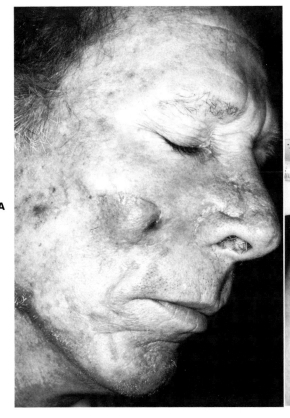
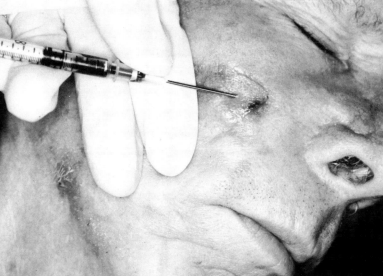

cytokines and growth factors, which stimulate fibroblasts to produce collagen and white cells to migrate and differentiate. After a lag time of approximately 1 week, inflammation decreases and collagen deposition occurs. Subsequently there is a steady gain in tensile strength as the newly deposited collagen is more effectively cross-linked, reoriented, and remodeled over the following weeks. However, usually at the time that sutures are removed, there is virtually no inherent tensile strength in the wound. Only 3% to 5% of unviolated normal skin tensile strength has accrued at the end of 2 weeks. It is not difficult to appreciate how precarious the early wound would be if it were not for the placement of buried absorbable sutures. Obviously there would not be enough innate strength to withstand the forces generated in the mobile, dynamic areas of the face. Surface antitension adhesive strips, placed after suture removal, add some protective insurance against wound separation.

In 1 month approximately 35% of maximum wound tensile strength has been gained. This is a crucial point because now the wound can withstand, for the most part, the forces of normal activity. This corresponds to the timeframe when the buried sutures have lost much of their strength and are in the process of dissolving. Over the succeeding months further contraction and maturation of the scar improve both the clinical appearance and the tensile strength to roughly 80% of the original unwounded skin.

Suture removal should follow a prescribed order. If any tension exists along the suture line, it may be prudent to first remove the sutures furthest from the tension and immediately replace them with antitension adhesive strips. Further removal then proceeds toward the higher tension stitches. If a split seems imminent, the remaining stitches may be left in place a few more days. With today's emphasis on physical fitness, instructions about the limitations on activities should be detailed, specific, and emphatic.

The management of a dehisced flap depends on both the cause and the timing of the separation. Uncomplicated, clean separations secondary to early suture removal or trauma may be immediately resutured without freshening the wound edges if it is performed within the first day. Fibroblasts are already poised and ready in the wound margins, and a second lag period can be avoided. The wound is remarkably resistant to infection at this point and quickly regains tensile strength. Complicated separations secondary to infection, hematoma, or necrosis or separations that have been present for greater than 24 hours are best left to heal by second intention, usually with the need for subsequent scar revision.

Case Examples

CASE 1

After removal of a recurrent basal cell carcinoma from the upper lip of a 52-year-old man, the defect (Fig. 24-19**A**) was repaired with an advancement flap, which used the remaining tissue of his upper lip (Fig. 24-19**B**). Following suture removal on postoperative day 7, the distal portion of the flap separated (Fig. 24-19**C**). The defect was relatively shallow and healed by granulation and epithelialization.

This case illustrates the tendency of advancement flaps to retract to their original position. It also demonstrates the problems attendant to flaps located on the mobile upper lip.

Figure 24-19 *A*, **Surgical defect of upper lip.** *B*, **Advancement flap is sutured into place.** *C*, **Dehisced wound after suture removal.** (*B* and *C* reprinted by permission of the publisher from Salasche SJ, Grabski WJ: Complications of flaps, *J Dermatol Surg Oncol* **17**:132–40, copyright 1991 by Elsevier Science Publishing Co, Inc.)

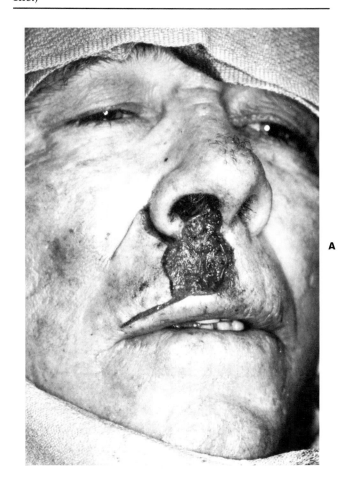

A

Figure 24-19, cont'd   For legend see opposite page.

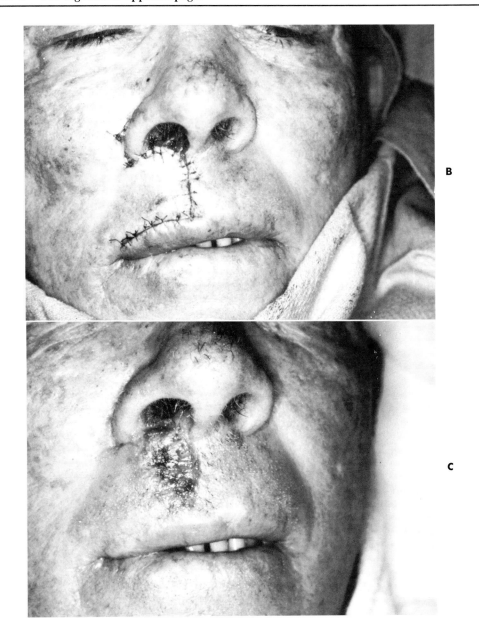

CASE 2

After a rotation flap repair of a defect of the cheek created by surgical extirpation of a recurrent basal cell carcinoma, a 60-year-old man developed a hematoma that was evacuated on the fifth postoperative day (Fig. 24-20**A**). After evacuation of the clot, the dehisced wound was allowed to heal by second intention (Fig. 24-20**B**). The resulting scar was thick and unsightly (Fig. 24-20**C**) and was ultimately revised by excision and resuturing of the scar (Fig. 24-20**D**).

When a hematoma becomes organized, it is often difficult to completely remove it from the flap bed. If the wound dehisces, healing must proceed by second intention. Daily care includes wet compresses to assist debridement. The final outcome is unpredictable, but, with a deformity such as in this case, scar revision is usually required. The timing of scar revision is not critical, but it is usually best to wait several months until wound maturation has occurred. Obviously, after a wound complication the patient is anxious and may not wish to wait that long but will usually go along with the surgeon's recommendation if the rationale for the delay is explained.

Figure 24-20 *A,* Hematoma under rotation flap. *B,* Dehisced flap 1 week after hematoma evacuation and debridement of wound with wet compresses. *C,* Bulky scar after healing by second intention. *D,* Three months later scar is excised and sutured.

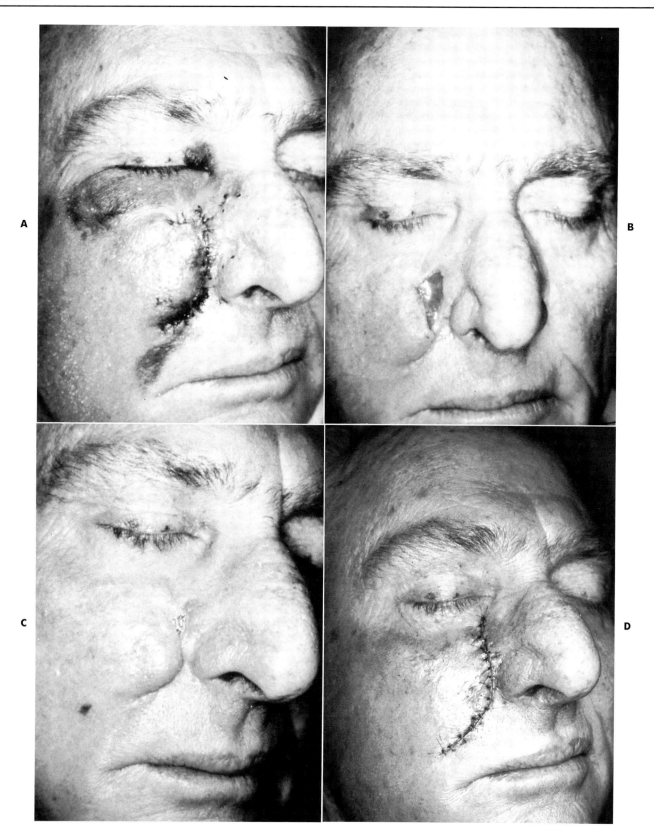

FLAP DESIGN PROBLEMS

The functions of a flap are to fill the surgical defect, restore anatomic continuity, maintain functional integrity, and provide an esthetic appearance. During rearrangement of adjacent available skin, complicated scar configurations are produced and unusual tension-stress relationships develop. If the flap is poorly designed or executed, scars may become accentuated instead of hidden, natural depressions may be obliterated, free margins may become distorted, or the natural boundaries of the units of the face may be unesthetically altered. Any of these mishaps will ruin the outcome of the flap.

Junction Lines and Esthetic Units

The face can be subdivided into esthetic units, which share common characteristics of skin texture, thickness, color, elasticity, pore size, hairiness, and so on. These units, such as the upper lip or chin, are bounded by strong natural lines referred to as junction or boundary lines, such as the melolabial sulcus or the vermilion border. Several principles of flap design are based on the concept of junction lines and esthetic units.[16,29,62-64] Closures should be confined to one unit if possible. If not, flaps should be designed so that tissue borrowed from one unit can be transferred to an adjacent unit that contains the defect in a manner that allows the resulting scars to fall into junction lines where they will be best camouflaged. Scars should not interrupt or cross at right angles to junction lines. Finally, if a significant portion of the unit is missing, it is usually best to sacrifice the remaining portion and repair the entire unit with the flap.

Case Examples

CASE 1

A 49-year-old woman with a recurrent basal cell carcinoma of the tip of the nose underwent resection of the tumor. The surgical defect was repaired with a dorsal nasal flap. The flap draped easily into place and was without undue wound-closure tension. However, the flap was designed with the incision lateral to rather than exactly in the nasal cheek groove, the junction line that divides the nose from the cheek. Shifting of this line laterally disrupted the harmony, symmetry, and midface proportions of the patient's face (Fig. 24-21). The nose appeared broadened, since the normal concavity of the groove was obliterated. The cosmetic result improved with scar revision and time.

Figure 24-21   Nasal tip defect is repaired with dorsal nasal flap. Nose appears broadened due to laterally placed scar.

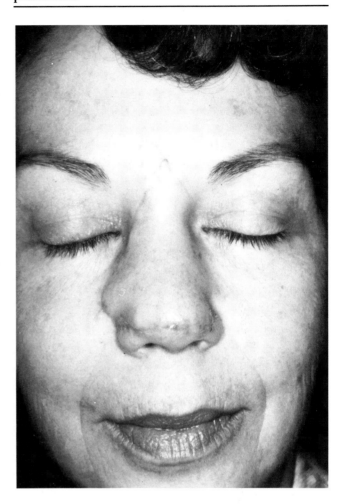

CASE 2

A morpheaform basal cell carcinoma was removed from the nasal cheek groove of a 51-year-old woman. The long axis of the defect was transverse and involved equal portions of the cheek and nasal sidewall (Fig. 24-22**A**). An inferiorly based transposition flap was designed with use of skin from the midlateral sidewall of the nose (Fig. 24-22**B**). Transposition of the flap placed the predominant scar lines across the concave nasal cheek groove (Fig. 24-22**C**). The ensuing thickened scar was quite noticeable as it so dramatically traversed and obliterated the natural vertical depression (Fig. 24-22**D**).

As a general principal it is better to move skin from the lateral to medial direction in the central part of the face rather than the opposite. There is more lax skin available in the cheek, and there is less tendency to disrupt cosmetically important midface landmarks.

Figure 24-22 *A,* Postoperative defect. *B,* Transposition flap is incised. *C,* Flap is sutured into place. *D,* Thick scar extends across junction line.

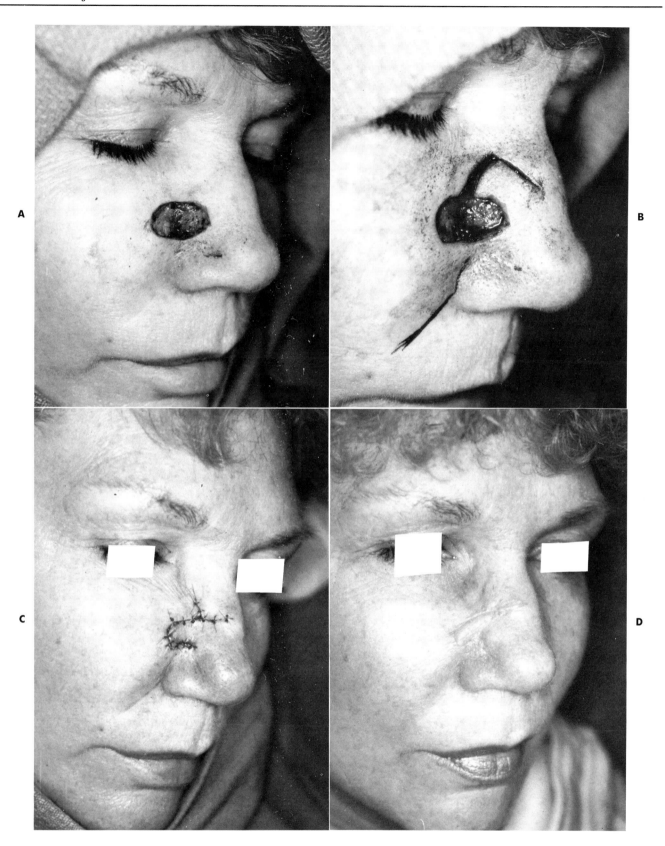

Crossing or disruption of midface junction lines is anathema, because these strong lines are anticipated as normal. If they are altered, one's attention is drawn to that point. This diverts attention away from looking into a person's eyes during conversation, a disconcerting situation for both parties. When the nasal cheek groove or other important junction lines of the central part of the face have been violated by scarring, a scar revision with multiple Z-plasties is often required. The best approach for repair of defects that traverse the nasal cheek groove, such as in the preceding case, is to repair the nose and cheek portions of the defect separately. Cheek skin can be advanced to the nasal facial junction and the nose defect closed with a similarly designed but smaller transposition flap, which also extends to the nasal cheek groove. The joint lines of the two flaps will then recreate the junction line and concavity rather than obliterate it.

CASE 3

A recurrent basal cell carcinoma was removed from the cutaneous upper lip of a 55-year-old man. This left a surgical defect that could not be closed without distortion of the corner of the mouth or the rim of the nostril (Fig. 24-23**A**). The defect was repaired with a superiorly based transposition flap (Fig. 24-23**B**), which resulted in a very noticeable fingerlike flap that "plugged" the defect but did little for the patient's appearance (Fig. 24-23**C**). A debulking revision of the flap (Fig. 24-23**D**) as well as corticosteroid injections, massage, and time improved the ultimate result (Fig. 24-23**E**).

There were several problems with this flap design. Most importantly it eliminated the melolabial fold and filled the upper melolabial and alar-facial sulcus. Also, because the flap replaced only a portion of the left upper cutaneous lip esthetic unit, it noticeably altered the expected pattern of the unit. Finally, the flap was a thickened, rounded blob that bore little resemblance to the tissue it replaced. Trapdoor or pincushion deformity, which some flaps develop, is a function of the flap's rounded contour, thicker donor site tissue, superiorly based design (persistent lymphedema), and contraction of the underlying wound bed scar. These factors will be discussed in more detail in a subsequent case example. Reconstruction of this defect might have been accomplished by an inferiorly based rotation flap incised along the melolabial fold, which would have confined the repair to the esthetic unit of the lip. Another solution would have been to design the cheek transposition flap with an inferior base and use several tacking sutures on the undersurface of the flap to recreate the melolabial sulcus.[65]

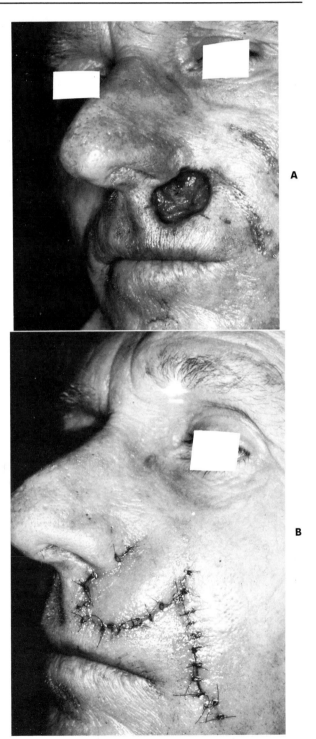

Figure 24-23   *A*, **Postoperative defect of cutaneous upper lip.** *B*, **Superior based transposition flap.** *C*, **Flap obliterates melolabial fold and sulcus and has significant trapdoor deformity.** *D*, **Debulking procedure removes excess fat and scar tissue.** *E*, **Outcome at 12 months.** (*C* **reprinted by permission of the publisher from Salasche SJ, Grabski WJ: Complications of flaps,** *J Dermatol Surg Oncol* **17:132–40, copyright 1991 by Elsevier Science Publishing Co, Inc.**)

Continued.

Figure 24-23, cont'd For legend see p. 575.

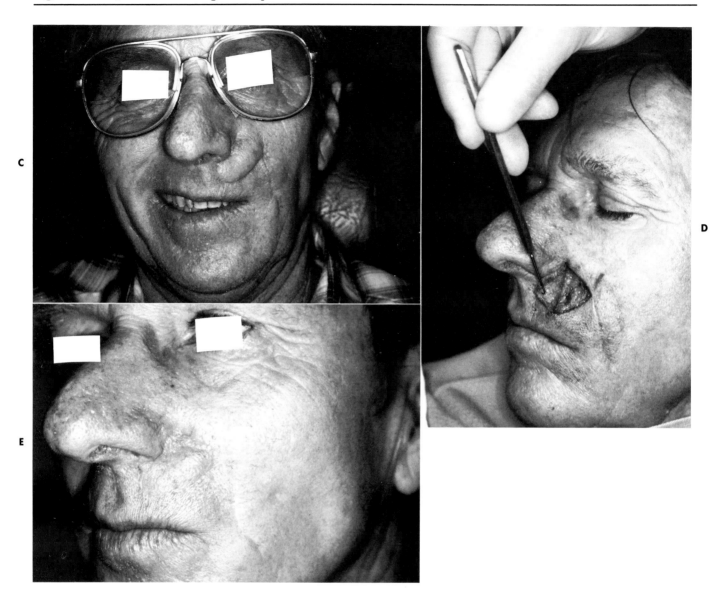

Free Margins

The free margins of the face are those discontinuities of the skin that occur near the orifices of the mouth, eyes, and ears.[29] They include the lips, eyelids, eyebrows, and helical rim. Whereas the free margins offer little resistance to an opposing force, they are easily distorted by scar contraction or tension vectors that pull perpendicular to the margin. While this may result in an asymmetry of the nostril rim, eyebrows (Fig. 24-24), or ears, the stakes are much higher around the eyes and mouth, where functional considerations are more important. An inadequate oral seal interferes with eating and drinking as well as phonation. If the lower eyelid is pulled away from the globe, excessive tearing or progressive symptoms of dry eye will supervene.

One of the most challenging aspects of facial reconstruction is to design esthetic and functional repairs of defects that impinge on one or more of the free margins. Surgical techniques devised to prevent free margin distortion include full-thickness skin grafts that reduce wound contraction, tacking (pexing or suspension) sutures that anchor the closure and redirect the tension to one point, and well-designed skin flaps whose tension vector shifts the pulling forces away from the margin.

Figure 24-24   Postoperative repair following removal of malignant fibrous histiocytoma in 38-year-old woman resulted in disturbing eyebrow asymmetry.

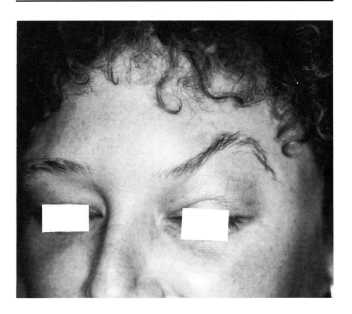

Figure 24-25   *A*, Defect after Mohs micrographic surgery to remove large squamous cell carcinoma. *B*, Large rotation flap at suture removal. *C*, Ectropion of lateral portion of lower eyelid, with chemosis, tearing, and inflammation.

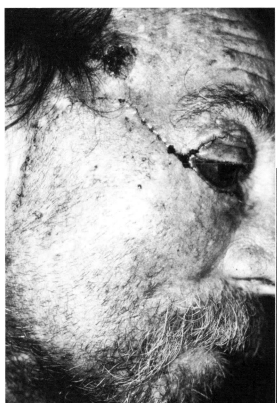

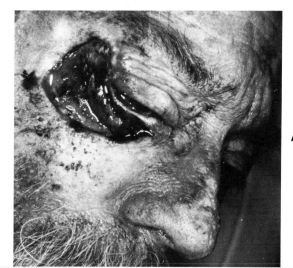

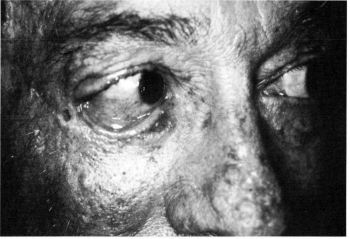

Case Examples

CASE 1

A 71-year-old recipient of a renal transplant was receiving several immunosuppressive agents and underwent excision of a rapidly growing primary squamous cell carcinoma of his lateral canthus and lower eyelid. The large postoperative defect, while imposing, did not involve full-thickness eyelid or lateral canthal tendons (Fig. 24-25**A**). A large rotation flap was fashioned to reconstruct the defect (Fig. 24-25**B**). Over the ensuing weeks a severe ectropion of the lower eyelid developed (Fig. 24-25**C**). This was ultimately repaired with a tarsorrhaphy. In the interim the patient complained of tearing and considerable ocular irritation and discomfort.

The strength and integrity of the lower eyelid must be taken into account when a wound repair impinges on this structure. Any innate laxity of the orbicularis oculi muscle or either canthal tendon should be assessed before surgery, and corrective measures must be incorporated into the reconstruction to compensate for the weakness. Similarly, any destruction of these structures during cancer extirpation requires the same considerations. Occasionally, large or heavy flaps will retract the lower eyelid because of their weight or due to wound contraction, as illustrated in Fig. 24-26**A** through **C**.

Exposure of the cornea from eyelid retraction or ectropion can have dire effects on vision if allowed to

persist. Interim care with frequent and regular use of artificial tears or ophthalmic antibiotic drops or ointment will generally protect the cornea until the protective function of the eyelid can be restored. Other temporizing measures include taping of the sagging eyelid, occlusion of the affected eye at night, or a simple suture tarsorrhaphy.

Figure 24-26 *A*, Large postoperative defect of cheek and portion of lower eyelid after removal of basal cell carcinoma in 30-year-old man. *B*, Large rotation flap used to reconstruct defect. *C*, Three months postoperatively there is wound contraction, resulting in thickened scar lines and scleral show. (Courtesy Shan R. Baker, M.D.)

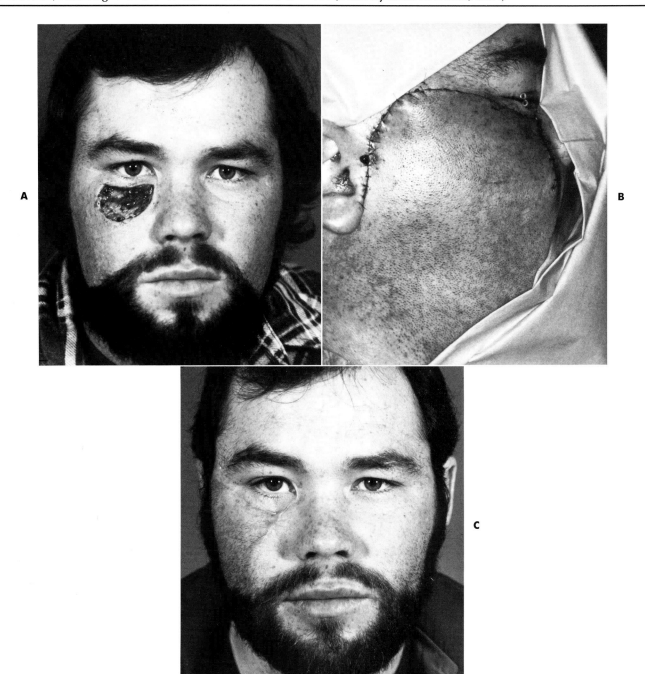

CASE 2

A small primary basal cell carcinoma was removed from the ala nasi of a 62-year-old man. Repair of the resultant defect was attempted with a transposition flap. When the transposition flap was elevated and sutured into place, the nostril rim was elevated (Fig. 24-27).

Examination of the flap design revealed that, when the secondary defect was closed, the tension vector was perpendicular to the nostril rim. Sufficient skin was mobilized to close the defect but at the expense of lifting the nostril upward. The defect was small enough to repair with adjacent nasal skin; however, the flap should have been designed so that the wound-closure tension was parallel to the nostril rim. Alternate approaches would have been a bilobe transposition flap or a full-thickness skin graft.

Figure 24-27   *A,* Postoperative ala nasi defect and incised flap. *B,* Flap transposition distorts nostril rim. (Courtesy of Theodore A. Tromovitch, M.D.)

CASE 3

The defect created by surgical removal of a basal cell carcinoma from the upper lip of a 68-year-old man was repaired with a bilateral advancement flap known as an A-T closure (Fig. 24-28**A** and **B**). Contraction of the vertical limb of the closure resulted in elevation of the upper lip near the commissure (Fig. 24-28**C**). Reexcision of the scar resulted in a satisfactory repair (Fig. 24-28**D**).

This case serves to demonstrate that scars contract in all directions.

Figure 24-28   *A,* **Defect of upper cutaneous lip.** *B,* **A-T closure of defect.** *C,* **Upward distortion of lip, with wound contraction.** *D,* **Postoperative result 3 months after scar revision.** (*B* through *D* courtesy John Zitelli, M.D.)

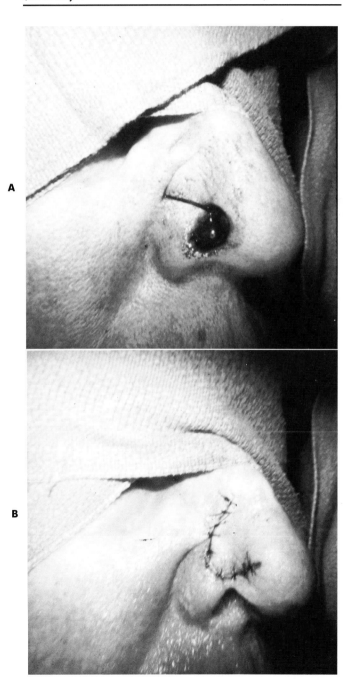

A

B

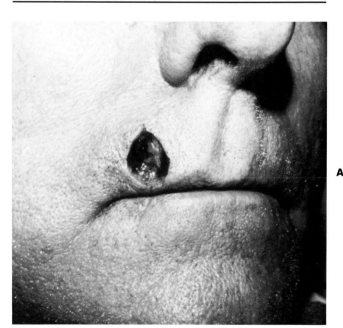

A

Continued.

Figure 24-28, cont'd For legend see p. 579.

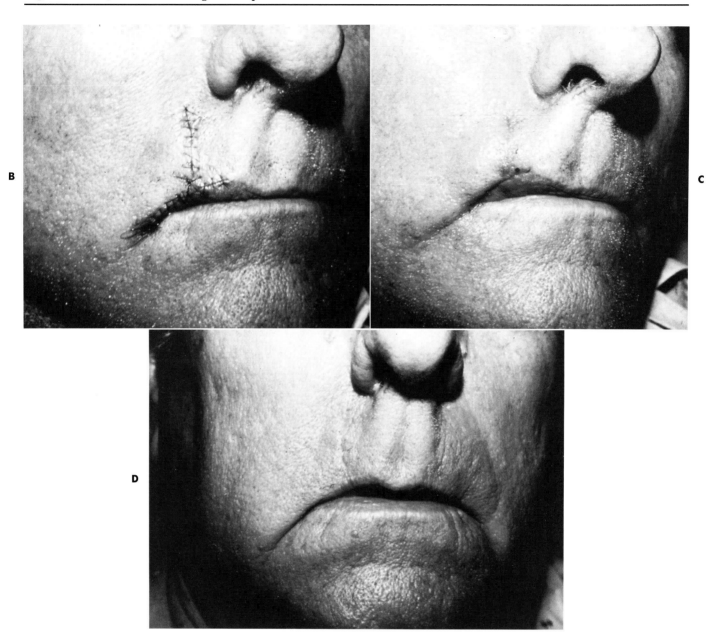

Trapdoor Deformity

As alluded to earlier, some flaps develop a U-shaped, bulky deformity known as trapdoor or pincushion deformity (Fig. 24-23**C**). Rounded or curved flap designs seem to be more prone to develop this distortion than sharply angulated ones. The flap appears to be pushed up within the confines of its borders, imparting thickness to the flap and giving the suture line an inverted appearance. The melolabial flap, transposed from the cheek to the nose, represents the prototypical example of a flap that is predisposed to pincushion deformity, the primary reason that this flap has been so maligned (Fig. 24-29**A** and **B**).[66-68] Contraction of a sheet of scar that forms between the wound bed and the undersurface of the flap is the primary cause of the deformity.[65,69] Contraction of this base scar, along with a similar shrinkage of the perimeter scar greatly limits the space the flap can fit into, and it buckles upward. Maneuvers designed to prevent trapdoor deformity include radical thinning and defatting of the flap, wide undermining beyond the recipient defect to produce a wider base scar, eversion of subcuticular or vertical mattress sutures, and use of postoperative intralesional corticosteroid injections.[69]

When an unsightly trapdoor deformity does develop, a secondary revision should be planned. The timing is optional, but it should probably be delayed at least several months until the wound has had an opportunity to mature. The flap is incised along one of the suture lines, and a wedge of scar and excess fat is removed. The flap is again draped into place, and any redundant skin should be trimmed before resuturing takes place.

CONCLUSION

The purpose of this chapter is not only to enumerate some of the pitfalls, disasters, and less than optimal sequelae attendant to performing flap surgery but also to imbue a sense that when complications arise, personal ego and medicolegal issues should become secondary to the fact that the patient is in trouble and needs help in a timely and skilled manner. Patients require prompt, continual, and accessible expert care to get them through their crisis. By the surgeon being available, caring, and knowledgeable, the complication will cause less distress to the patient. Patients who sense that their situation is being taken seriously and is being

Figure 24-29   *A,* Melolabial transposition flap for repair of alar defect. *B,* Pincushioning gives flap fingerlike appearance.

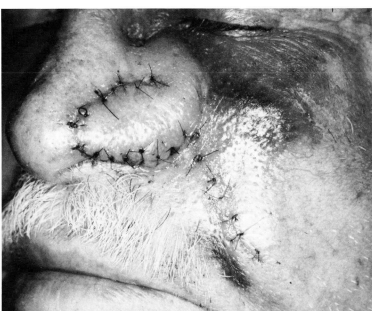

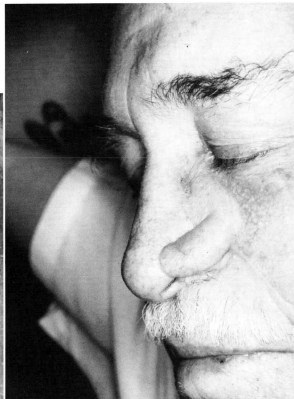

handled earnestly and compassionately are almost always willing to work with the physician for as long as it takes to successfully achieve the best possible outcome. On the other hand, patients who are made to feel guilty or abandoned are more likely to become frustrated, belligerent, and litigious.

It is of utmost importance that patients have clear and ready access to their physicians, particularly in the immediate postoperative period when surgery is performed in an outpatient setting. Written instructions on how to deal with emergencies along with phone numbers of the surgeon or a member of the surgical team are imperative. Although it is time consuming, a phone call by the surgeon on the evening of surgery or the next day allays the patient's fears, avoids problems, and establishes a positive rapport. If the patient finds it necessary to seek help from another physician, to report to an emergency room, or to suffer through a night without help, there is little chance that a trusting relationship can be reestablished. In a similar vein, if another physician's help is required to assist in management of a complication, it is wise to try to maintain overall control of the patient's management. If this is not possible, the surgeon should at least remain active in the case.

The onset of a complication always seems to produce feelings of blame and guilt for both the patient and the surgeon. An adversarial relationship is not usually a healthy one. There is a tendency on the part of physicians to try to assign blame to the patients when a flap is threatened. Why did they take aspirin or smoke? Why did they go back to work immediately instead of staying home and resting? It is probably best to just obtain and accurately record the sequence of events without insinuation of fault. A belligerent, defensive patient is not easy to care for and is certainly more likely to turn on the physician if the ultimate outcome is not deemed satisfactory.

Finally, the ultimate goal is prevention of complications. Hopefully, some of the lessons painfully learned and illustrated in this chapter will preclude their repetition in the reader's practice. Each complication that the practitioner encounters should serve as a mystery to be solved. What could have been better planned, what avoided, or what done differently to have averted the problem? To learn from one's experiences is certainly to gain wisdom.

REFERENCES

1. Goldwyn RM: *The unfavorable result in plastic surgery,* Boston, 1972, Little, Brown.
2. Salasche SJ: Acute surgical complications: cause, prevention, and treatment, *J Am Acad Dermatol* 15:1163, 1986.
3. Salasche SJ, Grabski WJ: Complications of flaps, *J Dermatol Surg Oncol* 17:132, 1991.
4. Leshin B, Whitaker DC, Swanson NA: An approach to patient assessment and preparation in cutaneous oncology, *J Am Acad Dermatol* 19:1081, 1981.
5. Nichols RL: Techniques known to prevent postoperative wound infection, *Infect Control* 3:34, 1982.
6. Sebben JE: Avoiding infection in office surgery, *J Dermatol Surg Oncol* 8:455, 1982.
7. Sebben JE: Sterile technique and the prevention of wound infection in office surgery: Part I. *J Dermatol Surg Oncol* 14:1364, 1988.
8. Sebben JE: Sterile technique and the prevention of wound infection in office surgery: Part II. *J Dermatol Surg Oncol* 15:38, 1989.
9. Myers B: Understanding flap necrosis, *Plast Reconstr Surg* 78:813, 1986 (editorial).
10. Cutting CB: Critical closing and perfusion pressures in flap survival, *Ann Plast Surg* 9:534, 1982.
11. Suzuki S, Isshiki N, Ogawa Y et al: The minimal requirement of circulation for survival of undelayed flaps in rats, *Plast Reconstr Surg* 78:221, 1986.
12. Daniel RK, Kerrigan CL: Skin flaps: an anatomical and hemodynamic approach, *Clin Plast Surg* 6:181, 1979.
13. Daniel RK, Kerrigan CL: Principles and physiology of skin flap surgery. In McCarthy JG, editor: *Plastic surgery, Vol 1,* Philadelphia, 1990, WB Saunders.
14. Pearl RM, Johnson D: The vascular supply to the skin: an anatomical and physiological reappraisal: Part I. *Ann Plast Surg* 11:99, 1983.
15. Pearl RM, Johnson D: The vascular supply to the skin: an anatomical and physiological reappraisal: Part II. *Ann Plast Surg* 11:196, 1983.
16. Salasche SJ, Berstein G, Senkarik M: *Surgical anatomy of the skin,* Norwalk, Conn, 1988, Appleton & Lange.
17. Kerrigan CL, Daniel RK: Monitoring acute skin flap failure, *Plast Reconstr Surg* 71:519, 1983.
18. Pang CY, Neligan PC, Forrest CR et al: Hemodynamics and vascular sensitivity to circulating norepinephrine in normal skin and delayed and acute random skin flaps in the pig, *Plast Reconstr Surg* 78:75, 1986.
19. Wu G, Calamel PM, Shedd DP: The hazards of injecting local anesthetic solutions with epinephrine into flaps: study, *Plast Reconstr Surg* 62:396, 1978.
20. Angel MR, Narayanan K, Swartz WM et al: Deferoxamine increases skin flap survival: additional evidence of free radical involvement in ischemic flap surgery, *Br J Plast Surg* 39:469, 1986.
21. Angel MF, Ramasastry SS, Swartz WM, et al: The critical relationship between free radicals and degree of ischemia: evidence for tissue intolerance of marginal perfusion, *Plast Reconstr Surg* 81:233, 1988.
22. McCord J: Oxygen-derived free radicals in postischemic tissue injury, *N Engl J Med* 312:159, 1985.

23. Angel MF, Kaufman T, Swartz WM et al: Studies of the nature of flap/bed interactions in rodents: Part I. *Ann Plast Surg* 17:317, 1986.

24. Angel MF, Ramasastry SS, Narayanan K et al: Studies on the nature of flap/bed interactions in rodents: Part II. *Ann Plast Surg* 17:434, 1986.

25. Kaufman T, Angel MF, Eichenlaub EH et al: The salutary effects of the bed on the survival of experimental skin flaps, *Ann Plast Surg* 14:64, 1985.

26. Larrabee WF Jr, Holloway GA Jr, Trachy RE et al: Skin flap tension and wound slough: correlation with laser Doppler velocimetry, *Otolaryngol Head Neck Surg* 90:185, 1982.

27. Larrabee WF Jr, Holloway FA Jr, Sutton D: Wound tension and blood flow in skin flaps, *Ann Otol Rhinol Laryngol* 93:112, 1984.

28. Myers MB, Combs B, Cohen G: Wound tension and wound sloughs: a negative correlation, *Am J Surg* 109:711, 1965.

29. Salasche SJ, Grabski WJ: *Flaps for the central face*, New York, 1990, Churchill Livingstone.

30. Winton GB, Salasche SJ: Wound dressings for dermatologic surgery, *J Am Acad Dermatol* 13:1026, 1985.

31. Angel MF, Ramasastry SS, Swartz WM et al: Augmentation of skin flap survival with allopurinol, *Ann Plast Surg* 18:494, 1987.

32. Arturson G, Khanna N: The effects of hyperbaric oxygen, dimethyl sulfoxide and complamim on the survival of experimental skin flaps, *Scand J Plast Reconstr Surg* 4:8, 1970.

33. Chu B, Deshmukh N: The lack of effect of pentoxifylline on random skin flap survival, *Plast Reconstr Surg* 83:315, 1989.

34. Collins TM, Caimi R, Lynch PR: The effects of nicotinamide and hyperbaric oxygen on skin flap survival, *Scand J Plast Hand Surg* 25:5, 1991.

35. Galla TJ, Saetzler R, Hammersen F: Increase in skin-flap survival by the vasoactive drug buflomedil, *Plast Reconstr Surg* 87:130, 1991.

36. Hira M, Tajima S, Sano S: Increased survival length of experimental flap by calcium antagonist nifedipine, *Ann Plast Surg* 24:45, 1990.

37. Hom D, Assefa G: The effects of endothelial cell growth factor on vascular compromised flaps, *Arch Otolaryngol Head Neck Surg* 118:950, 1992.

38. Kerrigan CL, Daniel RK: Pharmacologic treatment of the failing skin flap, *Plast Reconstr Surg* 70:541, 1982.

39. Knight KR, Kawabata H, Coe SA et al: Prostacyclin and prostanoid modifiers aid ischemic skin flap survival, *J Surg Res* 50:119, 1991.

40. Nichter L, Sobieski M, Edgerton M: Efficacy of topical nitroglycerin for random pattern skin-flap salvage, *Plast Reconstr Surg* 75:847, 1985.

41. Goldminz D, Bennett RG: Cigarette smoking and flap and full thickness graft failure, *Arch Dermatol* 127:1012, 1991.

42. Craig S, Rees TD: The effect of smoking on experimental flaps in hamsters, *Plast Reconstr Surg* 75:842, 1985.

43. Forrest C, Pang C, Lindsay W: Dose and time effects of nicotine treatment on the capillary blood flow and viability of random pattern flaps in the rat, *Br J Plast Surg* 40:295, 1987.

44. Jensen JA, Coodson WH, Hopf HW et al: Cigarette smoking decreases tissue oxygen, *Arch Surg* 126:1131, 1991.

45. Nolan J, Jenkins RA, Kurihara K et al: The acute effects of cigarette exposure on experimental skin flaps, *Plast Reconstr Surg* 75:544, 1985.

46. Pearl RM: A vascular approach to the prevention of infection, *Ann Plast Surg* 14:443, 1985.

47. Tran DT, Miller SH, Bucks D et al: Potentiation of infection by epinephrine, *Plast Reconstr Surg* 76:993, 1985.

48. Burke JF: Risk factors predisposing to wound infection and means of their prevention. In Dineen P, editor: *The surgical wound*, Philadelphia, 1981, Lea & Febiger.

49. Burke JF: The physiology of wound infection. In Hunt TK, editor: *Wound healing and wound infection*. East Norwalk, Conn, 1980, Appleton-Century-Crofts.

50. Adinolfi MF, Nichols RL: Postoperative wound infections, *Clin Dermatol* 2:86, 1984.

51. Edlich RF, Friedman HI, Haines PC et al: Biology of wound repair: its influence on surgical decision, *Facial Plast Surg* 1:169, 1984.

52. Klimek JJ: Treatment of wound infection, *Cutis* 36:21, 1985.

53. Nichols RL: Use of prophylactic antibiotics in surgical practice, *Am J Med* 70:686, 1981.

54. Sebben JE: Prophylactic antibiotics in cutaneous surgery, *J Dermatol Surg Oncol* 11:901, 1985.

55. Moake JL, Funicella T: Common bleeding disorders, *Clin Symp* 35:1, 1983.

56. Fisher HW: Surgery on patients receiving anticoagulants, *J Dermatol Surg Oncol* 3:210, 1977.

57. Amrein PC, Ellman L, Harris WH: Aspirin-induced prolongation of bleeding time and perioperative blood loss, *JAMA* 245:1825, 1981.

58. Mielke CH Jr: Influence of aspirin on platelets and the bleeding time, *Am J Med* 74:72, 1983.

59. Angel MF, Narayanan K, Swartz WM et al: The etiologic role of free radicals in hematoma-induced flap necrosis, *Plast Reconstr Surg* 77:795, 1986.

60. Mulliken JB, Healy NA: Pathogenesis of skin flap necrosis from an underlying hematoma, *Plast Reconstr Surg* 63:540, 1979.

61. Mulliken J, Im M: the etiologic role of free radicals in hematoma-induced flap necrosis, *Plast Reconstr Surg* 77:802, 1986 (discussion).

62. Burget GC: Aesthetic reconstruction of the nose, *Clin Plast Surg* 12:463, 1985.

63. Burget GC, Menick FJ: The subunit principle in nasal reconstruction, *Plast Reconstr Surg* 76:239, 1985.

64. Dzubow LM, Zack L: The principle of cosmetic junctions as applied to reconstruction of defects following Mohs surgery, *J Dermatol Surg Oncol* 16:353, 1990.

65. Zitelli JA: The nasolabial flap as a single-stage procedure, *Arch Dermatol* 126:1445, 1990.

66. Koranda FC, Webster RC: Trapdoor effect in nasolabial flaps, *Arch Otolaryngol* 111:421, 1985.

67. Walkinshaw MD, Chaffee HH: The nasolabial flap: a problem and its correction, *Plast Reconstr Surg* 69:30, 1982.

68. Webster RC, Benjamin RJ, Smith RC: Treatment of "trap door deformity," *Laryngoscope* 88:707, 1978.

69. Hosokawa K, Susuki T, Kikui T et al: Sheet of scar deformity: a hypothesis, *Ann Plast Surg* 25:134, 1990.

70. Clark RAF: Cutaneous tissue repair: I. Basic biologic considerations, *J Am Acad Dermatol* 13:701, 1985.

EDITORIAL COMMENTS

Shan R. Baker

As a result of improved techniques and advancement of technology, as well as enhanced awareness of the complications of our surgeries, clinicians have reduced the incidence of many complications of the past. Complications do occur in the hands of the best surgeons; however, they recognize them promptly and treat them effectively. Prevention is preferred, but when complications do occur recognition and timely treatment become the first priority. Complications and sequelae are separate entities. We strive to eliminate both by modifying our surgical techniques and improving methodologies, which provide better esthetic and functional form.

Dr. Salasche has provided a rather comprehensive discussion of various complications that may occur in reconstruction of facial defects with local flaps. Through his honesty and humility, he has provided insight into the prevention and management of a number of common complications. I agree in principle with all of the recommended methods to manage the complications discussed.

Dr. Salasche suggests that hematomas diagnosed several days after surgery are difficult to evacuate because of the organized adherent blood clot beneath the skin. He suggests treatment of larger hematomas by opening of the wound, removal of the fibrous clot, and treatment of the wound by mechanical debridement through the use of wound packing or compresses. Sometimes such a complication can be managed by making a small opening at the border of the wound and removing the clot by suctioning using a liposuction cannula or other suction device with a relatively large bore. The cannula is inserted and moved under the flap in multiple directions to mechanically break up the clot, which facilitates removal. Irrigation through the same wound opening and repeated suctioning are also helpful in removal of most of the clot. This approach reduces the need to open the wound widely to remove a clot and eliminates the need for healing by second intention. A similar technique is also useful in the treatment of early hematomas in which thrombis formation has not occurred. If active bleeding is not present, a drain can be inserted through the wound border and a compression dressing can be applied. The drain is usually removed the following day.

Dr. Salasche has discussed facial esthetic units and the importance of maintaining the integrity of the borders of these units. In my experience, obscuration or distortion of these borders is the most common sequela of use of local flaps to repair facial defects. This is particularly true of reconstruction of the nose or lip in which it is often necessary to use a cheek transposition or advancement flap, which by necessity crosses the alar-facial sulcus or melolabial sulcus. In nasal reconstruction, sequelae can frequently be avoided by use of an interpolation flap, which crosses over or under but not through the alar-facial sulcus. Although interpolation flaps have specific disadvantages, in recent years I have used the interpolation cheek flap more often because I believe the advantages of preservation of the alar-facial sulcus in its natural topography outweigh the disadvantages of the flap.

EDITORIAL COMMENTS

Neil A. Swanson

Dr. Salasche presents an excellent and concise discussion of the complications and related events of flap surgery. Several excellent case examples of the complication and its management are presented with each of the basic tetrad of complications.

There are a few points to emphasize. Once the blood supply to a flap becomes limited and the flap necrotic, do not debride the flap. As Dr. Salasche states, the eschar at worst is a biologic dressing. The surgeon will often be surprised when the eschar does separate to find at least a partial-thickness healing of the wound beneath that eschar. Surgeons who do not understand this often end up making a potentially less-than-optimal result worse.

Smoking and aspirin present my two biggest problems with flaps. As Dr. Salasche aptly describes and references, smoking is directly related to flap death. It is very real. If one can stop smoking for even a short period of time during the peri and postoperative period, flap survival can improve. In a heavy smoker, I often will modify my closure design with this in mind. Aspirin and aspirin-containing products create an ooze that is very difficult to control. I would personally much rather have a patient on Coumadin during a flap procedure than aspirin. As a bottom line, if I even think of placing a drain in these patients, I do so using a small Penrose drain and placing it across the entire wound surface exiting in a dependent position. It is sutured in place using a suture different than my skin

sutures to avoid confusion at the time of drain removal, usually in 24-36 hrs.

In my hands, the earliest symptom of infection is a patient who has significant concerns about pain. Remember, most infections do not begin until 4 to 8 days postoperatively. At that point a patient should have minimal pain. Therefore, when a phone call comes during this postoperative period from a patient complaining of pain, it should be respected.

Dr. Salasche gives some very nice examples of faulty flap design, crossing cosmetic and esthetic boundaries as well as not respecting free margins. A good understanding of these basic principles, especially that of secondary tissue movement and the tension vectors required to close the secondary defect of a flap, are critical. This is discussed in detail in Chapter 4.

This is a very thorough and honest chapter which should humble all surgeons.

25

SCAR REVISION AND CAMOUFLAGE

J. Regan Thomas

Timothy W. Frost

INTRODUCTION

Many of the principles of scar optimization can be employed at the time of flap selection and execution. Although careful planning of reconstruction of facial defects is important in the final outcome, in many cases it may not be possible to avoid certain sequelae of flap repair at the initial stage. Some techniques that are useful in scar camouflage are inappropriate during the initial reconstruction because the specific features that may require correction cannot be predicted accurately. The final result of facial reconstruction will often benefit from secondary scar refinement and camouflage. Scar camouflage is especially important for flaps and incisions on the face. Careful attention to detail, accurate scar analysis, and preoperative planning give the greatest likelihood of success.[1-4]

Every surgical incision results in scar formation. The goal of the reconstructive surgeon is not to reconstruct the face without scarring but rather to create scars that are as imperceptible as possible. This ideal scar, when fully matured, should possess the following characteristics[5]:

1. The scar should be flat and level with the surrounding skin. There should be no depression, or bulge, and there should be no step-off, or variation of height, from one side of the wound to the other that could cast a shadow.
2. There should be a good color and texture match across the scar and between the scar and the surrounding skin.
3. The scar should be narrow.
4. The scar should be parallel to the relaxed skin tension lines (RSTLs) and possibly should fall in a natural crease.

5. The scar should be sinuous, avoiding straight and unbroken lines, which can more easily be detected.

When a scar possesses properties that deviate greatly from these ideals, one or a combination of scar-camouflage techniques may be expected to improve its overall acceptability.

TIMING OF SCAR REVISION

Questions commonly arise about the appropriate timing of scar revision. Traditional teaching dictates that scar revision be delayed until 6 to 12 months after the initial surgery to allow for scar maturation. This timing is largely arbitrary, however, and more appropriately should take into consideration the location, skin type, and age of the patient.

Nearly all scars will tend to improve over a period of up to 1 to 3 years, and if a scar is expected to mature to acceptable appearance, it may be appropriate to wait for that period before deciding if additional revision is required. In many cases, however, it may be clear much sooner that various factors about the scar will not allow the scar to be truly optimal, such as a scar that is perpendicular to the RSTLs or that obviously has characteristics that deviate markedly from the ideal. In such a case it is acceptable to revise the scar sooner. If the underlying dermal scar is left undisturbed so as to provide support to the wound base during healing, a delay of 2 to 3 months is warranted to allow this deep scar to mature. If, on the other hand, the scar needs only the superficial smoothing or blending afforded by dermabrasion, 6 to 9 weeks is an appropriate wait; this is in accordance with the concept that healing wounds incorporate a high fibroblast activity at this time and dermabrasion healing would benefit from this wound stage.

SCAR ANALYSIS

Not every scar is amenable to improvement, but scars with the following properties are especially likely to benefit from revision: scars that are (1) widened; (2) perpendicular to RSTLs; (3) interrupting an esthetic unit of the face; (4) webbed; (5) hypertrophied; (6) pincushioned; (7) adjacent to, but not lying in, a favorable site; (8) long, unbroken, and not within RSTLs; or (9) causing distortion of facial features or anatomic function.

Many times a variety of alternatives are used in concert to gain optimum camouflage. Selection of the most appropriate technique or techniques depends on scar location and appearance. The patient should be informed at the time of scar revision that a variety of procedures may be required, with appropriate intervals between these steps. The patient should be aware that multiple steps are often required to gain the best possible result.

A variety of scar camouflage techniques are available to facial surgeons. The therapeutic steps and alternative techniques to be used in the surgical approach are based on scar position and location; skin type; proximity of the scar to vital structures; direction, width, and degree of contracture of the scar; and age of the patient. Techniques of scar revision may be subdivided as excision, irregularization, and epithelial abrasion. The optimum camouflage of a scar many times involves the application of selected techniques from each of these three categories in combination or in sequence, although some scars may not require all three. Certainly most scar camouflage techniques benefit from follow-up dermabrasion.

EXCISIONAL TECHNIQUES

Fusiform Excision

Scars with edges that are misaligned or perhaps too wide may sometimes be corrected by simple fusiform excision. The simplest procedure is generally the best, and those scars that fall within the RSTLs in favorable areas of the face may simply be reexcised in fusiform fashion and repaired with proper dermal approximation and equalization of wound edges. Fusiform excisions generally close without redundancy if they are created with angles that consist of 30° or less. Fusiform excisions that are greater than approximately 1 cm should be designed to render the ultimate scar line sinuously parallel to a contour line or RSTL. This

paralleling avoids a straight, predictable scar that is more apparent to the casual observer. Many times scars may be shifted to fall within normal skin creases or even behind hair-bearing areas to make them less apparent and more acceptable simply through the use of a fusiform excision technique. A typical example would be a scar on an exposed cheek area that may be shifted to fall within a fusiform excision along the melolabial sulcus.

Partial Serial Excision

Serial excisions may be used when the elasticity of the scar and surrounding tissue prohibits one-stage excision and closure without distortion of nearby anatomic landmarks. This technique essentially removes a portion of the scar by excision and allows the remaining scar edge to be closed to the adjacent normal skin to cover the defect. This partial excision avoids distortion while encouraging more elastic normal skin to stretch and accommodate and thus replaces that excised portion of scar. Subsequent additional excisions, which advance normal skin to cover the scar are used until eventually all of the scar has been excised. Recently the advent of tissue expanders allows this concept to be used with fewer necessary steps. This technique can be particularly applicable to broad burn scars. It is also a useful technique in excision of pigmented lesions of the face.[6]

SCAR IRREGULARIZATION

Z-Plasty

Z-plasty is the oldest and simplest technique used for scar irregularization. The central principle of Z-plasty is that by interposing triangular flaps rotated across the line of the scar, the length of the scar is increased and the line from one end of the scar to the other is interrupted. Z-plasty is especially helpful in effacing webbed scars or elongation of contracted scars, and for the so-called trapdoor scar.[7] The concept of multiple Z-plasties is used to irregularize and elongate a scar without rotation of large flaps of skin. Z-plasty is an important technique in scar revision and is dealt with extensively in Chapter 9. The important thing to remember about Z-plasty is that it is to be used when the scar requires elongation. If only irregularization of the scar is required, other techniques of irregularization and camouflage may be superior.

W-Plasty

W-plasty, which has at times been called "zigzag plasty," contains uniform interposed triangular advancement flaps and creates an irregular scar for better camouflage. W-plasty is particularly useful in reconstitution of scar lines to more nearly approximate RSTLs of the face.[8,9] This is a particularly helpful technique in areas of facial curvature, such as along the mandibular line, on the anterior surface of the ear, and at times on vertical scars of the forehead. Interruption or irregularization of a scar into its smaller components produces a camouflaging effect by interrupting the observer's recognition of the scar at each change of direction. This avoids the sharp demarcation between the scar and neighboring skin by intermingling the small scars with the normal unscarred tissue and thus camouflaging the site.

The scar is prepared by first injecting the scar and area to be undermined with local anesthetic, usually 1% lidocaine with a 1:100,000 concentration of epinephrine to enhance vasoconstriction. The skin and operative field are cleansed and draped in a sterile fashion.

The skin is then marked with a fine-tip marking pen, which is especially helpful to define the exact dimensions and fine details of the small flaps. First the portion of the scar that is widened, depressed, raised, or otherwise undesirable is outlined as the area of skin to be excised (Fig. 25-1**A**). Then the direction of the RSTLs where they cross the scar is identified at several locations along the scar. Lines running across the scar are then drawn at 5 mm intervals along its length. If the direction of the scar is less than approximately 45° from being perpendicular to the RSTLs, the crossing lines can be drawn parallel to the RSTLs; otherwise they may simply be slanted in the direction of the

RSTLs. The proposed W-shaped incision is then drawn on one side of the scar, with the bases falling midway between the previously drawn crossing lines and at the border of the area of scar to be excised. The apices of the triangles should fall on the crossing lines approximately 5 mm from the border of the scar. A mirror image of the first side is then drawn on the opposite side so that the tips will interdigitate when the skin is advanced perpendicular to the direction of the scar. The ends of the pattern must be tapered around the scar to allow for closure with an angle of 30° or less. These guidelines result in a series of triangles that are approximately 5 mm on each side with their tips separated by 5 mm. Each of the limbs is roughly aligned with the RSTLs. Limbs of 5 mm are optimal for camouflage, since limb lengths of 3 mm or less tend to be too small to irregularize the scar enough to keep it from appearing as a straight line, and limbs of more than 7 mm are long enough that they become visible individually.

With No. 11 surgical blade, the W-plasty incision is first scored superficially along its entire length so that its details will remain precisely defined during definitive excision. The incision is then deepened and the scar is excised (Fig. 25-1**B**). The deeper healed scar tissue is left intact to help resist contracture and depression of the scar during healing. The edges of the wound are undermined to allow for their advancement.

With use of a careful soft-tissue technique, the wound is closed in two layers. Dermal closure is accomplished by placement of several key 5-0 polyglactin (Vicryl) sutures through the dermis of the tip of a

Figure 25-1   **A,** Unacceptable scar. **B,** Multiple W-shaped figures running roughly parallel to RSTLs. **C,** Closure uses interrupted buried dermal sutures followed by running locked 6-0 rapidly absorbing gut suture.

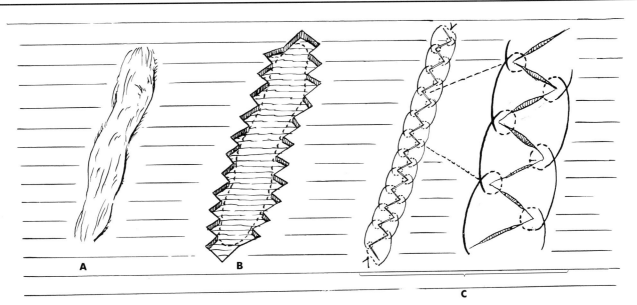

flap on one side and the corresponding angle between two flaps on the other side. Just enough of these sutures are placed so that the edges of the wound are advanced to interdigitate with little or no gap between the epithelium. The epithelial closure uses a running locking 6-0 rapidly absorbing gut suture. The suture generally runs from one end to the other, suturing all the tips of the flaps of one side into the angles of the other side. Then the tips of the other side are sewn into position as the suture proceeds back in the other direction (Fig. 25-1C). As always, careful attention to the exact alignment of the epithelial surface is critical.

Surgical adhesive is applied to the surrounding skin, and the incision is then stabilized with reinforced wound-closure tapes. The wound-closure tapes are left in place for 1 week. In most cases, one or more episodes of dermabrasion are applied beginning at 6 weeks to optimize scar camouflage and to smooth and blend the wound edges with surrounding skin.

Fig. 25-2A shows a highly visible straight-line scar.

Scar revision was accomplished using a W-plastic excision (Fig. 25-2B). The scar is included in the excision (Fig. 25-2C), and the flaps are fashioned in the direction of the RSTLs. A small Z-plasty has also been performed on a webbed portion of the scar in the medial canthal area. The wound is closed with a running locking 6-0 rapidly absorbing gut suture in the epithelial layer (Fig. 25-2D). Fig. 25-2E shows the early postoperative result 1 week after surgery. Two months postoperatively the wound is ready for dermabrasion (Fig. 25-2F and G).

The W-plasty technique has its greatest shortcoming in situations when it is used in a scar long enough to become "predictably irregular." Then the scar is somewhat more conspicuous. In these situations a better alternative might be the geometric broken-line closure (GBLC) technique, discussed next.

Figure 25-2 **A,** Depressed scar crossing path of RSTLs. **B,** Surgical plan outlined on skin using running W-plasty technique. **C,** Scar tissue has been excised. **D,** Wound closure with running locked 6-0 rapidly absorbing gut suture. **E,** Appearance 1 week postoperatively. **F and G,** Appearance 2 months postoperatively.

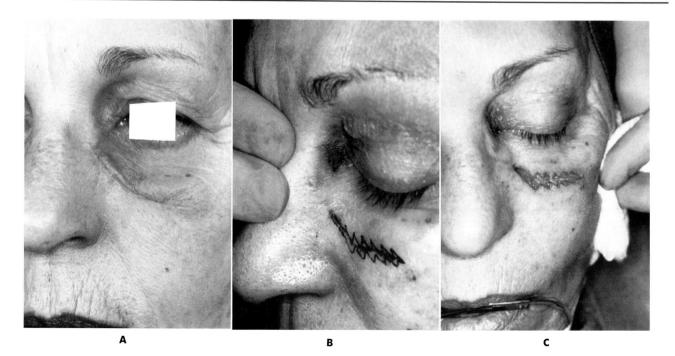

A   B   C

Figure 25-2 cont'd   For legend see opposite page.

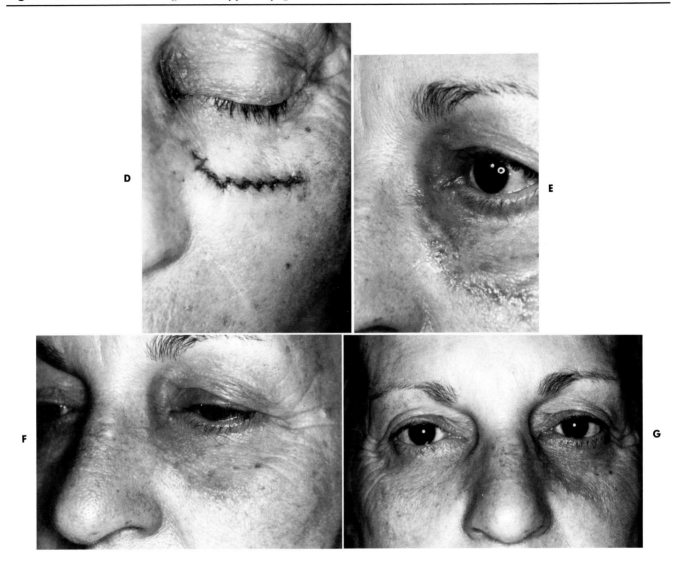

Geometric Broken-Line Closure

The GBLC is a scar irregularization technique with a bit more sophistication than the W-plasty.[10] The design of GBLC is composed of a series of random, irregular geometric shapes cut from one side of a wound and interdigitated with the mirror image of this pattern on the opposite side. The individual geometric components should be no more than 6 mm long in any dimension for best camouflage. The GBLC is most useful for long unbroken scars that cross RSTLs, such as those that run from one oral commissure diagonally up the cheek, or the mandible. As with Z-plasty and W-plasty, dermabrasion 6 or more weeks after GBLC provides optimal camouflage.

This technique is time consuming to execute. The steps of GBLC are virtually identical to those of W-plasty with the exception of the design of the shape of excised tissue (Fig. 25-3). In this case the lines drawn across the scar are simply placed perpendicular to the scar, since many of the lines of the new excision will have a variable relationship to the RSTLs. After the crossing lines are drawn at regular intervals, a series of randomly designed figures are created along one side of the scar. The purpose of this arrangement is to create a final scar with no regularity or predictable pattern. The figures used include triangles, various sized rectangles, and other combinations of shapes. Although they may vary slightly to give a random appearance, it is important to keep the lengths of the individual segments approximately 5 mm, for the reasons mentioned previously.

Once a random geometric line has been drawn on

Figure 25-3   **A,** Random geometric figures are designed around unacceptable scar. **B,** Scar is excised, leaving mirror-image wound edges of geometric figures. **C,** Wound edges are advanced and closed with running locking 6-0 rapidly absorbing gut suture.

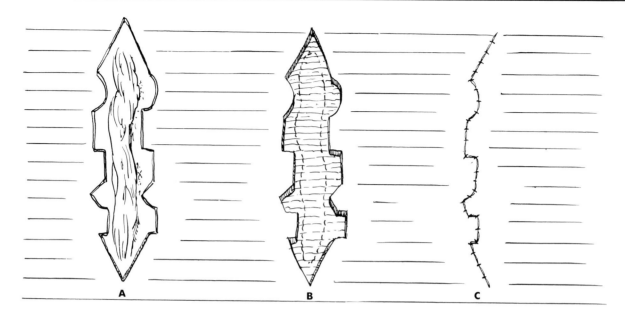

one side of the scar, a matching line is created on the opposite side using the crossing lines to align apices on one side with angles on the other and so forth.

Fig. 25-4**A** is an example of a scar treated with GBLC. A depressed vertical scar of the chin marked with lines at approximately every 1 cm is shown. Fig. 25-4**B** shows the superficial scar excised as outlined. The actual scar excised is seen in Fig. 25-4**C**. The wound is closed in two layers with absorbable dermal sutures. The epithelial closure is accomplished with a running locking 6-0 rapidly absorbing gut placed at the tips of the flaps (Fig. 25-4**D**). Fig. 25-4**E** shows the final result 6 months after scar revision and before dermabrasion.

EPITHELIAL ABRASION

Dermabrasion

Dermabrasion is an old technique and provides a superficial skin injury (to the level of the papillary dermis) that heals by reepithelialization from adnexal structures in the reticular dermis. Irregularities in the surface, such as a step-off between a flap and the surrounding skin, that are visible by their ability to cast shadows can be treated effectively by dermabrasion. The scar is not removed, but the scar and surface are brought to a more homogeneous level, reducing the amount of shadow. Another benefit is that dermabrasion creates a more subtle transition of color and texture from skin to scar to skin taken from possibly

another area by requiring newer, more homogeneous epithelium to form across all these areas.

Dermabrasion is also used in conjunction with other scar revision techniques in a sequential fashion. As stated previously, W-plasty and GBLC are generally followed by dermabrasion at 6 to 12 weeks postoperatively to better blend the new scar with the surrounding skin.

Several sessions may be necessary to achieve optimal results with dermabrasion, and the patient should be made aware of this at the outset. The best candidates for dermabrasion are individuals with fair hair and light skin because the risk of pigmentary changes after dermabrasion is greater in persons with darker skin. It may also be wise to avoid dermabrasion in pregnant women, patients who are receiving hormonal therapy, and patients with a history of perioral herpes infections because scarring and pigmentary changes are also more common in these individuals.

Shave Excision

For scars that are acceptably narrow but have contours that are elevated a few millimeters above the skin surface, shave excision may be quite helpful. Likewise, when the two edges of a scar are at unequal levels or when a flap has a small-standing cutaneous deformity (dog-ear), shave excision may be a useful means of revision. Using a thin scalpel blade or a flexible razor blade, superficial layers of skin and scar are shaved in a sawlike fashion, preserving an already well-healed

Figure 25-4   **A,** Vertical scar of chin, with GBLC designed. **B,** Scar has been excised and outlined. **C,** Excised scar tissue. **D,** Advancement and closure of wound edges. **E,** Six-month postoperative result; wound is now ready for dermabrasion.

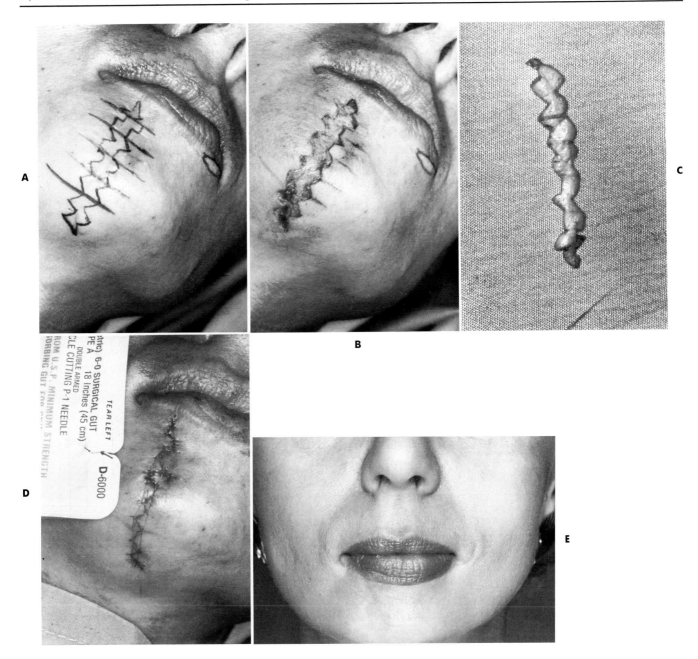

underlying dermis. Irregular elevation or elevated scars of sebaceous skin on the nose are particularly useful areas for this technique.

SUMMARY

Careful preoperative planning of facial flaps and incisions on the face can go a long way toward minimizing visible scar formation. In many cases, however, secondary revision may benefit scars resulting from the most meticulous surgery. An analysis of the particular problems related to a given scar will dictate the best approach. Techniques taken from three general categories—excision, irregularization, and epithelial abrasion—may be used alone or in combination. Those scars that are wide or are otherwise poor on the basis of their color or texture will benefit from excision and careful layered closure. Long, straight scars will also usually benefit from irregularization with W-plasty, geometric broken-line closure, or Z-plasty, the latter especially when the scar needs lengthening. Scars that are raised or contain step-offs or other surface irregularities will benefit from smoothing by shave excision or dermabrasion. This latter technique is almost always helpful in smoothing and blending scars and flaps as an adjunctive refinement to any of the previous techniques.

REFERENCES

1. Thomas JR: Face: examination and evaluation. In Cummings et al, editors: *Otolaryngology—head and neck surgery*, St Louis, 1986, CV Mosby.

2. Thomas JR: Scar analysis. In Thomas JR, Holt GR, editors: *Facial scars: incision, revision, and camouflage*, St Louis, 1989, CV Mosby.

3. Thomas JR: Wounds and scars. In Gates GA, editor: *Current therapy in otolaryngology-head and neck surgery*, Trenton, NJ, 1982, BC Decker.

4. Thomas JR, Mechlin DC: Scar revision. In Holt GR, et al, editors: *Decision making in otolaryngology*, Philadelphia, 1984, BC Decker.

5. Tardy ME, Thomas JR, Paschow MS: The camouflage of cutaneous scars, *Ear Nose Throat J* 60:61, 1981.

6. Tardy ME, Denneny J: Surgical alternatives in scar camouflage, *Facial Plast Surg* 1:209, 1984.

7. Holt GR: Treatment of trapdoor scars. In Thomas JR, Holt GR, editors: *Facial scars: incision, revision, and camouflage*, St Louis, 1989, CV Mosby.

8. Borges AF: Improvement of antitension lines scar by the "W-plastic" operation, *Br J Plast Surg* 12:29, 1959.

9. Borges AF: Principles of scar camouflage, *Facial Plast Surg* 1:181, 1984.

10. Webster RD, Davidson TM, Smith RC: Broken line scar revision, *Clin Plast Surg* 4:263, 1977.

EDITORIAL COMMENTS

Shan R. Baker

Scar revision is a crucial component in the final cosmetic result of any facial reconstruction. Although at times the result will not be enhanced by revision surgery, most scars will be improved with dermabrasion. The authors have provided indicators for scars that would benefit from revision and have discussed when one technique of scar revision is preferred over another. The surgeon can do much to improve his final cosmetic result after reconstructive surgery with the use of local flaps by selecting the flap that minimizes donor site deformity, planning incision lines that parallel or lie within natural skin creases, reconstructing entire facial esthetic units or subunits, and limiting the partial or total obliteration of critical esthetic junction zones by flaps and incisions.

EDITORIAL COMMENTS

Neil A. Swanson

It's very difficult to ask a person who has coedited an entire book on scar revision and camouflage to summarize thoughts in one chapter. This chapter should be used in conjunction with Chapter 9 on Z-plasty and Chapter 16 on Refinements and Revisions. It discusses in detail a few of the concepts of secondary scar revision and camouflage as well as details the techniques of W-plasty and GBLC. As the authors state, scar revision requires one or a combination of the three principles of (1) excision, (2) irregularization, and (3) abrasion. Where appropriate, simple excision of the scar with or without abrasion is the simplest means of scar revision. As shown in Chapter 9 by the myriad of examples given by Drs. Frodel and Wang, the Z-plasty provides excision and irregularization as well as a direction change and lengthening of scar. The W-plasty and geometric broken-line closure are two examples where all three techniques play a role.

I have a couple of technical comments. Abrasion is classically performed with dermabrasion. We now realize that dermabrasion of scars for esthetic reasons is best performed somewhere between 6 and 12 weeks. It can be performed around the scar itself and/or feathered into the entire esthetic unit. Care must be taken to blend the result because every dermabraded scar will have some degree of hypopigmentation. The dermabrasion can occur with or without local anesthesia, with or without freezing of the tissue using Frigiderm, and by an apparatus as simple as a battery-powered dermabrader or the Bell hand engine. One must be careful with the use of freezing agents because of the resultant hypopigmentation that can occur from too deep a freeze. When using a Bell hand engine, I usually will use a 2-mm fine diamond fraise, pear, or cone shaped and turn the speed down. It's much easier to start with low revolutions and increase than have to rerevise the scar because one dermabraded too deeply.

The shave technique described can also be done using a defocused carbon dioxide laser. This yields a very easy, regular, fine-tuning of uneven wound edges. Some surgeons will even use this method of fine abrasion (laserbrasion) for scars postoperatively.

INDEX